MICROBIAL FOOD CONTAMINATION

Second Edition

MICROBIAL
FOOD
CONTAMINATION

Second Edition

Edited by

CHARLES L. WILSON

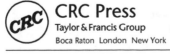

CRC Press
Taylor & Francis Group
Boca Raton London New York

CRC Press is an imprint of the
Taylor & Francis Group, an **informa** business

CRC Press
Taylor & Francis Group
6000 Broken Sound Parkway NW, Suite 300
Boca Raton, FL 33487-2742

First issued in paperback 2019

ISBN-13: 978-0-8493-9076-0 (hbk)
ISBN-13: 978-0-367-38851-5 (pbk)

Library of Congress Cataloging-in-Publication Data

Microbial food contamination / [edited by] Charles L. Wilson. -- 2nd ed.
    p. ; cm.
Includes bibliographical references and index.
ISBN-13: 978-0-8493-9076-0 (hardcover : alk. paper)
ISBN-10: 0-8493-9076-1 (hardcover : alk. paper)
    1. Food--Microbiology. 2. Food contamination. I. Wilson, Charles L.
    [DNLM: 1. Food Contamination. 2. Food Microbiology. WA 701 M626 2008]

QR115.M456 2008
664.001'579--dc22   2007015253

Visit the Taylor & Francis Web site at
http://www.taylorandfrancis.com

and the CRC Press Web site at
http://www.crcpress.com

To Miriam, my beloved wife,

whose love and warmth

sustain me

Contents

Section V   Bioterrorism and Microbial Food Contamination

Preface: Food—A Necessity and a Threat

The first section of the book is titled "Instances and Nature of Microbial Food Contamination." Microbial contamination is the most common cause of foodborne illnesses. The Centers for Disease Control and Prevention (CDC) estimates that foodborne diseases cause approximately 76 million illnesses, 325,000 hospitalizations, and 5,000 deaths in the United States each year. We are aware of more than five times the number of foodborne pathogens now than we were in 1942. Add to this the numerable toxins, allergens, and carcinogens that food may contain, and it gives you pause as you sit down to dinner. If this were not enough, we would now have to be concerned with the deliberate microbial contamination of our food by bioterrorists.

The globalization of the world's food supply has resulted in changing patterns of foodborne illnesses. Following the epidemiology of traditional and emerging foodborne pathogens has subsequently become a daunting task. Globalization reduces traditional geographic barriers that prohibited pathogens from spreading and increases the risk of outbreaks that stretch over many states or even countries. Great strides in tracking foodborne illnesses have been made, however, through the formation of the PulseNet molecular subtyping network. Dr. Efrain Ribot and his colleagues at the CDC show us the power of this network in Chapter 1.

Humans have been aware of potential threats accompanying their food since ancient times. There is historical evidence that food safety has always troubled humankind. Food safety rules can even be found in the Bible and in passages like these in the Qur'an:

> Forbidden unto you are: carrion and blood and swine flesh, and that which hath been dedicated unto any other than Allah, and the strangled, and the dead through beating, and the dead through falling from a height, and that which hath been killed by the goring of horns, and the devoured of wild beasts saving that which ye make lawful, and that which hath been immolated to idols. And that ye swear by the divining arrows. This is abomination. (Qur'an V:3)

The most comprehensive code of ancient laws concerning food safety can be found in the Bible, primarily the book of Leviticus. Some animals were described as unclean and unfit for consumption. The consumption of the blood of slaughtered animals was totally prohibited as the blood was considered the soul of the animal. Food safety laws of a sort can also be found in the writings of ancient Egypt. According to Plutarch, pigs were declared unhealthy animals and pork consumption was prohibited. Although they had no concept of microbial contamination, ancient societies did have a sense that meat could carry disease. The early admonishments in the Bible and Qur'an not to eat certain foods are still reflected in the kosher and halal food laws in modern societies, which are discussed in Chapter 11.

A range of microorganisms and their toxins can inhabit our food, including bacteria, fungi, viruses, parasitic protozoa, and helminthic parasites. All foods generally have a load of microorganisms that accumulate during harvest or during the postharvest period. These populations generally go unnoticed and are normal parts of the food we eat. However, when a "bad actor" emerges as a foodborne human pathogen, our awareness of the microbes in our food is heightened. *Escherichia coli*, for instance, is considered a normal constituent of the microflora of animals and humans. However, in recent years, a strain of *E. coli* (O157:H7) has proven to be devastating to certain human populations. Dr. Glen D. Armstrong in Chapter 2 provides us some new insights into this enterohemorrhagic bacterium.

Within the past 10 years, numerous outbreaks of foodborne illnesses have been associated with fresh vegetables (i.e., sprouts, tomatoes, lettuce, cabbage, celery, coleslaw, cucumbers, mushrooms, potatoes, radishes, green onions), fruit (i.e., cantaloupe, watermelon, raspberries, strawberries), and fruit juices (i.e., orange juice, apple juice). Increased demand for fresh fruits and vegetables has expanded production areas for these commodities and increased the importation of green vegetables from other countries. Both these phenomena have increased the opportunities for "exotic" microorganisms to hitch a ride on this produce. A recent example is the 2006 *E. coli* (O157:H7) contamination of spinach. Expansive spinach fields were in proximity to industrial animal farms. Researchers suspect that the *E. coli* on the spinach originated from the manure of the cattle on a nearby farm. Increased demand for fresh produce has also resulted in large-scale harvesting and processing practices that increase the risk that a small amount of a pathogen may infect a large amount of produce.

With all the publicity given to bacterial contamination of food by foodborne pathogens, we sometimes forget that viruses are considered to be preeminent causes of foodborne diseases in the United States. In 2006, a norovirus caused the closing of an Olive Garden restaurant in Indianapolis; the outbreak sickened over 400 patrons. Noroviruses and the virus causing hepatitis A are of greatest concern among those associated with food. The protozoan *Cryptosporidium* sp. in 1993 caused the largest outbreak of a waterborne disease on record. Approximately 403,000 persons who drank tap water processed in two water facilities in Milwaukee developed cryptosporidiosis. In Chapter 3, Dr. Dean O. Cliver discusses the incidence of virus- and protozoan-caused foodborne diseases and their implications in public health.

During the past two decades, transmissible spongiform encephalopathies (TSEs)—otherwise known as prion diseases—have received considerable public attention primarily because of the TSE known popularly as "mad cow disease." The first human disease recognized to be caused by a prion was Creutzfeldt–Jakob disease (CTD) and its variants. Although the incidence of prion-caused diseases is relatively small in humans, the severe neurological symptoms and fatal nature of these diseases induce fear. Since similar TSEs have been found in a number of animal species (cattle, sheep, goats, elk, deer, moose, and mink), there is confusion as to how consumption of meat from these animals might affect human health. Buchner and Asher sort all this out for us in Chapter 4.

Aflatoxins are powerful carcinogens that occur in our food. They are produced primarily by mold fungi belonging to the genera *Aspergillus* and *Penicillium*. Aflatoxins produced by these fungi have caused toxicity to animal and human populations worldwide. Approximately 4.5 billion people are exposed to uncontrolled amounts of aflatoxin B1 in third world countries. Dr. Stark discusses the molecular and biochemical mechanisms of action of acute toxicity and carcinogenicity induced by aflatoxin B1—as well as chemoprevention of liver cancer caused by aflatoxins—in Chapter 6.

An aflatoxin produced by the fungus *Fusarium verticillioides* causes sporadic outbreaks of equine leukoencephalomalacia and porcine pulmonary edema. The importance of *F. verticillioides* in human health is not clear. However, a correlation between high esophageal cancer rates and the consumption of corn contaminated with *F. verticillioides* has been recognized. Dr. Kenneth Voss and his colleagues, in Chapter 5, discuss the implications of the contamination of corn with *F. verticillioides* and the mycotoxin it produces.

The second section deals with the detection and monitoring of microbial food contaminants. In order to effectively combat microbial food contamination, it is necessary to rapidly and accurately detect contaminants. Dr. Fung, in Chapter 7, gives us an historical account of progress in this area and brings us up to date on recent developments. With regard to contaminant testing, Dr. Fung identifies three important epochs. The period from 1965 to 1985 was an era of miniaturization and diagnostic kit development. From 1985 to 1995, it was an era of genetic probes, molecular testing systems, and polymerase chain reaction (PCR) applications. Since 1995, we are in the biosensor, computer chip technology, and microarray-system development era. These modern tests arose partly in response to human genome projects and the evolving field of proteomics and related fields. The chapters following Dr. Fung's provide additional detail about the latest tests, and suggest where microbial testing may be headed in the future. In Chapter 9, Dr. Fratamico gives us an overview of applications of the polymerase chain reaction (PCR) for detection, identification, and typing of foodborne microorganisms. Drs. Rishpon and Neufeld tell us about rapid electrochemical biosensors for the identification and quantification of bacteria in Chapter 8.

The causal agent of prion diseases or transmissible spongiform encephalopathies (TSE's)—diseases that cause neurodegenerative diseases affecting humans and animals—are particularly difficult to detect in our food supply.

Prions are unconventional infectious agents with extraordinary physico-chemical features that give them the property to resist most common food antimicrobial treatments. The long incubation period between infection and disease expression in many prion diseases makes the detection of these diseases in infected tissues even more critical. Dr. Morales and his colleagues discuss the present status of our knowledge in this area and recent advances in prion detection in Chapter 10.

The third section deals with controlling microbial food contamination. Worldwide educational programs are underway to educate individuals on the prevention of foodborne illnesses. These programs emphasize certain fundamental practices including sanitation, pasteurization, the thorough cooking of foods, the proper storage of foods, and the avoidance of contact between raw foods and cooked foods. A basic tenant in these programs is the use of safe water and hand washing to prevent transference of human pathogens to food.

The hazard analysis critical control point (HACCP) system has been proposed and used worldwide to prevent contamination of food with foodborne pathogens. It is used by institutions to anticipate and prevent food safety violations before they occur. HACCP flowcharts allow food managers to identify the critical control points, which are operations (practice, preparation step, or procedure) in the production of a food product, and to make corrections as needed to prevent or eliminate hazards, or reduce them to acceptable levels. Criticism has been directed toward HACCP systems in some instances because their implementation has been left to the food industry itself with little outside supervision by independent food inspectors.

Once foods are contaminated with microorganisms, there are intervention technologies that can be applied. Drs. Regenstein and Chaudry in Chapter 11 provide a very useful examination of the implications of the kosher and halal food laws on food safety. Dr. Beuchat, in Chapter 12, explores how naturally occurring antimicrobial compounds in food can be used to control foodborne human pathogens. In Chapter 13, Dr. Juneja and his colleagues discuss how radiation, temperature, and pressure can be used to combat human foodborne pathogens in food. They also explore how these technologies affect the quality of food and its nutritional value.

Aflatoxins produced by several *Aspergillus* spp. occur in food and feed crops. These compounds are toxic and extremely carcinogenic when introduced into animal systems. A gene cluster in *Aspergillus* spp. has been identified where almost all the genes involved in aflatoxin biosynthesis reside. Deepak Bhatnagar and his colleagues discuss in Chapter 14 how aflatoxin production might be controlled by specifically targeting sites where aflatoxin production occurs. They also explore plant-derived metabolites that inhibit aflatoxin biosynthesis along with biocontrol methods to reduce aflatoxin production.

The fourth section is titled "Microbial Food Contamination and International Trade." Microbial food contaminants know no international borders. Although outbreaks of foodborne diseases are local, the increased importation of foods from other countries means that outbreaks can have an international origin. The interrelatedness of our food supply with that of other countries has been dramatized by outbreaks of mad cow disease (BSE) and the threat of avian flu. The mere threat of these diseases has caused restrictions on the exportation of meat products and has reduced consumption of beef and poultry by the public. With so much at stake economically, agricultural produces, scientists, and politicians find themselves in conflict. In Chapter 15, Robert and Edward LaBudde follow the history of mad cow disease from its appearance in Great Britain to Canada and the United States. They characterize the conflict that exists between science and economics in policy decisions concerning this disease, and they present a predictive model for anticipating future outbreaks.

Administrators, government officials, politicians, and business managers are being called upon to make policy decisions that deal with food safety as it impacts on public health and trade. Tools are being developed that will help them weigh the various factors that need to be considered in these decisions. Dr. Michael D. McElvaine discusses how risk assessment tools used in other areas can be applied to evaluating microbial food contaminants in Chapter 16. Human diseases that originate in animals—or zoonoses—have often proven particularly inscrutable when scientists try to predict their behavior. Dr. Moez Sanaa and Hussni O. Mohammed give us guidance on zoonotic disease risk assessment and mitigation in Chapter 17.

International institutions have been established to deal with the complexities of international trade and food safety. The Codex Alimentarius—Latin for food code or food law—is the preeminent commission in this regard. It is an international intergovernmental food standards organization whose importance increased substantially after the signing of the GATT Uruguay Round Trade Agreements and the rise of the World Trade Organization (WTO). In Chapter 18, Dr. Michael Wehr describes the history of Codex and how it develops and adopts food safety and quality standards internationally. He discusses how Codex deals with the complexities between threats from microbial foodborne human diseases and international trade policies.

Another international organization that deals with outbreaks of microbial foodborne human diseases is the International Food Safety Authorities Network (IFOSAN), which is part of the World Health Organization (WHO). IFOSAN has been set up as a global network in which participating countries notify IFOSAN of international food safety problems and accept shared responsibilities during food safety emergencies. Dr. Margaret Miller and her colleagues discuss the workings of IFOSAN in Chapter 19.

The last section deals with bioterrorism and microbial food contamination. Among the most recent challenges in dealing with microbial food contamination are the prospects that food may become deliberately contaminated by bioterrorists. Tommy G. Thompson, former secretary of Health and Human Services, said before his resignation in December 2004: "I, for the life of me, cannot understand why the terrorists have not, you know, attacked our food supply, because it is so easy to do," he said. "And we are importing a lot of food from the Middle East, and it would be easy to tamper with that."

In Chapter 20, Drs. Barbara Rasco and Gleyn E. Bledsoe explore the different chemical, radiological, and biological agents that could be employed by individuals intent on deliberately contaminating our food. They take a critical look at present food protection strategies and present a food defense plan that would reduce the vulnerabilities of our food supply to bioterrorism.

Keeping our food supply safe from microbial food contamination is a daunting task. Fortunately, as this book bears witness, important advances are being made in the detection and control of microbial food contamination. The establishment of national and international organizations such as PulseNet, Codex, and the International Food Safety Authorities Network is facilitating the rapid flow of information concerning food contamination and the implementation of appropriate responses. The editor is grateful to the authors of this volume for all they have done—and continue to do—to insure the safety of our food from microbial contamination.

Editor

Charles L. Wilson, PhD, is currently president and CEO of Wilson Associates International LLC, an international consulting group advising on the development of biologically-based technologies to preserve food. He recently retired from the USDA ARS Appalachian Fruit Research Station, in Kearneysville, West Virginia, after 37 years of service with the Federal government. Dr. Wilson's research and teaching career spans over 47 years, during which he has been at the forefront of research and thinking on the use of biological technologies to control plant diseases and weeds, and for the postharvest preservation of food.

In the early part of his career, Dr. Wilson was a professor at the University of Arkansas (1958–1968) where he received the Arkansas Alumni's award for distinguished teaching and research. He subsequently served on the faculty at Ohio State University from 1970 to 1979. Dr. Wilson joined the USDA ARS Appalachian Fruit Research Station in 1980, where he initiated a research program to find biologically-based alternatives to synthetic pesticides for the control of fruit diseases. This internationally recognized research program yielded a variety of innovative technologies for the control of postharvest diseases of fruits and vegetables, which include the use of antagonistic microorganisms, natural plant-derived fungicides, and the use of induced resistance.

Dr. Wilson and the Associates of Wilson Associates LLC are presently advising companies on the use of natural plant-derived and animal-derived antimicrobials for the control of plant diseases, weeds, and insect and foodborne human pathogens. His company is also advising other companies on the incorporation of natural antimicrobials into food packaging to extend the freshness of commodities placed in the package. In conjunction with investigators worldwide, Dr. Wilson has authored a series of international patents involving the use of antagonistic yeast and natural compounds to control postharvest diseases. Dr. Wilson has worked closely with industry to bring about the large-scale testing and commercialization of this technology and is presently consulting in this area.

In 1984, Dr. Wilson received the Washington Academy of Sciences Distinguished Service Award in the biological sciences for "pioneering research in understanding and manipulating plant diseases." He was also elected a fellow of the academy. In 1988, he received the ARS-NAA Scientist of the Year Award for "innovative research on biological control of postharvest diseases of fruit." In 1994, Dr. Wilson was named a fellow of the American

Phytopathology Society, and in 1996 he received the Award of Excellence from the Federal Laboratory Consortium for Technology Transfer for his role in developing the first EPA-registered antagonistic yeast biofungicide for the control of postharvest diseases of fruits and vegetables.

Dr. Wilson has authored or coauthored over 200 scientific publications, 18 patents, and 2 books on gardening. He has previously coedited books for Academic Press (*Exotic Plant Pests and North American Agriculture*) and CRC Press (*Biological Control of Postharvest Diseases—Theory and Practice; Microbial Food Contamination*).

Contributors

Glen D. Armstrong Department of Microbiology and Infectious Diseases, Faculty of Medicine, University of Calgary, Calgary, Canada

David M. Asher Center for Biologics Evaluation and Research, U.S. Food and Drug Administration, Rockville, Maryland

Larry R. Beuchat Center for Food Safety, University of Georgia, Griffin, Georgia

Deepak Bhatnagar Food and Food Safety Research Unit, U.S. Department of Agriculture, Southern Regional Research Center, New Orleans, Louisiana

Gleyn E. Bledsoe Institute of International Agriculture, Michigan State University, East Lansing, Michigan

Robert Brown Food and Food Safety Research Unit, U.S. Department of Agriculture, Southern Regional Research Center, New Orleans, Louisiana

Rebecca J. Buckner Center for Food Safety and Applied Nutrition, U.S. Food and Drug Administration, College Park, Maryland

Jeffrey W. Cary Food and Food Safety Research Unit, U.S. Department of Agriculture, Southern Regional Research Center, New Orleans, Louisiana

Joaquín Castilla Department of Neurology, University of Texas Medical Branch, Galveston, Texas

Muhammad M. Chaudry Islamic Food and Nutrition Council of America, Chicago, Illinois

Thomas E. Cleveland Food and Food Safety Research Unit, U.S. Department of Agriculture, Southern Regional Research Center, New Orleans, Louisiana

Dean O. Cliver Food Safety Laboratory and WHO Collaborating Center for Food Virology, Department of Population Health and Reproduction, University of California, Davis, California

Kara Cooper Division of Foodborne, Bacterial and Mycotic Diseases, PulseNet Methods Development Laboratory, Centers for Disease Control and Prevention, Atlanta, Georgia

Pina M. Fratamico U.S. Department of Agriculture, Agricultural Research Service—Eastern Regional Research Center, Wyndmoor, Pennsylvania

Daniel Y.C. Fung Department of Animal Sciences and Industry and Food Science Institute, Kansas State University, Manhattan, Kansas

Dennisse González Department of Neurology, University of Texas Medical Branch, Galveston, Texas

Eija Hyytia-Trees Division of Foodborne, Bacterial and Mycotic Diseases, PulseNet Methods Development Laboratory, Centers for Disease Control and Prevention, Atlanta, Georgia

Vijay K. Juneja Microbial Food Safety Research Unit, U.S. Department of Agriculture, Agricultural Research Service, Eastern Regional Research Center, Wyndmoor, Pennsylvania

Susumu Kawasaki National Food Research Institute, Food Hygiene Team, Kannondai, Tsukuba, Japan

Edward V. LaBudde Middle Thompson Lake, Libby, Montana

Robert A. LaBudde Least Cost Formulations, Ltd., Virginia Beach, Virginia

Michael D. McElvaine USDA, Office of Risk Assessment and Cost-Benefit Analysis, Washington, DC

Margaret Ann Miller Department of Food Safety, Zoonoses and Food-borne Diseases, World Health Organization, Geneva, Switzerland

Hussni O. Mohammed College of Veterinary Medicine, Cornell University, Ithaca, New York

Rodrigo Morales Department of Neurology, University of Texas Medical Branch, Galveston, Texas

Tova Neufeld Department of Molecular Microbiology, Tel Aviv University, Tel Aviv, Israel

Kanniah Rajasekaran   Food and Food Safety Research Unit, U.S. Department of Agriculture, Southern Regional Research Center, New Orleans, Louisiana

Barbara Rasco   Department of Food Science and Human Nutrition, Washington State University, Pullman, Washington

Carrie E. Regenstein   Carnegie Mellon University, Pittsburgh, Pennsylvania

Joe M. Regenstein   Cornell Kosher Food Initiative, Cornell University, Ithaca, New York

Efrain M. Ribot   Division of Foodborne, Bacterial and Mycotic Diseases, PulseNet Methods Development Laboratory, Centers for Disease Control and Prevention, Atlanta, Georgia

Ronald T. Riley   Toxicology and Mycotoxin Research Unit, USDA Agricultural Research Service, Athens, Georgia

Judith Rishpon   Department of Molecular Microbiology, Tel Aviv University, Tel Aviv, Israel

Moez Sanaa   National Veterinary School of Alfort, Maisons-Alfort, France

Jørgen Schlundt   Department of Food Safety, Zoonoses and Foodborne Diseases, World Health Organization, Geneva, Switzerland

Shiowshuh Sheen   Microbial Food Safety Research Unit, U.S. Department of Agriculture, Agricultural Research Service, Eastern Regional Research Center, Wyndmoor, Pennsylvania

Claudio Soto   Department of Neurology, University of Texas Medical Branch, Galveston, Texas

Avishay-Abraham Stark   Department of Biochemistry, Faculty of Life Sciences, Tel Aviv University, Israel

Gaurav Tewari   Tewari De-Ox Systems, Inc., San Antonio, Texas

Kristin Viswanathan   Department of Food Safety, Zoonoses and Foodborne Diseases, World Health Organization, Geneva, Switzerland

Kenneth A. Voss   Toxicology and Mycotoxin Research Unit, USDA Agricultural Research Service, Athens, Georgia

Janee B. Gelineau-van Waes Department of Genetics, Cell Biology & Anatomy, University of Nebraska, Nebraska Medical Center, Omaha, Nebraska

H. Michael Wehr U.S. Food and Drug Administration, Center for Food Safety and Applied Nutrition, College Park, Maryland

Jiujiang Yu Food and Food Safety Research Unit, U.S. Department of Agriculture, Southern Regional Research Center, New Orleans, Louisiana

Section I

Instances and Nature of Microbial Food Contamination

1

PulseNet and Emerging Foodborne Diseases

Efrain M. Ribot, Eija Hyytia-Trees, and Kara Cooper

CONTENTS

1.1 Introduction

Foodborne diseases cause an estimated 76 million illnesses each year in the United States with over 5.2 million of the infections attributed to foodborne bacterial pathogens (Mead et al. 1999). Of these, approximately 4.6 million infections are due to organisms currently tracked by the PulseNet system (Table 1.1). It is extremely important for the public health system to develop and implement new surveillance, outbreak detection, and response strategies geared toward reducing the number of foodborne illness in the United States and abroad (Spratt 1999; Swaminathan et al. 2001; Allos et al. 2004; CDC 2006c; Swaminathan et al. 2006). The future of foodborne disease control and prevention depends on the effectiveness and adaptability of

TABLE 1.1

Estimated Number of Cases per Year vs. Number of Patterns Submitted to the National Database for the Organisms Currently Tracked by PulseNet

Organism/Year Database Was Established	Estimated Number of Annual Cases	Number of Isolates Submitted to Databases (1996–2006)	Total Number of Patterns Submitted in 2005
Escherichia coli O157/1996	73,480	26,271	5,398
Salmonella/1998	1,412,498	143,009	33,305
Shigella spp./1998	448,240	25,290	4,864
Listeria monocytogenes/1998	2,518	7,725	2,182
Campylobacter/2004	2,453,926	4,578	853
Vibrio cholerae/2006	54	187	66

Note: The first column lists the foodborne organisms tracked by PulseNet and the year the database was established. The second column shows the number of estimated annual cases for each of the organisms (Mead et al. 1999). The third column shows the number of isolates represented in the national database as off the end of August, 2006. The last column lists the number of patterns submitted to the database in 2005. In some cases the number of patterns might be higher than the actual number of isolates represented in the database because some of them may have been analyzed with more than one enzyme.

the surveillance and outbreak detection strategies in place, in particular, in an era where clusters of illness associated with less traditional vehicles of transmission are becoming more common (Tauxe 1998). In the modern outbreak scenario described by Tauxe (1997), the control of clusters of illness is complicated by the fact that cases tend to be diffuse in nature, often spanning multiple localities, states, regions, or even countries. This new outbreak scenario emerges amidst changes in the food industry geared toward improving efficiency in the preparation, processing, and distribution of food products in an expanding global market (Swerdlow 1998; WHO 2004). It is now common for foods to be prepared in central plants, packaged in a different locality, often under many different brand names or labels, and distributed across large communities, states, and often countries. Contamination of food products at the farm or during the early stages of processing could lead to the distribution of a tainted food product to any location in the country. Multiple locality outbreaks present a formidable challenge for epidemiologists in the United States and abroad in particular in development and implementation of strategies for the rapid detection of clusters of illness that would allow for rapid intervention and ultimately prevention of additional infections from occurring (Tauxe 1997; Sobel et al. 2002). Although identifying the source of infection is absolutely important in the control of an outbreak, it is also of great importance to gain insight on how foodborne pathogens persist in animal reservoirs, survive, and adapt to environmental changes, and how different processing and distribution practices may enhance their ability to enter the human food chain.

The use of molecular subtyping tools in the area of epidemiologic investigations, along with advances in the field of informatics, has enhanced our ability to detect clusters of illness, by matching "like" isolates and disseminating data much more rapidly than previously possible (Swaminathan et al. 2001; Tauxe 2006). Molecular subtyping tools also provide us with the ability to link cases to the source or vehicle of infection strengthening our trace-back capabilities (Levin et al. 1999; Barrett et al. 2004). The sensitivity of some molecular subtyping tools is such that we are now capable of detecting widely dispersed clusters often involving very few cases (Laine et al. 2005; Gerner-Smidt et al. 2005). Interestingly, the benefits of utilizing molecular tools to aid in surveillance and epidemiologic investigations reach farther than rapid cluster detection. The accumulation of molecular subtypes could also be useful in detecting the emergence of new strains or strains that may have increased virulence or other phenotypic properties that could be considered a threat to public health (Johnson et al. 2004). Cataloging subtypes could also provide clues on attribution of illness to specific reservoirs, vehicles, or food preparation processes (CDC 2003; Wegener et al. 2003; Hald et al. 2004; Batz et al. 2005). The emergence of a subtype known to have caused an outbreak in the past can also be tracked and the characteristics leading to its reemergence studied to uncover similarities that might shed some light on the epidemiology and help with the implementation of effective preventive measures. Trends can also be detected by examining the frequency with which a particular subtype occurs in a given locality at a given time. This type of analysis can be expanded to include long-term (year to year) comparisons to show an increase or decrease of a particular subtype or track subtypes linked to other important characteristics, such as virulence or antimicrobial resistance markers (Kamal 1974; White et al. 2004; Wallmann 2006).

For a laboratory-based surveillance system to be effective at detecting clusters of illness it must provide as much coverage as possible of the population it is trying to protect. Also, isolates that enter the public heath system should be subtyped as close to real-time as possible and the information obtained should be shared immediately with the proper public health officials and organizations. For this to occur, the proper laboratory and communication infrastructure must be in place and operated by trained staff in the local public health laboratories. In addition, the strategic plan to be followed must have flexibility and adaptability as two of its core elements or it will run the risk of becoming too impractical to succeed in an ever-changing environment where pathogens are finding new ways to spread and cause illness in a population. To address this formidable challenge, we must continue to make improvements in the areas of surveillance, outbreak detection and response, and communication between public health agencies and the food industry.

1.2 Molecular Subtyping and Public Health

The term that best describes the symbiotic relationship between molecular subtyping techniques and public health is molecular epidemiology.

Molecular epidemiology, by definition, integrates two seemingly unrelated disciplines, molecular biology and epidemiology, to create one of the most powerful forces ever put together for the detection and prevention of human illness, infectious or otherwise. It is important to understand that molecular epidemiology is driven, primarily, by the principles of traditional epidemiology but makes use of molecular biology to study and define how disease is distributed in a population. The use of molecular tools can also enable us to identify etiologic agents, determinants, and potential risk factors associated with the disease and provide insight on how to treat it or what measures to implement in an attempt to prevent it from occurring again in the future.

Molecular epidemiology, at its best, employs subtyping approaches that correlate laboratory data with the epidemiological findings of the organism being investigated revealing links between cases and the determinants responsible for the illnesses. Sometimes the epidemiology drives molecular biologists to identify new ways to address important questions about a human pathogen or medical condition. In other instances, technology drives the epidemiology to change the approach used to analyze and interpret new types of data. Advances in the field of genomics have created quite a stir in the area of molecular epidemiology because of its seemingly endless potential in the area of strain differentiation. However, we would argue that not every approach derived from the genomics of an organism will translate into a successful tool for use in molecular epidemiology. Depending on the molecular strategy, it may be more suited for investigating possible evolutionary relationships between two or more organisms; a better understanding of the genetic dynamics of a given population (Heymann 1998; Reid et al. 2000; Donnenberg 2001; Morris 2003; Hyytia-Trees et al. 2006), or a study of the epidemiological relationships between bacterial pathogens belonging to the same genus, species, or serogroup (Graves and Swaminathan 2001; van Belkum 2003; Zhang et al. 2006).

The integration of molecular subtyping in the context of public health must lead to the collection of data that are epidemiologically relevant information and, therefore, can be used for the rapid detection of clusters of illness and not just for making inferences about possible genetic relationships from a strictly evolutionary or population genetics point of view. Often, claims are made about the high discriminatory power, high throughput, portability, and ease of use of many new tools as the main reasons to integrate them into the schemes used by public health laboratories. However, serious consideration should be given to their cost effectiveness and epidemiologic relevance. The use of molecular tools for laboratory-based surveillance and cluster detection must achieve a balance between discriminatory power and epidemiologic relevance, and not only ease of use or the ability to detect the largest number of differences between two or more isolates (Morse 1995; Tenover et al. 1997; Levin 1999; Foxman 2001; Barrett et al. 2004). Regardless of what the molecular data may suggest, it is important to keep in mind that establishing genetic relationships between isolates is only part of the picture and does not provide conclusive evidence that an outbreak may or may not be occurring (Barrett et al. 2004). It is safe to assume that no single molecular method will provide us with the 100% sensitivity and specificity needed to detect every outbreak and separate every sporadic isolate from the outbreak-related ones. In PulseNet, we recognize this as a practical truth, but continue to explore and evaluate other methods to overcome the limitations intrinsic to the methodology currently used by the network (Reid et al. 2000; Swaminathan et al. 2001; Gerner-Smidt et al. 2006). The ultimate goal is to develop a system that will achieve the proper balance between discriminatory power and epidemiologic relevance, and do so in an efficient and cost-effective manner.

1.3 PulseNet USA

PulseNet USA was established in 1996 as the national molecular subtyping network for the surveillance of foodborne bacterial infections (Swaminathan et al. 2001; Gerner-Smidt et al. 2006). PulseNet currently uses PFGE, the gold standard for the subtyping of most foodborne bacterial pathogens, for DNA fingerprint analysis of Shiga-toxin producing *E. coli* O157 (STEC O157), *Salmonella*, *Shigella* spp., *Campylobacter*, *Listeria monocytogenes*, and *Vibrio cholerae* (Ribot et al. 2001; Cooper et al. 2006; Ribot et al. 2006). The usefulness of PFGE as a subtyping tool has been confirmed by over 10 years worth of data accumulated in the national databases at the CDC. PulseNet's success as a laboratory-based surveillance system resides in the strong concordance between epidemiology and PFGE and the versatility (applicable for the subtyping of multiple organisms) and transfer-ability of this methodology to public health laboratories. Comparison of the PFGE data generated in multiple laboratories is facilitated by the use of highly standardized laboratory protocols, sophisticated analysis software (BioNumerics, Applied Maths, Sint-Martens-Latem, Belgium), and a web-based communication platform accessible on demand to participating laboratories and epidemiologists (Swaminathan et al. 2001; Gerner-Smidt et al. 2006). Currently, over 70 laboratories in the United States, including state, local, county, and federal public health laboratories, utilize the PulseNet-standardized PFGE protocols to perform laboratory-based surveillance on the isolates they receive. PFGE patterns are generated locally and uploaded to the PulseNet national database for comparison with patterns submitted by other laboratories (Swaminathan et al. 2001; Gerner-Smidt et al. 2006). Since PulseNet is a network (decentralized system), it is imperative for the methodology used to be strictly standardized to facilitate the comparison of data generated in different laboratories in different geographical locations. In general, standardization of protocols is a very complicated task since many variables need to be evaluated and subjected to a stringent validation process. PulseNet protocols are evaluated and validated by CDC and other laboratories to make sure that they will perform as expected in all the laboratories in the network.

PulseNet's success goes beyond the utility and versatility of PFGE as a subtyping tool. The philosophy upon which PulseNet was founded is as critical to the program as PFGE is. Very early in the development process, CDC recognized that for PulseNet to reach its potential it had to be sensitive to the needs of the participating members and focus on bridging the communication gaps that existed at the time between laboratorians and epidemiologists. This was accomplished by partnering with organizations such as the Association of Public Health Laboratories (APHL) and the Council for State and Territorial Epidemiologist (CSTE), the U.S. Department of Agriculture (USDA), and the Food and Drug Administration (FDA) (Swaminathan et al. 2001). The results of this multiagency collaboration have benefited public health by facilitating the early detection of clusters of foodborne illness and providing a Web-based communications platform where vital epidemiologic and laboratory information is shared instantaneously with all the network participants.

Success in any venture is often followed by increased expectations. In PulseNet, increased expectations have taken many forms; some of them are technical in nature, others logistical, but none are more significant than the ones in the area of data interpretation. In the end one must explain, or at least attempt to, what it means for two or more strains to be indistinguishable or different by a particular typing method. An honest attempt must be made to translate typing information into a language that clearly describes the epidemiological meaning of such a relationship. Ideally, the molecular subtyping tool used should provide unequivocal evidence that strains sharing a given profile are part of a common source outbreak, even in the absence of epidemiological data, while distinguishing among those that are not. Such a method would be 100% sensitive and 100% specific and, unfortunately, does not exist, at least not yet. PulseNet's efforts to identify the best possible and practical formula for subtyping foodborne pathogens is an ongoing endeavor that has led us to the establishment of a program referred to as "the next generation subtyping method," which is briefly described below.

1.4   PulseNet and the Concept of Strain Emergence

The classical meaning of the term "emerging pathogen" describes a disease-causing agent or pathogen as a newly recognized public health problem (Morse 1995; Struelens et al. 1998; Krause 2001). However, the use of the term "emerging" can also be used to describe less traditional scenarios such as a rise in a previously recognized pathogen because of new ways of transmission or a known pathogen that has acquired new pathogenic properties such as the acquisition of virulence or antimicrobial resistance markers (Threlfall et al. 1994; Glynn et al. 1998; von Baum 2005).

In PulseNet, the emergence of a strain can be established on the basis of its molecular fingerprint (PFGE pattern) or the link between a particular subtype and other phenotypic or genotypic characteristics. PFGE data can be used to determine emergence of clones or new strains by merely comparing their pattern against the patterns in the database for a given period or within a particular geographical area (Brooks et al. 2001; Karenlampi et al. 2003; Staples et al. 2006; Wetzel and Lejeune 2006). PFGE data can also be used to look for increases in the number of cases caused by a given pattern and to establish associations between patterns and vehicles of infections, in particular rare occurring or emerging vehicles.

In order to establish some relationships between a molecular subtype and any other marker, epidemiological or otherwise, a reliable bank of information must be available. PulseNet created such a data bank, known as the national PFGE fingerprint database, in which patterns are named using a standard nomenclature (Swaminathan et al. 2001; Gerner-Smidt et al. 2006). PulseNet's pattern naming system consists of a 10 character code with the generic structure XXXYYY.0000 where XXX is the code name of the bacterial pathogen, YYY denotes the restriction enzyme used to generate the PFGE pattern, and the last four characters represent the pattern number (Swaminathan et al. 2001). The scheme used to assign the pattern numbers denotes the order in which the patterns submitted to the database were named and not the degree of genetic similarity between any of the isolates represented therein. Once a pattern is uploaded to the PulseNet national database, it is named by the data manager and queries can be performed to determine if the submission corresponds to a previously seen pattern or if it is a new one. Queries to determine how frequently a particular pattern occurs can also be performed with ease.

Available epidemiologic information is linked to the patterns represented in the PFGE database via a series of data fields incorporated into the BioNumerics analysis software. These fields are customized for each of the pathogens tracked by PulseNet and contain important phenotypic and genotypic information, such as serotype, toxin type, antimicrobial susceptibility, source, and vehicle. These information fields can be queried to determine possible associations between specific PFGE subtypes and other epidemiologically or phenotypically relevant properties (Swaminathan et al. 2001; Gerner-Smidt et al. 2006). Queries can be expanded to identify clusters of isolates that share other genetic or phenotypic traits that might suggest the emergence of strains, clones, or trends among the patterns seen for any of the organisms tested. Queries can also be performed to determine whether the emergence of a pattern is associated with the geographical distribution of a particular food product.

1.5 Organisms Tracked by PulseNet

STEC O157 was first recognized as a serious health problem in 1982 after an epidemiologic investigation showed that patients experiencing hemorrhagic colitis had consumed undercooked hamburgers sold at a fast-food chain (Riley et al. 1983). Although outbreaks of STEC O157 associated with the consumption of contaminated ground beef and contact with infected animals still occur with a fairly high frequency; different vehicles of trans-mission have emerged (Table 1.2) since this human pathogen was first

TABLE 1.2

Selected Emerging Vehicles Associated with Outbreaks Seen since the Establishment of PulseNet in 1996

Vehicle	Pathogen	Year	Country	Reference
Alfalfa sprouts	*Salmonella* Muenchen	1999	United States	(Proctor et al. 2001)
	Salmonella Kottbus	2001	United States	(CDC 2002e)
	E. coli O157:H7	1997, 2003, 2004	United States	(Breuer et al. 2001; Ferguson et al. 2005)
	Salmonella Chester	2003	United States	
Lettuce	*E. coli* O157:H7	1996, 2002, 2004	United States	(Hilborn 1999)
	Salmonella Newport	2004	United States	
Parsley	*Shigella sonnei*	1998	United States/ Canada	(Naimi et al. 2003)
Tomatoes	*Salmonella* Baildon	2001	United States	(Cummings et al. 2001)
	Salmonella Javiana	2002	United States	(CDC 2002d)
	Salmonella Anatum	2004	United States	(CDC 2005a)
	Salmonella Typhimurium	2006	United States/ Canada	
Spinach	*E. coli* O157:H7	2003, 2006	United States	(CDC 2006b)
Almonds (raw)	*Salmonella* Enteritidis	2000, 2003	United States/ Canada	(CDC 2004; Isaacs et al. 2005)
Unpasteurized juice/cider	*E. coli* O157	1996	United States/ Canada	(CDC 1996b, 1997, 1999)
	Salmonella Muenchen	1999	United States/ Canada	
Cantaloupe/ honeydew	*Salmonella* Saphra	1997	United States	(CDC 2002a; Mohle-Boetani et al. 1999)
Melons	*Salmonella* Poona	2000–2002	United States	
	Salmonella Muenchen	2003		
	Shigella	2003	United States	
Ready-to-eat meats	*Listeria monocytogenes*	1998, 2000, 2002	United States	(CDC 2000b; Olsen et al. 2005)
Unpasteurized milk/cheese	*Campylobacter*	2001, 2003, 2004	United States	(CDC 2002b)

recognized (Morse 1995; Altekruse et al. 1997; Tauxe 1997; Krause 2001). Also, STEC serotypes other than O157 are increasingly recognized as a cause of severe gastrointestinal disease and outbreaks, mainly due to improved surveillance (CDC 2000a; Brooks et al. 2005). Because of the increased significance of the non-O157 serotypes, work is underway to optimize a standardized PFGE protocol for these pathogens.

Pathogenic *Salmonella* spp., in general, represent the most complex and difficult organisms for PulseNet to track, mainly because of the large number of cases identified and fingerprints submitted to the PulseNet USA database each year compared to other organisms tracked by PulseNet (Table 1.1). Still, the number of isolates submitted to the PulseNet database represents a fraction of the total 1.4 million estimated cases that occur in the United States each year (Mead et al. 1999). Over the past decade, PulseNet has provided useful subtyping information on the emergence of new vehicles of transmission (Table 1.2) and recognition of clonal strains with multidrug resistance (MDR) phenotypes (Evans 1996; Threlfall 2000; Herikstad et al. 2002; Ribot et al. 2002; Velge et al. 2005).

Of the bacterial pathogens tracked by PulseNet, Shigella is somewhat unique in that humans and other primates are the only known reservoir; outbreaks often occur from human-to-human transmission, via the fecal–oral route and often as the result of overcrowding and poor hygiene (Sur et al. 2004). Shigella is the third most common cause of bacterial gastroenteritis in the United States with most outbreaks caused by *Shigella sonnei* followed by *S. flexneri* and the recently emerged *S. boydii* (Kalluri et al. 2004; Woodward et al. 2005). *S. flexneri* and *S. dysenteriae* account for most of the cases identified in developing countries and endemic regions (Hale 1991; Sur et al. 2004). However, foodborne outbreaks of shigellosis occur with some frequency and are often associated with the consumption of food products contaminated by infected food-handlers (Trevejo et al. 1999) or fecal contamination of products, such as produce, on the field (Naimi et al. 2003).

Listeria monocytogenes can cause serious illness, often with symptoms such as high fever, neck stiffness, headaches, and nausea and, in some cases, septicemia and meningoencephalitis. Pregnant women (and their fetus), infants, the elderly, and individuals with a weakened immune system are typically the most severely affected group of the population. Listeriosis is particularly devastating in pregnant women, often resulting in miscarriages and stillbirths (CDC 2002c). Listeriosis caused by *L. monocytogenes* is also characterized by a high mortality (20%–25%) rate (Graves et al. 2005). Listeriosis outbreaks are difficult to detect partly because of the potentially long incubation times (3–70 days; median incubation time of 3 weeks) (Riedo et al. 1994). Molecular subtyping of *L. monocytogenes* has been instrumental in the detection of cluster of illness caused by this organism. The recent occurrence of several listeriosis outbreaks led regulatory agencies to establish a zero tolerance policy for *L. monocytogenes* in ready-to-eat foods. Since then, there has been a decline in the incidence of listeriosis, although outbreaks still occur sometimes leading to the recall of millions of pounds of the tainted product (CDC 1998, 2002c; Olsen et al.

2005; Shen et al. 2006). Queso fresco (Mexican style soft cheese), ready-to-eat turkey meat, and hot dogs have been some of the most frequent vehicles of transmission.

Of the estimated 2.5 million *Campylobacter* infections that occur each year, approximately 80% of them are attributable to foodborne transmission with *C. jejuni* causing most of the reported infections in the United States (Mead et al. 1999). It is believed that *Campylobacter* infections occur mainly as sporadic events and not as part of bona fide outbreaks with most of the cases (~99%) in the United States caused by *C. jejuni*. This idea is, in part, supported by molecular data that suggest a high degree of diversity among *Campylobacter* species. The benefits of using standardized subtyping methods for laboratory-based surveillance and epidemiologic investigations of *Campylobacter* remain unclear, primarily because isolates are seldom fully characterized by public health laboratories in the United States. However, outbreaks of campylobacteriosis do occur and they are often associated with the consumption of contaminated milk, particularly unpasteurized milk and untreated water (Harris et al. 1986; Deming et al. 1987; Fahey et al. 1995; Evans 1996; Friedman et al. 2000; Allos 2001; Oliver et al. 2005).

Vibrio cholerae remains an important pathogen that is endemic in many developing countries particularly in southern Asia, Africa, and Latin America, where it causes acute diarrheal disease often leading to rapid dehydration and estimated high rates of mortality (~120,000 deaths annually), particularly among untreated patients (Faruque et al. 1998). The vast majority of the cholera infections worldwide result from exposure to contaminated water resulting from inadequate sanitation or flooding (Ford 1999). The two *V. cholerae* serogroups that typically cause disease in human are O1 and O139, which emerged recently (Albert et al. 1993). *V. cholerae* O141 has recently emerged in the United States and has the potential to cause outbreaks of a cholerae-like illness (Dalsgaard et al. 2001; Crump et al. 2003). Although the epidemiology of *V. cholerae* O141 is not well under-stood, consumption of contaminated seafood appears to be a possible vehicle for foodborne transmission (Crump et al. 2003). Cholera is a public health concern also for developed countries to which cases could be imported via air or other forms of travel and where the disease could spread quickly resulting in an increase of sporadic cases or even outbreaks. The establishment of PulseNet PFGE standardized protocols stemmed from the need to enhance *V. cholerae* surveillance for the tracking illness as the result of natural and, potentially, intentional events (Swaminathan et al. 2006).

In contrast to the other organisms currently being tracked by PulseNet, *V. parahaemolyticus* and *V. vulnificus* have shown a significant increase in prevalence in recent years (CDC 2006c). Efforts are underway to develop, validate, and implement standardized PFGE protocols for both of these organisms. These organisms are ubiquitous in estuarine or marine environ-ments and share many of the characteristics associated with pathogenic vibrios (Kaneko 1973; Karaolis et al. 1994; Morris 2003). *V. parahaemolyticus* infections are primarily associated with the consumption of contaminated shellfish, particularly oysters, or foods cross-contaminated with shellfish. Skin infections can also occur from exposure of open wounds to saltwater (Kaneko 1973, 1974). *V. vulnificus* has recently emerged as a serious public health problem in the United States (CDC 1993; Strom 2000). This organism causes the most severe form of vibrio infections, often leading to septicemia, invasion of connective tissues, and death, and has the highest mortality rate for any foodborne bacterial pathogen (Blake et al. 1979; CDC 1993; Strom 2000).

1.6   PulseNet and Emergence of Foodborne Bacterial Pathogens

Routine subtyping of the organisms tracked by PulseNet has resulted in the detection of outbreaks that would have otherwise gone undetected or, at the very least, would have been difficult to identify (Laine et al. 2005). Molecular subtyping tools can help recognize the emergence of strains by finding associations, at the genome level, between a fingerprint or a subtype and other characteristics, such as phenotypic, clinical, or epidemi-ological, the organisms may possess. For instance, a strong association between a pathogen and a newly identified reservoir may indicate adaptive behavior on the part of the pathogen (Snoeyenbos et al. 1969; Borczyk et al. 1987; Chapman et al. 1993; Mishu et al. 1994; Morris 2003). The emergence or spread of strains with decreased sensitivity to antimicrobials is a direct result of antibiotics being used as prophylactics and growth promoters in food animals (Evans 1996; Glynn et al. 1998; Threlfall 2000; Gorbach 2001; Teale 2002; Shea 2003, 2004; White et al. 2004). The use of molecular tools can also help link cases from an outbreak to new vehicles of transmission or to identify the chain of events that led to the contamination of the food product. Expanding markets in the ready-to-eat-food industry, as well as increasing popularity of organic products such as fruits and vegetables, have also presented a formidable challenge for public health officials, mainly because these types of foods are usually not cooked before consump-tion (Altekruse et al. 1997; Tauxe 1997, 2006). As with outbreaks associated with traditional vehicles, subtyping helps us navigate through the ocean of cases and fish out those isolates that are likely to be part of the outbreak and to identify the likely source (contaminated item, label or company, distribu-tor, etc.). Emergence of a foodborne pathogen can also arise from changes in health-care practices, particularly in testing of clinical specimens with the goal of increasing efficiency and reducing costs (Mintz 2006). The role the movement and travel of food and people plays in the dissemination of pathogens from one city, country, or region to another must not be under-estimated either (Tauxe 1996; Gushulak 2000). Even changes in our social behavior can put us at risk of contracting an infection normally caused by a foodborne pathogen even when the implicated vehicle of infection is not food (CDC 1996a, 2005b). Natural disasters could also lead to the emergence or reemergence of a pathogen within a displaced population, in particular when the sanitation infrastructure is compromised and general hygiene is minimal or nonexistent (Drazen 2005; CDC 2006d; et al. 2007). Even isolates from sporadic cases can be subtyped to determine the presence of "hidden" clusters of illness and to ask questions about possible sources of such illness (Batz et al. 2005).

In the sections that follow, we will provide some examples of how PulseNet has contributed, directly or indirectly, to the recognition of emerging trends of foodborne pathogens. The accumulation of standardized molecular subtyping data and analysis with epidemiological information provide public health officials with new ways to evaluate clusters of illness, identify the source of the infection, and conduct epidemiological studies that focus not only on outbreak investigations but also identify the factors involved in sporadic illness (attribution) and establish and recognize emerging vehicles of transmission.

1.6.1 Emerging Vehicles

For years, it was considered that the majority of the recognized outbreaks were caused by STEC O157 and *Salmonella* resulted from the consumption of ground beef and poultry products, respectively. When a different vehicle was identified, it could often be linked to a cross-contamination event involving one of these traditional vehicles. In the past couple of decades, however, different vehicles have emerged, or are at least now recognized, for these foodborne bacterial pathogens ranging from fruits and vegetables to exotic pets (Ackman et al. 1995; Altekruse et al. 1997; Mermin et al. 1997; Tauxe 1997; Schroter et al. 2004). Contamination of produce is of particular public health importance because foods in this category are often consumed raw or exposed to cooking temperatures well below the levels needed to kill bacterial pathogens. For instance, outbreaks associated with lettuce, spinach, and other green leaf salad items appear to have become an emerging trend during the past 10–15 years (Tauxe 1997). Most recently, a multistate outbreak of STEC O157 was identified among patients who consumed contaminated baby spinach, resulting in over 200 illnesses, 1 fatality, and high rate of hospitalizations and HUS cases (CDC 2006b). Other examples of emerging vehicles are listed in Table 1.2. As the market and food production practices continue to change, the role of subtyping will become more important in the tracking and recognition of emerging vehicles. Pulse-Net's ability to recognize the emergence of new vehicles has been strengthened by partnering with programs and agencies, such as US Department of Agriculture (USDA), the National Antimicrobial Resistance Monitoring System (NARMS: www.cdc.gov/NARMS), and the Foodborne Diseases Active Surveillance Network (FoodNet: www.cdc.gov/foodnet), which have launched attribution studies designed to help identify links between sporadic cases and the source of infection by comparing subtypes in each of these databases (Gerner-Smidt et al. 2006).

1.6.2 Travel

The impact international travel and international distribution of foods has on a given population or region is best exemplified by the voyages of conquistadores between the Old and New (unknown) Worlds over 500 years ago. In the United States, children attending primary school learn, in great detail, about the five "seeds of change" (corn, potato, sugar, the horse, and disease) associated with the explorations that brought about the transformation of both the New and Old Worlds, transformation that still continues today (Wilson 1991; Wilson 1995; Gushulak 2000). Of these, diseases had the most devastating effect on the native cultures of the New World (Crosby 1972; Stauffer 1991), causing widespread death. Since then, the movement of populations and the commerce of international foods continue to play a major role in the spread of foodborne diseases, although at a much faster pace than what happened over 500 years ago. Nowadays, people can travel from one side of the globe to the other in about a day with foodstuff usually lagging not too far behind in speed of movement.

Travel-associated cases of foodborne illness can originate in the country of residence and be exported to the visiting country or countries, be acquired in the visiting country, or be acquired during actual travel from one location to the next. The latter was the case of an outbreak of shigellosis among Japanese travelers who had visited the Hawaiian Islands and were on their way back to their home country (Terajima et al. 2006). Although the actual vehicle of infection could not be confirmed, the epidemiologic investigation suggested that a salad served by the airline during the return flight could have been the vehicle of infection. PFGE data was used to confirm that all 15 cases, which were from different cities in Japan, were indeed part of the outbreak.

PFGE was also instrumental in tracking a prolonged outbreak of *S. sonnei* among members of several observant Jewish communities (Sobel et al. 1998). Interestingly, PFGE confirmed the following epidemiological findings: (1) the outbreak strains were not seen in non-Jewish neighboring communities and (2) community-to-community transmission occurred via travel of infected individuals. In some of these outbreaks, PFGE data were used to show that cases were linked to the contaminated product and also helped epidemiologists connect two seemingly distinct outbreaks occurring in different geographical locations in the United States.

The movement of people to different parts of the world increases the demand for traditional foods that must be shipped from various parts of the world. As the world gets smaller for travelers and food markets continue to expand, new strategies are needed to investigate the factors leading to the international spread of foodborne illness in order to establish effective preventive measures.

1.6.3   Changes in Public Health Practices: The Good and the Bad

Emergence of a pathogen can also be recognized because of a change in policies that affect public health. One of the changes that is currently impacting pathogen identification practices in the public health laboratories is the proliferation of non-culture identification methods (Klein et al. 2002; CDC 2006a). Use of non-culture identification methods in a clinical laboratory presents a challenge for subtyping networks such as PulseNet, because it could result in a decrease in the number of isolates available for subtyping, therefore reducing our ability to conduct laboratory-based surveillance and outbreak investigations. To address this concern, some commercial clinical laboratories are providing state public health laboratories with enrichment broths derived from the positive specimens they receive. Some state public health laboratories are now performing plating of these broths in various selective media aimed at selection of pathogens that are no longer cultured by clinical laboratories as well as pathogens that were not routinely cultured before (CDC 2006a). An example of an outbreak detected as the result of this change occurred in 2005 in the state of New York. By conducting tests beyond what a clinical laboratory would perform, the New York State Department of Health (NYSDOH) was able to identify the first outbreak of STEC O45 in the United States (CDC 2006a). Even though this STEC serotype is considered rare in the United States, this outbreak highlights the importance of culture confirmation and subtyping of not only well-known pathogens but also the ones that are less understood.

CDC and PulseNet USA in partnership with the Associated of Public Health Laboratories (APHL) and the Council of State and Territorial Epidemiologists (CSTE) is working with clinical laboratories in the US to ensure that samples that test positive with nonculture methods be forwarded to public health laboratories for further characterization and subtyping. The value of nonculture methods for detection should not overshadow the role culture-based techniques play in the study, characterization, and subtyping of emerging and re-emerging pathogens.

1.6.4   Natural Disasters

Natural disasters such as earthquakes, floods, hurricanes, and tsunamis have always been a challenge to public health. Survivors of a natural disaster are subject to illness as a result of injuries received during the incident or through exposure to disease that arise from the destruction of the public health infrastructure (Ivers 2006). One of the most significant causes of rapidly spreading disease following a natural disaster is contaminated drinking water (Drazen 2005). However, secondary effects of natural disasters, such as crowding and subsequent fecal–oral spread of gastrointestinal pathogens, may also contribute to the spread of diarrheal diseases (Ivers 2006). In the aftermath of two monsoon-related floods in 2004 in Bangladesh, over 17,000 patients were seen in one hospital with cholera being the most common cause of admission (Qadri et al. 2005). *V. cholerae* is also associated with the consumption of undercooked seafood. In fact, in the aftermath of hurricane Katrina, two cases of toxigenic *V. cholerae* O1 infection were attributed to the consumption of raw or undercooked shrimp (CDC 2003, 2006a). Luckily, the anticipated sharp increase in the number of cases with the consumption of contaminated water and wound infections never materialized.

1.6.5 Discovering Hidden Outbreaks

In some instances, the recognition of outbreaks in itself becomes an emerging trend as illustrated by the recent increase in the number of listeriosis outbreaks detected in the past 8 years. By all indications, *L. monocytogenes* was thought to cause primarily sporadic infections. The idea that *L. monocytogenes* did not cause many outbreaks was supported by the fact that only five outbreaks were recognized between the years 1978 and 1997. Ever since PulseNet implemented a standardized PFGE protocol for the subtyping of *L. monocytogenes* in 1998, the number of outbreaks detected in the United States has more than doubled the total seen in the previous 20 years (Gerner-Smidt et al. 2006). This suggests that many of the cases thought to be sporadic in nature before 1998 might have been indeed part of outbreaks if molecular subtyping had been available at the time.

1.7 Next Generation Subtyping

The high frequency of occurrence of certain patterns, particularly during outbreaks, presents a challenge to PulseNet. Although different molecular subtyping methods provide snapshot comparisons of two or more strains, none of the methods commonly used for subtyping of foodborne bacterial pathogens can claim 100% sensitivity and specificity. The most frequently seen problem is the so-called common and clonal PFGE patterns that may prevail in a state or a region but appear to have no connection to any particular outbreak (Borucki et al. 2004; Hedberg 2006; Threlfall 2000). Commonly occurring PFGE patterns may be confusing when compared with that of strains whose only link may be their indistinguishable fingerprint.

For a number of years PulseNet has recognized this problem and worked diligently to improve its subtyping capabilities. A project focusing on the development of the "next generation subtyping method" for PulseNet was launched in 2001 in collaboration with various public health partners including the Association of Public Health Laboratories (APHL) and three state public health laboratories (Minnesota Department of Public Health, Massachusetts Department of Public Health/State Laboratory Institute, and North Carolina State Laboratory of Public Health). The main objective of this project was to develop and evaluate sequence- or sequencing-based subtyping methodologies with higher sensitivity and specificity than PFGE, which also had a high level of epidemiologic concordance (Swaminathan et al. 2001; Gerner-Smidt et al. 2005; Gerner-Smidt et al. 2006).

In our present reality, we must concede that establishing genetic relatedness at any level, molecular or otherwise, cannot be used as an infallible predictor of epidemiologic relatedness. Accepting this truth is critical to our understanding of molecular epidemiology and for the steps that must be taken in order to use subtyping tools effectively. There are a number of DNA sequence-based subtyping tools that scientists have evaluated for establishing genetic relatedness between any given number of isolates or strains. Unfortunately, many of the studies have been made without testing an adequate number of isolates for which strong epidemiologic information is available. An evaluation of a new subtyping method must be performed on a large number of sporadic as well as outbreak-related isolates before inferences can be made about the method's ability to accurately discriminate between non-outbreak-related isolates while clustering those with a common source. The standardized method must then be tested in a prospective manner to determine how the subtyping data correlates to the epidemiologic findings in real time. More importantly, the method must also identify, when implemented in the context of a network, clusters of illness even when there is little or no epidemiologic information available.

Interrogation of whole genomic sequences has revealed that prokaryotic genomes contain a wide variety of repetitive DNA elements ranging from single-nucleotide repeats to large, complicated repeats consisting of dozens of nucleotides (van Belkum et al. 1998). Repeats organized in tandem and demonstrating individual unit number variability between strains are designated as variable-number tandem repeats (VNTRs). Multiple-locus VNTR analysis (MLVA) involves determination of the number of repeat copy units in multiple-loci PCR and capillary electrophoresis. MLVA has shown promise because of its ability to discriminate between otherwise indistinguishable subtypes within highly clonal organisms (Keim et al. 2000; Noller et al. 2003; Lindstedt et al. 2004; Keys et al. 2005). Therefore, PulseNet decided to invest in the development and evaluation of MLVA subtyping schemes for use in the PulseNet network as a second generation subtyping method. Much progress has been made on this front since the program was launched, resulting in a soon-to-be-released standardized protocol for MLVA subtyping of STEC O157 (Hyytia-Trees et al. 2006). The overall discriminatory power of this MLVA protocol appears to be equal to that of PFGE and has been shown to be particularly useful in discriminating epidemiologically unrelated isolates that possess some of the most commonly encountered PFGE patterns. MLVA subtyping schemes for *Salmonella* serotypes Typhimurium and Enteritidis and *L. monocytogenes* are also currently being developed and evaluated by CDC and its state health laboratory partners.

Some believe that nucleotide sequencing provides us with better genotypic answers, or at least data, than methods based on the analysis of DNA fragments, regardless of how they are generated (restriction analysis or

PCR). The advent of genome-sequencing projects and faster sequencing approaches continue to provide a seemingly endless source of information particularly in the area of comparative genomics (Fraser-Liggett 2005). PulseNet is currently working on the development of a method platform based on single nucleotide polymorphisms (SNPs) for STEC O157 as part of the third-generation subtyping methods to be integrated in the network in the future. In silico comparison of the two complete STEC O157 genomes (Sakai and EDL933; Hayashi et al. 2001; Perna et al. 2001) revealed potentially variable regions that could be used as subtyping targets. Comparative genome sequencing using microarrays for approximate 20% of the STEC O157 genome was performed on 11 isolates (Zhang et al. 2006). The genome regions sequenced comprised a total of 1199 chromosomal genes and the complete sequence of the large virulence plasmid (pO157). The resulting data revealed 906 SNPs in 523 chromosomal genes and a high level of DNA polymorphisms among the pO157 plasmids.

How these molecular tools will be used in PulseNet in the future remains to be seen. In addition to epidemiologic concordance, there are many other considerations that could allow these new tools to surpass PFGE as the new gold standard for subtyping foodborne pathogens or to simply be used as secondary tools to be employed under specific circumstances. On the basis of our experience we feel that in the near future foodborne bacterial subtyping will likely use these and other new tools in combination with already established ones, such as PFGE.

1.8 Concluding Remarks

The goal of public health surveillance is the prevention and control of illness in a specific population. Molecular subtyping has had a profound impact on public health by allowing for the rapid detection of clusters of foodborne illness, and thereby assisting in the recognition and investigation of outbreaks at the local, national, and international level. The main purpose of utilizing subtyping tools is to rapidly identify clusters and minimize the scope of an outbreak investigation by providing subtyping data that could be used in differentiating from those that are not. More focused outbreak investigation should allow for more rapid identification of the source, and reduction of the burden (cost and resources) placed on the epidemiologic investigation. However, care should be taken that regardless of the level of sophistication, discriminatory power, and epidemiologic concordance any particular method can offer, subtyping tools by themselves should not be used as absolute evidence that any number of like isolates are part of an outbreak. Subtyping tools must be used only as aids in the prospective detection of clusters of like strains to lead the epidemiologic investigation in the right direction and provide information to assist in linking the potential source, if possible, to the cases identified as part of an outbreak.

In addition to outbreak investigation, molecular subtyping can be used to answer different questions about the spread of foodborne illness. The first step is the recognition of a problem; but it is only after careful scientific investigations, often conducted during an outbreak, that the true nature of the problem may become apparent. The importance of these studies should not be underestimated because past experience has shown that the more that is known about a pathogen the better it can be controlled, and its prevalence declines (Tauxe 2002). Molecular subtyping provides a means to monitor the safety of the food production system, drive basic and public health research, and ultimately reveal clues about an outbreak that can be used by epidemiologists and public health officials to establish effective prevention measures.

Surveillance mechanisms are an integral part of the recognition of emergence. Truly emerging bacterial foodborne pathogens do not come around very frequently. However, the more likely scenario is the emergence of a new pathogen that has acquired new attributes, such as virulence factors or antimicrobial resistance. Since the establishment of PulseNet, there have been several examples of this type of emergence and PulseNet has been able to assist in the tracking and understanding of these organisms in the context of public health. The emergence of pathogens or emergence of patterns discussed in this chapter might be the result of the utilization of more sophisticated detection and identification tools and not due to de novo emergence within a population. Regardless of the mechanism behind their perceived emergence it is more important to acknowledge their impact on public health and the information they add to our understanding of the epidemiology of these foodborne pathogens.

The utility of PFGE as a subtyping tool and as a foundation of the PulseNet molecular subtyping network has been well documented. However, both technical and surveillance-related problems do exist with this technology. Although the epidemiological concordance of this method is usually very good, as databases expand and experience is gained, instances have been identified in which PFGE data did not provide useful epidemiologic information. Because of these factors, the search for new and better methodologies is something PulseNet has taken very seriously in the past several years. Care has been taken to identify a technique that could be efficiently employed in a network setting, while possessing sufficient sensitivity and specificity to provide epidemiologically relevant information.

The known repertoire of foodborne illnesses has changed dramatically over time. Therefore, the underlying theme in foodborne disease surveillance is to be on the lookout for the unusual as new pathogens, vehicles, and virulence properties continue to be recognized. Increases in international travel and the globalization of the food production and distribution practices will continue to complicate matters. However, enhancement of the existing system for detecting and investigating foodborne outbreaks will mean that the health of the public is better protected against illness.

References

Ackman, D. M., P. Drabkin, G. Birkhead, and P. Cieslak. 1995. Reptile-associated salmonellosis in New York State. *Pediatr. Infect. Dis. J.* 14 (11):955–959.

Albert, M. J., A. K. Siddique, M. S. Islam, A. S. Faruque, M. Ansaruzzaman, S. M. Faruque, and R. B. Sack. 1993. Large outbreak of clinical cholera due to *Vibrio cholerae* non-O1 in Bangladesh. *Lancet* 341 (8846):704.

Allos, B. M. 2001. *Campylobacter jejuni* infections: Update on emerging issues and trends. *Clin. Infect. Dis.* 32 (8):1201–1206.

Allos, B. M., M. R. Moore, P. M. Griffin, and R. V. Tauxe. 2004. Surveillance for sporadic foodborne disease in the 21st century: The FoodNet perspective. *Clin. Infect. Dis.* 38 (Suppl. 3):S115–S120.

Altekruse, S. F., M. L. Cohen, and D. L. Swerdlow. 1997. Emerging foodborne diseases. *Emerg. Infect. Dis.* 3 (3):285–293.

Barrett, T. J., E. M. Ribot, and B. Swaminathan. 2004. Molecular subtyping for epidemiology: Issues in comparability of patterns and interpretation of data. In *Molecular Microbiology: Diagnostic Principles and Practices*, edited by D. H. Dersing, F. C. Tenover, J. Vesalivic, Y. Tang, E. R. Unger, D. A. Relman, and T. White. Washington, DC: ASM Press.

Batz, M. B., M. P. Doyle, G. Morris, Jr., J. Painter, R. Singh, R. V. Tauxe, M. R. Taylor, and D. M. Lo Fo Wong. 2005. Attributing illness to food. *Emerg. Infect. Dis.* 11 (7):993–999.

Blake, P. A., M. H. Merson, R. E. Weaver, D. G. Hollis, and P. C. Heublein. 1979. Disease caused by a marine *Vibrio*. Clinical characteristics and epidemiology. *N. Engl. J. Med.* 300 (1):1–5.

Borczyk, A. A., M. A. Karmali, H. Lior, and L. M. Duncan. 1987. Bovine reservoir for verotoxin-producing *Escherichia coli* O157:H7. *Lancet* 1 (8524):98.

Borucki, M. K., J. Reynolds, C. C. Gay, K. L. McElwain, S. H. Kim, D. P. Knowles, and J. Hu. 2004. Dairy farm reservoir of *Listeria monocytogenes* sporadic and epidemic strains. *J. Food Prot.* 67 (11):2496–2499.

Breuer, T., D. H. Benkel, R. L. Shapiro, W. N. Hall, M. M. Winnett, M. J. Linn, J. Neimann, T. J. Barrett, S. Dietrich, F. P. Downes, D. M. Toney, J. L. Pearson, H. Rolka, L. Slutsker, and P. M. Griffin. 2001. A multistate outbreak of *Escherichia coli* O157:H7 infections linked to alfalfa sprouts grown from contaminated seeds. *Emerg. Infect. Dis.* 7 (6):977–982.

Brooks, J. T., S. Y. Rowe, P. Shillam, D. M. Heltzel, S. B. Hunter, L. Slutsker, R. M. Hoekstra, and S. P. Luby. 2001. *Salmonella typhimurium* infections transmitted by chlorine-pretreated clover sprout seeds. *Am. J. Epidemiol.* 154 (11):1020–1028.

Brooks, J. T., E. G. Sowers, J. G. Wells, K. D. Greene, P. M. Griffin, R. M. Hoekstra, and N. A. Strockbine. 2005. Non-O157 Shiga toxin-producing *Escherichia coli* infections in the United States, 1983–2002. *J. Infect. Dis.* 192 (8):1422–1429.

CDC. 1993. *Vibrio vulnificus* infections associated with raw oyster consumption—Florida, 1981–1992. *MMWR Morb. Mortal. Wkly. Rep.* 42 (21):405–407.

CDC. 1996a. Lake-associated outbreak of *Escherichia coli* O157:H7—Illinois, 1995. *MMWR Morb. Mortal. Wkly. Rep.* 45 (21):437–439.

CDC. 1996b. Outbreak of *Escherichia coli* O157:H7 infections associated with drinking unpasteurized commercial apple juice—British Columbia, California, Colorado, and Washington, October 1996. *MMWR Morb. Mortal. Wkly. Rep.* 45 (44):975.

CDC. 1997. Outbreaks of *Escherichia coli* O157:H7 infection and cryptosporidiosis associated with drinking unpasteurized apple cider—Connecticut and New York, October 1996. *MMWR Morb. Mortal. Wkly. Rep.* 46 (1):4–8.

CDC. 1998. Multistate outbreak of listeriosis—United States, 1998. *MMWR Morb. Mortal. Wkly. Rep.* 47 (50):1085–1086.

CDC. 1999. Outbreak of Salmonella serotype Muenchen infections associated with unpasteurized orange juice—United States and Canada, June 1999. *MMWR Morb. Mortal. Wkly. Rep.* 48 (27):582–585.

CDC. 2000a. *Escherichia coli* O111:H8 outbreak among teenage campers—Texas, 1999. *MMWR Morb. Mortal. Wkly. Rep.* 49 (15):321–324.

CDC. 2000b. Multistate outbreak of listeriosis—United States, 2000. *MMWR Morb. Mortal. Wkly. Rep.* 49 (50):1129–1130.

CDC. 2002a. Multistate outbreaks of Salmonella serotype Poona infections associated with eating cantaloupe from Mexico—United States and Canada, 2000–2002. *MMWR Morb. Mortal. Wkly. Rep.* 51 (46):1044–1047.

CDC. 2002b. Outbreak of *Campylobacter jejuni* infections associated with drinking unpasteurized milk procured through a cow-leasing program—Wisconsin, 2001. *MMWR Morb. Mortal. Wkly. Rep.* 51 (25):548–549.

CDC. 2002c. Outbreak of listeriosis—northeastern United States, 2002. *MMWR Morb. Mortal. Wkly. Rep.* 51 (42):950–951.

CDC. 2002d. Outbreak of Salmonella serotype Javiana infections—Orlando, Florida, June 2002. *MMWR Morb. Mortal. Wkly. Rep.* 51 (31):683–684.

CDC. 2002e. Outbreak of Salmonella serotype Kottbus infections associated with eating alfalfa sprouts—Arizona, California, Colorado, and New Mexico, February–April 2001. *MMWR Morb. Mortal. Wkly. Rep.* 51 (1):7–9.

CDC. 2003. Preliminary FoodNet data on the incidence of foodborne illnesses—selected sites, United States, 2002. *MMWR Morb. Mortal. Wkly. Rep.* 52 (15): 340–343.

CDC. 2004. Outbreak of Salmonella serotype Enteritidis infections associated with raw almonds—United States and Canada, 2003–2004. *MMWR Morb. Mortal. Wkly. Rep.* 53 (22):484–487.

CDC. 2005a. Outbreaks of *Salmonella* infections associated with eating Roma tomatoes—United States and Canada, 2004. *MMWR Morb. Mortal. Wkly. Rep.* 54 (13):325–328.

CDC. 2005b. *Shigella flexneri* serotype 3 infections among men who have sex with men—Chicago, Illinois, 2003–2004. *MMWR Morb. Mortal. Wkly. Rep.* 54 (33):820–822.

CDC. 2006a. Importance of culture confirmation of shiga toxin-producing *Escherichia coli* infection as illustrated by outbreaks of gastroenteritis—New York and North Carolina, 2005. *MMWR Morb. Mortal. Wkly. Rep.* 55 (38):1042–1045.

CDC. 2006b. Ongoing multistate outbreak of *Escherichia coli* serotype O157:H7 infections associated with consumption of fresh spinach—United States, September 2006. *MMWR Morb. Mortal. Wkly. Rep.* 55 (38):1045–1046.

CDC. 2006c. Preliminary FoodNet data on the incidence of infection with pathogens transmitted commonly through food—10 States, United States, 2005. *MMWR Morb. Mortal. Wkly. Rep.* 55 (14):392–395.

CDC. 2006d. Two cases of toxigenic *Vibrio cholerae* O1 infection after Hurricanes Katrina and Rita—Louisiana, October 2005. *MMWR Morb. Mortal. Wkly. Rep.* 55 (2):31–32.

Chapman, P. A., C. A. Siddons, D. J. Wright, P. Norman, J. Fox, and E. Crick. 1993. Cattle as a possible source of verocytotoxin-producing *Escherichia coli* O157 infections in man. *Epidemiol. Infect.* 111 (3):439–447.

Cooper, K. L., C. K. Luey, M. Bird, J. Terajima, G. B. Nair, K. M. Kam, E. Arakawa, A. Safa, D. T. Cheung, C. P. Law, H. Watanabe, K. Kubota, B. Swaminathan, and E. M. Ribot. 2006. Development and validation of a PulseNet standardized pulsed-field gel electrophoresis protocol for subtyping of *Vibrio cholerae*. *Foodborne Pathog. Dis.* 3 (1):51–58.

Crosby, A. W. 1972. *The Columbian exchange*. Vol. 291. Westport, CN: Greenwood Press.

Crump, J. A., C. A. Bopp, K. D. Greene, K. A. Kubota, R. L. Middendorf, J. G. Wells, and E. D. Mintz. 2003. Toxigenic *Vibrio cholerae* serogroup O141-associated cholera-like diarrhea and bloodstream infection in the United States. *J. Infect. Dis.* 187 (5):866–868.

Cummings, K., E. Barrett, J. C. Mohle-Boetani, J. T. Brooks, J. Farrar, T. Hunt, A. Fiore, K. Komatsu, S. B. Werner, and L. Slutsker. 2001. A multistate outbreak of *Salmonella enterica* serotype Baildon associated with domestic raw tomatoes. *Emerg. Infect. Dis.* 7 (6):1046–1048.

Dalsgaard, A., O. Serichantalergs, A. Forslund, W. Lin, J. Mekalanos, E. Mintz, T. Shimada, and J. G. Wells. 2001. Clinical and environmental isolates of *Vibrio cholerae* serogroup O141 carry the CTX phage and the genes encoding the toxin-coregulated pili. *J. Clin. Microbiol.* 39 (11):4086–4092.

Deming, M. S., R. V. Tauxe, P. A. Blake, S. E. Dixon, B. S. Fowler, T. S. Jones, E. A. Lockamy, C. M. Patton, and R. O. Sikes. 1987. *Campylobacter* enteritis at a university: Transmission from eating chicken and from cats. *Am. J. Epidemiol.* 126 (3):526–534.

Donnenberg, M. S. and T. S. Whittam. 2001. Pathogenesis and evolution of virulence in enteropathogenic and enterohemorrhagic *Escherichia coli*. *J. Clin. Invest.* 107 (5):539–548.

Drazen, J. M. and M. S. Klempner. 2005. Disaster, water, cholera, vaccines, and hope. *N. Engl. J. Med.* 352 (8):827.

Evans, S. and R. Davies. 1996. Case control study of multiple-resistant *Salmonella typhimurium* DT104 infection of cattle in Great Britain. *Vet. Rec.* 139 (23):557–558.

Fahey, T., D. Morgan, C. Gunneburg, G. K. Adak, F. Majid, and E. Kaczmarski. 1995. An outbreak of *Campylobacter jejuni* enteritis associated with failed milk pasteurisation. *J. Infect.* 31 (2):137–143.

Faruque, S. M., M. Asadulghani, N. Saha, A. R. Alim, M. J. Albert, K. M. Islam, and J. J. Mekalanos. 1998. Analysis of clinical and environmental strains of nontoxigenic *Vibrio cholerae* for susceptibility to CTXPhi: Molecular basis for origination of new strains with epidemic potential. *Infect. Immun.* 66 (12):5819–5825.

Ferguson, D. D., J. Scheftel, A. Cronquist, K. Smith, A. Woo-Ming, E. Anderson, J. Knutsen, A. K. De, and K. Gershman. 2005. Temporally distinct *Escherichia coli* O157 outbreaks associated with alfalfa sprouts linked to a common seed source—Colorado and Minnesota, 2003. *Epidemiol. Infect.* 133 (3):439–447.

Ford, T. E. 1999. Microbiological safety of drinking water: United States and global perspectives. *Environ. Health. Perspect.* 107 (Suppl. 1):191–206.

Foxman, B. and L. Riley. 2001. Molecular epidemiology: Focus on infection. *Am. J. Epidemiol.* 153 (12):1135–1141.

Fraser-Liggett, C. M. 2005. Insights on biology and evolution from microbial genome sequencing. *Genome Res.* 15 (12):1603–1610.

Friedman, C. R., J. Neimann, H. C. Wegener, and R. V. Tauxe. 2000. Epidemiology of *Campylobacter jejuni* infections in the United States and other industrialized nations. In *Campylobacter*, edited by I. Nachamkin and M. J. Blaser. Washington, DC: ASM Press.

Gerner-Smidt, P., J. Kincaid, K. Kubota, K. Hise, S. B. Hunter, M.-A. Fair, D. Norton, A. Woo-Ming, T. Kurzynski, M. J. Sotir, M. Head, K. Holt, and B. Swaminathan. 2005. Molecular surveillance of Shiga toxigenic *Escherichia coli* O157 by PulseNet USA. *J. Food Prot.* 68:1926–1931.

Gerner-Smidt, P., K. Hise, J. Kincaid, S. Hunter, S. Rolando, E. Hyytia-Trees, E. M. Ribot, and B. Swaminathan. 2006. PulseNet USA: A five-year update. *Foodborne Pathog. Dis.* 3 (1):9–19.

Glynn, M. K., C. Bopp, W. Dewitt, P. Dabney, M. Mokhtar, and F. J. Angulo. 1998. Emergence of multidrug-resistant *Salmonella enterica* serotype typhimurium DT104 infections in the United States. *N. Engl. J. Med.* 338 (19):1333–1338.

Gorbach, S. L. 2001. Antimicrobial use in animal feed—time to stop. *N. Engl. J. Med.* 345 (16):1202–1203.

Graves, L. M., S. B. Hunter, A. R. Ong, D. Schoonmaker-Bopp, K. Hise, L. Kornstein, W. E. DeWitt, P. S. Hayes, E. Dunne, P. Mead, and B. Swaminathan. 2005. Microbiological aspects of the investigation that traced the 1998 outbreak of listeriosis in the United States to contaminated hot dogs and establishment of molecular subtyping-based surveillance for *Listeria monocytogenes* in the PulseNet network. *J. Clin. Microbiol.* 43 (5):2350–2355.

Graves, L. M. and B. Swaminathan. 2001. PulseNet standardized protocol for subtyping *Listeria monocytogenes* by macrorestriction and pulsed-field gel electrophoresis. *Int. J. Food Microbiol.* 65 (1–2):55–62.

Gushulak, B. D. and D. W. MacPherson. 2000. Population mobility and infectious diseases: The diminishing impact of classical infectious diseases and new approaches for the 21st century. *Clin. Infect. Dis.* 31 (3):776–780.

Hald, T., D. Vose, H. C. Wegener, and T. Koupeev. 2004. A Bayesian approach to quantify the contribution of animal-food sources to human salmonellosis. *Risk. Anal.* 24 (1):255–269.

Hale, T. L. 1991. Genetic basis of virulence in *Shigella* species. *Microbiol. Rev.* 55 (2):206–224.

Harris, N. V., N. S. Weiss, and C. M. Nolan. 1986. The role of poultry and meats in the etiology of *Campylobacter jejuni/coli* enteritis. *Am. J. Public Health* 76 (4): 407–411.

Hayashi, T., K. Makino, M. Ohnishi, K. Kurokawa, K. Ishii, K. Yokoyama, C.-G. Han, E. Ohtsubo, K. Nakayama, T. Murata, M. Tanaka, T. Tobe, T. Iida, H. Takami, T. Honda, C. Sasakawa, N. Ogasawara, T. Yasunaga, S. Kuhara, T. Shiba, M. Hattori, and H. Shinagawa. 2001. Complete genome sequence of enterohemorrhagic *Escherichia coli* O157:H7 and genomic comparison with a laboratory strain K-12. *DNA Res.* 8 (1):11–22.

Hedberg, C. W. and J. M. Besser. 2006. Commentary: Cluster evaluation, PulseNet, and public health practice. *Foodborne Pathog. Dis.* 3 (1):32–35.

Herikstad, H., Y. Motarjemi, and R. V. Tauxe. 2002. Salmonella surveillance: A global survey of public health serotyping. *Epidemiol Infect* 129 (1):1–8.

Heymann, D. L. and G. R. Rodier. 1998. Global surveillance of communicable diseases. *Emerg. Infect. Dis.* 4 (3):362–365.

Hilborn, E. D., J. H. Mermin, P. A. Mshar, J. L. Hadler, A. Voetsch, C. Wojtkunski, M. Swartz, R. Mshar, M.-A. Lambert-Fair, J. A. Farrar, M. K. Glynn, and L. Slutsker. 1999. A multistate outbreak of *Escherichia coli* O157:H7 infections associated with consumption of Mesclun lettuce. *Arch. Intern. Med.* 159 (15):1758–1764.

Hyytia-Trees, E., S. C. Smole, P. A. Fields, B. Swaminathan, and E. M. Ribot. 2006. Second generation subtyping: A proposed PulseNet protocol for multiple-locus variable-number tandem repeat analysis of Shiga toxin-producing *Escherichia coli* O157 (STEC O157). *Foodborne Pathog. Dis.* 3 (1):118–131.

Isaacs, S., J. Aramini, B. Ciebin, J. A. Farrar, R. Ahmed, D. Middleton, A. U. Chandran, L. J. Harris, M. Howes, E. Chan, A. S. Pichette, K. Campbell, A. Gupta, L. Y. Lior, M. Pearce, C. Clark, F. Rodgers, F. Jamieson, I. Brophy, and A. Ellis. 2005. An international outbreak of salmonellosis associated with raw almonds contaminated with a rare phage type of *Salmonella enteritidis*. *J. Food Prot.* 68 (1):191–198.

Ivers, L. C. and E. T. Ryan. 2006. Infectious diseases of severe weather-related and flood-related natural disasters. *Curr. Opin. Infect. Dis.* 19 (5):408–414.

Johnson, J. R., M. A. Kuskowski, A. Gajewski, D. F. Sahm, and J. A. Karlowsky. 2004. Virulence characteristics and phylogenetic background of multidrug-resistant and antimicrobial-susceptible clinical isolates of *Escherichia coli* from across the United States, 2000–2001. *J. Infect. Dis.* 190 (10):1739–1744.

Kalluri, P., K. C. Cummings, S. Abbott, G. B. Malcolm, K. Hutcheson, A. Beall, K. Joyce, C. Polyak, D. Woodward, R. Caldeira, F. Rodgers, E. D. Mintz, and N. Strockbine. 2004. Epidemiological features of a newly described serotype of *Shigella boydii*. *Epidemiol. Infect.* 132 (4):579–583.

Kamal, A. M. 1974. The seventh pandemic of cholera. In *Cholera*, edited by D. B. N. W. Burrows. Philadelphia: Saunders.

Kaneko, T. and R. R. Colwell. 1973. Ecology of *Vibrio parahaemolyticus* in Chesapeake Bay. *J. Bacteriol.* 113 (1):24–32.

Kaneko, T. and R. R. Colwell. 1974. Distribution of *Vibrio parahaemolyticus* and related organisms in the Atlantic Ocean off South Carolina and Georgia. *Appl. Microbiol.* 28 (6):1009–1017.

Karaolis, D. K., R. Lan, and P. R. Reeves. 1994. Molecular evolution of the seventh-pandemic clone of *Vibrio cholerae* and its relationship to other pandemic and epidemic *V. cholerae* isolates. *J. Bacteriol.* 176 (20):6199–6206.

Karenlampi, R., H. Rautelin, M. Hakkinen, and M. L. Hanninen. 2003. Temporal and geographical distribution and overlap of Penner heat-stable serotypes and pulsed-field gel electrophoresis genotypes of *Campylobacter jejuni* isolates collected from humans and chickens in Finland during a seasonal peak. *J. Clin. Microbiol.* 41 (10):4870–4872.

Keim, P., L. B. Price, A. M. Klevytska, K. L. Smith, J. M. Schupp, R. Okinaka, P. J. Jackson, and M. E. Hugh-Jones. 2000. Multiple-locus variable-number tandem repeat analysis reveals genetic relationships within *Bacillus anthracis*. *J. Bacteriol.* 182 (10):2928–2936.

Keys, C., S. Kemper, and P. Keim. 2005. Highly diverse variable number tandem repeat loci in the *E. coli* O157:H7 and O55:H7 genomes for high-resolution molecular typing. *J. Appl. Microbiol.* 98 (4):928–940.

Klein, E. J., J. R. Stapp, C. R. Clausen, D. R. Boster, J. G. Wells, X. Qin, D. L. Swerdlow, and P. I. Tarr. 2002. Shiga toxin-producing *Escherichia coli* in children with diarrhea: A prospective point-of-care study. *J. Pediatr.* 141 (2):172–177.

Krause, R. M. 2001. Microbes and emerging infections: The compulsion to become something new. *ASM News* 67:15–20.

Laine, E. S., J. M. Scheftel, D. J. Boxrud, K. J. Vought, R. N. Danila, K. M. Elfering, and K. E. Smith. 2005. Outbreak of *Escherichia coli* O157:H7 infections associated with nonintact blade-tenderized frozen steaks sold by door-to-door vendors. *J. Food Prot.* 68 (6):1198–1202.

Levin, B. R., M. Lipsitch, and S. Bonhoeffer. 1999. Population biology, evolution, and infectious disease: Convergence and synthesis. *Science* 283 (5403):806–809.

Lindstedt, B. A., T. Vardund, L. Aas, and G. Kapperud. 2004. Multiple-locus variable-number tandem-repeats analysis of *Salmonella enterica* subsp. *enterica* serovar Typhimurium using PCR multiplexing and multicolor capillary electrophoresis. *J. Microbiol. Methods.* 59 (2):163–172.

Mead, P. S., L. Slutsker, V. Dietz, L. F. McCaig, J. S. Bresee, C. Shapiro, P. M. Griffin, and R. V. Tauxe. 1999. Food-related illness and death in the United States. *Emerg. Infect. Dis.* 5 (5):607–625.

Mermin, J., B. Hoar, and F. J. Angulo. 1997. Iguanas and Salmonella marina infection in children: A reflection of the increasing incidence of reptile-associated salmonellosis in the United States. *Pediatrics* 99 (3):399–402.

Mintz, E. D. 2006. Enterotoxigenic *Escherichia coli*: Outbreak surveillance and molecular testing. *Clin. Infect. Dis.* 42 (11):1518–1520.

Mishu, B., J. Koehler, L. A. Lee, D. Rodrigue, F. H. Brenner, P. Blake, and R. V. Tauxe. 1994. Outbreaks of *Salmonella enteritidis* infections in the United States, 1985–1991. *J. Infect. Dis.* 169 (3):547–552.

Mohle-Boetani, J. C., R. Reporter, S. B. Werner, S. Abbott, J. Farrar, S. H. Waterman, and D. J. Vugia. 1999. An outbreak of Salmonella serogroup Saphra due to cantaloupes from Mexico. *J. Infect. Dis.* 180 (4):1361–1364.

Morris, J. G., Jr. 2003. Cholera and other types of vibriosis: A story of human pandemics and oysters on the half shell. *Clin. Infect. Dis.* 37 (2):272–280.

Morse, S. S. 1995. Factors in the emergence of infectious diseases. *Emerg. Infect. Dis.* 1 (1):7–15.

Naimi, T. S., J. H. Wicklund, S. J. Olsen, G. Krause, J. G. Wells, J. M. Bartkus, D. J. Boxrud, M. Sullivan, H. Kassenborg, J. M. Besser, E. D. Mintz, M. T. Osterholm, and C. W. Hedberg. 2003. Concurrent outbreaks of *Shigella sonnei* and enterotoxigenic *Escherichia coli* infections associated with parsley: Implications for surveillance and control of foodborne illness. *J. Food Prot.* 66 (4):535–541.

Noller, A. C., M. C. McEllistrem, A. G. Pacheco, D. J. Boxrud, and L. H. Harrison. 2003. Multilocus variable-number tandem repeat analysis distinguishes outbreak and sporadic *Escherichia coli* O157:H7 isolates. *J. Clin. Microbiol.* 41 (12):5389–5397.

Oliver, S. P., B. M. Jayarao, and R. A. Almeida. 2005. Foodborne pathogens in milk and the dairy farm environment: Food safety and public health implications. *Foodborne Pathog. Dis.* 2 (2):115–129.

Olsen, S. J., M. Patrick, S. B. Hunter, V. Reddy, L. Kornstein, W. R. MacKenzie, K. Lane, S. Bidol, G. A. Stoltman, D. M. Frye, I. Lee, S. Hurd, T. F. Jones, T. N. LaPorte, W. Dewitt, L. Graves, M. Wiedmann, D. J. Schoonmaker-Bopp, A. J. Huang, C. Vincent, A. Bugenhagen, J. Corby, E. R. Carloni, M. E. Holcomb, R. F. Woron, S. M. Zansky, G. Dowdle, F. Smith, S. Ahrabi-Fard, A. R. Ong, N. Tucker, N. A. Hynes, and P. Mead. 2005. Multistate outbreak of *Listeria monocytogenes* infection linked to delicatessen turkey meat. *Clin. Infect. Dis.* 40 (7):962–967.

Perna, N. T., G. Plunkett, 3rd, V. Burland, B. Mau, J. D. Glasner, D. J. Rose, G. F. Mayhew, P. S. Evans, J. Gregor, H. A. Kirkpatrick, G. Posfai, J. Hackett,

S. Klink, A. Boutin, Y. Shao, L. Miller, E. J. Grotbeck, N. W. Davis, A. Lim, E. T. Dimalanta, K. D. Potamousis, J. Apodaca, T. S. Anantharaman, J. Lin, G. Yen, D. C. Schwartz, R. A. Welch, and F. R. Blattner. 2001. Genome sequence of enterohaemorrhagic *Escherichia coli* O157:H7. *Nature* 409 (6819):529–533.

Proctor, M. E., M. Hamacher, M. L. Tortorello, J. R. Archer, and J. P. Davis. 2001. Multistate outbreak of Salmonella serovar Muenchen infections associated with alfalfa sprouts grown from seeds pretreated with calcium hypochlorite. *J. Clin. Microbiol.* 39 (10):3461–3465.

Qadri, F., A. I. Khan, A. S. Faruque, Y. A. Begum, F. Chowdhury, G. B. Nair, M. A. Salam, D. A. Sack, and A. M. Svennerholm. 2005. Enterotoxigenic *Escherichia coli* and *Vibrio cholerae* diarrhea, Bangladesh, 2004. *Emerg. Infect. Dis.* 11 (7):1104–1107.

Reid, S. D., C. J. Herbelin, A. C. Bumbaugh, R. K. Selander, and T. S. Whittam. 2000. Parallel evolution of virulence in pathogenic *Escherichia coli*. *Nature* 406 (6791):64–67.

Ribot, E. M., C. Fitzgerald, K. Kubota, B. Swaminathan, and T. J. Barrett. 2001. Rapid pulsed-field gel electrophoresis protocol for subtyping of *Campylobacter jejuni*. *J. Clin. Microbiol.* 39 (5):1889–1894.

Ribot, E. M., R. K. Wierzba, F. J. Angulo, and T. J. Barrett. 2002. *Salmonella enterica* serotype Typhimurium DT104 isolated from humans, United States, 1985, 1990, and 1995. *Emerg. Infect. Dis.* 8 (4):387–391.

Ribot, E. M., M. A. Fair, R. Gautom, D. N. Cameron, S. B. Hunter, B. Swaminathan, and T. J. Barrett. 2006. Standardization of pulsed-field gel electrophoresis protocols for the subtyping of *Escherichia coli* O157:H7, Salmonella, and Shigella for PulseNet. *Foodborne Pathog. Dis.* 3 (1):59–67.

Riedo, F. X., R. W. Pinner, M. L. Tosca, M. L. Cartter, L. M. Graves, M. W. Reeves, R. E. Weaver, B. D. Plikaytis, and C. V. Broome. 1994. A point-source foodborne listeriosis outbreak: Documented incubation period and possible mild illness. *J. Infect. Dis.* 170 (3):693–696.

Riley, L. W., R. S. Remis, S. D. Helgerson, H. B. McGee, J. G. Wells, B. R. Davis, R. J. Hebert, E. S. Olcott, L. M. Johnson, N. T. Hargrett, P. A. Blake, and M. L. Cohen. 1983. Hemorrhagic colitis associated with a rare *Escherichia coli* serotype. *N. Engl. J. Med.* 308 (12):681–685.

Schroter, M., P. Roggentin, J. Hofmann, A. Speicher, R. Laufs, and D. Mack. 2004. Pet snakes as a reservoir for *Salmonella enterica* subsp. *diarizonae* (Serogroup IIIb): A prospective study. *Appl. Environ. Microbiol.* 70 (1):613–615.

Shea, K. M. 2003. Antibiotic resistance: What is the impact of agricultural uses of antibiotics on children's health? *Pediatrics* 112 (1 Pt 2):253–258.

Shea, K. M. 2004. Nontherapeutic use of antimicrobial agents in animal agriculture: Implications for pediatrics. *Pediatrics* 114 (3):862–868.

Shen, Y., Y. Liu, Y. Zhang, J. Cripe, W. Conway, J. Meng, G. Hall, and A. A. Bhagwat. 2006. Isolation and characterization of *Listeria monocytogenes* isolates from ready-to-eat foods in Florida. *Appl. Environ. Microbiol.* 72 (7):5073–5076.

Snoeyenbos, G. H., C. F. Smyser, and H. Van Roekel. 1969. Salmonella infections of the ovary and peritoneum of chickens. *Avian Dis.* 13 (3):668–670.

Sobel, J., D. N. Cameron, J. Ismail, N. Strockbine, M. Williams, P. S. Diaz, B. Westley, M. Rittmann, J. DiCristina, H. Ragazzoni, R. V. Tauxe, and E. D. Mintz. 1998. A prolonged outbreak of *Shigella sonnei* infections in traditionally observant Jewish communities in North America caused by a molecularly distinct bacterial subtype. *J. Infect. Dis.* 177 (5):1405–1409.

Sobel, J., P. M. Griffin, L. Slutsker, D. L. Swerdlow, and R. V. Tauxe. 2002. Investigation of multistate foodborne disease outbreaks. *Public Health Rep.* 117 (1):8–19.

Spratt, B. G. and M. C. Maiden. 1999. Bacterial population genetics, evolution and epidemiology. *Philos. Trans. R. Soc. Lond. B Biol. Sci.* 354 (1384):701–710.

Staples, J. E., K. A. Kubota, L. G. Chalcraft, P. S. Mead, and J. M. Petersen. 2006. Epidemiologic and molecular analysis of human tularemia, United States, 1964–2004. *Emerg. Infect. Dis.* 12 (7):1113–1138.

Stauffer, B. 1991. *The Columbian Exchange.* Westport, CT: Greenwood Press.

Strom, M. S. and R. N. Paranjpye. 2000. Epidemiology and pathogenesis of *Vibrio vulnificus. Microbes Infect.* 2 (2):177–188.

Struelens, M. J., Y. De Gheldre, and A. Deplano. 1998. Comparative and library epidemiological typing systems: Outbreak investigations versus surveillance systems. *Infect. Control Hosp. Epidemiol.* 19 (8):565–569.

Sur, D., T. Ramamurthy, J. Deen, and S. K. Bhattacharya. 2004. Shigellosis: Challenges and management issues. *Indian J. Med. Res.* 120 (5):454–462.

Swaminathan, B., T. J. Barrett, S. B. Hunter, and R. V. Tauxe. 2001. PulseNet: The molecular subtyping network for foodborne bacterial disease surveillance, United States. *Emerg. Infect. Dis.* 7 (3):382–389.

Swaminathan, B., P. Gerner-Smidt, L. K. Ng, S. Lukinmaa, K. M. Kam, S. Rolando, E. P. Gutierrez, and N. Binsztein. 2006. Building PulseNet International: An interconnected system of laboratory networks to facilitate timely public health recognition and response to foodborne disease outbreaks and emerging foodborne diseases. *Foodborne Pathog. Dis.* 3 (1):36–50.

Swerdlow, D. L. and S. F. Alterkruse. 1998. Foodborne diseases in the global village: What's on the plate for the 21st century? In *Emerging Infections 2*, edited by W. Scheld, W. Craig, and J. Hughes. Washington DC: ASM Press.

Taormina, P. J., L. R. Beuchat, and L. Slutsker. 1999. Infections associated with eating seed sprouts: An international concern. *Emerg. Infect. Dis.* 5 (5):626–634.

Tauxe, R. V. 1997. Emerging foodborne diseases: An evolving public health challenge. *Emerg. Infect. Dis.* 3 (4):425–434.

Tauxe, R. V. 1998. New approaches to surveillance and control of emerging foodborne infectious diseases. *Emerg. Infect. Dis.* 4 (3):455–456.

Tauxe, R. V. 2002. Emerging foodborne pathogens. *Int. J. Food Microbiol.* 78 (1–2): 31–41.

Tauxe, R. V. 2006. Molecular subtyping and the transformation of public health. *Foodborne Pathog. Dis.* 3 (1):4–8.

Tauxe, R. V. and J. M. Hughes. 1996. International investigation of outbreaks of foodborne disease. *Br. Med. J.* 313 (7065):1093–1094.

Teale, C. J. 2002. Antimicrobial resistance and the food chain. *J. Appl. Microbiol.* 92 Suppl.:85S–89S.

Tenover, F. C., R. D. Arbeit, and R. V. Goering. 1997. How to select and interpret molecular strain typing methods for epidemiological studies of bacterial infections: A review for healthcare epidemiologists. Molecular Typing Working Group of the Society for Healthcare Epidemiology of America. *Infect. Control Hosp. Epidemiol.* 18 (6):426–439.

Terajima, J., N. Tosaka, K. Ueno, K. Nakashima, P. Kitsutani, M. K. Gaynor, S. Y. Park, and H. Watanabe. 2006. *Shigella sonnei* outbreak among Japanese travelers returning from Hawaii. *Jpn. J. Infect. Dis.* 59 (4):282–283.

Threlfall, E. J. 2000. Epidemic *Salmonella typhimurium* DT 104—a truly international multiresistant clone. *J. Antimicrob. Chemother.* 46 (1):7–10.

Threlfall, E. J., J. A. Frost, L. R. Ward, and B. Rowe. 1994. Epidemic in cattle and humans of *Salmonella typhimurium* DT 104 with chromosomally integrated multiple drug resistance. *Vet. Rec.* 134 (22):577.

Trevejo, R. T., S. L. Abbott, M. I. Wolfe, J. Meshulam, D. Yong, and G. R. Flores. 1999. An untypeable *Shigella flexneri* strain associated with an outbreak in California. *J. Clin. Microbiol.* 37 (7):2352–2353.

van Belkum, A. 2003. High-throughput epidemiologic typing in clinical microbiology. *Clin. Microbiol. Infect.* 9 (2):86–100.

van Belkum, A., S. Scherer, L. van Alphen, and H. Verbrugh. 1998. Short-sequence DNA repeats in prokaryotic genomes. *Microbiol. Mol. Biol. Rev.* 62 (2):275–293.

Velge, P., A. Cloeckaert, and P. Barrow. 2005. Emergence of Salmonella epidemics: The problems related to *Salmonella enterica* serotype Enteritidis and multiple antibiotic resistance in other major serotypes. *Vet. Res.* 36 (3):267–288.

von Baum, H. and R. Marre. 2005. Antimicrobial resistance of *Escherichia coli* and therapeutic implications. *Int. J. Med. Microbiol.* 295:503–511.

Wallmann, J. 2006. Monitoring of antimicrobial resistance in pathogenic bacteria from livestock animals. *Int. J. Med. Microbiol.* 296 (Suppl. 41):81–86.

Watson, J. T., M. Gayer, and M. A. Connolly. 2007. Epidemics after natural disasters. *Emerg. Infect. Dis.* 13 (1):1–5.

Wegener, H. C., T. Hald, D. Lo Fo Wong, M. Madsen, H. Korsgaard, F. Bager, P. Gerner-Smidt, and K. Molbak. 2003. Salmonella control programs in Denmark. *Emerg. Infect. Dis.* 9 (7):774–780.

Wetzel, A. N. and J. T. LeJeune. 2006. Clonal dissemination of *Escherichia coli* O157:H7 subtypes among dairy farms in northeast Ohio. *Appl. Environ. Microbiol.* 72 (4):2621–2626.

White, D. G., S. Zhao, R. Singh, and P. F. McDermott. 2004. Antimicrobial resistance among gram-negative foodborne bacterial pathogens associated with foods of animal origin. *Foodborne Pathog. Dis.* 1 (3):137–152.

WHO. 2004. Globalization of infectious diseases: A review of linkages. In TDR/STR/SEB/ST/04.2. Geneva: World Health Organization.

Wilson, M. E. 1991. *A World Guide to Infections: Diseases, Distribution, Diagnosis*. New York: Oxford University Press.

Wilson, M. E. 1995. Travel and the emergence of infectious diseases. *Emerg. Infect. Dis.* 1 (2):39–46.

Woodward, D. L., C. G. Clark, R. A. Caldeira, R. Ahmed, G. Soule, L. Bryden, H. Tabor, P. Melito, R. Foster, J. Walsh, L. K. Ng, G. B. Malcolm, N. Strockbine, and F. G. Rodgers. 2005. Identification and characterization of *Shigella boydii* 20 serovar nov., a new and emerging Shigella serotype. *J. Med. Microbiol.* 54 (Pt 8):741–748.

Zhang, W., W. Qi, T. J. Albert, A. S. Motiwala, D. Alland, E. K. Hyytia-Trees, E. M. Ribot, P. I. Fields, T. S. Whittam, and B. Swaminathan. 2006. Probing genomic diversity and evolution of *Escherichia coli* O157 by single nucleotide polymorphisms. *Genome Res.* 16 (6):757–767.

2

Pathogenic Mechanisms of the Enterohemorrhagic Escherichia coli—Some New Insights

Glen D. Armstrong

CONTENTS

2.1 Introduction to the Enterohemorrhagic *Escherichia coli* Group of Organisms

The enterohemorrhagic *Escherichia coli* (*E. coli*) (EHEC) represent a subgroup of the enterovirulent bacteria known as Shiga toxin-producing *E. coli* or STEC.[1] What distinguishes the EHEC from other STEC is their etiologic association with two clinical conditions: hemorrhagic colitis (HC), and, occasionally, hemolytic uremic syndrome (HUS), in humans.[1,2] Although *E. coli* serotype O157:H7 causes the majority of cases of HC and HUS in North America and other parts of the developed World, numerous other less prevalent EHEC serotypes have been isolated from subjects afflicted by these pathogens.[3–5]

The clinical symptoms of HC include diarrhea, often but not always bloody, and abdominal pain. Fever is usually absent, or if present, is typically of a low grade. HUS, when it occurs, comprises a triad of clinical features, including hemolytic anemia, thrombocytopenia, and acute renal failure. The illness is associated with consuming EHEC-contaminated ground beef (hence its popular name, "hamburger disease") which has not been thoroughly cooked, or with ingesting untreated well water, unpasteurized milk, products produced from the same, or fruits and vegetables which have been washed in EHEC-contaminated water.[6–12]

Cattle represent a significant reservoir for these organisms[13–16] and the primary risk groups include young children and elderly individuals.[17–22] Additional risk factors include the proximity of one's dwelling to intensive agricultural operations involving cattle.[23,24,25] Because of the low infectious dose, person-to-person spread has also been documented in both sporadic and outbreak situations.[26]

The EHEC were first detected in patients presenting themselves to their physicians or hospital emergency rooms with signs of bloody diarrhea.[27] At that time, the most distinguishing EHEC feature was that cell-free extracts prepared from broth cultures were cytotoxic to African green monkey kidney (vero) cells. Hence, the term Verotoxin was originally used to describe this activity and EHEC were originally referred to as Verotoxigenic *E. coli* (VTEC).[28] This term is still commonly used in many articles related to these organisms. However, since the early days of their discovery, much has been learned about the complex pathogenic features associated with the EHEC group of bacteria. For example, it is now recognized that EHEC can express several serologically distinct Verotoxins which are structurally and functionally related to the potent cytotoxin, called Shiga toxin (Stx), expressed by *Shigella dysenteriae* type 1,[29] hence the alternate nomenclature of Shiga-toxigenic *E. coli* or STEC.

The first of the Shiga toxins to be identified, Stx1, Verotoxin 1 (VT1), is, for all purposes, identical to the Stx produced by *S. dysenteriae*.[30,31] The second, Stx2, (VT2), represents a family of Shiga toxins, which are genetically and antigenically unrelated to Stx1. This family includes the prototypic Stx2, as well as at least 10 Stx2-related variant forms.[32] Regardless, all these Shiga toxins are otherwise structurally and functionally identical. They are classified as AB_5-type multi-subunit toxins consisting of a single enzymatic A subunit and five identical B subunits (Figure 2.1A). The five Stx B subunits self-assemble into a pentameric ring-shaped structure displaying fivefold axial symmetry (Figure 2.1B).[33,34]

Except for one of the Stx2 variants, the pig edema toxin Stx2e,[35] all the remaining Stx B pentamers bind to the αGal(1,4)βGal(1,4)βGlc glycan sequence of globotriaosylceramide (Gb3) neutral glycolipid host cell receptors (Figure 2.1B). This lectin-like Gb3-dependent binding function of the Stx B pentamers subsequently activates endocytosis and facilitates delivery of the toxin's A subunit, via retrograde transport through the Golgi and endoplasmic reticulum membrane systems, to the cytoplasmic compartment of the host cell.[36] Once there, the Stx A subunit enzymatically depurinates

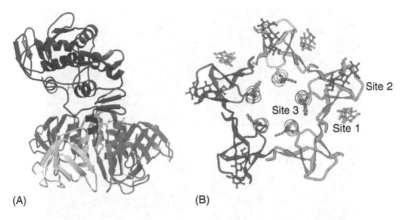

(A)   (B)

FIGURE 2.1
(A) X-ray crystal structure (From Fraser, M.E., Chernaia, M.M., Kozlov, Y.V., and James, M.N., *Nat. Struct. Biol.*, 1, 59, 1994. Reprinted by permission from Macmillan Publishers Ltd. Copyright 1994.) of Stx1 at 2.5 Å resolution showing the A subunit and the 5 B subunits in various shades of grey. (B) X-ray crystal structure (From Ling, H., Boodhoo, A., Hazes, B., Cummings, M.D., Armstrong, G.D., Brunton, J.L., and Read, R.J., *Biochemistry*, 37, 1777, 1998. Reprinted with permission from the American Chemical Society, Copyright 1998.) of the Stx1 B pentamer complexed with its glycan host cell receptors, (From Boyd, B. and Lingwood, C., *Nephron*, 51, 207, 1989.) the αGal(1,4)βGal(1,4)βGlc sequence of globotriaosylceramide (Gb3). 2.8 Å resolution.

the 28S rRNA component of the host cell ribosomes at a single location in its sequence. This prevents the 28S rRNA from participating in the chain elongation step in protein biosynthesis[29] and initiates the stress-activated programmed cell death (apoptosis) pathway in the affected host cell.[37]

The serological differences between Stx1 and Stx2 are reflective of differences in their primary amino acid sequences. The sequences of the Stx1 and prototypic Stx2 A and B subunits are 52% and 60% identical, respectively (Figure 2.2). Those of the prototypic Stx from *S. dysenteriae* and Stx1 are identical save for a single amino acid difference at position 45 in their respective A subunits.[31]

2.2   EHEC-Mediated Hemorrhagic Colitis

In addition to their ability to produce Shiga toxins, EHEC, like several other related gastrointestinal pathogens, reviewed in Refs. 38 and 39, express multiple virulence factors which contribute to their full pathogenic potential. Once ingested, the bacteria transit the stomach and small intestinal compartments to ultimately enter the lower regions of the gastrointestinal tract, primarily the terminal ileum and colon. The relative resistance of *E. coli* O157:H7 to acidic pH[40] may assist the bacteria as they transit through the stomach.

In the colon, the organisms initially adhere loosely to the mucosal side of the epithelium. The molecular details of this initial attachment process

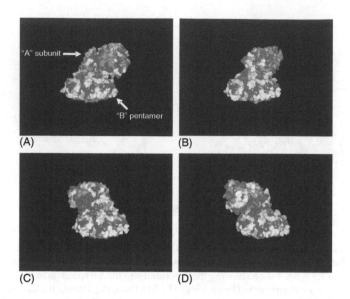

FIGURE 2.2

Primary amino acid sequence differences between Stx1 and Stx2 mapped onto the surface of the X-ray crystal structure of Stx2. Dark grey surfaces represent identical amino acid side chains, conserved and nonconserved amino acid side chains are represented by medium and light grey shading respectively. The four panels illustrate four different aspects of Stx2 each rotated by 90°. (Courtesy of Dr. Marie Fraser, University of Calgary.)

remain sketchy but multiple potential adhesins have been described and a large virulence-associated plasmid, pO157, may also influence this early stage of the infectious process.[41–48] It is possible, however, that the propensity for the EHEC to colonize the lower regions of the human intestine may be governed more by the lack of a specific adhesin for receptors expressed by epithelial cells lining the small intestine. This would facilitate the unimpeded passage of the bacteria through the small intestine on their way to the lower intestinal tract.

Regardless of the precise details of the initial adherence phase, contact with the host cell surface initiates a subsequent chain of pathogenic events ultimately leading to the intimate attachment of the bacteria to the intestinal epithelium.[39] This process requires the coordinated activity of multiple proteins whose expression is determined by genes located on a chromosomally located pathogenicity-associated island (PAI) called the locus of enterocyte effacement (LEE). These proteins include the structural and regulatory elements of a type III, contact-dependent, secretory system (TTSS), an afimbrial EHEC adhesin called intimin, as well as a protein called the translocated intimin receptor (Tir). Encoded by the LEE-associated genes as well are a group of *E. coli* secreted proteins (Esp), which are delivered to the cytoplasmic compartment of the host cell via the TTSS. Tir is also delivered, via the TTSS, into the host cell where it eventually becomes integrated across the host cell membrane, thereby providing a bacterial-encoded receptor for intimin.[49,50] Other TTSS-delivered effector proteins commandeer regulatory components, which govern the structural and functional integrity of the host cell cytoskeleton.

The net effect of the coordinated actions of all these LEE-encoded virulence factors is the intimate attachment of the organisms to cup-like structures on the apical side of the intestinal epithelial cell. These cup-like structures, or pedestals, are formed at the expense of the microvilli which normally adorn the surface of the intestinal epithelium. These two events, the disappearance of the microvilli and the intimate bacterial attachment to the host cell pedestals, are collectively referred to as the EHEC-attaching and -effacing phenotype. The pathological cascade of events that ultimately occur as a result of this elaborate EHEC colonization process include a reduction in the absorptive capacity of the infected region of the intestine in addition to a reduced epithelial barrier function,[51] the net effect being, diarrhea. In addition, one of the EHEC TTSS-delivered effector proteins, EspB, appears to exert an anti-inflammatory effect, thereby, thwarting any initial attempts by the host to eliminate the offending microbes, thereby, prolonging the diarrheal phase of the illness.[52,53]

2.3   Role of Shiga Toxins in EHEC Pathogenesis

The Shiga toxins appear to contribute to the pathogenesis of HC by collaborating with pro-inflammatory EHEC virulence factors thereby intensifying the mucosal inflammatory response to the infection[54-58] and the resulting collateral tissue damage which leads to bloody diarrhea. The clinical signs of HC, therefore, appear to result from a complex balance between multiple pro- and anti-inflammatory EHEC virulence factors. Presumably, host-specific factors related to regulation of the inflammatory response may also collaborate in a positive or negative sense with microbial factors in the pathogenesis of HC. Hence, depending on the particular set of circumstances, not all EHEC-infected subjects will develop bloody diarrhea or the Stx-associated extraintestinal complications of HUS.

HUS occurs when the Shiga toxins spread throughout the body via the circulatory system. How these toxins enter the circulation is not clear but it is possible this occurs through multiple pathways. In vitro, Stx1 appears to be able to access a trans-cellular trafficking pathway in polarized Caco-2 cell monolayers.[59-61] This implies that a portion of the Shiga toxins produced during an EHEC infection might be translocated across the undamaged intestinal epithelium. Stx1 and Stx2 may also gain access to the submucosal compartment via the paracellular channels created in the epithelial layer in response to EHEC colonization of the intestinal epithelium.[60] There is now a significant body of evidence that submucosal neutrophils may then transport Stx1 and Stx2 to extraintestinal tissues and target organs,[62-64] where the toxins appear to collaborate in a destructive cascade of micro-angiopathic, pro-inflammatory, and pro-thrombotic events.[65-71]   The complex pathogenesis of Stx-associated HUS has been nicely reviewed by Francois Proulx et al.[72]

Once in the circulation, glomerular capillaries are prime targets for the Shiga toxins because renal endothelial cells express high concentrations of Gb3 glycan receptors on their surfaces.[73] The blood vessels nourishing the brain also represent targets for the Shiga toxins.[67,74–77] Endotoxin, which is released as well during EHEC infections, may contribute to the pathogenesis of HUS by activating monocytes, leukocytes, and endothelial cells, thereby, intensifying the inflammatory response, as well as upregulating the expression of Stx Gb3 receptors on the endothelial cell surface.[78,79]

Surveillance data indicates that EHEC-expressing Stx2 alone or both Stx1 and Stx2 are more frequently associated with cases of severe HC and HUS.[80–83] This implies that Stx2 may be more toxic than Stx1 in humans. The greater involvement of Stx2 in HUS has also been observed in baboons challenged with purified endotoxin-depleted Stx1 or Stx2 thereby demonstrating that these toxins on their own can cause microangiopathic damage in the glomerular capillaries.[84] The reasons for the hypertoxicity of Stx2 are presently the subject of much conjecture.

2.4 Stx2 Binding to Human Serum Amyloid P Component

In a previous investigation directed at revealing possible risk factors for HUS, it was learned that human serum contained a nonimmunoglobulin-associated factor that effectively neutralized the Verocytotoxic activity of prototypic Stx2 but not Stx1, Stx2c, or Stx2e.[85] Although the mean concentration of this factor was lower in sera obtained from healthy infants than in adults, the range of values was considerable in both subject groups and, due to the study's limited statistical power, the differences were not deemed to be significant.[85] These authors concluded, therefore, that this nonimmunoglobulin Stx2-specific neutralizing factor was probably of no prognostic value in EHEC-infected patients. This early study, however, did not assess this relationship in age and sex-matched individuals who recovered from a relatively uncomplicated course of HC, as compared to ones who subsequently developed HUS as a complication of their EHEC infection.

Subsequently, Kimura et al.[86] reported that the serum factor described in the original article by Bitzan et al.[85] was serum amyloid P (SAP) component. Moreover, these investigators demonstrated that Stx2 bound only to human SAP (HuSAP) and not to SAP purified from the sera of a range of other nonhuman species.

SAP is a member of the "pentraxin" family of serum glycoporteins[87] which also includes C-reactive protein (CRP). HuSAP is a 25 kDa glycoprotein which self-assembles into pentamers (Figure 2.3A) displaying a fivefold axial symmetry very much akin to the Stx B pentamers.[88,89] The circulating concentration of SAP in healthy human serum ranges from 24 to 32 μg/mL but this can increase slightly during the acute phase of an infection.[90]

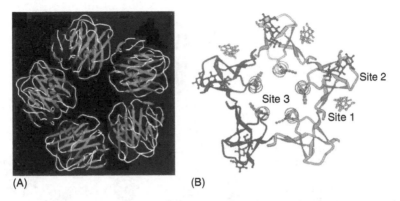

(A)　　　　　　　　　　　　(B)

FIGURE 2.3

X-ray crystal structures of (A) the pentameric form of HuSAP from the article in *Nature* by Emsley, J. et al. (From Emsley, J., White, H.E., O'Hara, B.P., Oliva, G., Srinivasan, N., Tickle, I.J., Blundell, T.L., Pepys, M.B., and Wood, S.P., *Nature*, 367, 338, 1994. Reprinted by permission from Macmillan Publishers Ltd. Copyright 1994.) and (B) the Stx1 B pentamer complexed with the Gb3 trisaccharide (From Ling, H., Boodhoo, A., Hazes, B., Cummings, M.D., Armstrong, G.D., Brunton, J.L., and Read, R.J., *Biochemistry*, 37, 1777, 1998. Reprinted with permission from the American Chemical Society, Copyright 1998.). In panel A, the view is of the "A" surface of the HuSAP pentamer. As depicted in these figures, the Stx B pentamer is about one-third the size of the HuSAP pentamer.

The biological role of SAP remains enigmatic. Data gleaned from in vitro studies suggest SAP may provide innate immunity to some infectious agents.[91,92] In vivo, however, SAP may have an antiphagocytic effect thereby contributing to the enhanced virulence of several pathogens.[93] Regardless, given the striking similarities in their X-ray crystal structures (Figure 2.3), we postulated that HuSAP binding to Stx2 might exploit the biochemical features of its shared symmetry with the Stx2 B pentamer. Consequently, we were intrigued to discover that peptide sequences from both the Stx2 A subunit and B pentamer were required for its binding to HuSAP.[94]

The recently published X-ray crystal structure of Stx2[95] reveals that, unlike Stx1, the penultimate four amino acids at the carboxy terminal end of the Stx2 A subunit extend from the opposing, receptor binding surface of its B pentamer. This finding prompted us to experimentally query the possibility that this extension of the A subunit might contribute to the formation of Stx2-HuSAP complexes. To test this postulate, we performed solution-phase competitive-binding inhibition assays using "Daisy," an enhanced derivative of "Starfish,"[96] the decavalent Gb3 receptor analog (Figure 2.4), which, as described in our previous article,[97] binds with an affinity in the submicromolar range to the receptor binding face of the Stx1 and Stx2 B pentamers.

We observed that Daisy, even at the highest concentration achievable in solution (10 mM), failed to competitively inhibit HuSAP binding to Stx2 holotoxin.[94] This observation implied that the penultimate four amino acids of the Stx2 A subunit do not contribute to HuSAP binding since Daisy, like Starfish, was designed to completely occlude the entire receptor binding

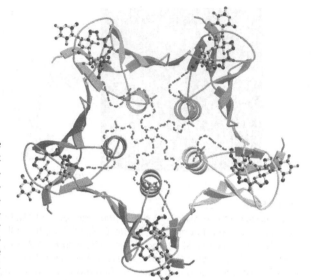

FIGURE 2.4
X-ray crystal structure of the Stx1 B pentamer Starfish complex (From Kitov, P.I., Sadowska, J.M., Mulvey, G., Armstrong, G.D., Ling, H., Pannu, N.S., Read, R.J., and Bundle, D.R., *Nature*, 403, 669, 2000. Reprinted by permission from Macmillan Publishers Ltd. Copyright 2000.). The core features of Starfish are depicted as dashed lines.

surface of the Stx2 B pentamer, including the central pore (Figure 2.4). The Daisy competitive binding inhibition studies also ruled out a role for the HuSAP glycan sequences in complex formation. Stx2 binding to HuSAP, therefore, represents an example of a Gb3-independent Stx interaction with a host factor.

Recently, the same Japanese investigators who discovered that Stx2 binds to HuSAP assessed its protective effect in Stx2-challenged mice.[98] These investigators concluded from their results that HuSAP probably did not represent a protective factor in human EHEC infections. However, these in vivo mouse experiments did not make provision for the continuous administration of HuSAP for the duration of the study. Given that the circulating half-life of HuSAP in mice is in the range of 3 h,[99] the single IV injection of only 2.5 or 5 mg/kg body weight given at the outset of the Stx2 challenge, would definitely not have been sufficient to protect the mice for the several days over which shigatoxemia subsequently developed in these animals.

We have since discovered that conventional Balb/C mice receiving twice daily IP injections of purified HuSAP, beginning at the outset, and continuing for the duration of the experiments, or better still, transgenic mice constitutively expressing HuSAP, were significantly protected from an LD_{100} (minimum dose required to kill 100% of the mice) challenge dose of Stx2 but not Stx1.[100] These findings imply that HuSAP binding to Stx2 is of sufficient affinity to provide in vivo protection, at least in mice, from a lethal dose of this toxin. We further discovered that HuSAP reduces the accumulation of ^{125}I-labeled Stx2 in target organs of HuSAP transgenic mice and inhibits ^{125}I-labeled Stx2 binding to ACHN (human kidney adenocarcinoma) cells (Figure 2.5). Therefore, the protective function of HuSAP in mice injected with a lethal dose of Stx2 may be related to its

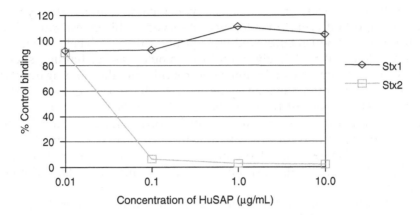

FIGURE 2.5

HuSAP inhibits binding of ^{125}I-labeled Stx2 but not ^{125}I-Stx1 to ACHN cells. Stx1 and Stx2 were labeled according to the protocol described in our previous report (From Mulvey, G.L., Marcato, P., Kitov, P.I., Sadowska, J., Bundle, D.R., and Armstrong, G.D., *J. Infect. Dis.*, 187, 640, 2003.). In this experiment, various concentrations of HuSAP were admixed with ^{125}I-labeled Stx1 or Stx2, each at a concentration of 10 ng/mL, and 15 min later these mixtures were added to ice-chilled confluent ACHN cell monolayers. After 30 min coincubation, the monolayers were washed with ice-cold PBS to remove unbound toxins. The monolayers were then solubilized in a 1% SDS/water solution and the bound radioactivity was recorded using a gamma counter. No HuSAP was added to the control monolayers.

ability to form complexes with this toxin in vivo; complexes which are diverted from the target organs, by an as yet undetermined mechanism.

These observations encouraged us to reexamine the concentration of HuSAP in sera obtained from sex- and age-matched EHEC-positive subjects suffering from HC or HC which subsequently developed into HUS, the hypothesis being that patients who experienced HUS as a consequence of their infection may, on average, display lower serum concentrations of HuSAP. Contrary to our hypothesis, we detected no significant difference in the circulating concentration of HuSAP in these different patient groups[100] thereby supporting the earlier[85] conclusion by Bitzan et al. that the serum concentration of HuSAP is of no prognostic value in this condition. The observation also suggested that, despite the encouraging mouse results, HuSAP, at least at normal physiological serum concentrations, appeared not to serve a protective function in EHEC-infected human subjects.

2.5 Gb3-Independent Stx1 and Stx2 Binding to Human Neutrophils

In 2000, te Loo and colleagues published an account[63] of a series of experiments in which they demonstrated that FITC-labeled Stx1 bound exclusively to the surface of human neutrophils in whole blood. No evidence for Stx1 binding to any other blood cell type, including monocytes, lymphocytes or importantly, erythrocytes, was observed in this investigation. Their studies, some of which employed biologically active ^{125}I-labeled toxin, also demonstrated that Stx1 likely bound to a single class of binding sites on freshly isolated nonactivated human neutrophils and, this binding event did not initiate toxin internalization by receptor-mediated endocytosis. Further, the dissociation constant (K_D) for Stx1 binding to the neutrophil receptors was determined to be approximately 10^{-8} mol/L which is about 100-fold lower than the affinity of Stx1 binding to Gb3 receptors.[63] Finally, these investigators also demonstrated that neutrophils could transfer their reversibly bound "cargo" of Stx1 to human glomerular microvascular endothelial cells in vitro.

In a follow-up publication,[64] te Loo et al. further demonstrated that neutrophils obtained from subjects suffering from *E. coli* O157-associated HUS had Stx2 bound to their surfaces. Based on these combined observations, te Loo et al. concluded that neutrophils may be responsible for transporting Stx1 and Stx2 from the intestinal mucosal compartment to blood vessels nourishing extraintestinal target organs and tissues. At these sites, they postulated that the Shiga toxins are capable of transferring from their Gb3-independent neutrophil receptors to the higher affinity Gb3 receptors on microvascular endothelial cells thereby initiating the subsequent cascade of microangiopathic events which are linked to the activation of the apoptosis program in these cells. The observations of te Loo and colleagues have more recently been independently corroborated by two groups[62,101] who concluded that the presence of circulating Stx-loaded neutrophils in whole human blood was of diagnostic and prognostic value in subjects suffering from an EHEC infection.

The te Loo findings are particularly interesting in light of observations related to leukocyte interactions with different populations of endothelial cells in the body. In this regard, leukocytes and endothelial cells respond to proinflammatory stimuli by producing complimentary adhesion molecules, referred to as selectins, on their surfaces. These complimentary adhesion molecules allow the leukocytes to identify activated endothelial cells thereby initiating the series of cellular and molecular events which ultimately result in the clinical signs of inflammation in the tissues. Intravital microscopic examination has revealed that the interactions of leukocytes with activated endothelial cells occur almost exclusively in postcapillary venules because the expression of selectins is restricted to these sites.[102,103]

Before arriving at the postcapillary venules, however, the leukocytes must first squeeze through the narrow blood vessels which form the capillaries. This brings the leukocyte surfaces into very close physical contact with the surface of the endothelial cells which form these narrow blood vessels. Despite this, however, the leukocytes rarely adhere to the walls of the capillaries. However, there is a growing body of evidence indicating that this paradigm of leukocyte recruitment to postcapillary venules does not apply to all capillary beds in the body. In fact, injurious leukocyte recruitment to capillary blood vessels has now been observed in the liver, the lungs, and significantly for this treatise, the glomeruli.[104–106]

In the glomerular capillaries, leukocytes become adherent to activated endothelial cells by a process of immediate arrest without demonstrating any of the prior rolling behavior which typifies their recruitment to activated endothelial cells in the postcapillary venules.[107] This suggests that a novel form of leukocyte adhesion to activated endothelial cells occurs in the glomerular capillary beds. Moreover, Kuligowski et al.[107] also recently reported that activated endothelial cells in the glomeruli increased their expression of P-selectin which also resulted in a P-selectin-dependent accumulation of platelets in these sites, an intriguing observation given the involvement of platelets and the resulting thrombocytopenia in the acute phase of HUS.

Taken together with the initial observations of te Loo et al.,[63] as well as those of other groups,[62,101] it is not difficult to imagine how circulating leukocytes might very well be capable of delivering their lethal cargo of reversibly bound Shiga toxins to glomerular endothelial cells as they attempt to squeeze through these exceedingly narrow blood vessels. The finding that glomerular endothelial cells in children are particularly well endowed with Stx Gb3 receptors would definitely facilitate this exchange reaction[108] which, because of the physical size of the capillaries, would not necessarily require prior activation of the endothelium. Subsequently, though, activation of glomerular endothelial cells, either in direct response to Stx binding,[65,109] or by additional proinflammatory bacterial products such as endotoxin, would only intensify the series of microangiopathic events, including the recruitment of platelets, which would then localize in the glomerular capillaries as opposed to the postcapillary venules.

Reports[110] indicating the presence of immobilized SAP in glomerular basement membranes also bear consideration in light of the observations, discussed earlier, of Stx2 binding to the soluble form of SAP. How the binding to this form of SAP might influence the toxic activity of Stx2, especially if the toxin is bound to Gb3-independent receptors on the surface of neutrophils, represents an intriguing question for additional study.

Although these observations provide additional insight into the pathogenic mechanisms of EHEC-mediated HUS, several questions remain. For example, the te Loo group also detected Shiga toxins on neutrophils obtained from household contacts of persons suffering from *E. coli* O157 infections[111] and some of these individuals were demonstrating no signs of clinical illness at the time. Therefore, other factors besides Stx binding to neutrophils must influence whether or not an EHEC-infected subject will develop HUS. Moreover, although te Loo et al. partially characterized the Gb3-independent neutrophil receptors for Stx1, no such data have ever appeared for the Stx2 receptor. There are also conflicting conclusions regarding the biochemical structure of the Gb3-independent neutrophil receptors for Stx1 and Stx2. In their first article,[63] the te Loo group reported that the neutrophil receptor for Stx1 was sensitive to proteolytic inactivation whereas in their second publication,[64] they implied that the Stx2 receptor is possibly a Gb3-related glycolipid.

2.6 Effects of Stx Binding on Neutrophil Function

In vitro at least, endotoxin-free preparations of Stx1 and Stx2 do not activate human neutrophils as assessed by the release of superoxide or elastase.[112] Further, priming human neutrophils with Stx1 caused a significant reduction in superoxide release when the cells were subsequently exposed to formyl-met-leu-phe (fMLP) or phorbol myristic acid (PMA). By contrast, Stx2 priming resulted in reduced production of superoxide when the neutrophils were subsequently treated with PMA but not fMLP and neither Stx1 nor Stx2 affected chemotaxis towards fMLP. In these in vitro experiments, therefore, the authors concluded that Stx1 and Stx2 do not activate but may impair neutrophil priming functions. This could prolong their effective lifetime in the circulation thereby enhancing their capacity to participate in Stx-mediated damage to the intestine and extraintestinal target organs. Indeed, there is a well-established positive prognostic link between marked leukocytosis and Stx-associated HUS in EHEC-infected individuals.[72] By contrast, Fendandez et al.[113] reported that neutrophils obtained from Stx-treated mice displayed an increased expression of CD11b, enhanced cytotoxic capacity, and greater adhesive properties, all signs of activation, than those isolated from the untreated animals. Preexposure to lipopolysaccharide (LPS) potentiated these Stx2-mediated effects on murine neutrophils. It is obvious, therefore, that human and murine neutrophils respond quite differently to Stx1 and Stx2 implying that these toxins either bind to different receptors on human and murine neutrophils or activate different signaling networks within them.

2.7 Treatment and Vaccination Strategies

Since their discovery, we have learned much about the complex pathogenic mechanisms elaborated by the EHEC group of organisms. Nonetheless, there is still no clear consensus on any intervention strategies in subjects suffering from HC and HUS. In this regard, certain antibiotics have been found to promote the release of greater amounts of the Shiga toxins by EHEC in vitro.[114–117] However, despite evidence that antibiotics are beneficial in murine models of EHEC infection,[118,119] there is no clear clinical evidence that antibiotics either increase or decrease the risk of HUS developing in subjects suffering from HC, unless they are provided later in the course of the illness or are coadministered with antimotility agents.[120,121] As a consequence, until there is some clear evidence supporting antibiotics in treating cases of EHEC, the prevailing recommendation is to avoid their use.

Human EHEC vaccination strategies involving various antigenic components of the organisms have focused on both active[122-129] and passive[32,130-132] approaches to the problem. Of these strategies, the therapeutic use of antibodies in the acutely ill patient may represent the most practical solution to the problem simply because of the practicalities of a mass immunization program designed to prevent an illness which, although devastating to the infected individuals, does not have nearly the same public health impact of the more common childhood diseases for which vaccines are available.

Another approach might be to use vaccination as a means of eliminating the organisms from cattle thereby limiting their entry into the human food chain.[133-137] However, developing a vaccine to eradicate what is essentially a commensal organism from cattle will require some finessing to achieve success. Nonetheless, it is an approach which deserves serious consideration.

Considering what is known about the central role of the Shiga toxins in EHEC-mediated disease, therapeutic strategies directed at neutralizing these key virulence factors are also worth consideration. Besides the therapeutic application of Stx-specific antibodies, high-affinity toxin binders have also been described.[96,138-141] Although one of these agents, Synsorb-Pk, failed to lessen the severity of HUS in pediatric subjects[142] and a deacylated version, lyso-Gb3, of the natural Stx receptor was reported to enhance the lethal effects of Stx2 in mice,[143] the more refined versions of these Stx-binding materials[97,139,141] may well prove to be more efficacious. Moreover, given the revelations of te Loo et al., innovative strategies directed at inhibiting the Gb3-independent binding of the Shiga toxins to human neutrophils may also now be well worth, considering as potential therapeutic options.

2.8 Concluding Remarks

The EHEC, at least *E. coli* O157:H7, appear to exist in a more or less commensal relationship with their bovine hosts and, there is some evidence[14] suggesting that the colorectal junction of the gastrointestinal tract might represent their primary colonization site in this species. If so, this would seem to be a very restricted environmental niche for the bacteria to arbitrarily choose as their preferred habitat. In humans, however, these organisms behave in a typically parasitic manner. Regardless of these opposing relationships, in both cases the bacteria have acquired the genetic resources which enable them to successfully interact with their hosts and many of the LEE-encoded proteins that are involved in the complex EHEC colonization strategy in humans are also expressed in cattle.[136]

These observations beg the fundamental question, has the bovine gastrointestinal tract been the only environmental niche which has influenced EHEC evolution? If so, are humans merely inconsequential hosts to these organisms? From an opposing perspective, have both humans and cattle provided selective environments which have directed the evolution of these bacteria? If one favors the position that is based on shear numbers, cattle might represent the preferred EHEC host; it is uncertain what selective pressures in these animals are at work in maintaining the genetic capacity of the bacteria to express Shiga toxins. Perhaps the answers to these thought-provoking questions will be revealed as we learn more about the pathogenic role of the Shiga toxins in human disease since it would now appear, based at least on the observation that Stx2 binds exclusively to HuSAP, that selective pressures may have played a hand in this as well. Comparative studies on the Gb3-independent binding of both Stx1 and Stx2 to neutrophils from the different species may also add more pieces to this intriguing puzzle.

References

1. Karmali, M.A. 2004. Infection by Shiga toxin-producing *Escherichia coli*: An overview. *Mol. Biotechnol.* 26:117–122.
2. Tarr, P.I., C.A. Gordon, and W.L. Chandler. 2005. Shiga-toxin-producing *Escherichia coli* and haemolytic uraemic syndrome. *Lancet* 365:1073–1086.
3. Banatvala, N., P.M. Griffin, K.D. Greene, T.J. Barrett, W.F. Bibb, J.H. Green, and J.G. Wells. 2001. The United States National Prospective Hemolytic Uremic Syndrome Study: Microbiologic, serologic, clinical, and epidemiologic findings. *J. Infect. Dis.* 183:1063–1070.
4. Besser, R.E., P.M. Griffin, and L. Slutsker. 1999. *Escherichia coli* O157:H7 gastroenteritis and the hemolytic uremic syndrome: An emerging infectious disease. *Annu. Rev. Med.* 50:355–367.
5. Goldwater, P.N. and K.A. Bettelheim. 2000. *Escherichia coli* 'O' group serology of a haemolytic uraemic syndrome (HUS) epidemic. *Scand. J. Infect. Dis.* 32:385–394.
6. Allerberger, F., A.W. Friedrich, K. Grif, M.P. Dierich, H.J. Dornbusch, C.J. Mache, E. Nachbaur, M. Freilinger, P. Rieck, M. Wagner, A. Caprioli, H. Karch, and L.B. Zimmerhackl. 2003. Hemolytic-uremic syndrome associated with enterohemorrhagic *Escherichia coli* O26:H infection and consumption of unpasteurized cow's milk. *Int. J. Infect. Dis.* 7:42–45.
7. Islam, M., M.P. Doyle, S.C. Phatak, P. Millner, and X. Jiang. 2004. Persistence of enterohemorrhagic *Escherichia coli* O157:H7 in soil and on leaf lettuce and parsley grown in fields treated with contaminated manure composts or irrigation water. *J. Food Prot.* 67:1365–1370.
8. Kasrazadeh, M. and C. Genigeorgis. 1995. Potential growth and control of *Escherichia coli* O157:H7 in soft hispanic type cheese. *Int. J. Food Microbiol.* 25:289–300.
9. Mayerhauser, C.M. 2001. Survival of enterohemorrhagic *Escherichia coli* O157:H7 in retail mustard. *J. Food Prot.* 64:783–787.
10. Reinders, R.D., S. Biesterveld, and P.G. Bijker. 2001. Survival of *Escherichia coli* O157:H7 ATCC 43895 in a model apple juice medium with different concentrations of proline and caffeic acid. *Appl. Environ. Microbiol.* 67:2863–2866.

11. Takeda, Y. 1999. Enterohemorrhagic *Escherichia coli* infection in Japan. *Pediatr. Int.* 41:198–201.
12. Wachtel, M.R., L.C. Whitehand, and R.E. Mandrell. 2002. Association of *Escherichia coli* O157:H7 with preharvest leaf lettuce upon exposure to contaminated irrigation water. *J. Food Prot.* 65:18–25.
13. Borczyk, A.A., M.A. Karmali, H. Lior, and L.M. Duncan. 1987. Bovine reservoir for verotoxin-producing *Escherichia coli* O157:H7. *Lancet* 1:98.
14. Low, J.C., I.J. McKendrick, C. McKechnie, D. Fenlon, S.W. Naylor, C. Currie, D.G. Smith, L. Allison, and D.L. Gally. 2005. Rectal carriage of enterohemorrhagic *Escherichia coli* O157 in slaughtered cattle. *Appl. Environ. Microbiol.* 71:93–97.
15. Renter, D.G. and J.M. Sargeant. 2002. Enterohemorrhagic *Escherichia coli* O157: Epidemiology and ecology in bovine production environments. *Anim. Health Res. Rev.* 3:83–94.
16. Van Donkersgoed, J., J. Berg, A. Potter, D. Hancock, T. Besser, D. Rice, J. LeJeune, and S. Klashinsky. 2001. Environmental sources and transmission of *Escherichia coli* O157 in feedlot cattle. *Can. Vet. J.* 42:714–720.
17. Carter, A.O., A.A. Borczyk, J.A. Carlson, B. Harvey, J.C. Hockin, M.A. Karmali, C. Krishnan, D.A. Korn, and H. Lior. 1987. A severe outbreak of *Escherichia coli* O157:H7-associated hemorrhagic colitis in a nursing home. *N. Engl. J. Med.* 317:1496–1500.
18. Cimolai, N., S. Basalyga, D.G. Mah, B.J. Morrison, and J.E. Carter. 1994. A continuing assessment of risk factors for the development of *Escherichia coli* 0157:H7-associated hemolytic uremic syndrome. *Clin. Nephrol.* 42:85–89.
19. Ostroff, S.M., P.M. Griffin, R.V. Tauxe, L.D. Shipman, K.D. Greene, J.G. Wells, J.H. Lewis, P.A. Blake, and J.M. Kobayashi. 1990. A statewide outbreak of *Escherichia coli* O157:H7 infections in Washington State. *Am. J. Epidemiol.* 132:239–247.
20. Panaro, L., D. Cooke, and A. Borczyk. 1990. Outbreak of *Escherichia coli* O157:H7 in a nursing home—Ontario. *Can. Dis. Wkly. Rep.* 16:90–92.
21. Rowe, P.C., E. Orrbine, H. Lior, G.A. Wells, E. Yetisir, M. Clulow, and P.N. McLaine. 1998. Risk of hemolytic uremic syndrome after sporadic *Escherichia coli* O157:H7 infection: Results of a Canadian collaborative study. Investigators of the Canadian Pediatric Kidney Disease Research Center. *J. Pediatr.* 132:777–782.
22. Ryan, C.A., R.V. Tauxe, G.W. Hosek, J.G. Wells, P.A. Stoesz, H.W. McFadden, Jr., P.W. Smith, G.F. Wright, and P.A. Blake. 1986. *Escherichia coli* O157:H7 diarrhea in a nursing home: Clinical, epidemiological, and pathological findings. *J. Infect. Dis.* 154:631–638.
23. Kistemann, T., S. Zimmer, I. Vagsholm, and Y. Andersson. 2004. GIS-supported investigation of human EHEC and cattle VTEC O157 infections in Sweden: Geographical distribution, spatial variation and possible risk factors. *Epidemiol. Infect.* 132:495–505.
24. Michel, P., J.B. Wilson, S.W. Martin, R.C. Clarke, S.A. McEwen, and C.L. Gyles. 1999. Temporal and geographical distributions of reported cases of *Escherichia coli* O157:H7 infection in Ontario. *Epidemiol. Infect.* 122:193–200.
25. Valcour, J.E., P. Michel, S.A. McEwen, and J.B. Wilson. 2002. Associations between indicators of livestock farming intensity and incidence of human Shiga toxin-producing *Escherichia coli* infection. *Emerg. Infect. Dis.* 8:252–257.
26. Rowe, P.C., E. Orrbine, H. Lior, G.A. Wells, and P.N. McLaine. 1993. Diarrhoea in close contacts as a risk factor for childhood haemolytic uraemic syndrome. The CPKDRC co-investigators. *Epidemiol. Infect.* 110:9–16.

27. Grandsen, W.R., M.A. Damm, J.D. Anderson, J.E. Carter, and H. Lior. 1985. Haemorrhagic cystitis and balanitis associated with verotoxin-producing *Escherichia coli* O157:H7. *Lancet* 2:150.
28. Karmali, M.A., M. Petric, C. Lim, P.C. Fleming, G.S. Arbus, and H. Lior. 1985. The association between idiopathic hemolytic uremic syndrome and infection by verotoxin-producing *Escherichia coli*. *J. Infect. Dis.* 151:775–782.
29. O'Brien, A.D., V.L. Tesh, A. Donohue-Rolfe, M.P. Jackson, S. Olsnes, K. Sandvig, A.A. Lindberg, and G.T. Keusch. 1992. Shiga toxin: biochemistry, genetics, mode of action, and role in pathogenesis. *Curr. Top. Microbiol. Immunol.* 180:65–94.
30. Calderwood, S.B., F. Auclair, A. Donohue-Rolfe, G.T. Keusch, and J.J. Mekalanos. 1987. Nucleotide sequence of the Shiga-like toxin genes of *Escherichia coli*. *Proc. Natl. Acad. Sci. U.S.A.* 84:4364–4368.
31. Strockbine, N.A., M.P. Jackson, L.M. Sung, R.K. Holmes, and A.D. O'Brien. 1988. Cloning and sequencing of the genes for Shiga toxin from *Shigella dysenteriae* type 1. *J. Bacteriol.* 170:1116–1122.
32. Tzipori, S., A. Sheoran, D. Akiyoshi, A. Donohue-Rolfe, and H. Trachtman. 2004. Antibody therapy in the management of shiga toxin-induced hemolytic uremic syndrome. *Clin. Microbiol. Rev.* 17:926–941.
33. Fraser, M.E., M.M. Chernaia, Y.V. Kozlov, and M.N. James. 1994. Crystal structure of the holotoxin from *Shigella dysenteriae* at 2.5 Å resolution. *Nat. Struct. Biol.* 1:59–64.
34. Stein, P.E., A. Boodhoo, G.J. Tyrrell, J.L. Brunton, and R.J. Read. 1992. Crystal structure of the cell-binding B oligomer of verotoxin-1 from *E. coli*. *Nature* 355:748–750.
35. DeGrandis, S., H. Law, J. Brunton, C. Gyles, and C.A. Lingwood. 1989. Globotetraosylceramide is recognized by the pig edema disease toxin. *J. Biol. Chem.* 264:12520–12525.
36. Sandvig, K., B. Spilsberg, S.U. Lauvrak, M.L. Torgersen, T.G. Iversen, and B. van Deurs. 2004. Pathways followed by protein toxins into cells. *Int. J. Med. Microbiol.* 293:483–490.
37. Cherla, R.P., S.Y. Lee, and V.L. Tesh. 2003. Shiga toxins and apoptosis. *FEMS Microbiol. Lett.* 228:159–166.
38. Donnenberg, M.S. and T.S. Whittam. 2001. Pathogenesis and evolution of virulence in enteropathogenic and enterohemorrhagic *Escherichia coli*. *J. Clin. Invest.* 107:539–548.
39. Nataro, J.P. and J.B. Kaper. 1998. Diarrheagenic *Escherichia coli*. *Clin. Microbiol. Rev.* 11:142–201.
40. Benjamin, M.M. and A.R. Datta. 1995. Acid tolerance of enterohemorrhagic *Escherichia coli*. *Appl. Environ. Microbiol.* 61:1669–1672.
41. Batisson, I., M.P. Guimond, F. Girard, H. An, C. Zhu, E. Oswald, J.M. Fairbrother, M. Jacques, and J. Harel. 2003. Characterization of the novel factor paa involved in the early steps of the adhesion mechanism of attaching and effacing *Escherichia coli*. *Infect. Immun.* 71:4516–4525.
42. Brunder, W., A.S. Khan, J. Hacker, and H. Karch. 2001. Novel type of fimbriae encoded by the large plasmid of sorbitol-fermenting enterohemorrhagic *Escherichia coli* O157:H(-). *Infect. Immun.* 69:4447–4457.
43. Doughty, S., J. Sloan, V. Bennett-Wood, M. Robertson, R.M. Robins-Browne, and E.L. Hartland. 2002. Identification of a novel fimbrial gene cluster related to long polar fimbriae in locus of enterocyte effacement-negative strains of enterohemorrhagic *Escherichia coli*. *Infect. Immun.* 70:6761–6769.

44. Tarr, P.I., S.S. Bilge, J.C. Vary, Jr., S. Jelacic, R.L. Habeeb, T.R. Ward, M.R. Baylor, and T.E. Besser. 2000. Iha: A novel *Escherichia coli* O157:H7 adherence-conferring molecule encoded on a recently acquired chromosomal island of conserved structure. *Infect. Immun.* 68:1400–1407.

45. Tatsuno, I., H. Kimura, A. Okutani, K. Kanamaru, H. Abe, S. Nagai, K. Makino, H. Shinagawa, M. Yoshida, K. Sato, J. Nakamoto, T. Tobe, and C. Sasakawa. 2000. Isolation and characterization of mini-Tn5Km2 insertion mutants of enterohemorrhagic *Escherichia coli* O157:H7 deficient in adherence to Caco-2 cells. *Infect. Immun.* 68:5943–5952.

46. Torres, A.G., J.A. Giron, N.T. Perna, V. Burland, F.R. Blattner, F. Avelino-Flores, and J.B. Kaper. 2002. Identification and characterization of lpfABCC'DE, a fimbrial operon of enterohemorrhagic *Escherichia coli* O157:H7. *Infect. Immun.* 70:5416–5427.

47. Torres, A.G. and J.B. Kaper. 2003. Multiple elements controlling adherence of enterohemorrhagic *Escherichia coli* O157:H7 to HeLa cells. *Infect. Immun.* 71:4985–4995.

48. Toth, I., M.L. Cohen, H.S. Rumschlag, L.W. Riley, E.H. White, J.H. Carr, W.W. Bond, and I.K. Wachsmuth. 1990. Influence of the 60-megadalton plasmid on adherence of *Escherichia coli* O157:H7 and genetic derivatives. *Infect. Immun.* 58:1223–1231.

49. DeVinney, R., M. Stein, D. Reinscheid, A. Abe, S. Ruschkowski, and B.B. Finlay. 1999. Enterohemorrhagic *Escherichia coli* O157:H7 produces Tir, which is translocated to the host cell membrane but is not tyrosine phosphorylated. *Infect. Immun.* 67:2389–2398.

50. Luo, Y., E.A. Frey, R.A. Pfuetzner, A.L. Creagh, D.G. Knoechel, C.A. Haynes, B.B. Finlay, and N.C. Strynadka. 2000. Crystal structure of enteropathogenic *Escherichia coli* intimin-receptor complex. *Nature* 405:1073–1077.

51. Howe, K.L., C. Reardon, A. Wang, A. Nazli, and D.M. McKay. 2005. Transforming growth factor-beta regulation of epithelial tight junction proteins enhances barrier function and blocks enterohemorrhagic *Escherichia coli* O157:H7-induced increased permeability. *Am. J. Pathol.* 167:1587–1597.

52. Hauf, N. and T. Chakraborty. 2003. Suppression of NF-kappa B activation and proinflammatory cytokine expression by Shiga toxin-producing *Escherichia coli*. *J. Immunol.* 170:2074–2082.

53. Sharma, R., S. Tesfay, F.L. Tomson, R.P. Kanteti, V.K. Viswanathan, and G. Hecht. 2006. Balance of bacterial pro- and anti-inflammatory mediators dictates net effect of enteropathogenic *Escherichia coli* on intestinal epithelial cells. *Am. J. Physiol. Gastrointest. Liver Physiol.* 290:G685-G694.

54. Aoki, Y. and T. Takeda. 2002. Effect of Shiga toxins on granulocyte function. *Microb. Pathog.* 32:279–285.

55. Jacewicz, M.S., D.W. Acheson, D.G. Binion, G.A. West, L.L. Lincicome, C. Fiocchi, and G.T. Keusch. 1999. Responses of human intestinal microvascular endothelial cells to Shiga toxins 1 and 2 and pathogenesis of hemorrhagic colitis. *Infect. Immun.* 67:1439–1444.

56. Morigi, M., G. Micheletti, M. Figliuzzi, B. Imberti, M.A. Karmali, A. Remuzzi, G. Remuzzi, and C. Zoja. 1995. Verotoxin-1 promotes leukocyte adhesion to cultured endothelial cells under physiologic flow conditions. *Blood* 86:4553–4558.

57. Thorpe, C.M., B.P. Hurley, L.L. Lincicome, M.S. Jacewicz, G.T. Keusch, and D.W. Acheson. 1999. Shiga toxins stimulate secretion of interleukin-8 from intestinal epithelial cells. *Infect. Immun.* 67:5985–5993.

58. Thorpe, C.M., W.E. Smith, B.P. Hurley, and D.W. Acheson. 2001. Shiga toxins induce, superinduce, and stabilize a variety of C-X-C chemokine mRNAs in intestinal epithelial cells, resulting in increased chemokine expression. *Infect. Immun.* 69:6140–6147.

59. Acheson, D.W., R. Moore, S. De Breucker, L. Lincicome, M. Jacewicz, E. Skutelsky, and G.T. Keusch. 1996. Translocation of Shiga toxin across polarized intestinal cells in tissue culture. *Infect. Immun.* 64:3294–3300.

60. Hurley, B.P., C.M. Thorpe, and D.W. Acheson. 2001. Shiga toxin translocation across intestinal epithelial cells is enhanced by neutrophil transmigration. *Infect. Immun.* 69:6148–6155.

61. Thorpe, C.M., B.P. Hurley, and D.W. Acheson. 2003. Shiga toxin interactions with the intestinal epithelium. *Methods Mol. Med.* 73:263–273.

62. Tazzari, P.L., F. Ricci, D. Carnicelli, A. Caprioli, A.E. Tozzi, G. Rizzoni, R. Conte, and M. Brigotti. 2004. Flow cytometry detection of Shiga toxins in the blood from children with hemolytic uremic syndrome. *Cytometry B Clin. Cytom.* 61:40–44.

63. te Loo, D.M.W.M., L.A. Monnens, T.J. Der Velden, M.A. Vermeer, F. Preyers, P.N. Demacker, L.P. van den Heuvel, and V.W. van Hinsbergh. 2000. Binding and transfer of verocytotoxin by polymorphonuclear leukocytes in hemolytic uremic syndrome. *Blood* 95:3396–3402.

64. te Loo, D.M.W.M., V.W. van Hinsbergh, L.P. van den Heuvel, and L.A. Monnens. 2001. Detection of verocytotoxin bound to circulating polymorpho-nuclear leukocytes of patients with hemolytic uremic syndrome. *J. Am. Soc. Nephrol.* 12:800–806.

65. Morigi, M., G. Micheletti, M. Figliuzzi, B. Imberti, M.A. Karmali, A. Remuzzi, G. Remuzzi, and C. Zoja. 1995. Verotoxin-1 promotes leukocyte adhesion to cultured endothelial cells under physiologic flow conditions. *Blood* 86:4553–4558.

66. Proulx, F., J.P. Turgeon, C. Litalien, M.M. Mariscalco, P. Robitaille, and E. Seidman. 1998. Inflammatory mediators in *Escherichia coli* O157:H7 hemor-rhagic colitis and hemolytic-uremic syndrome. *Pediatr. Infect. Dis. J.* 17:899–904.

67. Ruggenenti, P., M. Noris, and G. Remuzzi. 2001. Thrombotic microangiopathy, hemolytic uremic syndrome, and thrombotic thrombocytopenic purpura. *Kidney Int.* 60:831–846.

68. Sugatani, J., T. Igarashi, M. Munakata, Y. Komiyama, H. Takahashi, N. Komiyama, T. Maeda, T. Takeda, and M. Miwa. 2000. Activation of coagulation in C57BL/6 mice given verotoxin 2 (VT2) and the effect of co-administration of LPS with VT2. *Thromb. Res.* 100:61–72.

69. Yagi, H., N. Narita, M. Matsumoto, Y. Sakurai, H. Ikari, A. Yoshioka, E. Kita, Y. Ikeda, K. Titani, and Y. Fujimura. 2001. Enhanced low shear stress induced platelet aggregation by Shiga-like toxin 1 purified from *Escherichia coli* O157. *Am. J. Hematol.* 66:105–115.

70. Zoja, C., S. Angioletti, R. Donadelli, C. Zanchi, S. Tomasoni, E. Binda, B. Imberti, L.M. te, L. Monnens, G. Remuzzi, and M. Morigi. 2002. Shiga toxin-2 triggers endothelial leukocyte adhesion and transmigration via NF-kappaB dependent up-regulation of IL-8 and MCP-1. *Kidney Int.* 62:846–856.

71. Zoja, C., M. Morigi, and G. Remuzzi. 2001. The role of the endothelium in hemolytic uremic syndrome. *J. Nephrol.* 14 Suppl. 4:S58–S62.

72. Proulx, F., E.G. Seidman, and D. Karpman. 2001. Pathogenesis of Shiga toxin-associated hemolytic uremic syndrome. *Pediatr. Res.* 50:163–171.

73. Boyd, B. and C. Lingwood. 1989. Verotoxin receptor glycolipid in human renal tissue. *Nephron* 51:207–210.
74. Ergonul, Z., A.K. Hughes, and D.E. Kohan. 2003. Induction of apoptosis of human brain microvascular endothelial cells by shiga toxin 1. *J. Infect. Dis.* 187:154–158.
75. Fujii, J., Y. Kinoshita, T. Yutsudo, H. Taniguchi, T. Obrig, and S.I. Yoshida. 2001. Toxicity of Shiga toxin 1 in the central nervous system of rabbits. *Infect. Immun.* 69:6545–6548.
76. Kita, E., Y. Yunou, T. Kurioka, H. Harada, S. Yoshikawa, K. Mikasa, and N. Higashi. 2000. Pathogenic mechanism of mouse brain damage caused by oral infection with Shiga toxin-producing *Escherichia coli* O157:H7. *Infect. Immun.* 68:1207–1214.
77. Richardson, S.E., T.A. Rotman, V. Jay, C.R. Smith, L.E. Becker, M. Petric, N.F. Olivieri, and M.A. Karmali. 1992. Experimental verocytotoxemia in rabbits. *Infect. Immun.* 60:4154–4167.
78. Hughes, A.K., Z. Ergonul, P.K. Stricklett, and D.E. Kohan. 2002. Molecular basis for high renal cell sensitivity to the cytotoxic effects of shigatoxin-1: Upregulation of globotriaosylceramide expression. *J. Am. Soc. Nephrol.* 13:2239–2245.
79. Stricklett, P.K., A.K. Hughes, Z. Ergonul, and D.E. Kohan. 2002. Molecular basis for up-regulation by inflammatory cytokines of Shiga toxin 1 cytotoxicity and globotriaosylceramide expression. *J. Infect. Dis.* 186:976–982.
80. Hashimoto, H., K. Mizukoshi, M. Nishi, T. Kawakita, S. Hasui, Y. Kato, Y. Ueno, R. Takeya, N. Okuda, and T. Takeda. 1999. Epidemic of gastrointestinal tract infection including hemorrhagic colitis attributable to Shiga toxin 1-producing *Escherichia coli* O118:H2 at a junior high school in Japan. *Pediatrics* 103: E2(1)–E2(5).
81. Kleanthous, H., H.R. Smith, S.M. Scotland, R.J. Gross, B. Rowe, C.M. Taylor, and D.V. Milford. 1990. Haemolytic uraemic syndromes in the British Isles, 1985–1988: Association with verocytotoxin producing *Escherichia coli*. Part 2: Microbiological aspects. *Arch. Dis. Child* 65:722–727.
82. Ostroff, S.M., P.I. Tarr, M.A. Neill, J.H. Lewis, N. Hargrett-Bean, and J.M. Kobayashi. 1989. Toxin genotypes and plasmid profiles as determinants of systemic sequelae in *Escherichia coli* O157:H7 infections. *J. Infect. Dis.* 160:994–998.
83. Scotland, S.M., G.A. Willshaw, H.R. Smith, and B. Rowe. 1990. Properties of strains of *Escherichia coli* O26:H11 in relation to their enteropathogenic or enterohemorrhagic classification. *J. Infect. Dis.* 162:1069–1074.
84. Siegler, R.L., T.G. Obrig, T.J. Pysher, V.L. Tesh, N.D. Denkers, and F.B. Taylor. 2003. Response to Shiga toxin 1 and 2 in a baboon model of hemolytic uremic syndrome. *Pediatr. Nephrol.* 18:92–96.
85. Bitzan, M., M. Klemt, R. Steffens, and D.E. Muller-Wiefel. 1993. Differences in verotoxin neutralizing activity of therapeutic immunoglobulins and sera from healthy controls. *Infection* 21:140–145.
86. Kimura, T., S. Tani, Y.Y. Matsumoto, and T. Takeda. 2001. Serum amyloid P component is the Shiga toxin 2-neutralizing factor in human blood. *J. Biol. Chem.* 276:41576–41579.
87. Pepys, M.B. 2001. Pathogenesis, diagnosis and treatment of systemic amyloidosis. *Philos. Trans. R. Soc. Lond. Ser. B Biol. Sci.* 356:203–210.
88. Emsley, J., H.E. White, B.P. O'Hara, G. Oliva, N. Srinivasan, I.J. Tickle, T.L. Blundell, M.B. Pepys, and S.P. Wood. 1994. Structure of pentameric human serum amyloid P component. *Nature* 367:338–345.

89. Ling, H., A. Boodhoo, B. Hazes, M.D. Cummings, G.D. Armstrong, J.L. Brunton, and R.J. Read. 1998. Structure of the shiga-like toxin I B-pentamer complexed with an analogue of its receptor Gb3. *Biochemistry* 37:1777–1788.

90. Nelson, S.R., G.A. Tennent, D. Sethi, P.E. Gower, F.W. Ballardie, S. Amatayakul-Chantler, and M.B. Pepys. 1991. Serum amyloid P component in chronic renal failure and dialysis. *Clin. Chim. Acta* 200:191–199.

91. de Haas, C.J., Z.R. van der, B. Benaissa-Trouw, K.P. van Kessel, J. Verhoef, and J.A. van Strijp. 1999. Lipopolysaccharide (LPS)-binding synthetic peptides derived from serum amyloid P component neutralize LPS. *Infect. Immun.* 67:2790–2796.

92. Ying, S.C., A.T. Gewurz, H. Jiang, and H. Gewurz. 1993. Human serum amyloid P component oligomers bind and activate the classical complement pathway via residues 14–26 and 76–92 of the A chain collagen-like region of C1q. *J. Immunol.* 150:169–176.

93. Noursadeghi, M., M.C. Bickerstaff, J.R. Gallimore, J. Herbert, J. Cohen, and M.B. Pepys. 2000. Role of serum amyloid P component in bacterial infection: protection of the host or protection of the pathogen. *Proc. Natl. Acad. Sci. U.S.A.* 97:14584–14589.

94. Marcato, P., H.K. Vander, G.L. Mulvey, and G.D. Armstrong. 2003. Serum amyloid P component binding to Shiga toxin 2 requires both a subunit and B pentamer. *Infect. Immun.* 71:6075–6078.

95. Fraser, M.E., M. Fujinaga, M.M. Cherney, A.R. Melton-Celsa, E.M. Twiddy, A.D. O'Brien, and M.N. James. 2004. Structure of shiga toxin type 2 (Stx2) from *Escherichia coli* O157:H7. *J. Biol. Chem.* 279:27511–27517.

96. Mulvey, G.L., P. Marcato, P.I. Kitov, J. Sadowska, D.R. Bundle, and G.D. Armstrong. 2003. Assessment in mice of the therapeutic potential of tailored, multivalent Shiga toxin carbohydrate ligands. *J. Infect. Dis.* 187:640–649.

97. Kitov, P.I., J.M. Sadowska, G. Mulvey, G.D. Armstrong, H. Ling, N.S. Pannu, R.J. Read, and D.R. Bundle. 2000. Shiga-like toxins are neutralized by tailored multivalent carbohydrate ligands. *Nature* 403:669–672.

98. Kimura, T., S. Tani, M. Motoki, and Y. Matsumoto. 2003. Role of Shiga toxin 2 (Stx2)-binding protein, human serum amyloid P component (HuSAP), in Shiga toxin-producing *Escherichia coli* infections: Assumption from in vitro and in vivo study using HuSAP and anti-Stx2 humanized monoclonal antibody TMA-15. *Biochem. Biophys. Res. Commun.* 305:1057–1060.

99. Baltz, M.L., R.F. Dyck, and M.B. Pepys. 1985. Studies of the in vivo synthesis and catabolism of serum amyloid P component (SAP) in the mouse. *Clin. Exp. Immunol.* 59:235–242.

100. Armstrong, G.D., G.L. Mulvey, P. Marcato, T.P. Griener, M.C. Kahan, G.A. Tennent, C.A. Sabin, H. Chart, and M.B. Pepys. 2006. Human serum amyloid P component rotects against *Escherichia coli* O157:H7 Shiga toxin 2 in vivo: Therapeutic implications for Hemolytic-Uremic Syndrome. *J. Infect. Dis.* 193:1120–1124.

101. Brigotti, M., A. Caprioli, A.E. Tozzi, P.L. Tazzari, F. Ricci, R. Conte, D. Carnicelli, M.A. Procaccino, F. Minelli, A.V. Ferretti, F. Paglialonga, A. Edefonti, and G. Rizzoni. 2006. Shiga toxins present in the gut and in the polymorphonuclear leukocytes circulating in the blood of children with Hemolytic-Uremic Syndrome. *J. Clin. Microbiol.* 44:313–317.

102. Jung, U. and K. Ley. 1997. Regulation of E-selectin, P-selectin, and intercellular adhesion molecule 1 expression in mouse cremaster muscle vasculature. *Microcirculation* 4:311–319.
103. Ley, K. and P. Gaehtgens. 1991. Endothelial, not hemodynamic, differences are responsible for preferential leukocyte rolling in rat mesenteric venules. *Circ. Res.* 69:1034–1041.
104. De Vriese, A.S., K. Endlich, M. Elger, N.H. Lameire, R.C. Atkins, H.Y. Lan, A. Rupin, W. Kriz, and M.W. Steinhausen. 1999. The role of selectins in glomerular leukocyte recruitment in rat anti-glomerular basement membrane glomerulonephritis. *J. Am. Soc. Nephrol.* 10:2510–2517.
105. Downey, G.P., G.S. Worthen, P.M. Henson, and D.M. Hyde. 1993. Neutrophil sequestration and migration in localized pulmonary inflammation. Capillary localization and migration across the interalveolar septum. *Am. Rev. Respir. Dis.* 147:168–176.
106. Wong, J., B. Johnston, S.S. Lee, D.C. Bullard, C.W. Smith, A.L. Beaudet, and P. Kubes. 1997. A minimal role for selectins in the recruitment of leukocytes into the inflamed liver microvasculature. *J. Clin. Invest.* 99:2782–2790.
107. Kuligowski, M.P., A.R. Kitching, and M.J. Hickey. 2006. Leukocyte recruitment to the inflamed glomerulus: A critical role for platelet-derived p-selectin in the absence of rolling. *J. Immunol.* 176:6991–6999.
108. Lingwood, C.A. 1994. Verotoxin-binding in human renal sections. *Nephron* 66:21–28.
109. Morigi, M., M. Galbusera, E. Binda, B. Imberti, S. Gastoldi, A. Remuzzi, C. Zoja, and G. Remuzzi. 2001. Verotoxin-1-induced up-regulation of adhesive molecules renders microvascular endothelial cells thrombogenic at high shear stress. *Blood* 98:1828–1835.
110. Dyck, R.F., C.M. Lockwood, M. Kershaw, N. McHugh, V.C. Duance, M.L. Baltz, and M.B. Pepys. 1980. Amyloid P-component is a constituent of normal human glomerular basement membrane. *J. Exp. Med.* 152:1162–1174.
111. te Loo, D.M.W.M., A.E. Heuvelink, E. de Boer, J. Nauta, W.J. van der, C. Schroder, V.W. van Hinsbergh, H. Chart, N.C. van de Kar, and L.P. van den Heuvel. 2001. Vero cytotoxin binding to polymorphonuclear leukocytes among households with children with hemolytic uremic syndrome. *J. Infect. Dis.* 184:446–450.
112. Holle, J.U., J.M. Williams, L. Harper, C.O. Savage, and C.M. Taylor. 2005. Effect of verocytotoxins (Shiga-like toxins) on human neutrophils in vitro. *Pediatr. Nephrol.* 20:1237–1244.
113. Fernandez, G.C., C. Rubel, G. Dran, S. Gomez, M.A. Isturiz, and M.S. Palermo. 2000. Shiga toxin-2 induces neutrophilia and neutrophil activation in a murine model of hemolytic uremic syndrome. *Clin. Immunol.* 95:227–234.
114. Grif, K., M.P. Dierich, H. Karch, and F. Allerberger. 1998. Strain-specific differences in the amount of Shiga toxin released from enterohemorrhagic *Escherichia coli* O157 following exposure to subinhibitory concentrations of antimicrobial agents. *Eur. J. Clin. Microbiol. Infect. Dis.* 17:761–766.
115. Takahashi, K., K. Narita, Y. Kato, T. Sugiyama, N. Koide, T. Yoshida, and T. Yokochi. 1997. Low-level release of Shiga-like toxin (verocytotoxin) and endotoxin from enterohemorrhagic *Escherichia coli* treated with imipenem. *Antimicrob. Agents Chemother.* 41:2295–2296.

116. Walterspiel, J.N., S. Ashkenazi, A.L. Morrow, and T.G. Cleary. 1992. Effect of subinhibitory concentrations of antibiotics on extracellular Shiga-like toxin I. *Infection* 20:25–29.

117. Yoh, M., E.K. Frimpong, S.P. Voravuthikunchai, and T. Honda. 1999. Effect of subinhibitory concentrations of antimicrobial agents (quinolones and macrolide) on the production of verotoxin by enterohemorrhagic *Escherichia coli* O157:H7. *Can. J. Microbiol.* 45:732–739.

118. Isogai, E., H. Isogai, S. Hayashi, T. Kubota, K. Kimura, N. Fujii, T. Ohtani, and K. Sato. 2000. Effect of antibiotics, levofloxacin and fosfomycin, on a mouse model with *Escherichia coli* O157 infection. *Microbiol. Immunol.* 44:89–95.

119. Yoshimura, K., J. Fujii, H. Taniguchi, and S. Yoshida. 1999. Chemotherapy for enterohemorrhagic *Escherichia coli* O157:H infection in a mouse model. *FEMS Immunol. Med. Microbiol.* 26:101–108.

120. Fukushima, H., T. Hashizume, Y. Morita, J. Tanaka, K. Azuma, Y. Mizumoto, M. Kaneno, M. Matsuura, K. Konma, and T. Kitani. 1999. Clinical experiences in Sakai City Hospital during the massive outbreak of enterohemorrhagic *Escherichia coli* O157 infections in Sakai City, 1996. *Pediatr. Int.* 41:213–217.

121. Honda, T. 1999. Factors influencing the development of hemolytic uremic syndrome caused by enterohemorrhagic *Escherichia coli* infection: From a questionnaire survey to in vitro experiment. *Pediatr. Int.* 41:209–212.

122. Ahmed, A., J. Li, Y. Shiloach, J.B. Robbins, and S.C. Szu. 2006. Safety and immunogenicity of *Escherichia coli* O157 O-specific polysaccharide conjugate vaccine in 2–5-year-old children. *J. Infect. Dis.* 193:515–521.

123. Fukuda, T., T. Kimiya, M. Takahashi, Y. Arakawa, Y. Ami, Y. Suzaki, S. Naito, A. Horino, N. Nagata, S. Satoh, F. Gondaira, J. Sugiyama, Y. Nakano, M. Mori, S. Nishinohara, K. Komuro, and T. Uchida. 1998. Induction of protection against oral infection with cytotoxin-producing *Escherichia coli* O157:H7 in mice by shiga-like toxin-liposome conjugate. *Int. Arch. Allergy Immunol.* 116:313–317.

124. Horne, C., B.A. Vallance, W. Deng, and B.B. Finlay. 2002. Current progress in enteropathogenic and enterohemorrhagic *Escherichia coli* vaccines. *Expert Rev. Vaccines* 1:483–493.

125. Ishikawa, S., K. Kawahara, Y. Kagami, Y. Isshiki, A. Kaneko, H. Matsui, N. Okada, and H. Danbara. 2003. Protection against Shiga toxin 1 challenge by immunization of mice with purified mutant Shiga toxin 1. *Infect. Immun.* 71:3235–3239.

126. Konadu, E., A. Donohue-Rolfe, S.B. Calderwood, V. Pozsgay, J. Shiloach, J.B. Robbins, and S.C. Szu. 1999. Syntheses and immunologic properties of *Escherichia coli* O157 O-specific polysaccharide and Shiga toxin 1 B subunit conjugates in mice. *Infect. Immun.* 67:6191–6193.

127. Marcato, P., T.P. Griener, G.L. Mulvey, and G.D. Armstrong. 2005. Recombinant Shiga toxin B-subunit-keyhole limpet hemocyanin conjugate vaccine protects mice from Shigatoxemia. *Infect. Immun.* 73:6523–6529.

128. Marcato, P., G. Mulvey, R.J. Read, H.K. Vander, P.N. Nation, and G.D. Armstrong. 2001. Immunoprophylactic potential of cloned Shiga toxin 2 B subunit. *J. Infect. Dis.* 183:435–443.

129. Wen, S.X., L.D. Teel, N.A. Judge, and A.D. O'Brien. 2006. Genetic toxoids of Shiga toxin types 1 and 2 protect mice against homologous but not heterologous toxin challenge. *Vaccine* 24:1142–1148.

130. MacConnachie, A.A. and W.T. Todd. 2004. Potential therapeutic agents for the prevention and treatment of haemolytic uraemic syndrome in Shiga toxin producing *Escherichia coli* infection. *Curr. Opinion Infect. Dis.* 17:479–482.

131. Mukherjee, J., K. Chios, D. Fishwild, D. Hudson, S. O'Donnell, S.M. Rich, A. Donohue-Rolfe, and S. Tzipori. 2002. Human Stx2-specific monoclonal antibodies prevent systemic complications of *Escherichia coli* O157:H7 infection. *Infect. Immun.* 70:612–619.

132. Sheoran, A.S., S. Chapman-Bonofiglio, B.R. Harvey, J. Mukherjee, G. Georgiou, A. Donohue-Rolfe, and S. Tzipori. 2005. Human antibody against shiga toxin 2 administered to piglets after the onset of diarrhea due to *Escherichia coli* O157:H7 prevents fatal systemic complications. *Infect. Immun.* 73:4607–4613.

133. Dean-Nystrom, E.A., L.J. Gansheroff, M. Mills, H.W. Moon, and A.D. O'Brien. 2002. Vaccination of pregnant dams with intimin(O157) protects suckling piglets from *Escherichia coli* O157:H7 infection. *Infect. Immun.* 70:2414–2418.

134. Judge, N.A., H.S. Mason, and A.D. O'Brien. 2004. Plant cell-based intimin vaccine given orally to mice primed with intimin reduces time of *Escherichia coli* O157:H7 shedding in feces. *Infect. Immun.* 72:168–175.

135. Naylor, S.W., A.J. Roe, P. Nart, K. Spears, D.G. Smith, J.C. Low, and D.L. Gally. 2005. *Escherichia coli* O157: H7 forms attaching and effacing lesions at the terminal rectum of cattle and colonization requires the LEE4 operon. *Microbiology* 151:2773–2781.

136. Potter, A.A., S. Klashinsky, Y. Li, E. Frey, H. Townsend, D. Rogan, G. Erickson, S. Hinkley, T. Klopfenstein, R.A. Moxley, D.R. Smith, and B.B. Finlay. 2004. Decreased shedding of *Escherichia coli* O157:H7 by cattle following vaccination with type III secreted proteins. *Vaccine* 22:362–369.

137. Van Donkersgoed, J., D. Hancock, D. Rogan, and A.A. Potter. 2005. *Escherichia coli* O157:H7 vaccine field trial in 9 feedlots in Alberta and Saskatchewan. *Can. Vet. J.* 46:724–728.

138. Armstrong, G.D., P.C. Rowe, P. Goodyer, E. Orrbine, T.P. Klassen, G. Wells, A. MacKenzie, H. Lior, C. Blanchard, and F. Auclair. 1995. A phase I study of chemically synthesized verotoxin (Shiga-like toxin) Pk-trisaccharide receptors attached to chromosorb for preventing hemolytic-uremic syndrome. *J. Infect. Dis.* 171:1042–1045.

139. Nishikawa, K., K. Matsuoka, E. Kita, N. Okabe, M. Mizuguchi, K. Hino, S. Miyazawa, C. Yamasaki, J. Aoki, S. Takashima, Y. Yamakawa, M. Nishijima, D. Terunuma, H. Kuzuhara, and Y. Natori. 2002. A therapeutic agent with oriented carbohydrates for treatment of infections by Shiga toxin-producing *Escherichia coli* O157:H7. *Proc. Natl. Acad. Sci. U.S.A.* 99:7669–7674.

140. Olano-Martin, E., M.R. Williams, G.R. Gibson, and R.A. Rastall. 2003. Pectins and pectic-oligosaccharides inhibit *Escherichia coli* O157:H7 Shiga toxin as directed towards the human colonic cell line HT29. *FEMS Microbiol. Lett.* 218:101–105.

141. Watanabe, M., K. Matsuoka, E. Kita, K. Igai, N. Higashi, A. Miyagawa, T. Watanabe, R. Yanoshita, Y. Samejima, D. Terunuma, Y. Natori, and K. Nishikawa. 2004. Oral therapeutic agents with highly clustered globotriose for treatment of Shiga toxigenic *Escherichia coli* infections. *J. Infect. Dis.* 189:360–368.

142. Trachtman, H., A. Cnaan, E. Christen, K. Gibbs, S. Zhao, D.W. Acheson, R. Weiss, F.J. Kaskel, A. Spitzer, and G.H. Hirschman. 2003. Effect of an oral Shiga toxin-binding agent on diarrhea-associated hemolytic uremic syndrome in children: A randomized controlled trial. *JAMA* 290:1337–1344.

143. Takenaga, M., R. Igarashi, M. Higaki, T. Nakayama, K. Yuki, and Y. Mizushima. 2000. Effect of a soluble pseudo-receptor on verotoxin 2-induced toxicity. *J. Infect. Chemother.* 6:21–25.

3

Viruses and Protozoan Parasites in Food

Dean O. Cliver

CONTENTS

3.1 Introduction

Viruses are now considered to be preeminent causes of foodborne diseases in the United States[1] and some other countries. Protozoa are gaining recognition as causes of foodborne and waterborne diseases as well, though progress is somewhat slower. Prion diseases (transmissible spongiform encephalopathies) may well be the rarest of those transmitted via foods, but the majority of cases of new variant Creutzfeldt–Jakob disease (vCJD) are thought to have been foodborne (see Chapter 20),[2] and the impact of these on the food industry has been enormous. These groups have little in common, except that they all differ from the better-recognized bacterial causes of foodborne diseases. It is neither possible to describe them in detail here, nor possible to cite ultimate source references. Instead, general discussions will be based largely on reviews and secondary references, which the reader can resort to for more extensive information.

3.2 Viruses

The viruses of greatest concern with respect to transmission via foods are the noroviruses and the virus of hepatitis A.[3,4] The U.S. Centers for Disease Control and Prevention (CDC) propose that rotaviruses and astroviruses are often transmitted via foods in the United States,[1] but outbreaks caused by these agents are rarely reported. Hepatitis E virus causes significant outbreaks, especially via water, in some parts of the world.[4] Despite occasional allegations of zoonotic transmission, nearly all of the recorded foodborne and waterborne viral disease outbreaks have been caused by human-specific agents. Viruses are passed from person-to-person by a fecal–oral cycle, with food or water sometimes serving as a vehicle. Thus, any human virus that is transmitted via a fecal–oral cycle might be foodborne or waterborne, but some are more prominent than others in this regard. Most are small (<50 nm diameter), roughly spherical with a single strand of plus-sense RNA, and able to withstand pH 3 for perhaps an hour at room temperature. Again, because most are human specific, they have no animal reservoirs.

3.2.1 Gastroenteritis Viruses

The noroviruses are a genus within the family *Caliciviridae* that are estimated to cause two-thirds of foodborne illnesses in the United States.[1] They were formerly known as Norwalk-like or small, round, structured viruses.[4] The viral particle comprises a single strand of plus-sense RNA (~7.7 kb) coated with protein that, including protrusions, has a diameter of ca. 35 nm. Members of this family, including another genus called sapoviruses, are characterized by cup-shaped depressions on the surface of their protein coats. They occur in a wide variety of serological types, and the immunity gained from infection with one of them is apparently not durable, so there seems to be little prospect of a useful vaccine. Additionally, none of the noroviruses that infect humans has yet been propagated in cell culture, which complicates research dedicated to controlling them. Noroviruses may be transmitted via food or water, but they are highly contagious and may also be transmitted person-to-person and via fomites. The incubation period ranges from 24 to 48 h (extremes 10–50 h), and the duration of illness is usually from 24 to 48 h. Shedding in feces may continue for some days after recovery from the illness, but shedding of virus in vomitus is limited to the acute phase of the disease. If the infected person is a food handler, there are obviously various ways and opportunities for food to be contaminated with noroviruses, and many of these possibilities have been exemplified in recorded outbreaks. The other genus of the *Caliciviridae*, the sapoviruses, are less frequently transmitted via food and water.

The astroviruses are another genus of small, round RNA viruses with a distinctive surface appearance.[4] Seven or eight serotypes are known to infect humans and cause diarrhea, sometimes with vomiting; other types may only infect animals. Unlike the noroviruses, some human strains can be propagated in cell culture, particularly the Caco-2 line. Although Mead and coworkers estimate that astroviruses cause 39,000 foodborne illnesses annually (1% of total astrovirus illnesses that occur) in the United States,[1] foodborne outbreaks are seldom reported. At least one large outbreak has been reported in Japan.[5]

The rotaviruses are at least 70 nm in diameter and contain 11 segments of double-stranded RNA inside a double-layered protein coat.[3,4] CDC estimates for United States incidence (total and foodborne) are equal to those for the astroviruses;[1] the illness caused is also fairly similar. Three of seven known serogroups infect humans, and foodborne outbreaks have definitely been recorded. Symptomatic infections, not necessarily foodborne, are seen frequently in children in some parts of the world. Vaccines to prevent these are under development.

3.2.2 Hepatitis Viruses

Hepatitis A virus comprises a genus unto itself within the family *Picornaviridae*.[3,4] Although CDC says it causes fewer foodborne illnesses in the United States than the astroviruses or rotaviruses, several foodborne outbreaks are often reported per year. Hepatitis A is a reportable disease in the United States, which should favor the recording of foodborne outbreaks; but the incubation period ranges from roughly 2 to 7 weeks, with an average of about 4 weeks, which complicates the recognition of common sources, food, or other. Hepatitis A may entail a few weeks' debility, but death is rare; however, it is one of the more severe of foodborne viral diseases. In developing countries, where infection often occurs in early childhood, illness may be mild or imperceptible and confer lifelong immunity. The virus appears to be more resistant to heat and to drying than other *Picornaviridae*. Because a person who is incubating a case of hepatitis A may shed the virus 1–2 weeks before onset of illness, there are opportunities for apparently healthy food handlers to contaminate a great deal of food if their hygiene is poor. Vaccines are available to prevent the disease but are not universally administered in most countries, even those that are affluent. Persons known to have been exposed to hepatitis A, if they have not already been immunized, can be temporarily, passively protected by injection of pooled human immune serum globulin.

Hepatitis E virus seldom infects humans in North America, although a closely related agent is widespread in swine there.[4] Of the hepatitis viruses of humans, it is the only one other than the hepatitis A virus that is transmitted via a fecal–oral cycle. Clinically, it differs from hepatitis A in having a somewhat longer incubation period and in threatening the lives of pregnant women. The viral particle is somewhat larger than that of hepatitis A and has a coat protein organization similar to that of the noroviruses, but with a different organization of the RNA genome, whereby it has been assigned to a taxon unto itself. It is more often waterborne than foodborne and typically does not infect people early in life. Zoonotic transmission from raw or lightly cooked swine (including wild boar) and deer meat has been reported in Japan.

3.2.3   Possible Zoonoses

Tick-borne encephalitis is, as the name indicates, most often transmitted via a tick biological vector.[6] The tick species varies with the locale. In certain parts of the world, particularly Central and Eastern Europe, dairy animals (especially goats, but possibly also sheep and cattle) that are infected by tick bites shed the virus in their milk. If milk or milk products from these animals are ingested without pasteurization, people are at risk of undergoing a very serious virus infection.

Rabies virus infects cattle, and perhaps other dairy animals, with some frequency. Animals typically become infected via canid bites while grazing, but vampire bats are a source in some parts of the world. The virus has not been shown to be shed in the milk of infected animals, but it is common in the United States for people who may have ingested the milk to be urged to undergo rabies immunization. Although research to determine whether rabid cows shed the virus in their milk would present some hazards, the answer to this question might provide a very useful alternative to immunization of milk drinkers.

3.2.4   Human Enteroviruses

Enteroviruses of human origin (including polioviruses, coxsackieviruses, echoviruses, etc.) have long been known to be transmitted by a fecal–oral cycle. They are often detected in community wastewater and sometimes in shellfish or other food. In recent years, especially since the introduction of the polio vaccines, purported foodborne or waterborne outbreaks of enteroviral disease have not been reported in North America or Europe; whether such transmission is occurring in the less affluent world is unknown.

3.3   Protozoa

Protozoan genera that are associated with foodborne and waterborne human illness include *Cryptosporidium*, *Cyclospora*, *Entamoeba*, *Giardia*, and *Toxoplasma*.[7,8,9] These represent a broad range of host specificities, modes of transmission, and styles of pathogenesis. They are considered here in the order of their perceived significance to public health in the United States.

3.3.1 *Cryptosporidium* spp.

Cryptosporidium spp. distinguished itself in 1993 by causing the largest outbreak of waterborne disease on record. Approximately 403,000 persons who drank tap water processed in the southern of two drinking water facilities in Milwaukee developed cryptosporidiosis. At the time, the agent was assumed to be *C. parvum*; but the human-specific species, *C. hominis*, was later described and seems more likely to have been the cause of this outbreak. Milwaukee discharges its treated wastewater to Lake Michigan, one of the five Great Lakes of North America, and draws the raw water for its drinking water supply from the same source. *C. parvum* and *C. hominis* present special problems in the filtration stage of water purification because their oocysts are among the smallest (4–6 μm) of protozoan transmission forms. A possible triggering event was a change the city made in chemical coagulants, in an effort to produce a less-aggressive finished water and mobilize less lead from plumbing in the oldest section of the city. Although the coagulant used had performed successfully in other cities, there were temporary problems with it in Milwaukee that seem to have led to *C. hominis* passing the coagulation-and-settling treatment and then passing through the sand filters. Given that *C. hominis* is virtually refractory to chlorine, the agent was distributed throughout the south side area, to homes and business establishments. Although drinking water was the principal vehicle, various food processing establishments were thought to be at risk of contamination of their products via the water. Other waterborne and foodborne outbreaks have been recorded.

C. *hominis* and *C. parvum* invade the enterocytes lining the intestine and carry out a complex life cycle including a sexual reproduction phase. After incubation averaging 1 week, profuse diarrhea is common and usually lasts less than 30 days (with shedding continuing for 2–6 months). No treatment has yet been proven effective against *Cryptosporidium*. Cryptosporidiosis is diagnostic of AIDS in HIV-positive persons and will generally persist (with intermittent symptoms) for life. Both thick- and thin-walled oocysts are shed in feces, as well as sporozoites and other labile forms. Only the thick-walled oocysts represent a significant threat of persisting and being transmitted via the environment, including the food and water vehicles. Although *C. hominis* is human specific, *C. parvum* has some alternate hosts—especially cattle. Calves a few weeks old may show profuse, propulsive diarrhea that represents a threat to nearby humans. Other animals, particularly ruminants, may also be hosts and sources of zoonotic transmission to humans.

3.3.2 *Giardia lamblia*

Giardia lamblia (a.k.a. *duodenalis, intestinalis*) was generally regarded as a commensal in the United States until a group of tourists returned from what was then Leningrad with a highly characteristic form of diarrhea that evidently resulted from drinking the public water. *Giardia* trophozoites adhere to the mucosal surface of the intestinal lining and interfere with absorption of nutrients; clinicians learned to recognize the distinctive smell of fecal specimens from giardiasis patients. In subsequent years, giardiasis has been recognized as a widespread problem, especially among recreational campers who drink from surface waters. A variety of domestic and wild animals are reservoirs, in addition to humans; giardiasis is often called "beaver fever" in Canada. *Giardia* cysts are large enough (9–12 μm long) to be more readily removed in water treatment, but are somewhat chlorine resistant. Vehicles are unfiltered surface water, drinking water recontaminated with sewage, fruits, vegetables, salads, and other foods subject to direct or indirect fecal contamination. Like *Cryptosporidium*, *Giardia* can be transmitted directly among children in day care centers, causing explosive outbreaks.

3.3.3   *Toxoplasma gondii*

Toxoplasma gondii has the cat as its definitive host. An infected cat sheds oocysts for a few weeks and then is apparently immune for life. Meanwhile, other animals that accidentally ingest these oocysts become infected and develop tissue cysts in their muscles that contain large numbers of quiescent bradyzoites. These bradyzoites may be reactivated by events in the host's life or may cause infections in humans or other animals if they eat the host's muscle without prior cooking or freezing. Most *Toxoplasma* infections pass unnoticed; but the agent is a leading cause of congenital blindness, hydrocephalus, and retardation in babies infected in utero during the last trimester of gestation. Although the incidence of these birth defects is estimated at only 2090 cases with 42 deaths in the United States, the costs of caring for these infants are said to make this the costliest foodborne disease in the United States.[10]

3.3.4   *Cyclospora cayetanensis*

Cyclospora cayetanensis is a human-specific agent that differs from *Cryptosporidium hominis* in that its oocysts do not become infectious for some days to weeks (depending on conditions) after being shed in feces. Though fairly common in the developing world, cyclosporiasis first gained attention in the United States and Canada due to outbreaks associated with eating raspberries grown in Guatemala. These outbreaks occurred in successive years and inspired investigations by the United States but were never really explained—the shelf life of the raspberries is apparently shorter than the maturation period of the oocysts, so it was not possible to explain their infectivity. More recently, cyclosporiasis has been transmitted by basil and other herb vehicles.

3.3.5 *Entamoeba histolytica*

Entamoeba histolytica was once a frequent cause of waterborne disease in the United States; the agent is now fairly rarely heard from here, but continues to be a very significant threat in the poorer countries. *E. histolytica* causes amebic dysentery, sometimes with abscesses of the liver or other organs (trophozoites are invasive). This species infects only humans and is transmitted via fecally contaminated water and food.

3.4 Contamination

Most of the agents discussed above are transmitted via food and water as a result of contamination with feces (human or, in some instances, animal), so preventing fecal contamination will avoid these problems. Exceptions are the noroviruses, which may be shed copiously in vomitus and contaminate food by this route,[4] and *Toxoplasma gondii*, oocysts of which are shed in cat feces but which otherwise infect via tissue cysts in the muscles of infected animals.[8] Preventing *Toxoplasma* infections of food animals may not be entirely possible unless feral cats, free-range husbandry of the food animals, or both are eliminated. *Cyclospora* transmission seems to result from fecal contamination of food or water; since the oocysts need days or weeks to become infectious, fecal contamination must be indirect in the case of such short-lived vehicles as raspberries.[8]

3.5 Prevention

Since no treatment is available for the majority of foodborne diseases discussed in this chapter, prevention is an especially attractive goal. Viruses are much smaller, and protozoan transmission forms larger, than foodborne and waterborne bacteria. These agents are unable to multiply outside the host's body, which means they cannot multiply in food or water. Their inability to multiply outside the host also complicates detection, in that there are no procedures analogous to the enrichment that may be used in detecting foodborne and waterborne bacteria. Detection methods for protozoan transmission forms depend largely on skilled microscopy, assisted in some instances by serologic and genomic techniques. Viral detection methods that show the greatest promise are directed to the viral nucleic acid. These methods are exacting and expensive, so, they are typically applied only in the event that an outbreak has occurred. In the case of hepatitis A, food testing is further complicated by the long incubation period of the disease—appropriate samples are only rarely available 4–6 weeks after the event that led to an outbreak. Because of the difficulties of detecting viruses in food and water, indicators of fecal—and possibly viral—contamination have long been sought. Bacterial indicators of contamination, such as the coliform group, *Escherichia coli*, etc., are largely irrelevant. Coliphages (bacteriophages that infect *E. coli*), other bacteriophages, and cytopathic human enteroviruses are under continuing evaluation but apparently have limited application regarding the presence of noroviruses and hepatitis A virus, and probably none with regard to protozoa.

3.5.1 Sanitation

Fecal contamination can be largely prevented by composting waste material (human or animal) that is used as a soil amendment and by hand-washing before preparing food. Both composting and hand-washing must be done in technically sound fashion if they are to accomplish their purposes. Because much of the developed world uses the water-carriage toilet to dispose of feces, it is extremely important that wastewater be thoroughly treated and disinfected before being discharged or reused.

3.5.2 Inactivation

None of these agents can multiply in food or water, or indeed outside the body of the host in which they developed. If they occur in food or water, one hopes that they will be inactivated or killed before they can infect a consumer of the vehicle. Food that is cooked and then not recontaminated before being served is unlikely to serve as a vehicle for most of these agents. Thermal processes that are equivalent to milk pasteurization will apparently inactivate most viruses and prions completely. An exception is hepatitis A virus, which is somewhat more heat-resistant and also withstands drying better than most of the others. Freezing in food and water kills the transmission forms of protozoa with varying efficiency but preserves viruses. Viruses and the transmission forms of protozoa tend to be more resistant than bacteria to acid and chlorine; viruses are generally less resistant than *G. lamblia* cysts, which are far surpassed in chlorine resistance by *C. parvum*, and presumably *C. hominis*, oocysts. The viruses are generally susceptible to ultraviolet light and to strong oxidizing agents (e.g., chlorine and ozone), but not to quaternary ammonium compounds, in water and on exposed surfaces. Ionizing radiation is apparently effective against protozoa, but less so against viruses because of their relatively small target size.

3.6 Summary

Viruses and protozoa differ from bacterial pathogens in size and in their inability to multiply in food and water. Although these agents get less recognition because of difficulties of diagnosis and detection, noroviruses are said by CDC to cause most of the foodborne illnesses in the United States, and *Cryptosporidium hominis* apparently caused the largest waterborne disease outbreak in history. Most of the foodborne and waterborne viruses are human specific, whereas a significant portion of the protozoa are zoonotic. Even though viruses and protozoa cannot multiply outside of the host's body, inactivating or killing them in food and water presents some special problems.

References

1. Mead, P.S., Slutsker, L., Dietz, V., McCaig, L.F., Bresee, J.S., Shapiro, C., Griffin, P.M., and Tauxe, R.V. Food-related illness and death in the United States. *Emerg. Infect. Dis.*, 5, 607, 1999.
2. Erdtmann, R. and Sivitz, L.B., (Eds.). *Advancing Prion Science: Guidance for the National Prion Research Program*. Institute of Medicine of the National Academies, National Academies Press, Washington, DC, 2004.
3. Cliver, D.O. and Matsui, S.M. Viruses, in *Foodborne Diseases*, 2nd ed., Cliver, D.O. and Riemann, H.P., (Eds.), Academic Press, London, pp. 161–175, 2002, chapter 12.
4. Cliver, D.O., Matsui, S.M., and Casteel, M. Infections with viruses and prions, in *Foodborne Infections and Intoxications*, 3rd ed., Riemann, H.P. and Cliver, D.O., (Eds.), Academic Press (Elsevier), London, Amsterdam, pp. 367–448, 2006, chapter 11.
5. Oishi, I., Yamazaki, K., Kimoto, T., Minekawa, Y., Utagawa, E., Yamazaki, S., Inouye, S., Grohmann, G.S., Monroe, S.S., Stine, S.E., Carcamo, C., Ando, T., and Glass, R.I. A large outbreak of acute gastroenteritis associated with astrovirus among students and teachers in Osaka, Japan. *J. Infect. Dis.*, 170, 439, 1994.
6. Grešíková, M. Tickborne encephalitis, in *Foodborne Disease Handbook*, Vol. 2, Hui, Y.H., Gorham, J.R., Murrell, K.D., and Cliver, D.O., (Eds.), Marcel Dekker, New York, pp. 113–135, 1994, chapter 4.
7. Dubey, J.P., Murrell, K.D., and Cross, J.H. Parasites, in *Foodborne Diseases*, 2nd ed., Cliver, D.O. and Riemann, H.P., (Eds)., Academic Press, London, pp. 177–190, 2002, chapter 13.
8. Dubey, J.P., Cross, J.H., and Murrell, K.D. Foodborne parasites, in *Foodborne Infections and Intoxications*, 3rd ed., Riemann, H.P. and Cliver, D.O., (Eds.), Academic Press (Elsevier), London, Amsterdam, pp. 449–481, 2006, chapter 12.
9. Fayer, R. Waterborne zoonotic protozoa, in *Waterborne Zoonoses: Identification, Causes and Control*, Cotruvo, J.A., Dufour, A., Rees, G., Bartram, J., Carr, R., Cliver, D.O., Craun, G.F., Fayer R., and Gannon, V.P.J., (Eds.), IWA (International Water Association) Publishing, London, pp. 255–282, 2004, chapter 16.
10. Council for Agricultural Science and Technology (CAST). *Foodborne pathogens: Risks and consequences*. Task Force Report No. 122, CAST, Ames, IA, 1994.

4

Prions in the Food Chain

Rebecca J. Buckner and David M. Asher

During the past two decades, transmissible spongiform encephalopathies (TSEs or prion diseases) have garnered a great deal of attention due to the recognition, in 1986, of a new TSE called "mad cow disease" (known scientifically as bovine spongiform encephalopathy or BSE). The spread of BSE to cattle in at least 26 countries and the subsequent realization that BSE has been transmitted to humans had a great impact on food safety policy and affected international trade worldwide. When discussing food safety related to TSEs, we are mainly concerned with products from those ruminants widely used for food in North America: cattle, sheep, and, to a lesser extent, cervids. This chapter begins by discussing TSEs in general and then focuses on TSEs in the animals of interest and, especially, on measures to reduce the risk of TSE agents entering the food supply.

4.1 Transmissible Spongiform Encephalopathies

TSEs are fatal neurodegenerative disorders that affect humans and a number of animal species (cattle, sheep, goats, elk, deer, moose, cats, and mink); the animals currently of greatest concern are all ruminants (cattle, sheep, elk, and deer). TSEs are characterized by very long incubation periods—usually several years or even decades—followed by a relatively shorter course of neurological symptoms (though the duration of clinical illness in humans sometimes exceeds 2 years), inevitably ending in death [1]. TSEs of humans include kuru—the first human disease recognized to be a TSE because of its similarities to scrapie in sheep [2]—several forms of Creutzfeldt–Jakob disease (CJD) including variant CJD (vCJD), sporadic CJD, iatrogenic CJD and familial CJD, and the Gerstmann–Sträussler–Scheinker syndrome, which is also familial. The extremely rare fatal familial and sporadic insomnia syndromes [3] are also considered to be prion diseases. Nonhuman TSEs include scrapie in sheep and goats (the first recognized and best studied TSE), transmissible mink encephalopathy (TME), chronic wasting disease (CWD) in cervids, and feline spongiform encephalopathy (FSE) in domestic and exotic cats (presumably infected with BSE agent), as well as BSE in cattle and other ruminants [3]. BSE is the only TSE of animals known to have infected humans.

Brain tissues from humans and animals dying due to TSEs show a constellation of changes [4], including vacuoles causing a sponge-like (spongiform) appearance of the brain (Figure 4.1), an increase in size and number of astroglial cells (Figure 4.1B), and deposits of abnormal forms of a normal ubiquitous cell-associated protein called the prion protein or PrP; abnormal PrP is diffusely distributed in areas of the brain parenchyma but sometimes accumulates to form amyloid plaques as well (Figures 4.1C and 4.1D). (Amyloids—meaning starch-like—were originally defined as a heterogeneous group of filamentous proteins stained by iodine, Congo red,

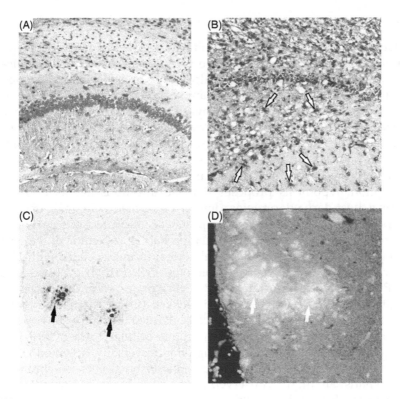

FIGURE 4.1

Constant and variable histopathological findings in brains with TSEs. (A) and (B): Spongiform change and astroytic hypertrophy are typical histopathological findings in brains with TSEs. Sections of hippocampus from brains of an uninfected control mouse (A) and a mouse experimentally infected with a TSE agent derived from a patient with Gerstmann–Sträussler–Scheinker (GSS) syndrome (B). Both sections were stained using a labeled antibody to the glial fibrillary acidic protein found in astrocytes and counterstained with hematoxylin. The brain with TSE (B) shows multiple vacuoles (spongiform change) and darkly stained hypertrophic astrocytes (arrows), not seen in the normal brain (A). (C) and (D): Amyloid plaques are sometimes found in brains with TSEs. A section from the cerebellum of a patient with GSS was stained as in the previous sections but with an antibody to prion protein (PrP) and without counterstain; the brain shows plaques (arrows) containing accumulations of PrP (C). An adjacent section (D) of the same area of brain as in (C) was incubated with thioflavine-S and photographed under UV light showing that that the plaques have fluorescence typical of amyloid proteins. (Images in (A) through (D) were kindly provided by Dr. Pedro Piccardo, FDA and Dr. Bernardino Ghetti, Indiana University, and modified for publication by Dr. Olga A. Maximova, FDA; images in (C) and (D) were previously published by Dr. Piccardo and others (From Piccardo, P., et al., *J. Neuropathol. Exper. Neurol.*, 54, 790, 1995.) and are shown here with his permission and that of the American Association of Neuropathologists, publishers).

thioflavine, and some other dyes.) In some TSEs, deposits of PrP are found in other nervous tissues, such as spinal cord and peripheral nerves, and in nonnervous tissues like intestine, spleen, lymph nodes, and bone marrow [5–9].

4.1.1 TSE Agents, Prion Proteins, and Disease Pathogenesis

The nature of the infectious agents and pathogenesis of TSEs are still poorly understood and are controversial. The TSE agents are clearly self-replicating and transmissible to other individuals of the same species and, sometimes with difficulty, to other species of mammals. The infectious TSE agents are unusually resistant to inactivation by high temperatures, including those achieved by traditional steam autoclaving, and to standard chemical sanitizing agents [10] that destroy most nucleic acids (and denature most proteins) of bacteria and viruses. So, whatever their molecular nature eventually proves to be, TSE agents are "unconventional" pathogens.

The prion hypothesis proposes that the infectious agents of TSEs are abnormal host-derived proteins devoid of nucleic acid [11]. (Prion is a term proposed by S.B. Prusiner for proteinaceous infectious particle [12].) The protein most often invoked as the probable progenitor of the agent is called the prion protein or PrP. The abnormal form associated with TSE has been variously designated as scrapie-type PrP (PrP^{Sc}), protease-resistant PrP (PrP^{res}), disease-associated PrP (PrP^d) or, as recently suggested by consultants to the WHO, TSE-associated PrP (PrP^{TSE}) [13]—the term that we will use in this chapter. PrP^{TSE} is derived by some poorly understood process from a normal noninfectious cellular form of PrP [PrP^C]). The prion hypothesis is widely, though not universally, accepted [11,14].

Normal prion proteins (encoded by an autosomal gene on chromosome 20 in humans) are highly conserved across various species including mammals, reptiles, fish, and amphibians [15–18]. In mammals, PrP^C is expressed in neurons and in other cells in smaller amounts, depending on the mammalian species [19]. In different species, PrP^C consists of 231–253 amino acid residues with high α-helix content (approximately 40%) and very little β-pleated-sheet content (approximately 3%). PrP^C is readily soluble in detergent–salt solutions, fully denatured by dilute chaotropic chemicals, and sensitive to digestion with the proteolytic enzyme proteinase K (PK). Although its functions are not understood, PrP^C binds copper and may play some role in cell signaling. Knock-out mice lacking expression of PrP^C have normal behavior and lifespan, so its function is clearly not essential [20]. PrP-knockout mice completely resist TSE infection by any route of exposure [21–23]. Although several aspects of the prion hypothesis remain controversial, it is clear that—at least in mice—prion protein must be expressed both for susceptibility to TSE infection and to develop overt disease.

The abnormal prion proteins, designated here as PrP^{TSE}, are insoluble in detergent–salt solutions and relatively protease-resistant, with higher β-pleated-sheet content (approximately 43%) and lower α-helix content (approximately 30%) than found in PrP^C [10,12,16,24,25]. It is not well understood how PrP^C conversion into PrP^{TSE} occurs; according to the prion hypothesis, the abnormal protein acts as a self-replicating template for the conversion of PrP^C into misfolded PrP^{TSE} [11]. Hosts are unable to dispose of PrP^{TSE} efficiently and, not recognizing the misfolded form of a normal protein as a foreign antigen, mount no protective immune response.

Although data support a role for PrP^{TSE} in the pathogenesis of prion diseases, how it causes disease and what other factors may be necessary are not entirely clear. PrP^{TSE} is a predominant macromolecule in fractions containing a semipurified infectious TSE agent. However, preparations of the infectious agent contain small nucleic acids as well, and cell-free in vitro conversion of PrP^C into PrP^{TSE} has not, thus far, generated infectivity [25,26], although it has been claimed recently in intriguing but unconfirmed reports [27–29]. In subclinical TSE infections, infectivity has been detected in central nervous system (CNS) tissue with no accompanying clinical signs of disease [30–33]. Alternative theories suggest that PrP^{TSE} must interact with other proteins both to replicate and cause disease [26,34–37]. Conversely, the protein may be neurotoxic and accelerate progression of disease but has only a limited capacity self-replication [38] insufficient to transmit true infection by the usual routes, implying the possible existence of another self-replicating infectious molecule [14,39]. Researchers agree that, whether or not PrP^{TSE} comprises the causative self-replicating agent of TSEs, finding of PrP^{TSE} in CNS tissue is generally a reliable indicator of TSE infection [33], though the absence of detectable PrP^{TSE} in tissue does not rule out the presence of infectivity [14,31,39,40].

4.1.2 Transmission of TSEs

Scrapie is the first TSE that was experimentally transmitted from naturally infected sheep to healthy sheep and goats by inoculation of tissue [41]. Scrapie is also the first TSE demonstrated to have contaminated a product—a veterinary vaccine derived from sheep tissue in the 1930s [42]. TSEs have since been transmitted accidentally via contaminated neurosurgical instruments, tissue grafts, injections of contaminated pharmaceuticals, blood transfusions and—most importantly for this chapter—by ingestion of contaminated food and feed. Kuru appears to have been transmitted exclusively by exposure to infected human tissues during cannibalism [43], BSE by contaminated cattle feed [44], and vCJD by human consumption of BSE-contaminated beef products [45], and later by blood transfusions [46–49]. Some TSEs of animals also appear to spread through environmental contamination, either from accidental ingestion or some other unknown means.

Efficiency of TSE transmission between species depends on presence or absence of a species barrier [14]. TSEs have generally been transmitted most readily between animals of the same species or closely related species. Most experimental transmissions of TSEs have involved mice, hamsters, rats, nonhuman primates, and a limited number of ruminants and other species. TSE agents can be adapted to infect hosts of new species, but that has usually required multiple attempts using high doses of infectivity, resulting in only a few successful transmissions after long incubation periods.

Serial passage of infectivity in a new host adapts the agent to more efficient propagation in that species and stabilizes the incubation period, which also depends upon the dose of infectivity and the route of exposure.

4.1.3   TSE Agent Strains

Like other infectious agents, TSE agents exhibit stable differences in biological behavior suggesting strain variations [50]. When TSE agents had been adapted to infect lines of inbred mice, different strains elicited unique syndromes with different constellations of incubation period and the type, severity, and distribution of histopathology in the brain [51]; those characteristics have been maintained on serial passages in mice of the same line and even after passage from mice into a new host species (encoding PrP with a different amino acid sequence) and then back into mice. Most notable has been the effect of TSE agent strain on incubation period—time from inoculation until onset of overt illness. For example, one scrapie strain injected at high dose into mice resulted in TSE after a mean incubation period with a standard error of less than 2%, whereas inoculation of the same dose of infectivity from a different TSE strain into mice of the same genotype resulted in disease with a significantly different mean incubation period that was just as consistent [51]. Therefore, TSE strains have been conveniently distinguished by mean incubation periods after intracranial (IC) inoculation of a high dose, by neuropathological lesion profiles and lesion scores (e.g., semiquantitative intensity of vacuolation in nine different anatomic regions of the brain [52]) in standard lines of inbred mice, and by the presence or absence of amyloid plaques induced in those mice [51]. Experimental evidence indicates that there may be more than 20 strains of scrapie agent. Early studies first suggested that there might be only a single strain of BSE agent, though the recent descriptions of a new bovine amyloidotic spongiform encephalopathy (BASE, see below) having characteristics somewhat different from those of BSE now call that conclusion into question. Though, for many years, animal models have been useful for strain typing, several authorities have proposed that molecular characteristics of PrP^{TSE} (as visualized by Western blotting, sometimes called glycotyping) elicited by a TSE agent might better define strains of agent. PrP glycotypes have been classified both by the molecular mass of PK-treated de-glycosylated PrP^{TSE} (either 19 kDa or 21 kDa, depending on the number of amino acids cleaved from the N-terminus of the molecule by PK) and by the relative abundance of diglycosylated, monoglycosylated, and nonglycosylated forms (resulting from differences in cleavage of the two carbohydrate side chains). Although glycotyping has been especially useful for presumptive identification of BSE-derived strains of agent [53] and has served as a basis to classify clinical variants of CJD [54], recent findings that mixtures of PrP^{TSE} glycotypes are present both in vCJD [55] and other clinical forms of CJD [56]—albeit with one type predominating—suggest that coding for a single unique PrP^{TSE}

glycotype is unlikely to explain TSE strain variation or to define a strain of agent uniquely.

4.1.4   Pathogenesis of TSEs

The portals through which the infectious agents enter and leave the body and pathways by which infection spreads within the body during natural TSEs, particularly after infections by the oral route, are only partially understood. One important pathway involves spread of infectivity from the digestive tract to the lymphoreticular system and then by way of the peripheral nervous system, blood stream, or both to the spinal cord and brain [18]. Direct spread of infection from the digestive tract to the nervous system by way of the autonomic nervous system has also been described [57].

4.1.5   TSE Testing

The "gold-standard" test for a TSE has been detection of infectivity by bioassay—transmitting disease to susceptible animals, originally to animals of the same or closely related species (sheep and goats for scrapie and nonhuman primates for kuru and CJD) and later to conventional rodents and to transgenic mice engineered to express various ruminant PrPs or human PrP. Amounts of infectious agent have generally been defined operationally by determining the dilution of material containing a 50% infectious or lethal dose (ID_{50} or LD_{50}) in each inoculum by a given route of exposure; oral ingestion of infectivity is generally a relatively inefficient route of transmission—about 10^4 times less efficient than intraperitoneal (IP) injection and 10^9 times less efficient than direct IC inoculation, which has generally provided the most sensitive assay [58,59]. Infectivity content can also be roughly estimated based on the linear relationship between the number of LD_{50} injected and the resulting incubation period (time to onset of illness) or time to death, though that dose–response relationship is not linear at very high concentrations of infectivity and near the endpoint dilution.

There is currently no generally accepted feasible antemortem diagnostic test for TSEs in either humans or animals. Antemortem tests for PrP^{TSE} in lymphoid tissues have shown some promise for early diagnosis of some ruminant TSEs (nictitating membrane) [60,61] and for vCJD in humans (tonsil) [62,63]. Brain biopsies are sometimes performed for antemortem diagnosis of humans with dementing illnesses, but are not feasible for animals. Abnormalities in magnetic-resonance images of the midbrain [64,65] and elevations of various spinal fluid proteins (though not PrP [66]) have been useful to discriminate CJD from other encephalopathies of humans, but those methods are not applicable to antemortem diagnosis of TSEs of animals.

Postmortem tests are based on detection of histopathologic changes in brain tissue, or by detection of PrP^{TSE} using immunohistochemical (IHC)

FIGURE 4.2
Western blot of normal PrP (PrP^C) and the protease-resistant form of PrP found in TSEs (PrP^TSE). Detergent-treated extracts of hamster brain tissue were incubated with either the proteolytic enzyme proteinase K (PK) or with plain diluent (No PK). Extracts of normal control (left) and scrapie-infected (right) hamster brain were subjected to electrophoresis in polyacrylamide gel, transferred to a nitrocellulose membrane, incubated with chromagen-labeled antibody to PrP, and then exposed to photographic film. Note that PK treatment completely eliminated all detectable PrP^C from normal brain while leaving PrP^TSE from scrapie-infected brain. The change in electrophoretic mobility of PrP^TSE after PK treatment results from cleavage of part of the amino-terminal end of the protein. (The image was kindly provided by Dr. Igor Bacik and Dr. Olga A. Maximova, FDA.)

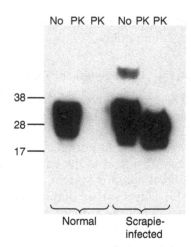

staining (Figure 4.1C), Western blot (Figure 4.2), enzyme-linked immuno-sorbant assay (ELISA), or other immunoassays [16]. In the past, along with bioassays, IHC was considered to be a gold-standard test for confirming diagnosis of a TSE. More recently, a combination of IHC and Western blot has been used to confirm BSE. Several rapid tests, most based on ELISA, are currently licensed for postmortem diagnosis of BSE, though reactive results are usually confirmed by another type of test, such as IHC or Western blot. Rapid tests for TSE may be unreliable early in infection, when PrP^TSE is not yet detectable in brain tissue. Novel tests, like conformation-dependent immunoassay (CDI) [67–70] and protein misfolding cyclical amplification (PMCA) [71,72], are claimed to have greatly increased sensitivity, but this remains to be independently confirmed.

4.2 Bovine Spongiform Encephalopathy

BSE is a TSE of cattle with long incubation periods (from 2 to more than 8 years), most likely acquired by consumption of feed containing an animal product contaminated with the BSE agent [73,74], especially meat-and-bone meal. The U.K. Ministry of Agriculture, Fisheries and Food (MAFF, now renamed the Department for Environment, Food and Rural Affairs [DEFRA]) first recognized BSE as a distinct disease in November 1986 [75]. The clinical signs of BSE include abnormalities in behavior, gait, and posture. Affected cattle usually first show increased apprehension, abnormal reactions to sound and touch, a swaying gait, and other more subtle changes in normal behavior, including separation from the herd while at pasture, disorientation, blank staring, and excessive licking of the nose or flanks. Within weeks after onset of clinical BSE, animals may begin to stumble and fall; and when allowed to progress, the disease typically ends with seizures, coma, and death [75].

The main histopathological indicator of BSE is the finding of spongiform change in brain tissue, most prominent in the obex but also seen in other areas of the brain. The brains of cows with BSE have rarely contained significant numbers of amyloid plaques [76], but diffuse deposits of PrP^{TSE} can usually be demonstrated in the parenchyma of the obex. In cases of atypical BSE, so-called BASE, reported from Italy [16], accumulations of PrP^{TSE} in amyloid plaques were present in cerebral white matter, and pathological changes were not as prominent in the obex as they are in typical BSE. Atypical cases of BSE have also been reported from France, Japan, and the United States. The explanation for such atypical cases is not clear; they might either be unusual manifestations of infection with the original BSE agent or due to infections with new strains of TSE agent arising either from BSE agent after serial passages in bovines or from scrapie agent of small ruminants. It has also been proposed that BASE might result from a de novo spontaneous generation of TSE agent in cattle, a proposal also favored by proponents of the prion hypothesis to explain the origin of sporadic CJD and Nor98-type atypical scrapie.

4.2.1 Origin of BSE

Epidemiological studies have characterized the outbreak of BSE in the United Kingdom as a prolonged extended epidemic arising at various locations, all due to a common original point source, and have suggested that feed contaminated by a TSE agent—likely during the 1970s—probably started the outbreak [77]. Although the origin of BSE may never be known with certainty, one popular theory suggests that contaminated cattle feed containing rendered material from sheep with scrapie was the probable culprit. Another theory holds that—as postulated for BASE—BSE arose spontaneously in cattle in the United Kingdom. Whatever the origin of BSE, it is widely acknowledged that infection subsequently spread via BSE-contaminated bovine materials rendered into meat-and-bone meal added to the feed of cattle [78] before the United Kingdom banned that practice in 1988 [73], first for the feeding of ruminants and later for all farmed animals.

Since BSE was first identified, over 186,000 cattle have been diagnosed with the disease in the United Kingdom [79], though estimates put the probable total number of cases there between 1 million and 3 million [80]. The precautionary slaughter of millions of British cows and increasingly stringent prohibitions on animal feeding practices appear to have markedly slowed the epidemic in the United Kingdom, but have not yet eradicated BSE. In 1992 (the peak year of the epidemic), more than 36,000 cases of BSE were confirmed in the United Kingdom; in 2005, 225 confirmed cases of BSE were reported by United Kingdom authorities (Figure 4.3) [79].

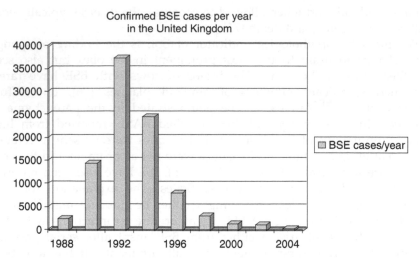

FIGURE 4.3
Confirmed BSE cases per year in the United Kingdom.

The measures used to control BSE in the United Kingdom failed to prevent its spread to cattle in other countries importing BSE-infected cattle, beef products, and animal feed or feed additives [73]. In addition to the United Kingdom, BSE has been reported in native-born cattle in 25 other countries: Austria, Belgium, Canada, Croatia, the Czech Republic, Denmark, Finland, France, Germany, Greece, Israel, Italy, Japan, Liechtenstein, Luxembourg, the Netherlands, Poland, Portugal, the Republic of Ireland, Slovakia, Slovenia, Spain, Sweden, Switzerland, and the United States (Table 4.1) [79].

The epidemiology of BSE in the United Kingdom and a limited number of experimental studies suggest that there has been little if any cow-to-calf or horizontal (cow-to-cow) transmission of BSE [81,82]. The within-herd incidence of BSE during the height of the epidemic in the United Kingdom never exceeded 2.7% [79].

4.2.2 Distribution of Infectivity in Tissues of Cattle after Infection with BSE Agent

After BSE was recognized to be zoonotic—the only TSE recognized to pass from animals to humans—considerable work began to study infectivity in various bovine tissues in order to improve the understanding of the risk to humans [5–9,13]. Three pathogenesis studies have been initiated in which cattle tissues were assayed for infectivity by IC inoculation of mice or calves with suspensions of tissues from cattle that were fed the BSE agent. Tissue infectivity can be categorized as high infectivity, lower infectivity, and no infectivity detected (Tables 4.2 through 4.5) [13]. High-infectivity tissues are

TABLE 4.1

Incidence of BSE—Indigenous Cases

Country	1985–1989	1990–1994	1995–1999	2000	2001	2002	2003	2004	2005	Total
United Kingdom	10,188	136,574	32,640	1,443	1,202	1,144	425	343	225	184,939
Ireland	10	78	342	149	246	333	183	126	69	1,539
France		10	69	161	274	239	137	54	18	962
Portugal		12	362	149	110	86	133	92	37	981
Switzerland		118	215	33	42	24	21	3	3	459
Belgium			10	9	46	38	15	11	2	131
Netherlands			6	2	20	24	19	6	...	77
Liechtenstein			2	0	0	0	0	0	...	2
Luxembourg			1	0	0	1	0	0	1	3
Germany				7	125	106	54	65	...	357
Spain				2	82	127	167	137	75	590
Denmark				1	6	3	2	1	...	13
Italy					48	38	29	7	7	129
Slovakia					5	6	2	7	...	20
Japan					3	2	4	5	7	20
Czech Republic				2	2	4	7	8	23	
Slovenia					1	1	1	2	1	7
Austria					1	0	0	0	1	2
Finland					1	0	0	...		1
Greece					1	0	0	0	...	1
Poland						4	5	11	19	40
Israel							1	0	0	1
Canada							2	1	1	4
United States								1	1	4

Note: Table constructed from data obtained at http://www.oie.int.

... No data available.

TABLE 4.2

Key to Entries in Tables 4.3 through 4.5
(Summary of Distribution of Infectivity
and PrP^{TSE} in Tissues: vCJD, Other
Human TSEs, BSE, and Scrapie)

+	Infectivity or PrP^{TSE} detected
−	No detectable infectivity or PrP^{TSE}
NT	Not tested
NA	Not applicable
( )	Limited or preliminary data
?	Controversial results

Source: Adapted from World Health Organization Guidelines on Tissue Infectivity Distribution in Transmissible Spongiform Encephalopathies, Proceedings of a Consultation Convened by WHO, Geneva 14–16 September 2005, published 2006, and accessed at http://www.who.int/ bloodproducts/ TSEREPORT-LoRes.pdf

CNS tissues that contain high titers of infectivity in the clinical phases of all TSEs and certain other tissues anatomically associated with these CNS tissues. Lower infectivity tissues harbor infectivity or PrP^{TSE} in at least one

TABLE 4.3

High-Infectivity Tissues in TSEs. CNS Tissues and Certain Tissues Anatomically Associated with CNS Having High Titers of Infectivity

	Human TSEs				Cattle		Sheep and Goats	
	vCJD		Other TSEs		BSE		Scrapie	
Tissues	Infectivity	PrP^{TSE}	Infectivity	PrP^{TSE}	Infectivity	PrP^{TSE}	Infectivity	PrP^{TSE}
Brain	+	+	+	+	+	+	+	+
Spinal cord	+	+	+	+	+	+	+	+
Retina	NT	+	+	+	+	NT	NT	+
Optic nerve	NT	+	NT	+	+	NT	NT	+
Spinal ganglia	+	+	NT	+	+	NT	NT	+
Trigeminal ganglia	+	+	NT	+	+	NT	NT	+
Pituitary gland	NT	+	+	+	−	NT	+	NT
Duramater	NT	−	+	−	NT	NT	NT	NT

Source: Adapted from World Health Organization Guidelines on Tissue Infectivity Distribution in Transmissible Spongiform Encephalopathies, Proceedings of a Consultation Convened by WHO, Geneva 14–16 September 2005, published 2006, and accessed at http://www.who.int/bloodproducts/TSEREPORT-LoRes.pdf

TABLE 4.4

Lower-Infectivity Tissues in TSEs. Peripheral Tissues Testing Positive for Infectivity and PrP^{TSE} in at Least One Form of TSE

Tissues	Human TSEs				Cattle		Sheep and Goats	
	vCJD		Other TSEs		BSE		Scrapie	
	Infectivity	PrP^{TSE}	Infectivity	PrP^{TSE}	Infectivity	PrP^{TSE}	Infectivity	PrP^{TSE}
Peripheral nervous system								
Peripheral nerves	+	+	(-)	+	+	+	+	+
Enteric plexuses	NT	+	NT	(-)	NT	+	NT	+
Lymphoreticular tissues								
Spleen	+	+	+	+	-	-	+	+
Lymph nodes	+	+	+	-	-	-	+	+
Tonsil	+	+	NT	-	+	-	+	+
Nictitating membrane	NA	NA	NA	NA	+	-	NT	+
Thymus	NT	+	NT	-	-	NT	+	NT
Alimentary tract								
Esophagus	NT	-	NT	-	-	NT	NT	+
Fore-stomach (ruminants only)	NA	NA	NA	NA	-	NT	NT	+
Stomach/abomasum	NT	-	NT	NT	-	NT	NT	+
Duodenum	NT	-	NT	NT	-	NT	NT	+
Jejunum	NT	+	NT	-	-	NT	NT	+
Ileum	NT	+	NT	-	+	+	+	+
Appendix	-	+	NT	-	NA	NA	NA	NA
Large intestine	+	+	NT	-	-	NT	+	+
Reproductive tissues								
Placenta	NT	-	(-)	-	-	NT	+	+
Other tissues								
Lung	NT	-	+	-	-	NT	-	-
Liver	NT	-	+	-	-	NT	+	NT
Kidney	NT	-	+	-	-	-	-	-
Adrenal	NT	+	-	-	NT	NT	+	NT
Pancreas	NT	-	NT	-	-	NT	+	NT
Bone marrow	-	-	(-)	-	(+)	NT	+	NT
Skeletal muscle	NT	+	(-)	+	(+)	NT	-	-
Tongue	NT	-	NT	-	-	NT	NT	+
Blood vessels	NT	+	NT	+	-	NT	NT	+
Nasal mucosa	NT	NT	NT	+	-	NT	+	+
Salivary gland	NT	-	NT	NT	-	NT	+	NT
Cornea	NT	-	+	-	NT	NT	NT	NT
Body fluids								
CSF	-	-	+	-	-	NT	+	NT
Blood	+	?	-	?	-	?	+	?

Source: Adapted from World Health Organization Guidelines on Tissue Infectivity Distribution in Transmissible Spongiform Encephalopathies, Proceedings of a Consultation Convened by WHO, Geneva 14–16 September 2005, published 2006, and accessed at http://www.who.int/bloodproducts/TSEREPORT-LoRes.pdf

type of TSE. Finally, some tissues contain no infectivity detectable by current assay techniques in any of the recognized TSEs.

The first pathogenesis study of BSE was started in the United Kingdom by the Veterinary Laboratory Administration (VLA) in 1991 [6,7]. Thirty calves were each dosed orally with 100 g of BSE-contaminated brain containing $10^{3.5}$ IC LD_{50} units/g by infectivity titration in RIII mice. (A comparative titration of another BSE-infected suspension showed that RIII mice were about 500-fold less sensitive than calves to infection by the IC route, and each of five cattle inoculated IC with samples from this same brain pool developed BSE between 23 and 30 months later, confirming that the material selected for the first oral dosing experiment contained a substantial amount

TABLE 4.5

Tissues with No Infectivity Detected in TSEs. Tissues Examined for Infectivity and PrP^{TSE} in Any TSE with Negative Results

| | Human TSEs | | | | Cattle | | Sheep and Goats | |
| | vCJD | | Other TSEs | | BSE | | Scrapie | |
Tissues	Infectivity	PrP^{TSE}	Infectivity	PrP^{TSE}	Infectivity	PrP^{TSE}	Infectivity	PrP^{TSE}
Reproductive tissues								
Testis	NT	–	(-)	–	–	NT	–	NT
Prostate/epididymis/seminal vesicle	NT	–	(-)	–	–	NT	–	NT
Semen	NT	–	(-)	–	–	NT	NT	NT
Ovary	NT	–	NT	–	–	NT	–	NT
Uterus (non-gravid)	NT	–	NT	–	–	NT	–	NT
Placenta fluids	NT	NT	(-)	NT	–	NT	NT	NT
Fetus	NT	NT	NT	NT	–	NT	–	–
Embryos	NT	NT	NT	NT	–	NT	?	NT
Musculo-skeletal tissues								
Bone	NT	NT	NT	NT	–	NT	NT	NT
Heart/pericardium	NT	–	–	–	–	NT	–	NT
Tendon	NT	NT	NT	NT	–	NT	NT	NT
Other tissues								
Gingival tissue	NT	–	–	–	NT	NT	NT	NT
Dental pulp	NT	–	NT	–	NT	NT	NT	NT
Trachea	NT	–	NT	–	–	NT	NT	NT
Skin	NT	–	NT	–	–	NT	–	NT
Adipose tissue	NT	–	(-)	–	–	NT	NT	NT
Thyroid gland	NT	–	(-)	–	NT	NT	–	NT
Mammary gland/udder	NT	NT	NT	NT	–	NT	–	NT
Body fluids, secretions, and excretions								
Milk	NT	NT	(-)	NT	–	–	–	NT
Colostrum	NT	NT	(-)	NT	(-)	–	–	NT
Cord blood	NT	NT	(-)	NT	(-)	NT	NT	NT
Saliva	NT	–	–	NT	NT	NT	–	NT
Sweat	NT	NT	–	NT	NT	NT	NT	NT
Tears	NT	NT	–	NT	NT	NT	NT	NT
Nasal mucus	NT	–	–	NT	NT	NT	NT	NT
Bile	NT	NT	NT	NT	NT	NT	NT	NT
Urine	NT	NT	–	–	–	NT	NT	NT
Feces	NT	NT	–	NT	–	NT	–	NT

Source: Adapted from World Health Organization Guidelines on Tissue Infectivity Distribution in Transmissible Spongiform Encephalopathies, Proceedings of a Consultation Convened by WHO, Geneva 14–16 September 2005, published 2006, and accessed at http://www.who.int/bloodproducts/TSEREPORT-LoRes.pdf

of BSE agent.) Several of the orally dosed animals were sequentially killed at intervals from 2 months through 40 months after exposure, and a wide variety of their tissues were collected for infectivity assays in RIII or C57Bl mice—two inbred lines of conventional mice susceptible to BSE infection. (The limit of detection of infectivity by the cattle assay has been approximately 10 cattle IC LD$_{50}$ units or 10$^{3.7}$ mouse IC + IP LD$_{50}$ units/g.) Selected tissues from cattle in the first VLA study were later inoculated IC into calves to increase the sensitivity of detecting infectivity. The earliest detection of infectivity in the first VLA study was in a pool of distal ileum from three animals 6 months postexposure; PrP^{TSE} was detected in Peyer's patches at the same time. At 32 months, a spinal cord sample contained infectivity. CNS tissues tested (brain, spinal cord, dorsal root ganglia [clusters of nerve cells lying within bone of the vertebral column and attached to spinal cord] and trigeminal ganglia [similar clusters of nerve cells connected to brain and close to the skull surface]) from animals killed from 32 to 40 months after exposure contained the BSE agent, months before anticipated onset of clinical of illness. (Although no infectivity was detected in neural tissues collected 26 months after dosing, the experimental design permits no estimate of when during the interval between 26 and 32 months infectivity might have first appeared in the CNS.)

A second experimental oral exposure pathogenesis study was initiated by the United Kingdom VLA in 1997. Three groups of 100 cattle were either dosed with 100 g or 1 g of BSE-infected brain or were left undosed as controls. As in the first study, small numbers of animals were sequentially killed at 3 month intervals starting 3 months after exposure through more than 66 months. A preliminary report of this study described infectivity in tonsils collected 10 months after dosing; a more detailed report on this study is forthcoming.

A third experimental BSE pathogenesis study began at the end of 2002 in Germany. BSE-infected brain stem material provided by the United Kingdom VLA was used to orally dose 56 calves with 100 g, while 18 controls received the same dose of normal brain. Samples of blood, cerebrospinal fluid (CSF), and urine have been collected from the animals at intervals of 2–4 months and stored. Serial kills of four BSE-exposed cows and one control take place every 4 months, and more than 150 tissues and fluids from each necropsy are to be studied. In addition to IHC and Western blots to detect PrP^{TSE} in the tissues, infectivity is being assayed by injection of transgenic mice overexpressing bovine PrP^C [Tgbov mice] known to be very sensitive to the BSE agent. Their relative sensitivity was estimated by comparing results of infectivity titrations with the same reference BSE brain stem pool assayed in Tgbov mice and RIII conventional mice: $10^{7.7}$ LD_{50} in Tgbov mice versus only $10^{3.3}$ in the RIII mice. Tgbov mice seemed to be slightly more sensitive than cattle in detecting the BSE agent [83].

Limitations of all three pathogenesis studies result from the relatively small number of cattle originally exposed to the BSE agent (because of logistical difficulties in working with cattle and limited resources, experiments using larger numbers of calves were not feasible). There are also limitations imposed by tissue sampling: infectivity might not be uniformly distributed through tissues of interest; only limited volumes of tissue can be injected IC into animals, reducing the sensitivity of bioassays for detecting infectivity; and the pooling of tissues from several animals, though increases the chances of detecting inconsistent infections, further decreases assay sensitivity because of dilution.

There also remains a concern that the experimental pathogenesis studies might not faithfully mimic natural BSE-infections of cattle—perhaps because the experimental studies have administered unrealistically large doses of infectivity. In contrast to results of the experimental BSE pathogenesis studies, PrP^{TSE} has never been detected in the ileum of bovines with natural cases of BSE. One pool of lymph nodes and one pool of spleen from five BSE cases were negative on assay in mice and cattle, implying a maximum infectivity content less than 0.1 IC LD_{50} units/g in cattle. One pool of tonsils from three calves was positive 10 months after dosing (one of five assay cattle inoculated IC with the pooled tonsils developed BSE after 45 months on test). A pool of nictitating membrane (rich in lymphoid tissue) from 10 clinically suspect cases of BSE (nine subsequently confirmed) was positive (incubation period 31 months) implying an approximate infectivity titer between 10 and 100 $\log_{10}$ IC LD_{50} units/g for cattle [13]. Assays in RIII mice for infectivity in naturally infected clinical BSE cases found infectivity only in CNS, including brain, spinal cord, and retina [13,84].

The same group of investigators conducting the third experimental pathogenesis study of BSE recently reported an important investigation of the ninth naturally acquired German BSE case, assaying tissues for infectivity by injections of both conventional RIII mice and Tgbov mice. No infectivity was detected in spleen or lymph nodes of this BSE case, and all reproductive tissues of this animal, which was in late pregnancy, were also free of detectable infectivity. However, infectivity was detected in the Peyer's patches of the distal ileum by assay in Tgbov mice after a very long mean incubation period (540 days) while the RIII mice injected with the same material remained negative even after a mouse-to-mouse subpassage of brain material. Infectivity was also found in peripheral nerves (sciatic and facial but not radial nerve) in Tgbov mice—also after long incubation times of 438 and 538 days. It is interesting to note that a single Tgbov mouse among a total of 10 inoculated with semitendinosus muscle was positive after an incubation period of 520 days [83]; that finding, if confirmed, is potentially important because it represents the reported detection of BSE agent in a bovine muscle [85]. However, contamination of the sample with neural tissue remains a possible alternative explanation for the finding. Experiments feeding muscle from BSE-infected cattle have failed to transmit infectivity [86].

Infectivity has also been detected in blood and blood components from infected mice and hamsters [87]. Though blood from cattle naturally infected with BSE has not transmitted infectivity to mice, whole blood taken from a sheep experimentally infected with BSE and whole blood from a sheep naturally infected with scrapie transmitted disease when large volumes were transfused into sheep [88–90]. Other studies on the potential for muscle and blood to transmit infection are ongoing.

Several studies have been conducted to determine the potential for bovine milk and milk products to transmit BSE infectivity. In one experiment, milk was collected from cows showing signs of BSE and then was either fed to or inoculated into the brains of mice. The mice were then observed for almost 2 years for signs of neurological disease. None of the mice exposed to milk from BSE-infected cows by either route developed encephalopathy or other signs of TSE [91]. However, those studies did not consider the species barrier between conventional mice and cattle (described above) that reduces sensitivity of the BSE infectivity assay, which might warrant repeating with Tg mice more susceptible to BSE agent. However, in later studies, calves allowed to suckle BSE-infected cows failed to get BSE despite the absence of a species barrier [92,93], providing reassurance that milk is not likely to provide an efficient vector for transmitting infection. The overall pattern of dramatic decline in BSE cases in the United Kingdom after 1992 also seems inconsistent with transmission of BSE from cows to calves by milk.

The Scientific Steering Committee of the European Union has reported on the proportion of total infectivity in various tissues [94]. The Committee estimates that, in an animal with clinical disease, approximately 64% of the infectivity is in the brain, 26% in the spinal cord, 4% in the dorsal root ganglia, 2.5% in the trigeminal ganglia, and 3% in the distal ileum. In 2003, another review reported generally similar estimates of infectivity (i.e., 60.2% in brain, 24.1% in the spinal cord, 3.6% in the dorsal root ganglia, 2.4% in the trigeminal ganglia, and 9.6% in the distal ileum) [95].

Unlike experimental studies, it is not possible to determine distribution of infectivity during incubation periods of natural BSE, because healthy infected cattle cannot be identified.

Cases of atypical BSE (or BASE) have been reported among the animals screened positive with systematic testing of cattle over 30 months of age in Europe: such cases have been described in Italy, France, the Netherlands, Denmark, Germany, Japan, and the United States [96,97]. BASE is said to display a specific pattern of distribution of PrP^{TSE} accumulation, mainly in frontal cortex instead of obex as in typical cases. In both Europe and the United States, animals with atypical BSE were much older than those with typical BSE, whereas the Japanese BASE cases were, in very young asymptomatic animals (20 and 23 months old), detected by universal rapid tests of obex tissues collected from clinically healthy cattle at the slaughterhouse. An agent has recently been transmitted to mice from the tissue of a cow with BASE [98], but the pathogenesis of BASE—if different from typical BSE—remains unknown.

4.2.3 Age of Cattle and Clinical Disease

Clinical cases of BSE in cattle younger than 30 months of age are relatively rare. According to the U.K. DEFRA, among cattle born in the United Kingdom with highest incidence of BSE infection (i.e., those born in 1987–1988, 5 years before the peak in confirmed cases), cattle under 3 years old represented less than 0.16% of BSE cases (61 of 39,140 cattle with BSE) [79]. Another report, evaluating selected herds with animals of known ages in the first 6 months of 1989 and 1990, found that BSE incidence in 2 year old cattle (0.04% in 1989 and 0.05% in 1990) was approximately 15-fold lower than in 3 year old cattle (0.56% in 1989 and 0.86% in 1990), and 45-fold to 75-fold lower than the incidence in 4 year old cattle (2.83% in 1989 and 2.76% in 1990) [44]. Two year old cattle with BSE represented only about 0.5% of all BSE cases in the selected herds during those 6 month periods. The incidence of BSE in 2 year old cattle (0.01%) decreased considerably in 1991, presumably because they were born after the United Kingdom implemented prohibition for meat-and-bone meal in cattle feed in 1988.

Infectivity has been detected in CNS just before expected onset of clinical BSE in cattle, usually at age 30 months or older [13], although, as noted above, limitations in study design leave uncertainties regarding the earliest time at which the brain might have become infectious. On the basis of experimental rather than naturally occurring cases, palatine tonsils of infected calves harbored small amounts of infectivity 10 months postexposure, and distal ileum of the small intestine as early as 6 months postexposure.

4.2.4 Slaughter Techniques and Potential for Contamination of Meat with BSE Agent

Certain methods used to stun cattle (render them unconscious before slaughter) may force visible pieces of brain tissue into the circulatory system. The frequency with which fragments of CNS tissue might enter the circulatory system of stunned cattle and the size of fragments depended on the method of stunning used. When air-injection pneumatic stunners were used, CNS tissue fragments were seen in the right ventricle of the heart and in the pulmonary artery and identified microscopically in the jugular vein [99–102]. The European Commission's Scientific Steering Committee (SSC) concluded that any type of penetrative stunning that damages the brain can disseminate CNS fragments into the blood of the great veins, right-heart chambers, pulmonary arteries, and lungs [103]. The SSC concluded that the risk of contaminating other tissues with CNS was negligible unless small particles entered the systemic circulation. Should that happen, any risk to consumers from contamination of tissues and organs with CNS tissue would depend on the level of BSE infectivity in the brain of the stunned animal.

4.2.5 BSE in Species Other Than Cattle

In addition to cattle, BSE has been detected in other species. BSE has occurred naturally in bison, eland, gemsbok, kudu, nyala, oryx (all in the same family Bovidae as domestic cattle), exotic felines and domestic cats [3], and in at least one goat. Naturally acquired BSE has not been reported in sheep, although sheep have been experimentally infected with BSE agent both by feeding and injection. In all these cases, consumption of feed contaminated with the BSE agent was the probable source of infection. The diagnosis of BSE in a goat in January 2005 was of particular concern because it was the first case of naturally acquired BSE described in a small ruminant [16]. (An earlier goat that might also have been naturally infected by BSE was reported later [104,105].) Strain typing by lesion profile in mice experimentally inoculated with brain suspension confirmed that the sick goat had been infected with BSE agent rather than with scrapie or some other atypical TSE. The detection of BSE in a goat indicates that there might be some low prevalence of infection in small ruminants in Europe, and sheep and goats were both exposed to the same kind of contaminated feed believed to have caused BSE in cattle. There has been an early concern that both sheep and goats might harbor a BSE infection clinically and histopathologically indistinguishable from scrapie; however, there is no evidence for a significant epidemic of BSE with scrapie-like manifestations in either sheep or goats, because annual cases of scrapie diagnosed in Europe have not increased since the inception of the BSE epidemic.

4.2.6 Creutzfeldt–Jakob Disease, Variant Creutzfeldt–Jakob Disease, and Other TSEs of Humans

Sporadic CJD (sCJD) affects humans throughout the world with an annual incidence of approximately one case per million population [11]. The highest death rates from sCJD in the United States and the United Kingdom occur in individuals between the ages of 60 and 70 years [106]. Death generally occurs less than a year after onset of progressive neurological deterioration [11]. Typical early symptoms of sCJD include changes in sleeping and eating patterns, and inappropriate behavior and confusion, eventually progressing to frank dementia, akinetic mutism and, finally, stupor or coma. Many cases also show early loss of coordination, ataxia; sCJD and most other forms of CJD are accompanied by periodic myoclonic spasms. All forms of CJD are invariably fatal [106]. The origin of sCJD is not understood; genetic susceptibility must play some role, because persons homozygous for methionine at codon 129 of the prion-protein-encoding gene are greatly overrepresented [11], though persons with other genotypes are not completely spared the disease.

In April 1996, British scientists reported a previously unrecognized new variant of CJD (vCJD) in 10 young patients having symptoms somewhat different from those of sporadic CJD [45,107]. All cases of vCJD had histopathologic evidence of spongiform changes in the brain but also showed formation of unique "florid" plaques (flower-like cores of amyloid protein surrounded by halos of vacuoles) not typical of other forms of CJD [11]. Clinically, vCJD usually begins with psychiatric changes, such as depression, anxiety, nightmares, or hallucinations. These symptoms are followed by memory impairment, progressing to dementia in the late stages of illness. The clinical course may last up to 2 years or even longer before death occurs [108].

The unique epidemiology (geographic distribution concentrated in United Kingdom and France), clinical presentation (unusually young age, psychiatric complaints at onset), and histopathological features (florid plaques) of vCJD suggested almost immediately that it was probably a new TSE attributable to human infection with BSE agent [63,109–111]. Resemblance of TSE lesion profiles in mice inoculated with suspensions of brain tissues from patients with vCJD to those in mice inoculated with suspensions from cattle with BSE [112] supported that inference, as did the observation that PrP^{TSE} extracted from both sources shared an unusual electrophoretic pattern. Monkeys (genetically close to humans) inoculated with samples of brain from BSE-infected cattle developed a TSE histopathologically very similar to vCJD in humans [113]. Most authorities are persuaded that vCJD in humans is an infection caused by consumption of cattle products contaminated with the BSE agent [94,106,114]. Attempts to match consumption of particular diets in the United Kingdom with development of vCJD have been only partially informative [115–117]. They reported suggestive but inconclusive evidence of differences observed in consumption of products containing ground beef and mechanically recovered meat (including head meat) between vCJD cases and controls in Britain.

As of November 2006, CDC reported that a total of 200 patients had been diagnosed with vCJD worldwide, including 164 in United Kingdom, 21 in France, 4 in the Republic of Ireland, 3 in the USA, 2 in the Netherlands, and 1 each in Canada, Italy, Japan, Portugal, Saudi Arabia, and Spain. All except 10 of the 200 reported vCJD patients had resided either in the United Kingdom (170 cases) or in France (20 cases) for more than 6 months during the period 1980–1996, peak of the large United Kingdom BSE outbreak. All four North American vCJD cases were probably infected with the BSE agent while living abroad; the Canadian case and two of the United States cases were longtime residents of United Kingdom, while the most recent United States case was in a person who had, except for relatively short periods of travel, lived in Saudi Arabia until 2005 [19,118]. The Japanese case is of special interest, affecting a person who spent less than 1 month in the United Kingdom 12 years before onset of illness, suggestive of a possible point exposure to BSE agent. Based on probable incubation periods for vCJD in humans that might range from 5 to more than 20 years, epidemiological models have projected that many more (600 to more than 3000) cases of vCJD caused by consumption of BSE-contaminated cattle products might be expected to occur in the United Kingdom in the future [112,119]. A recent survey of archived appendix samples in the United Kingdom using IHC staining for PrP^{TSE} suggested that prevalence might be even greater [120,121]. In recent years, the number of new vCJD cases detected each year has declined in the United Kingdom but has not yet declined in France [118]. To date, all diagnosed cases of vCJD have occurred in persons homozygous for the gene encoding methionine at codon 129 of the PrP-encoding gene—a genotype overrepresented in cases of other forms of CJD as well. However, the finding of PrP^{TSE} in lymphoid tissues of three United Kingdom residents with other PrP genotypes suggests that all persons must be considered potentially susceptible to infection with the BSE agent and that the possibility of a later "second wave" of vCJD cases cannot be dismissed.

The oral infectious dose of BSE-contaminated material for humans is not known. Despite widespread exposure of the British population to BSE-contaminated meat products, only a very small percentage of the exposed population has been diagnosed with vCJD to date. However, experiments indicate that the oral infectious dose for cattle is very low. Seven of 10 calves fed 1 g samples of infected brain came down with BSE. Six years after oral consumption of even lower doses of brain material, 3 of 15 calves fed 0.1 gram, 1 of 15 calves fed 0.01 gram, and 1 of 15 calves fed 0.001 gram (1 mg) brain samples had already developed the disease. This experiment is on-going [122]. It has been speculated that, because of a human–bovine species barrier, 10–10,000 times more BSE-infected material might be needed to transmit disease to humans, although direct confirmation of that assumption is not possible.

4.2.7 BSE Agent in the Food Supply

Since the route of oral infection in humans is not well understood and the infectious dose is unknown, it has been considered prudent policy worldwide to limit exposure of the human population to material containing the BSE agent. This has been accomplished primarily by attempting to determine BSE prevalence through surveillance of cattle, prohibiting certain ruminant feeding practices and slaughter techniques, controlling imports of ruminants and ruminant-derived products, and removing the highest-risk tissues from the food supply.

Foods that present a risk of contamination with the BSE agent are primarily those that might contain CNS tissue or other potentially infectious tissue. In addition to brains and spinal cords themselves (occasionally consumed intact as food), other foods that may contain CNS include mechanically deboned meat, bone-derived gelatin, dietary supplements containing organs or organ extracts, natural sausage casings made from bovine intestine, and rendered products such as protein meals for animal feed and tallow for food and feed. Other than certain processing for gelatin and tallow derivative production mentioned later, there is very little information available on the ability of food processing methods to destroy the BSE agent in contaminated foods.

4.2.7.1 International Recommendations on BSE

4.2.7.1.1 World Health Organization

The World Health Organization (WHO) is the United Nations specialized agency for health with the objective of the attainment by all peoples with the highest possible level of health. Since 1991, the WHO has convened 11 scientific consultations on TSE issues and offered a number of published recommendations on BSE. The WHO recommends that all countries prohibit the use of most ruminant-derived materials in ruminant feed and exclude tissues that are likely to contain the BSE agent from any animal feed or human food.

4.2.7.1.2   World Organization for Animal Health

The World Organization for Animal Health (acronym OIE for previous name Office International des Epizooties) is an international standards setting body that, among other things, develops science-based recommendations to guide decision makers in ensuring the safety of food of animal origin. OIE is a sister organization to the Codex Alimentarius Commission, an international intergovernmental body that develops science-based food safety and commodity standards, guidelines, and recommendations. Codex has not developed specific recommendations on BSE, in part because the OIE recommendations for BSE were intended to protect human health as well as animal health. OIE develops recommendations in the Terrestrial Animal Health Code [123]. The code includes chapter 2.3.13 on BSE with recommendations intended to manage the human and animal health risks associated with the presence of the BSE agent in cattle. The following sections highlight the 2006 BSE recommendations in the code; more recent versions of the code may be available at http://www.oie.int.

4.2.7.1.2.1   Risk Assessment   The OIE recommends that the BSE risk status of the cattle population of a country be determined based on a risk assessment identifying all potential factors for BSE occurrence and their historical perspective. Factors affecting the potential occurrence of BSE include (1) the presence or absence of animal TSE agents in a country and, if present, their prevalence based on the outcome of surveillance, (2) use of meat-and-bone meal from the indigenous ruminant population, (3) use of imported meat-and-bone meal, (4) imported live animals, (5) imported animal feeds and feed ingredients, (6) other imported products of ruminant origin intended for human consumption that might have contained certain tissues and might have been fed to cattle, and (7) other imported products of ruminant origin used in live cattle. If any of these factors is present, OIE recommends that the likelihood of exposure of cattle to the BSE agent be assessed. In addition to a risk assessment, OIE recommends that educational programs be implemented for veterinarians, farmers, and other workers to encourage reporting of suspected cases of BSE; the compulsory notification and investigation of all cattle showing clinical signs consistent with BSE; and, within the framework of a BSE surveillance and monitoring system, the examination of brain and other tissues collected from suspect animals.

4.2.7.1.2.2   BSE Risk Status   Based on the results of the risk assessment and ongoing surveillance appropriate for the size of the cattle population, OIE categorizes a country as having negligible BSE risk if the country has reported no BSE or only reported BSE in imported animals or if the last indigenous case of BSE was reported more than 11 years ago; a ban on feeding ruminant-derived meat-and-bone meal has been enforced for at least 8 years; and the country has had requirements for compulsory notification and investigation of BSE cases, has had educational programs in place, and has required the obligatory examination of brain or other tissues from a surveillance program for at least 7 years.

Based on the results of the risk assessment and ongoing surveillance program appropriate for the size of the cattle population, OIE categorizes a country as having controlled BSE risk if the country has reported no BSE or one or more cases of BSE in an imported animal or indigenous cases of BSE; has a ban on feeding ruminant-derived meat-and-bone meal that has been enforced for less than 8 years, and has requirements for compulsory notification and investigation of BSE cases; and has educational programs in place, and has requirements for the obligatory examination of brain or other tissues from a surveillance program that have been complied with for less than 7 years. OIE categorizes a country as having an undetermined BSE risk if the country has not been demonstrated to meet the requirements for a BSE lower-risk category.

4.2.7.1.2.3 Recommended Trade Restrictions Based on BSE Risk OIE recommends that certain commodities be freely traded regardless of the country of origin. These products include the following:

- Milk and milk products
- Gelatin and collagen derived from hides and skins
- Protein-free tallow (containing a maximum level of insoluble impurities of 0.15% by weight) and derivatives made from this tallow
- Dicalcium phosphate
- Deboned skeletal muscle meat (excluding mechanically separated meat) from cattle 30 months of age or less, which were not subjected to a stunning process, prior to slaughter, with a device injecting compressed air or gas into the cranial cavity, or subjected to a pithing process; which were subject to antemortem and postmortem inspections and were not suspect or confirmed BSE cases; and which have been prepared in a manner to avoid contamination with high-risk tissues
- Blood and blood by-products from cattle that were not subjected to a stunning process, prior to slaughter, with a device injecting compressed air or gas into the cranial cavity, or to a pithing process

For all cattle-derived commodities not listed above, the OIE recommends that trade depend on the BSE risk status of the country of origin.

4.2.7.1.2.4 Trade in Cattle For trade in cattle from negligible-risk countries, documentation is recommended indicating that the country has in place and enforces requirements for compulsory notification and investigation of BSE cases, educational programs, and the examination of brain or other tissues from a surveillance program.

For trade in cattle from controlled-risk countries, documentation is recommended indicating that the country has in place and enforces requirements for compulsory notification and investigation of BSE cases, educational programs, and the examination of brain or other tissues from a surveillance program; that the cattle selected for export are identified by a permanent identifier that allows tracing of the animal; and, in case of a country with an indigenous case of BSE, that cattle selected for export were born after the date on which a ban on feeding ruminant-derived meat-and-bone meal was effectively enforced.

For trade in cattle from undetermined-risk countries, documentation is recommended indicating that the country has an effectively enforced ban on feeding ruminant-derived meat-and-bone meal and that cattle selected for export were born at least 2 years after implementation of the ban; that any BSE cases in the country are identified, slaughtered, and the carcasses completely destroyed; and that cattle selected for export are identified by a permanent identifier that allows tracing of the animal.

4.2.7.1.2.5 Trade in Fresh Meat and Meat Products   For trade in fresh meat and meat products from negligible-risk countries, documentation is recommended indicating that the country enforces requirements for compulsory notification and investigation of BSE cases, educational programs, and the examination of brain or other tissues from a surveillance program. The document should also indicate that all fresh meat and meat products for export are sourced from cattle that undergo antemortem and postmortem inspections.

For trade in fresh meat and meat products from controlled-risk countries, documentation is recommended indicating that the country enforces requirements for compulsory notification and investigation of BSE cases, educational programs, and the examination of brain or other tissues from a surveillance program. The document should also indicate that all fresh meat and meat products for export are sourced from cattle that undergo antemortem and postmortem inspection and were not subjected to a stunning process, prior to slaughter, with a device injecting compressed air or gas into the cranial cavity, or subjected to a pithing process. Finally, the document should indicate that the exported meat and meat products do not contain and were not contaminated by

- mechanically separated meat;
- tonsils and distal ileum of the small intestine and products derived from them from cattle of any age; and
- brains, eyes, spinal cord, skull, vertebral column, and products derived from them from cattle over 30 months of age.

For trade in fresh meat and meat products from undetermined-risk countries, documentation is recommended indicating that the cattle from which the products were derived were not suspect or confirmed BSE cases, were not fed meat-and-bone meal, were subject to antemortem and postmortem inspection, and were not subjected to a stunning process, prior to slaughter, with a device injecting compressed air or gas into the cranial cavity, or subjected to a pithing process. In addition, the document should indicate that the fresh meat and meat products do not contain, and were not contaminated by

- tonsils and distal ileum of the small intestine and products derived from them from cattle of any age;
- brains, eyes, spinal cord, skull, vertebral column, and products derived from them from cattle over 12 months of age;
- mechanically separated meat from the skull and vertebral column from cattle over 12 months of age; and
- nervous and lymphatic tissues exposed during the deboning process.

Finally, the OIE recommends specific processing for gelatin and collagen prepared from bones and for tallow derivatives not sourced from protein-free tallow; a study demonstrated that the acid and alkaline processes used in gelatin production will clear certain amounts of BSE infectivity [124]. For tallow (other than protein-free tallow) or dicalcium phosphate, OIE recommends that it not be sourced from brains, eyes, spinal cords, skulls, vertebral columns, or products derived from them from cattle over 30 months of age.

4.2.7.2 National Requirements for BSE in the Food Supply

In June 1988, the United Kingdom adopted the first official regulations to control BSE in the food supply with an order prohibiting the use of certain ruminant proteins in ruminant feed. In 1989, it issued another order prohibiting the use in human food of certain tissues already prohibited for use in animal feed. In 1994, the European Community (EC) prohibited the feeding of most mammalian proteins to ruminants for its member states, and in 2001 the EC promulgated TSE Regulation 999/2001 prohibiting, among other things, the use of certain bovine, ovine, and caprine tissues for human food. As research on TSEs progressed, EC has amended its rules many times. Initially, United Kingdom legislation was more stringent than EC legislation, but the two have become harmonized over the years as the BSE epidemic in the United Kingdom diminished and BSE risk in the United Kingdom became more similar to the risk posed by BSE in some other Member States of the EC.

The EC has established measures for control of TSEs through Regulation (EC) No. 999/2001 (http://www.europa.eu.int) and its amendments, and the United Kingdom has established complementary controls for TSEs in the Transmissible Spongiform Encephalopathies Regulations 2006 (http://www.defra.uk.co).

The United States and Canada have tried to harmonize their BSE requirements because of the large amount of trade in live animals and beef products between the countries, especially before the discovery of BSE in both countries. The United States and Canada were proactive in establishing rules to prohibit the feeding of most mammalian protein to ruminants by imposing feed bans in 1997, 6 years before BSE was detected in either country. (The United Kingdom, EC, and Japan enacted feed bans only after BSE had already become established in their national cattle herds.) The proactive feed ban is considered the most important of several regulatory firewalls protecting animals and humans in North America from BSE.

Regulations defining BSE requirements in Canada can be found in its Food and Drug Regulations and its Health of Animals Regulations (http://www.inspection.gc.ca). Regulations defining BSE requirements in the United States can be found for animal health and most meat products under the U.S. Department of Agriculture (http://www.usda.gov) and for certain meat-containing products, dietary supplements, and animal feed under the U.S. Food and Drug Administration (http://www.fda.gov).

Europe and North America are not the only regions having national regulations for BSE. Many other countries have also prohibited the feeding of ruminant protein to ruminants and implemented surveillance and monitoring programs for BSE. To date, however, only countries or regions that have already identified an actual case of BSE have put in place measures to remove high-risk materials from the food supply.

4.3 Scrapie

Scrapie is a TSE of sheep and goats. Scrapie was the first recognized TSE, described in sheep in the 1700s. Its origin is unknown, and it was originally thought to be a genetic disease. Scrapie was demonstrated to be experimentally transmissible in the 1930s [41]. The minimum incubation period appears to be 1–2 years, and the disease most often affects animals 2–5 years old [62]. Clinical signs of scrapie include behavioral changes, loss of coordination, pruritus (itching), weakness, tremors, recumbency, and, in sheep, weight loss despite normal appetite. Pruritis gave scrapie its common English name, because animals with clinical disease tend to rub or scrape themselves against objects. Clinical signs vary somewhat from animal to animal, but neurological deterioration is inexorable.

Histopathological study of the brain in typical cases of scrapie reveals spongiform changes in a variety of locations, including the medulla, pons, cerebellum, substantia nigra, mesencephalon, hypothalamus, thalamus, septal area, corpus striatum, and neocortex. Anatomic distribution of vacuolation in particular areas of the brain depends on the scrapie strain and the genotype of the sheep affected; in some cases, amyloid plaques may also be found in brains of sheep with scrapie. It may be difficult to diagnose scrapie by histopathology alone [125]. In 1981, scrapie-associated fibrils (SAF) were first described in detergent-treated extracts of scrapie brains [126]. The protein comprising SAF was later found to be PrP^{TSE} [127]—the same misfolded form of protein contained in amyloid plaques. Aggregates of PrP^{TSE} can often be detected in the preclinical phase of disease and PrP^{TSE}/SAF concentrations are often correlated closely with scrapie infectivity titers [125].

In 1998, cases of atypical scrapie were described in Norway. Nor98-type atypical scrapie has now been reported from other countries; its wide geographic distribution in isolated areas has reinforced a theory that it might be a spontaneous TSE of sheep [16,98,128]—a controversial theory, not universally accepted, that has also been invoked to explain the occurrence of sCJD in humans and both BSE and BASE in cattle. Sheep with atypical scrapie usually show no signs of pruritus; PrP^{TSE} accumulates primarily in the cerebellar cortex instead of the cerebrum and demonstrates an unusual banding pattern on Western blot [129].

Certain genotypes of sheep seem especially susceptible to scrapie; the amino acids at positions 136, 154, and 171 of the prion protein appear to be the primary determining factor for susceptibility to many strains of agent [130]. Sheep with the homozygous VRQ genotype (single-letter amino acid code denoting valine^{136}, arginine^{154}, glutamine^{171}) appear to be the most susceptible, while sheep with the homozygous ARR (A = alanine) genotype are highly resistant to infection with most strains of scrapie agent. When compared to VRQ, alleles encoding other combinations of amino acids at the same three positions seem to confer somewhat increased resistance to scrapie, but not as high as ARR. The genetic factor in susceptibility has led some regions and countries to attempt control of scrapie using selective breeding of flocks to increase resistance to infection. That practice poses a theoretical risk of maintaining the silent propagation of scrapie agent through inapparent infections with exceptionally long incubation periods [131].

4.3.1 Transmission of Scrapie

Unlike BSE, scrapie appears to spread among animals horizontally, though no more than 5% of a herd is generally affected. The infection spreads most commonly from ewe to lamb and to other members in the same birthing groups, presumably through contact with infected placentas and placental fluids [132,133]. There may also be some environmental contamination with scrapie agent leading to transmission of infection. Research has shown that scrapie infectivity has survived in soil for at least 3 years with only 50% loss of infectivity titer [134]; it has also been proposed that the agent can adhere to minerals in soil that preserve infectivity. There is a possibility that scrapie agent might escape from tissues of infected animals—perhaps after death—persist in soil, and infect grazing animals as they feed [135]. Infected urine, saliva, or feces might theoretically contaminate the environment with the scrapie agent as well [18,136,137].

4.3.2   Distribution of Infectivity in Sheep and Goats with Scrapie

Scrapie agent is more widely distributed in the tissues of infected sheep and goats than is BSE agent in cattle (see Tables 4.2 through 4.5). Peripheral nerves and lymphoid tissues are often infected in scrapie, even during early stages of the disease. In sheep and goats that are genetically susceptible to scrapie, infectivity in lymphoid tissue has first been detected approximately 2 months after infection, whereas infectivity appeared in CNS tissues approximately 10 months after infection. Time of appearance of scrapie infectivity seems to depend on the amino acids at positions 136, 154, and 171 of PrP (described above). No infectivity has been detected in sheep milk, but these data are limited. The presence of PrP^{TSE} in sheep muscle has been reported [133]. As mentioned previously, Houston et al. and Hunter found that both BSE and scrapie were efficiently transmitted between sheep by blood transfusions [88–90].

4.3.3   Scrapie Agent in the Food Supply

Prevalence of scrapie varies greatly according to region [125]. Certain countries, such as Australia and New Zealand, are considered to be scrapie-free, whereas in other areas, such as Northern Europe, it has been estimated that 5%–6% of flocks are infected. In the United States, estimated national prevalence of scrapie in sheep is less than 1%. In general, scrapie appears to be more prevalent in the northern hemisphere than in the southern hemisphere. Scrapie is not classified as a zoonotic disease, because no epidemiological evidence has suggested that scrapie agent has infected humans. Nonetheless, for precautionary reasons, most countries—including the United States—have attempted to keep scrapie-infected animals from entering the human food chain or their use in other products, not least of all because of the recent concern that BSE in sheep and goats might be indistinguishable from scrapie.

4.4   Chronic Wasting Disease

Chronic wasting disease (CWD) was first described as a disease of captive deer in the late 1960s. Originally thought to be a metabolic disorder, the disease was eventually recognized as a TSE about 20 years later. CWD has been found in mule deer, white-tailed deer, Rocky Mountain elk, and moose [3,138,139]. CWD is the only TSE known to exist in wild animal populations. To date, CWD has been found naturally only in North America, though there have been cases in deer exported to South Korea from North America. CWD is endemic in wild cervid populations in north central Colorado and southeastern Wyoming (the original CWD-endemic area). CWD has also been found in wild cervid populations in Illinois,

Nebraska, New Mexico, South Dakota, Utah, Wisconsin, West Virginia, New York, and in Canada. In addition, CWD has been identified in farmed deer and elk in Colorado, Nebraska, Wyoming, Montana, Oklahoma, South Dakota, Wisconsin, Minnesota, Kansas, New York, and in Canada [140]. CWD prevalence has been estimated at less than 1% in the wild and in some farmed herds, but has been as high as 30% in deer from the original endemic area [141]. Prevalence in elk populations is believed to be lower than in deer populations. The incubation period of CWD is not precisely known. Most affected cervids have been 3–5 years old, though some were older. The youngest cervid known to have died of CWD was 17 months old and the oldest was 15 years old [142].

As for other TSEs, during the early stages of CWD infection, there are no clinical signs of disease [138]. Early signs of disease include subtle behavioral changes, including periods of depression and staring. Weight loss, without apparent loss of appetite, progresses throughout the disease, explaining why CWD was originally attributed to a metabolic disorder. In the final stages of disease, clinical signs of CWD may include increased drinking and urinating, excessive salivation, lack of coordination, and trembling. CWD is invariably fatal. CWD often presents as aspiration pneumonia caused by difficulty swallowing; in many cases, the pneumonia causes death [142].

Examination of brain tissue of cervids with CWD usually reveals spongiform changes typical of other TSEs. Lesions can be found in the medulla oblongata, pons, mesencephalon, and telencephalon in cervids with clinical disease. In animals with preclinical and clinical disease, the lesions are most striking in the parasympathetic vagal nucleus in the dorsal portion of the medulla oblongata at the obex [142,143]; the finding of typical lesions in the obex is generally sufficient to confirm a diagnosis of CWD. When the obex is not available for testing, negative results for CWD based on histopathology may be inconclusive. Accumulations of PrP^{TSE} can often be detected both later in the incubation period of CWD and during clinical illness by IHC in the brain (where PrP^{TSE} sometimes accumulates in florid plaques resembling those of vCJD (Figure 4.4)), tonsils, lymph nodes and lymphoid tissues, Peyer's patches of the small intestine, and spleen. In fact, tonsillar biopsies have proven useful to diagnose CWD in live deer though not in elk. In mule deer and white-tailed deer, immunostaining detected PrP^{TSE} in tonsils as long as 14 months before onset of clinical illness [61].

The origin of CWD is unknown, though, as for other TSEs, there are several theories [142]. CWD might be cervid-adapted scrapie from infected sheep or have resulted from a spontaneous mutation-like change in properties of the prion protein that then transmitted naturally. CWD might have come from some still unrecognized TSE of other wild animals. No evidence supports or refutes any of these theories, and, as for BSE, scrapie, and most other TSEs, the origin of CWD may never be known.

Similar to scrapie, there may be genetic differences in susceptibility to CWD in elk. In one study genotyping the PrP-encoding genes of 43 CWD-positive

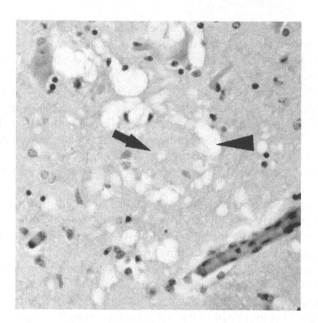

FIGURE 4.4
Multiple vacuoles in a hematoxylin–eosin-stained section from the brain of a white-tailed deer with chronic wasting disease (CWD). Note the presence of a flower-like (florid) plaque (arrow indicating core of the plaque) comprised of amorphous eosinophilic material surrounded by a halo of vacuoles (arrow head). Florid plaques have rarely been seen in most TSEs, but they are common in both CWD and variant Creutzfeldt–Jakob disease (vCJD). The similarity between florid plaques in CWD and vCJD, while intriguing, is probably coincidental. (The late Dr. Elizabeth Williams, University of Wyoming, kindly provided the original image, modified by Dr. Olga A. Maximova, FDA.)

elk, most of the ill animals were homozygous for methionine at codon 132; a few methionine/leucine heterozygotes were also discovered, but no animal with CWD was homozygous for leucine/leucine at that locus [60,141]. However, since that study, CWD has been detected naturally in elk of all three genotypes, though ill animals encoding M/M at codon 132 were clearly over-represented in herds studied. It appears that elk with M/L or L/L genotypes at codon 132 had longer incubation periods for CWD than did M/M homozygotes. There is also some evidence that the alleles at other codons of the PrP-encoding gene may influence incubation periods for CWD in deer, though no genotype appears to confer complete resistance [141]. Research is ongoing to determine if selective breeding for a CWD-resistant genotype in cervids would be useful for disease management.

4.4.1 Transmission of CWD

Of all the TSEs recognized to date, CWD seems to be the most infectious and is very efficiently transmitted from cervid to cervid. The horizontal transmission has recently been mainly attributed to saliva [144], explaining early observations suggesting spread of CWD by casual contact among cervids—exposures at common feeding and watering stations and reuse of pastures previously grazed by CWD-infected cervids [136,145]. Unlike BSE, CWD does not appear to have been transmitted through contaminated feed, an unlikely mechanism for natural transmission of an infectious disease in vegetarian animals. Studies of the placentas, ovaries, and fetal tissues of two pregnant mule deer revealed no PrP^{TSE}, and it appears unlikely from that observation and the patterns of occurrence of CWD that maternal transmission contributes significantly to the spread of infection [146]. In fact, in one study, CWD was transmitted with equal effectiveness (89%) to two birth cohorts, only one from an infected mother; the only identifiable source of CWD for both cohorts was contaminated pasture [145]. (The pastures involved were in a Colorado research facility that tried and failed to eradicate CWD after the land was first contaminated in the 1960s. Despite rigorous measures taken by the facility to eradicate CWD in 1985, 10 of 57 deer placed in the pens in 1990 had developed CWD by 1997. Note that the extremely high levels of CWD contamination found in pens used for experimental research can probably not be extrapolated to predict natural conditions in the field.)

Though CWD appears to spread easily among cervids, efforts to transmit the disease orally to noncervids have not been successful thus far [142]. After the recognition that BSE caused a human illness, there was concern that CWD might spread to cattle grazing with cervids. Ongoing research indicates that cattle have developed CWD after experimental IC inoculation with CWD-infected mule deer brain. However, simultaneous experiments with cattle dosed orally with similar material have not shown any evidence of disease during more than 7 years of observation [141]; the cattle were to be observed for at least three more years. Another experiment in which cattle were housed together with CWD-infected deer failed to transmit any illness suggestive of TSE to the cattle, though all the deer involved—both CWD-infected and control—have since died. Examination of brain tissue from several cattle demonstrated no changes characteristic of TSE, and others are still under observation. A survey of 262 adult cattle residing in a CWD-endemic area for at least 4 years demonstrated no evidence of a TSE [141]. In addition to cattle, CWD has also been transmitted experimentally by IC inoculation of infected cervid brain suspensions to sheep, goats, mice, ferrets, mink, hamsters, and squirrel monkeys [141,147,148].

4.4.2 Distribution of Infectivity in Cervids with CWD

Similar to scrapie agent, CWD agent accumulates in lymphoid tissues, central and peripheral nervous tissues, and other organs of cervids. The particular tissues that harbor infectivity depend on the species of cervid [141]. In mule deer with CWD, infectivity has been found in the brain, spinal cord, retina, peripheral nervous system, enteric nervous system, endocrine organs, and lymphatic tissues, including tonsils, retropharyngeal lymph nodes, nodes associated with the alimentary tract, peripheral lymph nodes, and spleen. In white-tailed deer and elk, infectivity has been found in brain, spinal cord, tonsil, and retropharyngeal lymph node. During the incubation period, it appears that PrP^{TSE} develops first in tonsil and lymphoid tissue (as early as 10–80 days postinoculation in mule deer fawns [149]), followed by deposition in the dorsal vagal nucleus in the medulla oblongata with little spongiform change, then at about the same time as clinical disease occurs, spongiform change appears in the medulla oblongata, and finally widespread deposition of PrP^{TSE} and spongiform change in brain tissue outside the medulla oblongata [141].

Williams [141] postulated that infectivity in blood could be the route by which peripheral tissues are infected in deer; a recent report described transmission of CWD by transfusion of blood to healthy deer from CWD-infected animal [144]. Another study demonstrated infectivity in muscle of CWD-infected mule deer by bioassay in Tg mice [150]. The findings of infectivity in muscles and blood of cervids with CWD has renewed concern about the safety of cervid tissues, although limited preliminary studies have not revealed any evidence suggesting transmission of the infection to humans consuming venison from endemic areas (see below).

Aside from venison, the other most commonly consumed cervid product is "velvet antler," extracts of which are used in dietary supplements, consumed primarily in Asia. There is no indication to date that antler velvet harbors CWD infectivity.

4.4.3 CWD Agent in the Food Supply

There is currently no evidence that the CWD agent has infected humans. A study of the in vitro conversion of PrP^C to PrP^{TSE} found that PrP^{TSE} from brain of a cervid with CWD readily converted normal cervid PrP^C into its abnormal form, while its efficiency converting PrP^C from normal sheep, cattle, and humans into PrP^{TSE} was significantly lower than conversion from cervid PrP^C [151]. In another study [152], investigators attempted to transmit CWD by IC injections of infected cervid brain suspensions into transgenic mice expressing either bovine or human PrP; none of those mice developed spongiform encephalopathy or accumulated detectable PrP^{TSE} during 750 days of observation (normal lifespan for the mice). Similar transgenic mice expressing cervid PrP developed TSE within 118 days after inoculation with CWD agent.

Because of concerns over the increasing prevalence of CWD in wild cervids and the possibility that it could cause a human disease, the Centers for Disease Control and Prevention (CDC) in the United States investigated three reported cases of sporadic CJD in young persons who had eaten venison [153]. After evaluating the histopathologic profiles and studying Western blots of PrP^{TSE} extracted from brains from the three cases, CDC concluded that each patient had died with typical sporadic CJD rather than any unusual TSE that might have been expected from a human CWD infection. Since approximately 40% of the U.S. population reports having eaten hunter-harvested deer or elk meat, these cases of sporadic CJD were probably coincidental.

Though there is no evidence that CWD is linked to human illness, authorities in both the United States and Canada do not recommend consumption of venison from CWD-infected cervids. Many regions in which CWD has been detected have cervid management programs including increased surveillance for the disease. Hunters are advised to avoid harvesting deer and elk that appear ill, to wear gloves when field-dressing animals, and to avoid contact with highest-risk materials from the carcasses: brain, spinal cord, and lymphoid tissues. Both the United States and Canada have CWD surveillance and eradication programs for farmed cervids, including testing and depopulation of herds found to contain CWD-positive animals.

Prior to the increase in detection of CWD in North American herds, there was a large export market for antler velvet. However, some countries banned the import of North American antlers because of concerns over CWD [10].

4.5 Conclusion

TSEs have had a significant effect on food safety policy and trade in the past decade. Measures taken thus far to prevent exposure of animals and humans to tissues that may transmit BSE have clearly proven effective The Food and Agriculture Organization of the United Nations recently reported that BSE is on the decline worldwide, with cases dropping about 50% a year during each of the last 3 years. As research adds to knowledge about tissue infectivity and the risk to humans from animal TSEs, approaches that industry and regulators take to keep prions from entering the food chain must adapt accordingly.

References

1. Johnson, R.T. and Gibbs, C.J. 1998. Creutzfeldt–Jakob disease and related transmissible spongiform encephalopathies. *N. Engl. J. Med.* 339(27): 1994–2004.
2. Hadlow, W.J. 1959. Scrapie and kuru. *Lancet* 2(7097): 289–290.
3. Council for Agricultural Science and Technology. 2000. Transmissible spongiform encephalopathies in the United States, Task Force Report No. 136.
4. Ironside, J., B. Ghetti, M. Head, P. Piccardo, and R. Will. Prion diseases. *Greenfield's Neuropathology*, Eds. S. Love, D. Louis, and D. Ellison. London, Edward Arnold Limited. (In Press).
5. Herzog, C, N. Sales, N. Etchegaray, A. Charbonnier, S. Freire, D. Dormont, J.-P. Deslys, and C.I. Lasmezas. 2004. Tissue distribution of bovine spongiform encephalopathy agent in primates after intravenous or oral infection. *Lancet* 363(9407): 422–428.

6. Wells, G.A.H., S.A.C. Hawkins, R.B. Green, A.R. Austin, I. Dexter, Y.I. Spencer, M.J. Chaplin, M.J. Stack, and M. Dawson. 1998. Preliminary observations on the pathogenesis of experimental bovine spongiform encephalopathy (BSE): An update. *Vet. Rec.* 142: 103–106.
7. Wells, G.A.H., M. Dawson, S.A.C. Hawkins, R.B. Green, I. Dexter, M.E. Francis, M.M. Simmons, A.R. Austin, and M.W. Horigan. 1994. Infectivity in the ileum of cattle challenged orally with bovine spongiform encephalopathy. *Vet. Rec.* 135: 40–41.
8. Wells, G.A.H., S.A.C. Hawkins, R.B. Green, Y.I. Spencer, I. Dexter, and M. Dawson. 1999. Limited detection of sternal bone marrow infectivity in the clinical phase of experimental bovine spongiform encephalopathy (BSE). *Vet. Rec.* 144: 292–294.
9. Brown, K.L., D.L. Ritchie, P.A. McBride, and M.E. Bruce. 2000. Detection of PrP in extraneural tissues, *Microsc. Res. Tech.* 50: 40–45.
10. Janka, J. and F. Maldarelli. 2004. Prion diseases: Update on mad cow disease, variant Creutzfeldt–Jakob disease, and the transmissible spongiform encephalopathies. *Curr. Infect. Dis. Rep.* 6(4): 305–315.
11. Prusiner, S.B. 2001. Shattuck lecture-neurodegenerative diseases and prions. *N. Engl. J. Med.* 344(20): 1516–1526.
12. Prusiner, S.B. 1982. Novel proteinaceous infectious particles cause scrapie. *Science* 216(4542): 136–144.
13. World Health Organization. 2005. *WHO Guidelines on Tissue Infectivity in Transmissible Spongiform Encephalopathies*, Geneva, WHO.
14. Chesebro, B. 2003. Introduction to the transmissible spongiform encephalopathies or prion diseases. *Br. Med. Bull.* 66: 1–20.
15. Oesch, B., D.B. Teplow, N. Stahl, D. Serban, L.E. Hood, and S.B. Prusiner. 1990. Identification of cellular proteins binding to the scrapie prion protein. *Biochemistry* 29(24): 5848–5855.
16. Gavier-Widen, D., M.J. Stack, T. Baron, A. Balachandran, and M. Simmons. 2005. Diagnosis of transmissible spongiform encephalopathies in animals: A review. *J. Vet. Diagn. Invest.* 17(6): 509–527.
17. van Rheede, T., M.M. Smolenaars, O. Madsen, and W.W. de Jong. 2003. Molecular evolution of the mammalian prion protein. *Mol. Biol. Evol.* 20(1): 111–121.
18. Novakofski, J., M.S. Brewer, N. Mateus-Pinilla, J. Killefer, and R.H. McCusker. 2005. Prion biology relevant to bovine spongiform encephalopathy. *J. Anim. Sci.* 83(6): 1455–1476.
19. Collins, S.J., V.A. Lawson, and C.L. Masters. 2003. Transmissible spongiform encephalopathies. *Lancet* 363(9402): 51–61.
20. Bueler, H., M. Fischer, Y. Lang, H. Bluethmann, H.P. Lipp, S.J. DeArmond, S.B. Prusiner, M. Aguet, and C. Weissmann. 1992. Normal development and behaviour of mice lacking the neuronal cell-surface PrP protein. *Nature* 356(6370): 577–582.
21. Bueler, H., A. Aguzzi, A. Sailer, R.A. Greiner, P. Autenried, M. Aguet, and C. Weissmann. 1993. Mice devoid of PrP are resistant to scrapie. *Cell* 73(7): 1339–1347.
22. Weissmann, C., H. Bueler, M. Fischer, A. Sailer, A. Aguzzi, and M. Aguet. 1994. PrP-deficient mice are resistant to scrapie. *Ann. N.Y. Acad. Sci.* 724: 235–240.
23. Weissmann, C., H. Bueler, M. Fischer, A. Sauer, and M. Aguet. 1994. Susceptibility to scrapie in mice is dependent on PrPC. *Philos. Trans. R. Soc. Lond. B Biol. Sci.* 343(1306): 431–433.
24. Prusiner, S.B. 1998. Prions. *Proc. Natl. Acad. Sci. U.S.A.* 95(23): 13363–13383.

25. Caughey, B.W., A. Dong, K.S. Bhat, D. Ernst, S.F. Hayes, and W.S. Caughey. 1991. Secondary structure analysis of the scrapie-associated protein PrP 27–30 in water by infrared spectroscopy. *Biochemistry* 30(31): 7672–7680.

26. Hill, A.F., M. Antoniou, and J. Collinge. 1999. Protease-resistant prion protein produced in vitro lacks detectable infectivity. *J. Gen. Virol.* 80(Pt 1): 11–14.

27. Legname, G., I.V. Baskakov, H.O. Nguyen, D. Riesner, F.E. Cohen, S.J. DeArmond, and S.B. Prusiner. 2004. Synthetic mammalian prions. *Science* 305(5684): 673–676.

28. Legname, G., H.O. Nguyen, I.V. Baskakov, F.E. Cohen, S.J. Dearmond, and S.B. Prusiner. 2005. Strain-specified characteristics of mouse synthetic prions. *Proc. Natl. Acad. Sci. U.S.A.* 102(6): 2168–2173.

29. Castilla, J., P. Saa, C. Hetz, and C. Soto. 2005. In vitro generation of infectious scrapie prions. *Cell* 121(2): 195–206.

30. Race, R., K. Meade-White, A. Raines, G.J. Raymond, B. Caughey, and B. Chesebro. 2002. Subclinical scrapie infection in a resistant species: Persistence, replication, and adaptation of infectivity during four passages. *J. Infect. Dis.* 186(Suppl. 2): S166–S170.

31. Race, R., A. Raines, G.J. Raymond, B. Caughey, and B. Chesebro. 2001. Long-term subclinical carrier state precedes scrapie replication and adaptation in a resistant species: Analogies to bovine spongiform encephalopathy and variant Creutzfeldt–Jakob disease in humans. *J. Virol.* 75(21): 10106–10112.

32. Manuelidis, L., W. Fritch, and Y.G. Xi. 1997. Evolution of a strain of CJD that induces BSE-like plaques. *Science* 277(5322): 94–98.

33. Hill, A.F. and J. Collinge. 2003. Subclinical prion infection in humans and animals. *Br. Med. Bull.* 66: 161–170.

34. Tatzelt, J., J. Zuo, R. Voellmy, M. Scott, U. Hartl, S.B. Prusiner, and W.J. Welch. 1995. Scrapie prions selectively modify the stress response in neuroblastoma cells. *Proc. Natl. Acad. Sci. U.S.A.* 92(7): 2944–2948.

35. Telling, G.C., M. Scott, J. Mastrianni, R. Gabizon, M. Torchia, F.E. Cohen, S.J. DeArmond, and S.B. Prusiner. 1995. Prion propagation in mice expressing human and chimeric PrP transgenes implicates the interaction of cellular PrP with another protein. *Cell* 83(1): 79–90.

36. Rieger, R., F. Edenhofer, C.I. Lasmezas, and S. Weiss. 1997. The human 37-kDa laminin receptor precursor interacts with the prion protein in eukaryotic cells. *Nat. Med.* 3(12): 1383–1388.

37. Saborio, G.P., C. Soto, R.J. Kascsak, E. Levy, R. Kascsak, D.A. Harris, and B. Frangione. 1999. Cell-lysate conversion of prion protein into its protease-resistant isoform suggests the participation of a cellular chaperone. *Biochem. Biophys. Res. Commun.* 258(2): 470–475.

38. Nazor, K.E., F. Kuhn, T. Seward, M. Green, D. Zwald, M. Purro, J. Schmid, K. Biffiger, A.M. Power, B. Oesch, A.J. Raeber, and G.C. Telling. 2005. Immunodetection of disease-associated mutant PrP, which accelerates disease in GSS transgenic mice. *EMBO. J.* 24(13): 2472–2480.

39. Manuelidis, L. 2003. Transmissible encephalopathies: Speculations and realities. *Viral. Immunol.* 16(2): 123–139.

40. Lasmezas, C.I., J.P. Deslys, O. Robain, A. Jaegly, V. Beringue, J.M. Peyrin, J.G. Fournier, J.J. Hauw, J. Rossier, and D. Dormont. 1997. Transmission of the BSE agent to mice in the absence of detectable abnormal prion protein. *Science* 275(5298): 402–405.

41. Cuillé, J. and P.-L. Chelle. 1936. La tremblante du mouton est elle inoculable? *Comptes Redus de l' Academie des Sciences* 203: 1552–1554.

42. Asher, D.M. 1999. The transmissible spongiform encephalopathy agents: Concerns and responses of United States regulatory agencies in maintaining the safety of biologics. *Dev. Biol. Stand.* 100: 103–118.

43. Collinge, J., J. Whitfield, E. McKintosh, J. Beck, S. Mead, D.J. Thomas, and M.P. Alpers. 2006. Kuru in the 21st century—An acquired human prion disease with very long incubation periods. *Lancet* 367(9528): 2068–2074.

44. Wilesmith, J.W., G.A. Wells, M.P. Cranwell, and J.B. Ryan. 1988. Bovine spongiform encephalopathy: Epidemiological studies. *Vet. Rec.* 123(25): 638–644.

45. Will, R.G., J.W. Ironside, M. Zeidler, S.N. Cousens, K. Estibeiro, A. Alperovitch, S. Poser, M. Pocchiari, A. Hofman, and P.G. Smith. 1996. A new variant of Creutzfeldt–Jakob disease in the UK. *Lancet* 347(9006): 921–925.

46. Peden, A.H., M.W. Head, D.L. Ritchie, J.E. Bell, and J.W. Ironside. 2004. Preclinical vCJD after blood transfusion in a PRNP codon 129 heterozygous patient. *Lancet* 364(9433): 527–529.

47. Peden, A.H., D.L. Ritchie, and J.W. Ironside. 2005. Risks of transmission of variant Creutzfeldt–Jakob disease by blood transfusion. *Folia Neuropathol.* 43(4): 271–278.

48. Llewelyn, C.A., P.E. Hewitt, R.S. Knight, K. Amar, S. Cousens, J. Mackenzie, and R.G. Will. 2004. Possible transmission of variant Creutzfeldt–Jakob disease by blood transfusion. *Lancet* 363(9407): 417–421.

49. Hewitt, P.E., C.A. Llewelyn, J. Mackenzie, and R.G. Will. 2006. Creutzfeldt–Jakob disease and blood transfusion: Results of the UK Transfusion Medicine Epidemiological Review study. *Vox. Sang.* 91(3): 221–230.

50. Bruce, M.E. 2003. TSE strain variation. *Br. Med. Bull.* 66: 99–108.

51. Bruce, M.E., I. McConnell, H. Fraser, and A.G. Dickinson. 1991. The disease characteristics of different strains of scrapie in Sinc congenic mouse lines: Implications for the nature of the agent and host control of pathogenesis. *J. Gen. Virol.* 72(Pt 3): 595–603.

52. Fraser, H. and A.G. Dickinson. 1968. The sequential development of the brain lesions of scrapie in three strains of mice. *J. Comp. Pathol.* 78(3): 301–311.

53. Collinge, J., K.C. Sidle, J. Meads, J. Ironside, and A.F. Hill. 1996. Molecular analysis of prion strain variation and the aetiology of 'new variant' CJD. *Nature* 383(6602): 685–690.

54. Parchi, P., R. Castellani, S. Capellari, B. Ghetti, K. Young, S.G. Chen, M. Farlow, D.W. Dickson, A.A. Sima, J.Q. Trojanowski, R.B. Petersen, and P. Gambetti. 1996. Molecular basis of phenotypic variability in sporadic Creutzfeldt–Jakob disease. *Ann. Neurol.* 39(6): 767–778.

55. Yull, H.M., D.L. Ritchie, J.P. Langeveld, F.G. van Zijderveld, M.E. Bruce, J.W. Ironside, and M.W. Head. 2006. Detection of type 1 prion protein in variant Creutzfeldt–Jakob disease. *Am. J. Pathol.* 168(1): 151–157.

56. Minor, P., J. Newham, N. Jones, C. Bergeron, L. Gregori, D. Asher, F. van Engelenburg, T. Stroebel, M. Vey, G. Barnard, and M. Head. 2004. Standards for the assay of Creutzfeldt–Jakob disease specimens. *J. Gen. Virol.* 85(Pt 6): 1777–1784.

57. Kimberlin, R.H., S.M. Hall, and C.A. Walker. 1983. Pathogenesis of mouse scrapie. Evidence for direct neural spread of infection to the CNS after injection of sciatic nerve. *J. Neurol. Sci.* 61(3): 315–325.

58. Kimberlin, R.H. and C.A. Walker. 1978. Pathogenesis of mouse scrapie: Effect of route of inoculation on infectivity titres and dose-response curves. *J. Comp. Pathol.* 88(1): 39–47.

59. Prusiner, S.B. 1999. *Prion Biology and Diseases*. New York, Cold Springs Harbor Laboratory Press.

60. O'Rourke, K.I., T.V. Baszler, T.E. Besser, J.M. Miller, R.C. Cutlip, G.A. Wells, S.J. Ryder, S.M. Parish, A.N. Hamir, N.E. Cockett, A. Jenny, and D.P. Knowles. 2000. Preclinical diagnosis of scrapie by immunohistochemistry of third eyelid lymphoid tissue. *J. Clin. Microbiol.* 38(9): 3254–3259.

61. Wild, M.A., T.R. Spraker, C.J. Sigurdson, K.I. O'Rourke, and M.W. Miller. 2002. Preclinical diagnosis of chronic wasting disease in captive mule deer (*Odocoileus hemionus*) and white-tailed deer (*Odocoileus virginianus*) using tonsillar biopsy. *J. Gen. Virol.* 83(Pt 10): 2629–2634.

62. Schreuder, B.E., L.J. van Keulen, M.E. Vromans, J.P. Langeveld, and M.A. Smits. 1998. Tonsillar biopsy and PrPSc detection in the preclinical diagnosis of scrapie. *Vet. Rec.* 142(21): 564–568.

63. Hill, A.F., M. Desbruslais, S. Joiner, K.C. Sidle, I. Gowland, J. Collinge, L.J. Doey, and P. Lantos. 1997. The same prion strain causes vCJD and BSE. *Nature* 389(6650): 448–450, 526.

64. Zeidler, M., R. Knight, G. Stewart, J.W. Ironside, R.G. Will, A.J. Green, and M. Pocchiari. 1999. Diagnosis of Creutzfeldt–Jakob disease. Routine tonsil biopsy for diagnosis of new variant Creutzfeldt–Jakob disease is not justified. *Br. Med. J.* 318(7182): 538.

65. Zeidler, M., R.J. Sellar, D.A. Collie, R. Knight, G. Stewart, M.A. Macleod, J.W. Ironside, S. Cousens, A.C. Colchester, D.M. Hadley, and R.G. Will. 2000. The pulvinar sign on magnetic resonance imaging in variant Creutzfeldt–Jakob disease. *Lancet* 355(9213): 1412–1418.

66. Wong, B.S., A.J. Green, R. Li, Z. Xie, T. Pan, T. Liu, S.G. Chen, P. Gambetti, and M.S. Sy. 2001. Absence of protease-resistant prion protein in the cerebrospinal fluid of Creutzfeldt–Jakob disease. *J. Pathol.* 194(1): 9–14.

67. Safar, J. and S.B. Prusiner. 1998. Molecular studies of prion diseases. *Prog. Brain. Res.* 117: 421–434.

68. Safar, J., H. Wille, V. Itri, D. Groth, H. Serban, M. Torchia, F.E. Cohen, and S.B. Prusiner. 1998. Eight prion strains have PrP(Sc) molecules with different conformations. *Nat. Med.* 4(10): 1157–1165.

69. Safar, J.G., M.D. Geschwind, C. Deering, S. Didorenko, M. Sattavat, H. Sanchez, A. Serban, M. Vey, H. Baron, K. Giles, B.L. Miller, S.J. Dearmond, and S.B. Prusiner. 2005. Diagnosis of human prion disease. *Proc. Natl. Acad. Sci. U.S.A.* 102(9): 3501–3506.

70. Bellon, A., W. Seyfert-Brandt, W. Lang, H. Baron, A. Groner, and M. Vey. 2003. Improved conformation-dependent immunoassay: Suitability for human prion detection with enhanced sensitivity. *J. Gen. Virol.* 84(Pt 7): 1921–1925.

71. Saborio, G.P., C. Soto, R.J. Kascsak, E. Levy, R. Kascsak, D.A. Harris, and B. Frangione. 1999. Cell-lysate conversion of prion protein into its protease-resistant isoform suggests the participation of a cellular chaperone. *Biochem. Biophys. Res. Commun.* 258(2): 470–475.

72. Saa, P., J. Castilla, and C. Soto. 2006. Ultra-efficient replication of infectious prions by automated protein misfolding cyclic amplification. *J. Biol. Chem.* 281: 35245–35252.

73. Collee, J.G. and R. Bradley. 1997. BSE: A Decade on-Part I. *Lancet* 349: 636–641.

74. Anderson, R.M., C.A. Connelly, N.M. Ferguson, M.E.J. Woolhouse, C.J. Watt, H.J. Udy, S. MaWhinney, S.P. Dunstan, T.R.E. Southwood, J.W. Wilesmith, J.B.M. Ryan, L.J. Hoinville, J.E. Hillerton, A.R. Austin, and G.A.H. Wells.

1996. Transmission dynamics and dpidemiology of BSE in British Cattle. *Nature* 382: 779–788.

75. Wells, G.A., A.C. Scott, C.T. Johnson, R.F. Gunning, R.D. Hancock, M. Jeffrey, M. Dawson, and R. Bradley. 1987. A novel progressive spongiform encephalopathy in cattle. *Vet. Rec.* 121(18): 419–420.

76. Jeffrey, M. and L. Gonzalez. 2004. Pathology and pathogenesis of bovine spongiform encephalopathy and scrapie. *Curr. Top. Microbiol. Immunol.* 284: 65–97.

77. Wilesmith, J.W., G.A. Wells, M.P. Cranwell, and J.B. Ryan. 1988. Bovine spongiform encephalopathy: Epidemiological studies. *Vet. Rec.* 123(25): 638–644.

78. Kimberlin, R.H. and J.W. Wilesmith. 1994. Bovine spongiform encephalopathy: Epidemiology, low dose exposure, and risks, *Ann. N.Y. Acad. Sci.* 724: 210–220.

79. DEFRA. 2006. Department of Environment, Food, and Rural Affairs, United Kingdom. http://www.defra.gov.uk

80. Smith, P.G. and R. Bradley. 2003. Bovine spongiform encephalopathy (BSE) and its epidemiology. *Br. Med. Bull.* 66: 185–198.

81. The BSE Inquiry. 2000. www.bseinquiry.gov.uk/index.htm

82. Donnelly, C.A., N.M. Ferguson, A.C. Ghani, M.E. Woolhouse, C.J. Watt, and R.M. Anderson. 1997. The epidemiology of BSE in cattle herds in Great Britain. I. Epidemiological processes, demography of cattle and approaches to control by culling. *Philos. Trans. R. Soc. Lond. B Biol. Sci.* 352(1355): 781–801.

83. Buschmann, A. and M.H. Groschup. 2005. Highly bovine spongiform encephalopathy-sensitive transgenic mice confirm the essential restriction of infectivity to the nervous system in clinically diseased cattle. *J. Infect. Dis.* 192(5): 934–942.

84. Fraser, H. and J. Foster. 1993. Transmission to mice, sheep and goats and bioassay of bovine tissues. In *Transmissible Spongiform Encephalopathies.* R. Bradley, and B. Marchant eds. A Consultation on BSE with the Scientific Veterinary Committee of the Commission of the European Communities held in Brussels, September 14–15 1993. Document VI/4131/94-EN. Brussels, European Commission Agriculture: 145–159.

85. Bosque, P.J., C. Ryou, G. Telling, D. Peretz, G. Legname, S.J. DeArmond, and S.B. Prusiner. 2002. Prions in skeletal muscle. *Proc. Natl. Acad. Sci. U.S.A.* 99(6): 3812–3817.

86. Scientific Steering Committee, European Commission. 2002. Prions in muscles, A statement adopted by the scientific steering committee at its Meeting of 4–5 April 2002. Accessed online at http://www.europa.eu.int

87. Scientific Steering Committee, European Commission. 2002. The implications of the recent papers on transmission of BSE by blood transfusion in sheep (Houston et al., 2000; Hunter et al., 2002). Accessed online at http://www.europa.eu.int

88. Houston, F., J.D. Foster, A. Chong, N. Hunter, and C.J. Bostock. 2000. Transmission of BSE by blood transfusion in sheep. *Lancet* 356(9234): 999–1000.

89. Hunter, N. 2003. Scrapie and experimental BSE in sheep. *Br. Med. Bull.* 66: 171–83.

90. Hunter, N., J. Foster, A. Chong, S. McCutcheon, D. Parnham, S. Eaton, C. MacKenzie, and F. Houston. 2002. Transmission of prion diseases by blood transfusion. *J. Gen. Virol.* 83(Pt 11): 2897–2905.

91. Taylor, D.M., C.E. Ferguson, C.J. Bostock, and M. Dawson. 1995. Absence of disease in mice receiving milk from cows with bovine spongiform encephalopathy. *Vet. Rec.* 136: 592.

92. Wilesmith, J.W. and J.B. Ryan. 1997. Absence of BSE in the offspring of pedigree suckler cows affected by BSE in Great Britain. *Vet. Rec.* 141: 250–251.

93. Donnelly, C.A. 1998. Transmission of BSE: Interpretation of the data on the offspring of BSE-affected pedigree suckler cows. *Vet. Rec.* 142: 579–580.

94. Scientific Steering Committee, European Commission. 1999. Opinion of the Scientific Steering Committee on the human exposure risk (HER) via food with respect to BSE, accessed online at http://ec.europa.eu/food/fs/sc/ssc/out67_en.html

95. Comer, P.J. and P.J. Huntly. 2003. TSE risk assessments: A decision support tool. *Stat. Methods Med. Res.* 12(3): 279–291.

96. Casalone, C., G. Zanusso, P. Acutis, S. Ferrari, L. Capucci, F. Tagliavini, S. Monaco, and M. Caramelli. 2004. Identification of a second bovine amyloidotic spongiform encephalopathy: Molecular similarities with sporadic Creutzfeldt–Jakob disease. *Proc. Natl. Acad. Sci. U.S.A.* 101: 3065–3070.

97. Biacabe, A.G., J.L. Laplanche, S. Ryder, and T.G. Baron. 2004. Distinct molecular phenotypes in bovine prion diseases. *EMBO Rep.* 5(1): 110–115.

98. Buschmann, A., A. Gretzschel, A.G. Biacabe, K. Schiebel, C. Corona, C. Hoffmann, M. Eiden, T. Baron, C. Casalone, and M.H. Groschup. 2006. Atypical BSE in Germany—Proof of transmissibility and biochemical characterization. *Vet. Microbiol.* 117(2–4): 103–116.

99. Garland, T., N. Bauer, and M. Bailey, Jr. 1996. Brain emboli in the lungs of cattle after stunning. *Lancet* 348(9027): 610.

100. Schmidt, G.R., K.L. Hossner, R.S. Yemm, and D.H. Gould. 1999. Potential for disruption of central nervous system tissue in beef cattle by different types of captive bolt stunners. *J. Food. Prot.* 62(4): 390–393.

101. Anil, M.H., S. Love, C.R. Helps, J.L. McKinstry, S.N. Brown, A. Philips, S. Williams, A. Shand, T. Bakirel, and D. Harbour. 2001. Jugular venous emboli of brain tissue induced in sheep by the use of captive bolt guns. *Vet. Rec.* 148(20): 619–620.

102. Anil, M.H., S. Love, S. Williams, A. Shand, J.L. McKinstry, C.R. Helps, A. Waterman-Pearson, J. Seghatchian, and D.A. Harbour. 1999. Potential contamination of beef carcases with brain tissue at slaughter. *Vet. Rec.* 145(16): 460–462.

103. Scientific Steering Committee, European Commission. 2001. Scientific Report on Stunning Methods and BSE Risks, Prepared by the TSE BSE ad hoc Group at its Meeting of 13 December 2001 and Including the Outcome of a Public Consultation via Internet Between 10 September and 26 October 2001. Accessed online at http://www.europa.eu.int

104. Anonymous. 2005. BSE agent in goat tissue: First known naturally occurring case confirmed. *Euro Surveill.* 10(2): E050203 1.

105. Anonymous. 2005. Possible case of BSE agent in a UK goat that died in 1990. *Euro Surveill.* 10(2): E050210 2.

106. Brown, P. 1997. The risk of bovine spongiform encephalopathy (mad cow disease) to human health. *J. Am. Med. Assoc.* 278(12): 1008–1011.

107. Chazot, G., E. Broussolle, C. Lapras, T. Blattler, A. Aguzzi, and N. Kopp. 1996. New variant of Creutzfeldt–Jakob disease in a 26-year-old French man. *Lancet* 347(9009): 1181.

108. Collinge, J. 2001. Prion diseases of humans and animals: Their causes and molecular basis. *Ann. Rev. Neurosci.* 24: 519–550.

109. Almond, J. and J. Pattison. 1997. Human BSE. *Nature* 389(6650): 437–438.

110. Scott, M.R., R. Will, J. Ironside, H.O. Nguyen, P. Tremblay, S.J. DeArmond, and S.B. Prusiner. 1999. Compelling transgenetic evidence for transmission of bovine spongiform encephalopathy prions to humans. *Proc. Natl. Acad. Sci. U.S.A.* 96(26): 15137–15142.

111. Collinge, J. 1999. Variant Creutzfeldt–Jakob Disease. *Lancet* 354: 317–323.

112. Brown, P. 2001. Bovine spongiform encephalopathy and variant Creutzfeldt–Jakob disease. *Br. Med. J.* 322(7290): 841–844.

113. Lasmezas, C.I., J.G. Fournier, V. Nouvel, H. Boe, D. Marce, F. Lamoury, N. Kopp, J.J. Hauw, J. Ironside, M. Bruce, D. Dormont, and J.P. Deslys. 2001. Adaptation of the bovine spongiform encephalopathy agent to primates and comparison with Creutzfeldt–Jakob disease: Implications for human health. *Proc. Natl. Acad. Sci. U.S.A.* 98(7): 4142–4147.

114. Brown, P., R.G. Will, R. Bradley, D.M. Asher, and L. Detwiler. 2001. Bovine spongiform encephalopathy and variant Creutzfeldt–Jakob disease: Background, evolution and current concerns. *Emerg. Infect. Dis.* 7(1): 6–16.

115. Ward, H.J., D. Everington, S.N. Cousens, B. Smith-Bathgate, M. Leitch, S. Cooper, C. Heath, R.S. Knight, P.G. Smith, and R.G. Will. 2006. Risk factors for variant Creutzfeldt–Jakob disease: A case-control study. *Ann. Neurol.* 59(1): 111–120.

116. Van Duijn, C.M., N. Delasnerie-Laupretre, and C. Masullo. 1998. Case-control study of risk factors of Creutzfeldt–Jakob disease in Europe during 1993–1995. *Lancet* 351: 1081–1085.

117. Beghi, E., C. Gandolfo, C. Ferrarese, N. Rizzuto, G. Poli, M.C. Tonini, G. Vita, M. Leone, G. Logroscino, E. Granieri, G. Salemi, G. Savettieri, L. Frattola, G. Ru, G.L. Mancardi, and C. Messina. 2004. Bovine spongiform encephalopathy and Creutzfeldt–Jakob disease: Facts and uncertainties underlying the causal link between animal and human diseases. *Neurol. Sci.* 25: 122–129.

118. The Centers for Disease Control and Prevention, U.S. Department of Health and Human Services. 2006. Accessed at http://www.cdc.gov/ncidod/dvrd/vcjd/other/vCJD_112906.htm

119. Clarke, P. and A. Ghani. 2005. Projections of the future course of the primary vCJD epidemic in the UK: Inclusion of subclinical infection and the possibility of wider genetic susceptibility. *J. R. Soc. Interface* 2: 19–31.

120. Hilton, D.A., A.C. Ghani, L. Conyers, P. Edwards, L. McCardle, D. Ritchie, M. Penney, D. Hegazy, and J.W. Ironside. 2004. Prevalence of lymphoreticular prion protein accumulation in UK tissue samples. *J. Pathol.* 203(3): 733–739.

121. Hilton, D.A., J. Sutak, M.E. Smith, M. Penney, L. Conyers, P. Edwards, L. McCardle, D. Ritchie, M.W. Head, C.A. Wiley, and J.W. Ironside. 2004. Specificity of lymphoreticular accumulation of prion protein for variant Creutzfeldt–Jakob disease. *J. Clin. Pathol.* 57(3): 300–302.

122. Vossen, P., J. Kreysa, and M. Goll. 2003. Overview of the BSE risk assessments of the European Commission's Scientific Steering Committee (SSC) and its TSE/BSE ad hoc group. Accessed online at http://www.europa.eu.int/comm/food/fs/sc/ssc/out364_en.pdf

123. The World Organisation for Animal Health. 2006. Terrestrial animal health code. Accessed at http://www.oie.int/eng/Normes/mcode/en_sommaire.htm

124. Grobben, A.H., P.J. Steele, R.A. Somerville, and D.M. Taylor. 2004. Inactivation of the bovine-spongiform-encephalopathy (BSE) agent by the acid and alkaline processes used in the manufacture of bone gelatine. *Biotechnol. Appl. Biochem.* 39: 329–338.

125. Laplanche, J., N. Hunter, M. Shinagawa, and E.S. Williams. 1999. Scrapie, chronic wasting disease, and transmissible mink encephalopathy. In *Prion Biology and Diseases*, Ed. S.B. Prusiner. New York, Cold Springs Harbor Laboratory Press.

126. Mertz, P.A., R.A. Somerville, H.M. Wisniewski, and K. Iqbal. 1981. Abnormal fibrils from scrapie-infected brain. *Acta Neuropathol. (Berl)* 54: 63–74.

127. Bolton, D.C., M.P. McKinley, and S.B. Prusiner. 1982. Identification of a protein that purifies with the scrapie prion. *Science* 218(4579): 1309–1311.

128. Orge, L., A. Galo, C. Machado, C. Lima, C. Ochoa, J. Silva, M. Ramos, and J.P. Simas. 2004. Identification of putative atypical scrapie in sheep in Portugal. *J. Gen. Virol.* 85: 3487–3491.

129. Benestad, S.L., P. Sarradin, and B. Thu. 2003. Cases of scrapie with unusual features in Norway and designation of a new type, Nor98. *Vet. Rec.* 153: 202–208.

130. Dawson, M., L.J. Hoinville, B.D. Hosie, and N. Hunter. 1998. Guidance on the use of PrP genotyping as an aid to the control of clinical scrapie. *Vet. Rec.* 142: 623–625.

131. Ronzon, F., A. Bencsik, S. Lezmi, J. Vulin, A. Kodjo, and T. Baron. 2006. BSE inoculation to prion diseases-resistant sheep reveals tricky silent carriers. *Biochem. Biophys. Res. Commun.* 350: 872–877.

132. Race, R., A. Jenny, and D. Sutton. 1998. Scrapie infectivity and proteinase K-resistant prion protein in sheep placenta, brain, spleen, and lymph node: Implications for transmission and antemortem diagnosis. *J. Infect. Dis.* 178(4): 949–953.

133. Andreoletti, O., C. Lacroux, A. Chabert, L. Monnereau, G. Tabouret, F. Lantier, P. Berthon, F. Eychenne, S. Lafond-Benestad, J.M. Elsen, and F. Schelcher. 2002. PrP(Sc) accumulation in placentas of ewes exposed to natural scrapie: Influence of foetal PrP genotype and effect on ewe-to-lamb transmission. *J. Gen. Virol.* 83(Pt 10): 2607–2616.

134. Brown, P. and D.C. Gajdusek. 1991. Survival of scrapie virus after 3 years' interment. *Lancet* 337(8736): 269–270.

135. Johnson, C.J., K.E. Phillips, P.T. Schramm, D. McKenzie, and J.M. Aiken. 2006. Prions adhere to soil minerals and remain infectious. *PLoS Pathog.* 2(4):e32.

136. Miller, M.W., E.S. Williams, N.T. Hobbs, and L.L. Wolfe. 2004. Environmental sources of prion transmission in mule deer. *Emerg. Infect. Dis.* 10: 1003–1006.

137. Shaked, G.M., Y. Shaked, Z. Kariv-Inbal, M. Halimi, I. Avraham, and R. Gabizon. 2001. A protease resistant prion protein isoform is present in urine of animals and humans affected with prion diseases. *J. Biol. Chem.* 276: 31479–31482.

138. Miller, M.W., M.A. Wild, and E.S. Williams. 1998. Epidemiology of chronic wasting disease in captive Rocky Mountain elk. *J. Wildl. Dis.* 34(3): 532–538.

139. Gross, J.E. and M.W. Miller. 2001. Chronic wasting disease in mule deer: Disease dynamics and control. *J. Wildl. Manage.* 65(2): 205–215.

140. The Animal and Plant Health Inspection Service, U.S. Department of Agriculture. 2006. Chronic wasting disease. Accessed at http://www.aphis.usda.gov/vs/nahps/cwd/

141. Williams, E.S. 2005. Chronic wasting disease. *Vet. Pathol.* 42: 530–549.

142. Salman, M.D. 2003. Chronic wasting disease in deer and elk: Scientific facts and findings. *J. Vet. Med. Sci.* 65(7): 761–768.

143. Peters, J., J.M. Miller, A.L. Jenny, T.L. Peterson, and K.P. Carmichael. 2000. Immunohistochemical diagnosis of chronic wasting disease in preclinically affected elk from a captive herd. *J. Vet. Diagn. Invest.* 12: 579–582.
144. Mathiason, C.K., J.G. Powers, S.J. Dahmes, D.A. Osborn, K.V. Miller, R.J. Warren, G.L. Mason, S.A. Hays, J. Hayes-Klug, D.M. Seelig, M.A. Wild, L.L. Wolfe, T.R. Spraker, M.W. Miller, C.J. Sigurdson, G.C. Telling, and E.A. Hoover. 2006. Infectious prions in the saliva and blood of deer with chronic wasting disease. *Science* 314(5796): 133–136.
145. Miller, M.W. and E.S. Williams. 2003. Horizontal prion transmission in mule deer. *Nature* 425: 35–36.
146. Spraker, T.R., R.R. Zink, B.A. Cummings, C.J. Sigurdson, M.W. Miller, and K.I. O'Rourke. 2002. Distribution of protease-resistant prion protein and spongiform encephalopathy in free-ranging mule deer (*Odocoileus hemionus*) with chronic wasting disease. *Vet. Pathol.* 39: 546–556.
147. Hamir, A.N., R.A. Kunkle, R.C. Cutlip, J.M. Miller, K.I. O'Rourke, E.S. Williams, M.W. Miller, M.J. Stack, M.J. Chaplin, and J.A. Richt. 2005. Experimental transmission of chronic wasting disease agent from mule deer to cattle by the intracerebral route. *J. Vet. Diagn. Invest.* 17: 276–281.
148. Marsh, R.F., A.E. Kincaid, R.A. Bessen, and J.C. Bartz. 2005. Interspecies transmission of chronic wasting disease prions to squirrel monkeys (*Saimiri sciureus*). *J. Virol.* 79(21): 13794–13796.
149. Sigurdson, C.J., E.S. Williams, M.W. Miller, T.R. Spraker, K.I. O'Rourke, and E.A. Hoover. 1999. Oral transmission and early lymphoid tropism of chronic wasting disease PrP^{res} in mule deer fawns (*Odocoileus hemionus*). *J. Gen. Virol.* 80: 2757–2764.
150. Angers, R.C., S.R. Browning, T.S. Seward, C.J. Sigurdson, M.W. Miller, E.A. Hoover, and G.C. Telling. 2006. Prions in skeletal muscles of deer with chronic wasting disease. *Science* 311(5764): 1117.
151. Raymond, G.J., A. Bossers, L.D. Raymond, K.I. O'Rourke, L.E. McHolland, P.K. Bryant III, M.W. Miller, E.S. Williams, M. Smits, and B. Caughey. 2000. Evidence of a molecular barrier limiting susceptibility of humans, cattle and sheep to chronic wasting disease. *EMBO J.* 19(17): 4425–4430.
152. Kong, Q., S. Huang, W. Zou, D. Vanegas, M. Wang, D. Wu, J. Yuan, M. Zheng, H. Bai, H. Deng, K. Chen, A.L. Jenny, K. O'Rourke, E.D. Belay, L.B. Schonberger, R.B. Peterson, M.-S. Sy, S.G. Chen, and P. Gambetti. 2005. Chronic wasting disease of elk: Transmissibility to humans examined by transgenic mouse models. *J. Neurosci.* 25(35): 7944–7949.
153. Belay, E.D., P. Gambetti, L.B. Schonberger, P. Parchi, D.R. Lyon, S. Capellari, J.H. McQuiston, K. Bradley, G. Dowdle, J.M. Crutcher, and C.R. Nichols. 2001. Creutzfeldt–Jakob disease in unusually young patients who consumed venison. *Arch. Neurol.* 58: 1673–1678.

5

Toxicity of Fumonisins, Mycotoxins from Fusarium verticillioides

Kenneth A. Voss, Ronald T. Riley, and Janee B. Gelineau-van Waes

CONTENTS

5.1 Introduction

Fusarium verticillioides (formerly *F. moniliforme* Sheldon) causes sporadic outbreaks of equine leukoencephalomalacia (ELEM)[1-4] and porcine pulmonary edema (PPE).[4-6] *F. verticillioides* is nephrotoxic and hepatotoxic to multiple species and causes liver tumors in rats.[4,7-9] The importance of *F. verticillioides* to human health is not clear although a correlation between high esophageal cancer rates and consumption of corn contaminated with *F. verticillioides* has long been recognized.[10,11] More recent observations suggest that fumonisins might increase the risk of neural tube defects under some conditions.[12,13]

The discovery of fumonisins B_1 (FB_1), FB_2, FA_1, and FA_2[14] was a major advance in understanding the toxicity of *F. verticillioides* and *F. proliferatum*, the other major fumonisin-producing fungus, and the list of fumonisin homologues and reaction products continues to grow.[15] Fumonisins, like *F. verticillioides*, have worldwide distribution in corn. They are relatively stable under most cooking conditions and are therefore found in corn-based foods.[11,15] While found in low amounts, generally <1 ppm, in commercial corn-based products from industrialized countries, fumonisin concentrations in corn intended for human consumption in some regions can be high,[11,15] at times exceeding levels that are toxic to animals. Persons consuming high amounts of corn for cultural or medical (for example, those who must avoid wheat) considerations are potentially subject to relatively high fumonisin intakes.

FB_1, the most common and thoroughly studied fumonisin, reproduces *F. verticillioides* toxicity when given to horses (ELEM),[16,17] swine (PPE),[18-20] and laboratory animals (hepato- and nephrotoxicity).[9,11,14] FB_1 is also a liver and kidney carcinogen in rodents.[21,22] The International Agency for Research on Cancer[23] classified FB_1 as "possibly carcinogenic" (Group 2B) to humans and the FAO/WHO Joint Expert Committee for Food Additives[11] recommended a maximum tolerable daily intake of 2 μg/kg body weight. The FDA industry guidance for fumonisins ($FB_1 + FB_2 + FB_3$) in corn intended for human consumption varies from 2 (degermed dry-milled maize products) to 4 (corn for masa production) ppm[24,25] and the maximum allowable fumonisin ($FB_1 + FB_2$) levels in foods proposed by the European Union range from 0.2 (processed maize-based foods for babies, infants, and young children) to 2 (unprocessed maize) ppm.[26] The FDA has also issued guidelines for fumonisins in animal feeds that vary by species.[27] The aforementioned recommendations and guidance levels were established after consideration of fumonisin's mode of action and its toxicity to farm and laboratory animal species.

5.2 Fumonisins and Sphingolipid Metabolism

5.2.1 Ceramide Synthase Inhibition

FB_1 inhibits ceramide synthase (sphinganine (sphingosine)-*N*-acyl transferase) thus preventing the de novo synthesis of ceramide[28,29] (Figure 5.1).

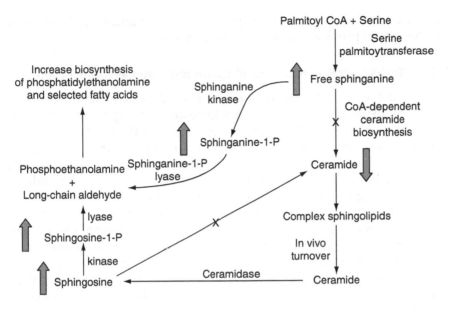

FIGURE 5.1
De novo sphingolipid biosynthetic pathway and degradation pathway showing point of disruption by fumonisin B_1 (FB_1). Since sphinganine is an intermediate and not a product of de novo biosynthesis its elimination is termed degradation. Gray arrows indicate the known effects on the metabolite pools in vivo as a result of disruption by FB_1. (From Riley, R.T. and Voss, K.A., *Toxicol. Sci.*, 92, 335, 2006. With permission.)

A correlation between disruption of sphingolipid metabolism and hepato-toxic or nephrotoxic end points has been demonstrated in rats, mice, horses, swine, and other species as reviewed by Bolger et al.[11] and Riley et al.[29] and inhibition occurs at doses equal to or less than those that cause overt toxicity. The immediate consequences of ceramide synthase inhibition include accumulation of the sphingoid bases sphinganine (Sa) and, to a lesser extent, sphingosine (So) and an increase in the Sa/So ratio in tissues, serum, and urine.[30,31] Complex sphingolipids, which are downstream meta-bolites of ceramide, decrease in tissues.[30] Accumulation of the 1-phosphate metabolites of Sa or So has also been demonstrated in the serum and kidney of rats,[31] the liver of ducks,[32] and the serum of pigs[33] after fumonisin exposure. Increased tissue, serum or urine Sa, and Sa/So are useful biomar-kers of fumonisin exposure in laboratory experiments; however, the overall extent of sphingolipid metabolism disruption might be underestimated if Sa-1-phosphate and So-1-phosphate are also not considered.[31]

Fumonisin-induced changes in Sa and Sa/So are reversible as Sa and So concentrations return to control levels upon removal of the exposure source.[34,35] However, Sa concentrations remain somewhat elevated, although well below peak levels, in animals given a relatively high dose of fumonisin followed by a continuous low-level exposure.[28,34] Due to these and other considerations, the use of Sa concentration and Sa/So as biomarkers in animal "field" experiments and human epidemiological studies can be problematic and has not been extensive.

5.2.2 Toxicological Implications of Sphingolipid Metabolism Disruption

The physiological consequences of sphingolipid metabolism disruption in fumonisin-exposed animals are likely to be far reaching. Sphingolipids are structural components of cell membrane-associated lipid rafts,[28] are signaling molecules for a diverse array of physiological functions,[28,29,36] and, in this regard, their concentrations in cells change in response to extracellular signaling stimuli[28,37] affecting cell survivability. Sa, So, and ceramide are proapoptotic, growth inhibitory and cytotoxic whereas So-1-phosphate is progrowth, antiapoptotic, and promotes cell differentiation.[28,36,38] The ratio of So-1-phosphate to ceramide is likely a critical determinant of cell survival.[38] While sphingolipid metabolism disruption has been correlated with the onset of organ-specific pathological effects of fumonisins, proving a direct connection between specific sphingolipid concentration changes, such as increased Sa or decreased complex sphingolipids, and specific toxicological end points has been elusive. Nonetheless, there is ample evidence consistent with the hypothesis that disruption of sphingolipid metabolism disrupts the balance between apoptosis and mitosis in tissues and that this imbalance is a critical component of fumonisin's carcinogenic mode of action.[11,29,39] FB$_1$ also inhibits cell adhesion (cell–cell and cell–matrix) and affects membrane permeability, likely through mechanisms that are sphingolipid dependent.[40–42] Moreover, So blocks L-type calcium channels,[43] an effect which might contribute to PPE (see below).

So-1-P is now recognized as a ligand for a family of membrane bound G-protein-coupled sphingosine-1-phosphate receptors (S1PR, formerly designated endothelial growth and differentiation or Edg receptors)[36,44,45] that are involved in multiple physiological processes including cell proliferation and survival, cell differentiation, apoptosis, cell mobility, cell adhesion, and angiogenesis. So-1-P has been shown to decrease renal blood flow in rats via a mechanism that likely involves S1PR.[45]

There are only a few reports concerning the effect of ceramide synthase inhibition on ceramide and complex sphingolipid concentrations in vivo. Liver and kidney complex sphingolipids decreased in a dose-dependent manner in rats fed diets containing 15–150 ppm FB$_1$ for 4 weeks[30] as did sphingosine-containing complex sphingolipids in the liver of pigs fed with 39–175 ppm fumonisins (FB$_1$ + FB$_2$) for up to 14 days.[46] Serum complex sphingolipids of ponies were also decreased within days after the animals were put on feed containing 15–44 ppm fumonisins.[47] It is hypothesized that complex sphingolipid depletion is mechanistically involved in some aspects of fumonisin toxicity. A likely example is that a reduction of complex sphingolipids found in membrane-associated lipid rafts disrupts processes that are dependent on these structures, such as pathogen recognition[11,28,48] and vitamin uptake.[49]

5.3   Diseases in Farm Animals

Equine leukoencephalomalacia and PPE are recognized toxicoses of fumonisins in farm animals. The clinical course and pathology of these diseases are reviewed in detail[11,50–53] and are summarized below.

5.3.1   Equine Leukoencephalomalacia

5.3.1.1   *Clinical Course and Pathology*

Equine leukoencephalomalacia (ELEM) is a hemorrhagic and liquefactive lesion of the white matter. Clinically, the syndrome has rapid onset and affected animals present with loss of appetite, listlessness, ataxia, "head pressing," paralysis of facial muscles, recumbency, and death. There may be liver involvement (hepatotoxic ELEM) and, in advanced cases, the liver becomes small, pale, and firm. Apoptosis, necrosis, and fibrosis are found microscopically.

5.3.1.2   *Experimental Findings*

Cerebral edema and focal hemorrhagic lesions were found in a horse that was given seven intravenous injections of 0.125 mg/kg body weight over 9 days.[17] Clinical signs and brain lesions indicative of ELEM were also induced in a horse orally dosed with 1.25–4 mg FB_1/kg body weight over 33 days and in a second horse orally given 1–4 mg FB_1/kg body weight over 29 days.[16] In other studies, a no observed effect level of 0.01 mg/kg body weight was observed in horses given intravenous injections of FB_1 for 28 days.[54] Doses of $\geq$0.05 FB_1 elicited mild clinical signs of neurotoxicity after 6 days with more severe neurological effects developing about day 9. Spinal taps revealed changes in the cerebrospinal fluid of the horses exhibiting neurologic signs (elevated IgG, cerebrospinal protein, and albumin concentrations and increased albumin quotients [ratio of albumin in cerebrospinal fluid/serum]) that suggested fumonisin treatment caused vasogenic cerebral edema. As in other species, fumonisins disrupt sphingolipid metabolism in Equidae.[47,55,56] Smith et al.[55] gave intravenous injections of 0, 0.01, or 0.2 mg FB_1/kg body weight to horses for up to 28 days and found that serum and right ventricular Sa and So were increased in the treated horses. Those animals having clinical signs of neurotoxicity also showed cardiovascular effects including decreased heart rates, cardiac outputs, and right ventricular contractility as well as increased systemic vascular resistance leading the authors to suggest that impaired cardiovascular function might play a role in ELEM. FB_2 and FB_3 also affect sphingolipid profiles in Equidae. Feed contaminated with *F. proliferatum* culture material providing 75 ppm FB_2 ($\leq$3 ppm FB_1 or FB_3) caused hepatotoxic ELEM and disrupted sphingolipid metabolism in ponies.[56] In the same experiment, feed contaminated with 75 ppm FB_3 (<1 ppm FB_1 or FB_2) provided by another *F. proliferatum* isolate did not cause ELEM but did disrupt sphingo-lipid metabolism, albeit less effectively than the feed contaminated with FB_2.[56] FDA guidance levels[27] indicate that total fumonisin ($FB_1 + FB_2 + FB_3$) concentrations in corn and corn by-product components of rations for Equidae should not exceed 5 ppm and the finished product should not contain more than 1 ppm.

5.3.2 Porcine Pulmonary Edema

5.3.2.1 Clinical and Pathological Findings

Porcine pulmonary edema is a sporadic syndrome of swine that, like ELEM, is associated with the consumption of *F. verticillioides* or *F. proliferatum*-molded corn. The disease has been reproduced by intravenous injection of purified FB_1[18] and by feeding fumonisin-contaminated diets.[19,50] The intoxicated animals lose their appetite and become listless, suffer respiratory distress, and ultimately succumb to respiratory failure. Fluid-filled, often markedly distended lungs are typically found at necropsy. Brain lesions are absent and the liver might be involved. The FDA guidance for swine feed is that the corn and corn by-products therein should contain no more than 20 ppm total fumonisins and that the finished feed should contain no more than 10 ppm.[27]

5.3.2.2 Mechanistic Aspects

Sauviat et al.[57] reported that FB_1 blocked calcium current and inhibited mechanical contractility of isolated frog heart atria. This is significant in that it suggests PPE could be secondary to left-sided cardiac insufficiency. Indeed, experiments have shown that exposure to FB_1 or *F. verticillioides* culture materials decreased cardiac output, heart rate, and mean arterial pressure while at the same time increasing pulmonary artery pressure and pulmonary resistance in pigs.[43,58] Sa and So concentrations in the left ventricle and plasma of these animals were elevated[43,58] and, in another experiment, increased serum So-1-P (and Sa-1-P)[33] concentrations were found in fumonisin-exposed pigs. These observations have mechanistic implications because So blocks L-type calcium channels, thereby, potentially inhibiting myocardial contractility by interfering with calcium ion transport in heart muscle.[43,58] As in rats,[45] there is evidence suggesting that sphingolipids can affect vascular tone in pigs. Sa and So relaxed phenylephrin-contracted and -uncontracted porcine thoracic aortic or pulmonary arterial rings (So only) in vitro.[59] So-1-P exerted a minimal affect on the aortic and phenylnephrin-treated pulmonary arterial rings, but increased the tension of untreated pulmonary arterial rings. Further in vivo experiments are needed to further explore the effects of sphingolipids on vascular resistance and determine the relevance of these in vitro observations in the pathophysiology of PPE.

5.3.3 Other Species

Reports on the toxicity of fumonisins to other agriculturally important animals including poultry, ruminants, mink, and catfish have been summarized by the FDA Center for Veterinary Medicine.[27] The liver is the main target organ and, as in other species, sphingolipid metabolism is disrupted. With the exception of catfish, however, the aforementioned species are less sensitive to fumonisins than horses, pigs, laboratory rodents, or rabbits. Accordingly, the guidance levels that have been issued for these species are higher than those for horses and swine and range from 15 (breeding stock, all species) to 50 (poultry) ppm total fumonisins in finished feed rations. Rabbits are extremely sensitive to fumonisins and develop liver and kidney pathologies similar to those of laboratory rodents at low doses. The FDA guidance for total fumonisins in formulated rabbit feeds is 1 ppm and fumonisins should not exceed 5 ppm in the corn and corn by-product component (not to exceed 20% w/w) of the ration. The guidance for catfish is 10 ppm.

5.4 Toxicological Effects in Laboratory Animals

5.4.1 Subchronic Toxicity and Pathological Findings

A series of studies showed that the liver and kidney are the two major target organs in rodents.[9,11] Moreover, the pathology induced by *F. verticillioides*, *F. verticillioides* culture materials, and purified FB_1 were similar,[9,14,60] thus establishing the connection between *F. verticillioides* toxicity and FB_1. Culture materials prepared from fungal isolates that produce FB_2 or FB_3 (but not FB_1)[35] induced lesions in rats similar to those caused by FB_1, although the findings also suggested that FB_2 and FB_3 were less potent. Howard et al.[61] fed a series of diets with equivalent amounts (ranging up to 140 μmol/kg diet = 101 ppm FB_1 equivalents) of FB_1, FB_2, FB_3, and hydrolyzed FB_1 to female mice for 28 days. They found altered tissue sphingolipid profiles and hepatic lesions only in those animals fed diets with 70 and 140 μmol/kg FB_1 and concluded that FB_1 is the major hepatotoxic fumonisin in mice. That ELEM developed in ponies given feed contaminated with 75 ppm FB_2 but not in ponies given feed containing 75 ppm FB_3[56] provides further evidence that differences exist in the potency of FB_1, FB_2, and FB_3.

The microscopic liver and kidney pathology in rats exposed to fumonisins is well documented.[11,35,50,60–66] The initial microscopic finding in liver is usually scattered apoptotic hepatocytes (or "single cell necrosis" in early reports). As injury progresses, the number of apoptotic cells increases and cytoplasmic vacuolation, mitosis, cytomegaly, anisocytosis, and anisokaryosis appear. Bile duct proliferation, focal (oncotic or coagulative) necrosis, fibrosis, oval cell proliferation, and hepatocellular hyperplasia are seen in advanced lesions, giving the severely affected liver a nodular or cirrhotic appearance. Choleangiofibrosis and foci of cellular alteration (morphological assessment) and enzyme (γ-glutamyl-transpeptidase [GGT] or glutathione sulfotransferase [GST])-positive foci have also been reported.[14,65] Serum chemical indicators of hepatotoxicity including alanine and aspartate aminotransferase, and alkaline phosphatase activities; as well as cholesterol, triglycerides, and bilirubin concentrations are increased. There is a sex-dependent difference in response, with no observed effect levels (NOEL) being somewhat lower in females[9,61,63,64] (Table 5.1).

The hepatic effects in mice are similar to those reported for rats and include apoptosis and increased mitosis.[9,62,67] A dietary no observed effect level of 27 ppm FB_1 was established for female $B6C3F_1$ mice in a 90 day feeding study.[62] Hepatotoxicity (apoptosis and serum chemical indications of liver injury) were found at 81 ppm. In contrast, no evidence of hepatotoxicity was found in male mice fed diets supplemented with 81 ppm FB_1, the highest dietary concentration tested.

In Sprague-Dawley and F344 rats, the kidney is a more sensitive target organ than liver: the NOEL (studies $\leq$90 days) for nephropathy in males is lower than both the NOEL for nephropathy in females and the NOEL for hepatopathy in either sex[35,61–64,66] (Table 5.1). As in liver, apoptosis is an early finding. The apoptotic epithelial cells are scattered throughout the proximal tubules of the outer medulla (or corticomedullary junction). Only a few are present at low doses, but, with increased exposure, apoptotic cells become more numerous and detach from the basement membrane while the number of mitotic figures increase. Additional features appearing in more severely affected kidneys are tubular hyperplasia with cytoplasmic basophilia, decreased epithelial height, cytoplasmic vacuolation, and variation in the size of cell and nucleus. Focal tubular atrophy with hyaline deposition or interstitial fibrosis may be present but interstitial inflammation is generally absent or minimal, except in the most severe cases. Taken together, this spectrum of changes can be summarized as simultaneous cell loss (apoptosis and tubular atrophy) and replication (mitotic figures and tubular hyperplasia). Decreased kidney weights, which are often found in fumonisin-exposed rats, suggest that the overall balance between apoptosis and regeneration is shifted in favor of cell loss.[61,62,66] It has been proposed that constant compensatory regeneration in response to apoptosis is an important component of FB_1's epigenetic mechanism of renal carcinogenesis in male rats,[39,66] allowing critically damaged cells to escape apoptosis. Functional indications of fumonisin-induced renal toxicity in rats include increased urinary enzyme levels (GGT, lactate dehydrogenase, N-acetyl-β-D-glucosamine), increased urine volume, proteinuria, and reduced anion (p-aminohippuric acid) and cation (tetraethylammonium) transport.[68] While less sensitive than rats, apoptosis also occurs in the kidney tubules of fumonisin-exposed mice.[9,11,67,69]

TABLE 5.1

Summary of Dose-Response in Male and Female Rats Subchronically Fed with Diets Containing FB_1

Strain	Exposure Duration	FB_1 in the Diet (ppm)	Males		Females		Reference
			Liver	Kidney	Liver	Kidney	
Sprague-Dawley	28 days	0,15,50,150	NOEL = 50 LOEL = 150	NOEL <15	NOEL = 50 LOEL = 150	NOEL = 15 LOEL = 50	[60]
F344	28 days	0,99,163, 234,484	NOEL = 163 LOEL = 234	NOEL <99	NOEL = 99 LOEL = 163	NOEL = 99 LOEL = 163	[66]
F344	90 days	0,3,9,27,81	NOEL = >81	NOEL = 3 LOEL = 9	NOEL = 27 LOEL = 81	NOEL = 27 LOEL = 81	[62]

Note: NOEL, no observed effect level, ppm; LOEL, lowest observed effect level, ppm.

5.4.2 Carcinogenicity

F. verticillioides culture material[7] and corn naturally contaminated with fumonisins[70] were hepatocarcinogenic when fed to rats. Gelderblom et al., using a rat liver bioassay based on the induction of GGT-positive foci, reproduced the liver cancer promoting activity of *F. verticillioides* strain MRC 826 (MRC 826; which has since become a widely used fungal isolate for fumonisin research) with FB_1[14] and then demonstrated that FB_1 is hepatocarcinogenic.[21] In the chronic feeding study,[21] in which BD IX male (the only sex tested) rats were fed 50 ppm FB_1, all animals examined after 18 months developed cirrhosis and 10 of 15 rats examined between 18 and 26 months had primary hepatocellular carcinoma. FB_1 was not nephrocarcinogenic in this study, although chronic interstitial nephritis was found at 26 weeks. Proliferative lesions of the type previously found in the esophagus or forestomach of rats after chronic dietary exposure to fungal culture materials[8] were not present in the FB_1-exposed rats, indicating that FB_1 was not the cause of these lesions in the earlier experiments.

Two-year feeding studies of FB_1 in F344/Nctr rats and B6C3F$_1$ mice were conducted by Howard et al.[22] Dietary FB_1 concentrations for the rat study were 0, 5, 15, 50, and either 100 (females) or 150 (males) ppm. FB_1 was nephrocarcinogenic in males fed $\geq$50 ppm FB_1. The neoplastic lesions consisted of tubular adenomas and carcinomas. Among the 18 carcinomas identified in the 50 and 150 ppm groups,[71] the majority represented a highly malignant, anaplastic phenotype and, among these, one displayed a sarcomatous appearance previously unknown in rodents. Other renal lesions included (proximal) tubular apoptosis, regeneration and hyperplasia, and interstitial hyalinization in males fed 50 or 150 ppm and, to a lesser degree, in the females fed 100 ppm FB_1. No other neoplastic effects were found. FB_1 dietary concentrations for the chronic mouse study were 0, 5, 15, 50 (females only), 80, or 150 (males only) ppm. FB_1 was hepatocarcinogenic to the female mice at concentrations $\geq$50 ppm. The combined incidences of hepatocellular adenomas and carcinomas in the groups fed 50 or 80 ppm FB_1 were 40% and 87%, respectively, and ranged from 2% (15 ppm) to 11% (controls) in the other groups. No neoplastic effects were found in males.

It is not known why the target organs in the rat feeding studies of Gelderblom et al.[21] and Howard et al.[22] differed. Strain- and sex-dependent differences in sphingolipid metabolism, fumonisin accumulation, or other physiological factors might play a role or, as discussed by Gelderblom et al.,[70] compositional differences in the diets used in these studies might have been critical. In any event, the chronic feeding studies clearly demonstrated that FB_1 is a rodent carcinogen at dietary concentrations $\geq$50 ppm, but provided no evidence that FB_1 caused neoplastic esophageal lesions. Gelderblom et al.[72] reported on the clinical chemistry, sphingoid base profile, and other indications of liver and kidney toxicity that were found in vervet monkeys fed MRC 826 that provided estimated doses of 0.35–0.39 (high dose) or 0.15 (low dose) mg/kg body weight FB_1 over 13.5 years.

Liver biopsies revealed apoptosis, fibrosis, nodular hyperplasia, mild to scant bile duct proliferation, and in some cases, inflammatory infiltrates. No neoplastic effects were reported.

Simultaneous exposure to fumonisins and other mycotoxins, especially aflatoxin, is a potential concern. FB_1 promoted cancer in the liver of aflatoxin-initiated rainbow trout and in multiple organs of *N*-methyl-*N'*-nitro-nitrosoguanidine-initiated trout when fed to the fish for 34 weeks.[73] FB_1 disrupted sphingolipid metabolism and the sphingoid base profile changes were correlated with the mycotoxin's cancer promoting effect in the aflatoxin-initiated group. This suggests that sphingolipid-dependent signaling might have a mechanistic role in liver cancer promotion and that additive or synergistic effects in other species concurrently exposed to aflatoxin and fumonisins are possible. Results of an experiment utilizing a short-term carcinogenicity assay support this supposition. Specifically, the number and size of enzyme (GSTP)-positive foci in the liver of rats sequentially treated with aflatoxin B_1 and FB_1 was increased compared to animals receiving only aflatoxin or FB_1.[74] Due to the potential for coexposure,[74–77] further experiments are needed to determine the extent to which these mycotoxins act additively or synergistically, especially in regard to their carcinogenic potential.

5.5 Neural Tube Defects

5.5.1 Observations Implicating Fumonisins as a Risk Factor

Neural tube defects (NTDs) are congenital malformations that include the phenotypes spina bifida, exencephaly, and craniorhachischisis[12,13] and are a consequence of a failure of the neural tube to close properly during gestation. They are relatively common birth defects, having an average incidence of about 10/10,000 live births. Except for most mild manifestations, NTDs are either not compatible with life or the newborn dies from infection of the exposed tissue.

NTD rates among Mexican-American women in the Texas–Mexico border region increased from their average of about 15/10,000 to 27/10,000 live births in 1990–1991 and a possible link between fumonisins and NTDs was suggested.[12,78] Relatively high rates of NTD-affected pregnancies are also seen in parts of southern Africa (35–61/10,000), northern China (57–73/10,000), and Guatamala (up to 106/10,000 in some areas) where the population depends on maize as a food source and where the maize is likely contaminated with fumonisins.[78] NTD etiology is not well understood but is clearly a multifactoral process involving genetic, nutritional, and environmental factors.[79,80] The role of fumonisins as a risk factor for NTDs remains uncertain; however, laboratory studies have provided the basis for a mechanistic hypothesis for further investigations.

5.5.2　Mechanistic Hypothesis

Folate is an important nutritional factor for reducing the risk of NTD-affected pregnancies.[79] FB_1 inhibited carrier-mediated transport of folate in Caco-2 cells[49] in vitro and in pregnant LM/Bc mice in vivo.[13] Because the high-affinity placental folate carrier (a GPI-anchored protein known as folate binding protein 1 or *folbp*1 in mice and folate receptor α in humans) is associated with sphingolipid-rich lipid rafts in cell membranes, the following chain of events leading to an increased risk of an NTD affected pregnancy were hypothesized: (1) ceramide synthase is inhibited by fumonisin; (2) complex sphingolipids in lipid rafts are decreased; (3) *folbp*1 function is disrupted; and (4) folate transport is inhibited at the critical time for neural tube closure.

5.5.3　Mouse Models

Rodent and rabbit reproductive and teratology studies of *F. verticillioides* indicated that fumonisins were fetotoxic at high, maternally toxic doses but showed no evidence of teratogenicity (reviewed in[9,11]). A dose-dependent increase in NTDs (exencephaly) was induced; however, intraperitoneal injections of ≥ 5 mg/kg body weight FB_1 were given to pregnant LM/Bc mice.[13] The timing of the doses, which were given during gestation days 7.5 and 8.5, the critical time for neural tube closure, was important. A NOEL was not found. All litters were NTD positive at doses ≥ 15 mg/kg body weight and, at the highest dose of 20 mg/kg body weight, 80% of the embryos were affected. Furthermore, ^{14}C-FB_1 biodistribution experiments and sphingolipid measurements indicated that FB_1 crossed the placenta of LM/Bc mice. These findings are in contrast to those of earlier experiments in rodents and rabbits[9,11] that provided no evidence for in utero exposure. These apparently contradictory results have not yet been reconciled. The gestation day (stage of placental development) on which the experiments were carried out (earlier in the LM/Bc studies of Gelineau-van Waes et al.[13]) or species-/strain-related differences in placental physiology are possible explanations.

Additional findings in LM/Bc mice support the hypothesis that fumonisin-exposure increases the risk of NTDs by disrupting folate transport. These findings are: (a) FB_1 exposure decreased the accumulation of radiolabel in the embryos of dams injected with ^3H-folate; (b) treating the FB_1-exposed (20 mg/kg body weight) dams with folate (50 mg/kg body weight) during gestation significantly reduced (ca. 50% reduction) the incidence of NTDs; and (c) administration of the complex sphingolipid ganglioside GM_1 (10 mg/kg body weight) during gestation reduced the incidence (ca. 95% reduction) of NTDs even more effectively than did folate.[13]

Reddy et al.[81] found no evidence of NTDs or other teratogenic effects when maternally toxic doses of FB_1 were given by gavage to pregnant CD1 mice. To determine if they are refractory to NTD induction by FB_1, pregnant CD1 mice were given FB_1[82] according to the intraperitoneal dosing protocol of Gelineau-van Waes et al.[13] Doses ranged from 15 to 45 mg/kg body weight in the first and from 10 to 100 mg/kg body weight in the second trial. Dose-related increases in the incidence of NTD-positive litters were found in both experiments. Approximately 40% of the litters were positive at 45 mg/kg body weight FB_1 (both trials) and the highest incidence of affected litters, 55%, was found at 100 mg/kg body weight FB_1 (trial 2). Furthermore, a NOEL was not established as 11% (1 of 9 litters, trial 1)–8% (1 of 12 litters, trial 2) of the low-dose litters in the two trials were NTD positive. Thus, FB_1 does induce NTDs in CD1 mice, although they are less sensitive than the LM/Bc strain. Comparative studies, using these and other mouse strains, will be useful models for elucidating the mechanism(s) underlying NTD induction in mice and ascertaining their relevance to humans.

5.6 Summary and Conclusion

FB_1 is the most thoroughly studied of the *Fusarium* mycotoxins known as fumonisins. While the human health effects of fumonisins are unclear, FB_1 has been established as a cause of the animal diseases resulting from the ingestion of *F. verticillioides* and *F. proliferatum* contaminated feed. These include equine leukoencephalomalacia, porcine pulmonary edema, liver and kidney toxicity in multiple species, and liver and kidney cancer in rodents. FB_1 and other fumonisins inhibit the enzyme ceramide synthase in vivo, an event that disrupts sphingolipid metabolism and is the trigger underlying the molecular events mediating fumonisin toxicity. These events include disruption of sphingolipid-dependent and other signaling pathways, altering the balance between apoptotic cell death and cell proliferation in target tissues, interfering with nutrient transport, inhibition of cell-to-cell or cell to substrate adhesion, or other key functions. While the general toxicology of fumonisins is well characterized, efforts to better understand the toxicology and mechanism of action of these common mycotoxins continue. Determining the mechanistic roles that sphingoid base 1-phosphates and complex sphingolipids play in fumonisin toxicity and the relationships between fumonisins, sphingolipids, and neural tube defects in mouse models are two areas of ongoing research to determine the extent to which these mycotoxins are risk factors for human health.

References

1. Haliburton, J.C. and Buck, W.B. Equine leucoencephalomalacia: An historical review, *Curr. Top. Vet. Med. Anim. Sci.*, 33, 75, 1986.
2. Haliburton, J.C., Vesonder, R.F., Lock, T.F., and Buck, W.B. Equine leucoencephalomalacia (ELEM): A study of *Fusarium moniliforme* as an etiological agent, *Vet. Hum. Toxicol.*, 21, 348, 1979.

3. Wilson, B.J. and Maronpot, R.R. Causative fungus agent of leukoencephaloma-lacia in equine animals, *Vet. Record*, 88, 484, 1971.
4. Kriek, N.P.J., Kellerman, T.S., and Marasas, W.F.O. Comparative study of the toxicity of *Fusarium verticillioides* (= *F. moniliforme*) to horses, primates, pigs, sheep and rats, *Onderstepoort J. vet. Res.*, 48, 129, 1981.
5. Diaz, G.J. and Boermans, H.J. Fumonisin toxicosis in domestic animals: A review, *Vet. Hum. Toxicol.*, 36, 548, 1994.
6. Palyusik, M. and Moran, E.M. Porcine pulmonary edema with hydrothorax: A review, *J. Environ. Pathol. Toxicol. Oncol.*, 13, 63, 1994.
7. Jaskiewicz, K., van Rensburg, S.J., Marasas, W.F.O., and Gelderblom, W.C.A. Carcinogenicity of *Fusarium moniliforme* culture material in rats, *J. Natl. Cancer Inst.* 78, 321, 1987.
8. Marasas, W.F.O., Kriek, N.P.J., Finchem, J.E., and van Rensburg, S.J. Primary liver cancer and oesophageal basal cell hyperplasia in rats caused by *Fusarium moniliforme*, *Int. J. Cancer*, 34, 383, 1984.
9. Voss, K.A., Riley, R.T., Norred, W.P., Bacon, C.W., Meredith, F.I., Howard, P.C., Plattner, R.D., Collins, T.F.X., Hansen, D.K., and Porter, J.K. An overview of rodent toxicities: Liver and kidney effects of fumonisins and *Fusarium moniliforme*, *Environ. Health Perspect.*, 109 (Suppl. 2), 259, 2001.
10. Marasas, W.F.O. Fumonisins: Their implications for human and animal health, *Nat. Toxins*, 3, 193, 1995.
11. Bolger, M., Coker, R.D., DiNovi, M., Gaylor, D., Gelderblom, W.C.A., Olsen, M., Paster, N., Riley, R.T., Shephard, G., and Speijers, G.J.A. Fumonisins. In: *Safety Evaluation of Certain Mycotoxins in Foods. FAO Food and Nutrition Paper 74*, World Health Organization, Geneva, pp. 103–279, 2001.
12. Missmer, S.A., Suarez, L., Felkner, M., Wang, E., Merrill, A.H., Jr., Rothman, K.J., and Hendricks, K.A. Exposure to fumonisins and the occurrence of neural tube defects along the Texas-Mexico border, *Environ. Health Perspect.*, 114, 237, 2006.
13. Gelineau-van Waes, J.B., Starr, L., Maddox, J.R., Aleman, F., Voss, K.A., Wilberding, J., and Riley, R.T. Maternal fumonisin exposure and risk for neural tube defects: Mechanisms in an *in vivo* mouse model. *Birth Defects Res. Part. A Clin. Mol. Teratol.*, 73, 487, 2005.
14. Gelderblom, W.C.A., Jaskiewicz, K., Marasas, W.F.O., Thiel, P.G., Horak, R.M., Vleggaar, R., and Kriek, N.P.J. Fumonisins-novel mycotoxins with cancer pro-moting activity produced by *Fusarium moniliforme*, *Appl. Environ. Microbiol.*, 54, 1806, 1988.
15. Humpf, H.U. and Voss, K.A. Effects of food processing on the chemical structure and toxicity of fumonisin mycotoxins. *Mol. Nutr. Food Res.*, 48, 255, 2004.
16. Kellerman, T.S., Marasas, W.F.O., Thiel, P.G., Gelderblom, W.C.A., Cawood, M., and Coetzer, J.A.W. Leukoencephalomalacia in two horses induced by oral dosing of fumonisin B_1, *Onderstepoort J. vet. Res.*, 57, 269, 1990.
17. Marasas, W.F.O., Kellerman, T.S., Gelderblom, W.C.A., Coetzer, J.A.W., Thiel, P.G., and van der Lugt, J.J. Leukoencephalomalacia in a horse induced by fumo-nisin B_1 isolated from *Fusarium moniliforme*, *Onderstepoort J. vet. Res.*, 55, 197, 1988.
18. Harrison, L.R., Colvin, B.M., Greene, J.T., Newman, L.E., and Cole, Jr. J.R. Pulmonary edema and hydrothorax in swine produced by fumonisin B_1, a toxic metabolite of *Fusarium moniliforme*, *J. Vet. Diagn. Invest.*, 2, 217, 1990.
19. Haschek, W.M., Motelin, G., Ness, D.K., Harlin, K.S., Hall, W.F., Vesonder, R.F., Peterson, R.E., and Beasley, V.R. Characterization of fumonisin toxicity in orally and intravenously dosed swine, *Mycopathologia*, 117, 83, 1992.

20. Colvin, B.M., Cooley, A.J., and Beaver, R.W. Fumonisin toxicosis in swine: Clinical and pathologic findings, *J. Vet. Diagn. Invest.*, 5, 232, 1993.
21. Gelderblom, W.C.A., Kriek, N.P.J., Marasas, W.F.O., and Thiel, P.G. Toxicity and carcinogenicity of the *Fusarium moniliforme* metabolite, fumonisin B_1 in rats, *Carcinogenesis*, 12, 1247, 1991.
22. Howard, P.C., Eppley, R.M., Stack, M.E., Warbritton, A., Voss, K.A., Lorentzen, R.J., Kovach, R.M., and Bucci, T.J. Fumonisin B_1 carcinogenicity in a two-year feeding study using F344 rats and B6C3F₁ mice, *Environ. Health Perspect.* 109 (Suppl. 2), 277, 2002.
23. International Agency for Research on Cancer. IARC Monographs on the Evaluation of Carcinogenic Risks to Humans, IARC Press, Lyon, 301, 2002.
24. Center for Food Safety and Nutrition, US Food and Drug Administration. Final guidance for industry, fumonisins in foods and animal feeds (November 9, 2001), http://www.cfsan.fda.gov/~dms/fumongu2.html, 2001.
25. Center for Food Safety and Nutrition, U.S. Food and Drug Administration. Background paper in support of fumonisin levels in corn and corn products intended for human consumption (November 9, 2001), http://www.cfsan.fda.gov/~dms/fumongu3.html, 2001.
26. Commission of European Communities. Commission Regulation (EC) No. 856/2005 of 6 June 2005 amending Regulation (EC) No. 466/2001 as regards *Fusarium* toxins. *Off. J. Eur. Union* 48, 3, 2005.
27. Center for Food Safety and Nutrition, U.S. Food and Drug Administration. Background paper in support of fumonisin levels in animal feed: Executive summary of this scientific document (November 9, 2001) http://www.cfsan.fda.gov/~dms/fumonbg4.html, 2001.
28. Merrill, Jr., A.H., Sullards, M.C., Wang, E., Voss, K.A., and Riley, R.T. Sphingolipid metabolism: Roles in signal transduction and disruption by fumonisins, *Environ. Health Perspect.*, 109 (Suppl. 2), 283, 2001.
29. Riley, R.T., Enongene, E.N., Voss K.A., Norred, W.P., Meredith, F.I., Sharma, R.P., Spitsbergen, J., Williams, D.E., Carlson, D.B., and Merrill, Jr., A.H. Sphingolipid perturbations as mechanisms for fumonisin carcinogenesis, *Environ. Health Perspect.*, 109 (Suppl. 2), 301, 2001.
30. Riley, R.T., Hinton, D.M., Chamberlain, W.J., Bacon, C.W., Wang, E., Merrill, Jr., A.H., and Voss, K.A. Dietary fumonisin B_1 induces disruption of sphingolipid metabolism in Sprague-Dawley rats: A new mechanism of nephrotoxicity, *J. Nutr.*, 124, 594, 1994.
31 Riley, R.T. and Voss, K.A. Differential sensitivity of rat kidney and liver to fumonisin toxicity: Organ-specific differences in toxin accumulation and sphingoid base metabolism, *Toxicol. Sci.*, 92, 335, 2006.
32. Tardieu, D., Tran, S.T., Auvergne, A., Babile, R., Benard, G., Bailly, J.D., and Guerre, P. Effects of fumonisins on liver and kidney sphinganine and the sphinganine to sphingosine ratio during chronic exposure in ducks, *Chem. Biol. Interact.*, 160, 51, 2006.
33. Piva, A., Casadei, G., Pagliuga, G., Cabassi, E., Galvano, F., Solfrizzo, M., Riley, R.T., and Diaz, D.E. Activated carbon does not prevent the toxicity of culture material containing fumonisin B_1 when fed to weanling piglets, *J. Anim. Sci.*, 83, 1939, 2005.
34. Enongene, E.N., Sharma, R.P., Bhandari, N., Miller, J.D., Meredith, F.I., Voss, K.A., and Riley, R.T., Persistence and reversibility of the elevation in free sphingoid bases induced by fumonisin inhibition of ceramide synthase, *Toxicol. Sci.*, 67, 173, 2002.

35. Voss, K.A., Plattner, R.D., Riley, R.T., Meredith, F.I., and Norred, W.P. *In vivo* effects of fumonisin B_1-producing and fumonisin B_1-nonproducing *Fusarium moniliforme* isolates are similar: Fumonisins B_2 and B_3 cause hepato- and nephrotoxicity in rats, *Mycopathologia*, 141, 45, 1998.
36. Chalfant, C.E. and Spiegel, S. Sphingosine 1-phosphate and ceramide 1-phosphate: Expanding roles in cell signaling, *J. Cell Sci.*, 118, 4605, 2005.
37. Neumeyer, J., Hallas, C., Merkel, O., Winoto-Morbach, S., Jakob, M., Thon, L., Adam, D., Schneider-Brachert, W., and Schütze, S. TNF-receptor I defective in internalization allows for cell death through activation of neutral sphingomyelinase, *Exp. Cell Res.*, 312, 2142, 2006.
38. Payne, S.G., Milstien, S., and Spiegel, S. Sphingosine-1-phosphate: Dual messenger functions. *FEBS Lett.*, 30, 54, 2002.
39. Dragan, Y.P., Bidlack, W.R., Cohen, S.M., Goldsworthy, T.L., Hard, G.C., Howard, P.C., Riley, R.T., and Voss, K.A. Implications of apoptosis for toxicity, carcinogenicity, and risk assessment: Fumonisin B_1 as an example, *Toxicol. Sci.*, 61, 6, 2001.
40. Gon, Y., Wood, M.R., Kiosses, W.B., Jo, E., Germanna Sanna, M., Chun, J., and Rosen, H. $S1P_3$ receptor-induced reorganization of epithelial tight junctions compromises lung barrier integrity and is potentiated by TNF, *PNAS*, 102L, 9270, 2005.
41. Pelagalli, A., Belisario, M.A., Squillacioti, C., Morte, R.D., d'Angelo, D., Tafuri, S., Lucisano, A., and Staiano, N. The mycotoxin fumonisin B_1 inhibits integrin-mediated cell-matrix adhesion, *Biochimie*, 81, 1003, 1999.
42. Ramasamy, S., Wang, E., Henning, B., and Merrill, Jr., A.H. Fumonisin B_1 alters sphingolipid metabolism and disrupts the barrier function of endothelial cells in culture, *Toxicol. Appl. Pharmacol.*, 133, 343, 1995.
43. Smith, G.W., Constable, P.D., Eppley, R.M., Tumbleson, M.E., Gumprecht, L.A., and Haschek-Hock, W.M. Purified fumonisin B_1 decreases cardiovascular function but does not alter pulmonary capillary permeability in swine, *Toxicol. Sci.*, 56, 240, 2000.
44. Pyne, S. and Pyne, N.J. Sphingosine 1-phosphate signaling in mammalian cells, *Biochem. J.*, 349, 385, 2000.
45. Bischoff, A., Czyborra, P., Meyer zu Heringdorf, D., Jakobs, K.H., and Michel, M.C. Sphingosine 1-phosphate reduces rat renal and mesenteric blood flow *in vivo* in a pertussis toxin-sensitive manner, *Br. J. Pharmacol.*, 130, 1878, 2000.
46. Riley, R.T., An, N.H., Showker, J.L., Yoo, H.-S., Norred, W.P., Chamberlain, W.J., Wang, E., Merrill, A.H., Jr., Motelin, G., Beasley, V.R., and Haschek, W.M. Alteration of tissues and serum sphinganine to sphingosine ratio: An early biomarker of exposure to fumonisin-containing feeds in pigs. *Toxicol. Appl. Pharmacol.*, 118, 105, 1993.
47. Wang, E., Ross, P.F., Wilson, T.M., Riley, R.T., and Merrill, Jr., A.H. Increases in serum sphingosine and sphinganine and decreases in complex sphingolipids in ponies given feed containing fumonisins, mycotoxins produced by *Fusarium moniliforme. J. Nutr.*, 122, 1706, 1992.
48. Dresden Obsborne, C., Pittman Noblet, G., Enongene, E.N., Bacon, C.W., Riley, R.T., and Voss, K.A. Host resistance to *Trypanosoma cruzi* infection is enhanced in mice fed *Fusarium verticillioides* ($=F.$ *moniliforme*) culture material containing fumonisins, *Food Chem. Toxicol.*, 40, 1789, 2002.
49. Stevens, V.L. and Tang, J. Fumonisin B_1-induced sphingolipid depletion inhibits vitamin uptake via the glycosylphosphatidylinositol-anchored folate receptor, *J. Biol. Chem.*, 272, 18020, 1997.

50. Haschek, W.M., Voss, K.A., and Beasley, V.R. Selected mycotoxins affecting animal and human health. In: *Handbook of Toxicologic Pathology*, 2nd Edition, Vol. 1, Haschek, Rousseaux, and Wallig, (Eds.), Academic Press, San Diego, pp. 645–699, 2002.

51. Voss, K.A., Riley, R.T., Plattner, R.D., Norred, W.P., Meredith, F.I., Porter, J.K., and Bacon, C.W. Toxicity associated with fumonisin contaminated corn. In: *Microbial Food Contamination*, Wilson and Droby, (Eds.), CRC Press, Boca Raton, FL, pp. 27–45, 2001.

52. Buck, W.B., Haliburton, J.C., Thilsted, J.P., Lock, T.F., and Vesonder, R.F. Equine leucoencephalomalacia: Comparative pathology of naturally occurring and experimental cases, *Am. Assoc. Vet. Lab. Diag.*, 239, 1979.

53. Wilson, T.M., Ross, P.F., Owens, D.L., Rice, L.G., Green, S.A., Jenkins, S.J., and Nelson, H.A. Experimental reproduction of ELEM. A study to determine the minimum toxic dose in ponies, *Mycopathologia*, 117, 115, 1992.

54. Foreman, J.H., Constable, P.D., Waggoner, A.L., Levy, M., Eppley, R.M., Smith, G.W., Tumbleson, M.E., and Haschek, W.M. Neurologic abnormalities and cerebrospinal fluid changes in horses administered fumonisin B_1 intravenously, *J. Vet. Intern. Med.*, 18, 223, 2004.

55. Smith, G.W., Constable, P.D., Foreman, J.H., Eppley, R.M., Waggoner, A.L., Tumbleson, M.E., and Haschek, W.M. Cardiovascular changes associated with intravenous administration of fumonisin B_1 in horses, *Am. J. Vet. Res.*, 63, 538, 2002.

56. Riley, R.T., Showker, J.L., Owens, D.L., and Ross, P.F. Disruption of sphingolipid metabolism and induction of equine leukoencephalomalacia by *Fusarium proliferatum* culture material containing fumonisin B_2 of B_3, *Environ. Toxicol. Pharmacol.*, 3, 221, 1997.

57. Sauviat, M.P., Laurent, D., Kohler, F., and Pellegrin, F. Fumonisin, a toxin from the fungus *Fusarium moniliforme* Sheld blocks both the calcium current and the mechanical activity in frog atrial muscle, *Toxicon*, 29, 1025, 1991.

58. Constable, P.D., Smith, G.W., Rottinghaus, G.E., Tumbleson, M.E., and Haschek, W.M. Fumonisin-induced blockade of ceramide synthase in sphingolipid biosynthetic pathway alters aortic input impedance spectrum of pigs, *Am. J. Physiol. Heart Circ. Physiol.*, 284, H2034, 2003.

59. Hsiao, S.H., Constable, P.D., Smith, G.W., and Haschek, W.M. Effects of exogenous sphinganine, sphingosine, and sphingosine-1-phosphate on relaxation and contraction of porcine thoracic aortic and pulmonary arterial rings, *Toxicol. Sci.*, 86, 194, 2005.

60. Voss, K.A., Chamberlain, W.J., Bacon, C.W., and Norred, W.P., A preliminary investigation on renal and hepatic toxicity in rats fed purified fumonisin B_1. *Nat. Toxins*, 1, 222, 1993.

61. Howard, P.C., Couch, L.H., Patton, R.E., Eppley, R.M., Doerge, D.R., Churchwell, M.I., Marques, M.M., and Okerberg, C.V. Comparison of the toxicity of several fumonisin derivatives in a 28-day feeding study with female $B6C3F_1$ mice, *Toxicol. Appl. Pharmacol.*, 185, 153, 2002.

62. Voss, K.A., Chamberlain, W.J., Bacon, C.W., Herbert, R.A., Walters, D.B., and Norred, W.P. Subchronic feeding study of the mycotoxin fumonisin B_1 in $B6C3F_1$ mice and Fischer 344 rats, *Fundam. Appl. Toxicol.*, 24, 102, 1995.

63. Bondy, G., Barker, M., Mueller, R., Fernie, S., Miller, J.D., Armstrong, C., Hierlihy, S.L., Rowsell, P., and Suzuki, C. Fumonisin B_1 toxicity in male Sprague-Dawley rats, *Adv. Exper. Med. Biol.*, 392, 251, 1996.

64. Bondy, G.S., Suzuki, C.A.M., Mueller, R.W., Fernie, S.M., Armstrong, C.L., and Hierlihy, S.L. Gavage Administration of the fungal toxin fumonisin B_1 to female Sprague-Dawley rats, *J. Toxicol. Environ. Health*, Part A, 53, 135, 1998.

65. Mehta, R., Lok, E., Rowsell, P.R., Miller, J.D., Suzuki, C.A., and Bond, G.S. Glutathione S-transferase-placental form expression and proliferation of hepatocytes in fumonisin B_1-treated male and female Sprague-Dawley rats. *Cancer Lett.*, 128, 31, 1998.

66. Howard, P.C., Warbritton, A., Voss, K.A., Lorentzen, R.J., Thurman, J.D., Kovach, R.M., and Bucci, T.J. Compensatory regeneration as a mechanism for renal tubule carcinogenesis of fumonisin B_1 in the F344/N/Nctr BR rat, *Environ. Health Perspect.*, 109 (Suppl. 2), 309, 2001.

67. Sharma, R.P., Dugyala, R.R., and Voss, K.A. Demonstration of *in-situ* apoptosis in mouse liver and kidney after short-term repeated exposure to fumonisin B_1, *J. Comp. Pathol.*, 117, 371, 1997.

68. Suzuki, C.A.M., Hierlihy, L., Barker, M., Curran, I., Mueller, R., and Bondy, G.S. The effects of fumonisin B_1 on several markers of nephrotoxicity in rats, *Toxicol. Appl. Pharmacol.*, 133, 207, 1995.

69. Bucci, T.J., Howard, P.C., Tolleson, W.H., Laborde, J.B., and Hansen, D.K. Renal effects of fumonisin mycotoxins in animals, *Toxicol. Pathol.*, 26, 160, 1998.

70. Gelderblom, W.C.A., Rheeder, J.P., Leggott, N., Stockenstrom, S., Humphreys, J., Shepard, G.S., and Marasas, W.F.O. Fumonisin contamination of a corn sample associated with the induction of hepatocarcinogenesis in rats-role of dietary deficiencies, *Food Chem. Toxicol.*, 42, 471, 2004.

71. Hard, G.C., Howard, P.C., Kovatch, R.M., and Bucci, T.J. Rat kidney pathology induced by chronic exposure to fumonisin B_1 includes rare variants of renal tubule tumor, *Toxicol. Pathol.*, 29, 379, 2001.

72. Gelderblom, W.C.A., Seier, J.V., Snijman, P.W., Van Schalkwyk, D.J., Shephard, G.S., and Marasas, W.F. Toxicity of a culture material of *Fusarium verticillioides* strain MRC 826 to nonhuman primates, *Environ. Health Perspect.*, 109 (Suppl. 2), 267, 2001.

73. Carlson, D.B., Williams, D.E., Spitsbergen, J.M., Ross, P.F., Bacon, C.W., Meredith, F.I., and Riley, R.T. Fumonisin B_1 promotes aflatoxin B_1 and N-methyl-N'-nitro-nitrosoguanidine-initiated liver tumors in rainbow trout, *Toxicol. Appl. Pharmacol.*, 172, 29, 2001.

74. Gelderblom, W.C., Marasas, W.F., Lebepe-Mazur, S., Swanevelder, S., Vessey, C.J., and Hall Pde, L. Interaction of fumonisin B_1 and aflatoxin B_1 in a short-term carcinogenesis model in rat liver. *Toxicology*, 17, 161, 2002.

75. Chamberlain, W.J., Bacon, C.W., Norred, W.P., and Voss, K.A. Levels of fumonisin B_1 in corn naturally contaminated with aflatoxins, *Food Chem. Toxicol.*, 12, 995, 1993.

76. Bankole, S.A. and Mabekoje, O.O. Occurrence of aflatoxins and fumonisins in preharvest maize from south-western Nigeria. *Food Addit. Contam.*, 21, 251, 2004.

77. Pacin, A.M., Gonzalez, H.H., Etcheverry, M., Resnik, S.L., Vivas, L., and Espin, S. Fungi associated with food and feed commodities from Ecuador. *Mycopathologia*, 156, 87, 2003.

78. Marasas, W.F., Riley, R.T., Hendricks, K.A., Stevens, V.L., Sadler, T.W., Gelineau-van Waes, J., Missmer, S.A., Cabrera, J., Torres, O., Gelderblom, W.C., Allegood, J., Martinez, C., Maddox, J., Miller, J.D., Starr, L., Sullards, M.C., Roman, A.V., Voss, K.A., Wang, E., and Merrill, Jr., A.H. Fumonisins disrupt sphingolipid metabolism, folate transport, and neural tube development in

embryo culture and *in vivo*: A potential risk factor for human neural tube defects among populations consuming fumonisin-contaminated corn, *J. Nutr.,* 134, 711, 2004.

79. Cabrera, R.M., Hill, D.S., Etheredge, A.J., and Fennell, R.H. Investigations into the etiology of neural tube defects, *Birth Defects Res. C Embryo Today,* 72, 330, 2004.

80. Greene, N.D.E. and Copp, A.J. Mouse models of neural tube defects: Investigating preventive mechanisms. *Am. J. Med. Gen. Part C (Semin. Med. Genet.)* 135C, 31, 2005.

81. Reddy, R.V., Johnson, G., Rottinghaus, G.E., Casteel, S.W., and Reddy, C.S. Developmental effects of fumonisin B_1 in mice. *Mycopathologia,* 134, 161, 1996.

82. Voss, K.A., Gelineau-van Waes, J.B., and Riley, R.T. Fumonisins: Current research trends in developmental toxicology, *Mycotoxin Res.,* 22, 61, 2006.

6

Molecular and Biochemical Mechanisms of Action of Acute Toxicity and Carcinogenicity Induced by Aflatoxin B_1, and of the Chemoprevention of Liver Cancer

Avishay-Abraham Stark

CONTENTS

6.1 Acute Toxicity and Carcinogenicity of Aflatoxin to Humans

Aflatoxins (AFs) are products of *Aspergillus* and *Penicillium* species. They are highly potent in the induction of acute toxicity in animals and in humans. Approximately 4.5 billion people are exposed to uncontrolled amounts of AFB_1 in the third world.[1]

The liver is the prime target organ for acute toxicity and carcinogenicity in all species in that the predominant route of exposure is via the alimentary tract.[2] Acute aflatoxicosis outbreaks in Uganda and Taiwan resulted in vomiting, abdominal pain, pulmonary edema, and fatty infiltration and necrosis of the liver. Consumption of AF-contaminated corn (6–16 ppm) in 200 Indian villages resulted in over 25% fatalities, for which the primary cause of death was gastrointestinal hemorrhage.[3–5]

The symptoms of acute aflatoxicosis are indistinguishable from those of Reye's syndrome; vomiting, convulsions, coma, and death were associated with cerebral edema and fatty involvement of the liver, kidney, and heart. Aflatoxin B_1 was detected in the liver, kidney, brain, bile, and gastrointestinal content of 22 out of 23 fatalities attributed to Reye's syndrome in Thailand[6] and the United States.[7]

In addition to their prevalence in crops, foods, and feedstuff, AFs are frequently at high levels in airborne, respirable grain dust particles. They may represent an occupational and environmental hazard. For example, a significant increase in mortality from total cancer and respiratory cancer has been observed in peanut-processing workers exposed to AF-contaminated dust.[8–11] The lung is also at risk after dietary AF exposure.[12] Immunosuppression is another feature of acute AF intoxication. Exposure of lungs to aerosolic AF resulted in suppression of phagocytosis by alveolar macrophages that persisted for 2 weeks.[13] The amount of DNA adducts was proportional to the concentration of AF and to the time of exposure.[14] Although seemingly impractical, AF-containing bombs have been loaded and deployed by the Iraqis.[15]

Aflatoxin B_1 is carcinogenic to many organs in many species. It is one of the most potent hepatocarcinogens in animals and humans. Very strong correlation exists between the daily dietary intake of AFB_1 and the incidence of primary liver cancer in humans (Figure 6.1). The slope of the log–log curve is close to unity, indicating that at these low doses the mutagenic AFB_1 acts predominantly as an initiator and has little effect on cell proliferation, similar to hepatocarcinogenesis induced in mice by low doses of N-acetyl-2-aminofluorene.[16]

Hepatocellular carcinoma is the fifth most frequent cancer in men and the eighth in women. Food contaminated with AF is the most important risk factor in South East Africa and South East Asia. Other important risk factors in Western countries are chronic infections with HBV and HCV and alcoholism that lead to liver cirrhosis that is associated with 90% of HCC.[17]

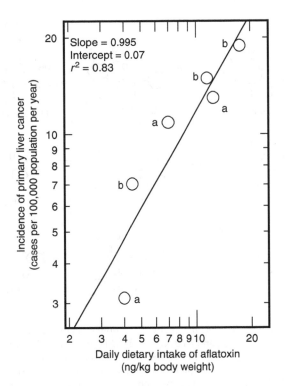

FIGURE 6.1

Correlation between ingestion of aflatoxins and the incidence of primary liver cancer in humans. The daily dietary intake of aflatoxins was calculated from the concentration of aflatoxins in foods and the daily intake of these foods (a) in Kenya (From Peers, F.G., et al., *Int. J. Cancer*, 17, 167, 1976.) and (b) in Swaziland (From Peers, F.G. and Linsel C.A., *Br. J. Cancer*, 27, 473, 1973.). In Mozambique, a calculated daily intake of 222 ng aflatoxins per kg body weight was associated with a primary liver cancer incidence of 35.5 cases per 100,000 population per year (From van Rensburg, S.J. et al., *S. Afr. Med. J.*, 48, 2508a, 1974.).

6.1.1 Biochemical Activation of Aflatoxins

Aflatoxins must undergo oxidative metabolism in order to be converted into acutely toxic and carcinogenic reactive species. AF toxicity and carcinogenicity are exerted by covalent binding of reactive AF metabolites to cellular macromolecules: DNA, RNA, and protein.[2,18–21]

6.1.2 Biochemical Activation in the Liver

Aflatoxin metabolism has been studied most extensively in the liver. In the liver, metabolism involves the NADPH-dependent cytochrome P-450 (CYP). The levels of activation, DNA binding, mutant frequency, and sensitivity to the acute toxic effects in a certain cell type depend on the types of cytochrome P-450 and their levels in these cells.[22] Activation of AFs toward toxicity, mutagenicity, and carcinogenicity results from oxidation at the 8,9

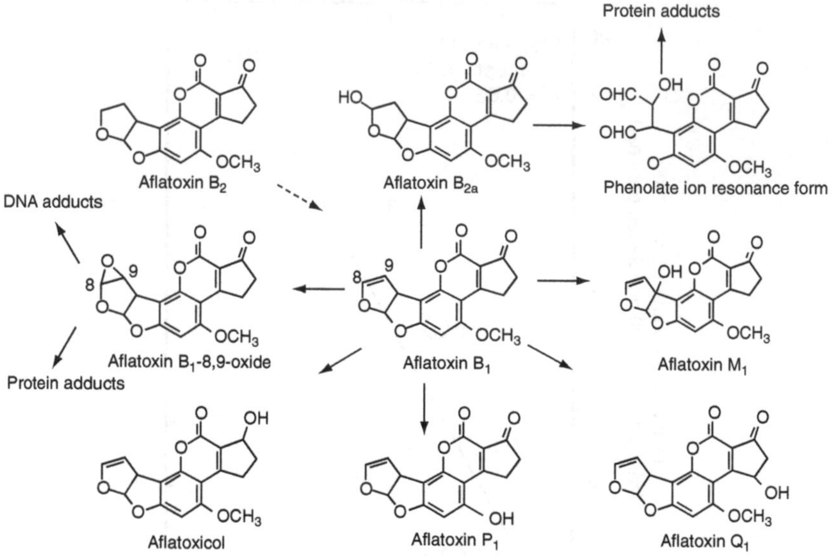

FIGURE 6.2

Metabolism of aflatoxin B_1. Oxidation by microsomal cytochrome P-450 leads to the formation of AFM_1, AFP_1, AFQ_1, and AFB_1-8,9-oxide. Unidentified oxidative reactions lead to the formation of AFL and AFB_{2a}. AFB2 can be converted to AFB_1 by a microsomal dehydrogenase. Addition of water to AFB_1-8,9-oxide (probably by epoxide hydrolase or a similar enzyme) yields AFB_1-8,9-diol. AFB_1-8,9-diol and AFB_{2a} are converted nonenzymatically to the phenolate ion, which covalently binds proteins by formation of Schiff bases with amino moieties. AFB_1-8,9-oxide can react with nucleophilic centers in proteins, such as thiols in cysteine and methionine, and N-3 and N-7 in histidine to give other protein adducts. Addition of glutathione to AFB_1-8,9-oxide by glutathione transferase is the primary detoxification reaction of AFB_1.

position that forms AF-8,9-oxide. The latter binds covalently to DNA, RNA, and protein. Hydroxylation of AF at other positions yields AFM_1, AFP_1, AFQ1, AFB_{2a}, and aflatoxicol (AFL) (Figure 6.2). These are less toxic and less carcinogenic than AF-8,9-oxide. Although threefold less carcinogenic than AFB_1, AFM_1 is an important food contaminant in that it appears in milk of cows fed with AFB_1-containing grains, and is concentrated in cheese and other milk products. AFM_1 appears also in the milk of lactating mothers in AF-infested areas.[23]

AF-8,9-oxide is converted by the detoxification enzyme epoxide hydrolase to 8,9-dihydrodiol. The latter metabolite and other hydroxylated AFs are converted to their glutathione (GSH) conjugates by GSH-S-transferase (GST) and are excreted in the urine as mercapturic acids.[24,25] AFB_2 contains a saturated 8,9 bond. Its weak mutagenicity and carcinogenicity may be due to a dehydrogenase that converts it to AFB_1 by desaturation of the 8,9 bond.[26]

Ingested AF that escapes the liver is distributed to other organs, where it can be metabolized and exert toxicity and carcinogenicity. The resistance of a certain species to AFB_1-induced carcinogenicity is usually correlated with the capability to detoxify AFB_1, predominantly by conjugation to glutathione.

6.1.3 Biochemical Activation in the Lung

As compared to the liver, only a few studies have been conducted on the activation/inactivation metabolism in the lung. Activation of AF in the rat and rabbit lung is carried out by CYP2B4 or CYP4B1, and CYP1 detoxifies AF by its conversion to AFM_1.[27-29] Most of the lung metabolism occurs in the nonciliated tracheal and bronchiolar epithelial (Clara) cells,[28,30,31] which are also the prime targets of the acute toxicity of AF.[31] Detoxification by GSH conjugation of AF, however, is sixfold lower in the rabbit lung as compared to the liver.[32] The lung activates AF to a mutagen more efficiently than benzo(a)pyrene, a known lung carcinogen.[33] Clara cells in the human lung are more rare and do not contain high concentrations of the activating enzymes as compared to those in the rodent lung; thus, they are unlikely to be the center of bioactivation of AFs. Surfactant-secreting alveolar type II cells in the human lung contain high P-450 activities and are capable of bioactivation.[34,35]

In addition to cytochrome P-450, microsomal prostaglandin H synthase and cytosolic lipoxygenase are involved in xenobiotic metabolism. The process is termed cooxidation, because metabolism depends on the oxidation of arachidonic acid. Cooxidation is more important in extrahepatic tissues, where the overall P-450 activity is relatively low. In the Guinea pig, for example, considerable P-450-independent activation of AF occurs in the presence of indomethacin, an inhibitor of prostaglandin H synthase, but is inhibited by a lipoxygenase inhibitor, indicating that lipoxygenase is responsible for AF activation.[36-38] The human lung is typically low in cytochrome P-450[39,40] and rich in prostaglandin H synthase and lipoxygenase. Studies with sorted lung cells revealed that AF activation is carried out primarily by lung macrophages where cooxidation was the predominant pathway.[35,41,42] AF activation[40] and DNA binding[43] by the human lung show great interindividual variability. A significant fraction of inhaled AF is translocated to the blood and the liver, resulting in binding to liver DNA.[44,45]

6.1.4 Photoactivation

In addition to microsomal metabolism, AFs are photoactivated by ultraviolet light (e.g., sunlight) to yield reactive-DNA-binding species, which form DNA adducts that are indistinguishable from those produced by microsomal metabolism. Chemically reactive (singlet) molecular oxygen, formed upon energy transfer from the photoexcited coumarin moiety of AF, oxidizes the 8,9-unsaturated bond in the furan moiety of AFB_1. AFB_2 lacks the 8,9-unsaturated bond, but its coumarin moiety readily forms singlet oxygen. Thus, photoactivated mixtures of AFB_1 and AFB_2 act synergistically in DNA binding.[46-51] Contamination of exposed skin with AFs in the sunlight may thus be hazardous.

6.2   Molecular Mechanism of Action of Aflatoxins

6.2.1   Relationship between Carcinogenicity, Mutagenicity, and Acute Toxicity and AF Binding to Cellular Macromolecules

Carcinogenicity[2] and mutagenicity[52,53] of AFs are associated with their DNA binding properties. Acute toxicity may be associated also with AF-protein binding.[54] The synthesis of DNA and RNA is rapidly inhibited by AF. Protein synthesis, mitochondrial electron transport, and lipid biosynthesis are also inhibited.

The typical symptoms of acute aflatoxicosis in mammals are hypolipidemia, hypocholesterolemia and hypocarotenaemia, severe hepatic steatosis, and weight loss. These perturbations in the metabolism of lipids have been recently suggested to stem from binding of AF to amino groups of lysyl residues on the LDL protein B-100, rendering the LDL unrecognizable by their receptors, and thus are not absorbed by peripheral cells. Upon return to the liver, the modified LDL particles return to the liver and bind to the sinusoidal cells, leading to accumulation of fat in the liver and starvation for lipids in the periphery.[55] Bacterial endotoxins (lipopolysaccharides) augment the acute hepatotoxicity by activation of the coagulation system; the latter is required for injury of hepatic parenchymal cells.[56]

Ingestion of AF leads also to the breakdown of lysosomes in parenchymal liver cells and to the release of degradative enzymes. The latter causes acute damage to the liver (hemorrhage and necrosis).[2] The susceptibility of a certain organ or a species to AFB_1-induced carcinogenicity is correlated with the frequency of AFB_1 adducts in the DNA of the organ or species in question. For example, in Fischer rats, AFB_1 is carcinogenic to the liver but not the kidney. AFB_1 adducts are tenfold more frequent in the liver DNA as compared to kidney DNA. Mice, hamsters, and monkeys are resistant to AFB_1-induced hepatocarcinogenesis, whereas rats, ducks, and trout are highly susceptible.[57] The level of AFB_1–DNA adduct in mouse liver is 80-fold lower than that found in rat liver.[19] The resistance of a species to AF carcinogenicity is correlated with the ability to detoxify AF, primarily by conjugation to GSH. In a study aimed to determine whether there is a genetic variability in the detoxification of AF in humans by genotyping detoxifying enzymes, GSTA4 was significantly related to excess risk in males.[58]

6.2.2   Molecular Aspects of AFB_1–DNA Binding

Oxidation of AFB_1 at the 8,9-position forms AFB_1-8,9-oxide (Figure 6.2). The electrophilic C-8 sustains a nucleophilic attack by N^7 of guanine, resulting in 8,9-dihydro-8-(N^7-guanyl)-9-hydroxy AFB_1 (Figure 6.3). Excluding two reports about in vitro binding of chemically activated AFB_1 to cytosine[59] and formation of alkali labile (apurinic) sites at adenine residues,[60]

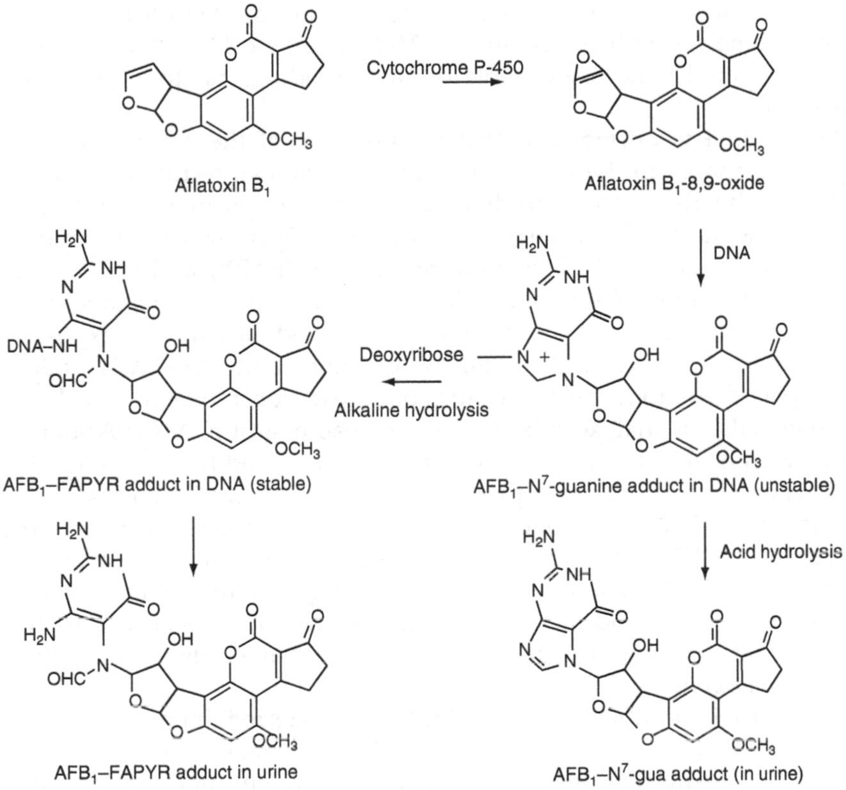

FIGURE 6.3

Covalent binding of aflatoxin B_1 to DNA. The electrophilic C-8 of AFB_1-9-oxide is attacked by the nucleophilic N^7 atom of guanine, where the leaving group is the oxygen, resulting in a covalent bond between AFB_1 and guanine, and in a positive charge on the imidazole moiety of guanine. The latter weakens the glycosidic bond between guanine and deoxyribose, leading to facile depurination and shedding of the adduct, which ultimately appears in the urine. In case an opening of the imidazole moiety occurs by alkaline hydrolysis, there is no positive charge and the glycosidic bond becomes stable. Such formamido pyrimidine (FAPYR)–AFB_1 adducts are also removed and appear in the urine. The appearance of N^7-guanine and FAPYR adducts are indicative of exposure to aflatoxins, and their quantity reflects the severity of the exposure.

the reaction of metabolically activated AFB_1 in vitro or in vivo[61,62] is unique among DNA-binding carcinogens in that it exclusively binds N^7 of guanine. Other carcinogens bind a variety of nucleophilic atoms in DNA. The high specificity of AFB_1 for N^7 guanine is most probably due to steric constraints of the noncovalent intercalation of the furan moiety of AFB_1 in the major groove of DNA, bringing the reactive C-8 of AFB_1-8,9-oxide into close proximity to N^7 of guanine. Dependence of AFB_1–DNA binding on the flanking sequences (see below) and inhibition of binding by covalently linked, intercalated benzofuran indicate that precise noncovalent intercalation of AFB_1-8,9-oxide must precede binding with N^7 guanine.[63] Metabolites of AFB_1 that contain the 8,9-unsaturated bond are capable of DNA binding, but to a lesser extent than AFB_1.[64]

The adduct is unstable, in that modification of the N^7 position forms a positive charge in the imidazol moiety of guanine, resulting in destabilization of the glycosidic bond that leads to facile depurination of the AFB_1-N^7-guanine adduct[65] and strand scission.[66] Opening of the imidazole ring forms a stable AF–formamidopyrimidine (FAPY) adduct.[61,67,68] Due to their instability, N^7-guanine adducts of AFB_1 or of its metabolites are excreted in the urine and are used to monitor and measure the exposure of humans to aflatoxins.[25,69] AFB_1-N^7-guanine and AF–FAPY adducts are repaired predominantly by nucleotide excision repair in *E. coli*[70] and in mammals, in that xeroderma pigmentosum group A (XPA)-deficient human cell lines fail to repair AF–DNA adducts[71] and XPA-deficient mice and are more prone to AFB_1 hepatocarcinogenesis.[72] Tissue specificity of AFB_1 carcinogenesis is inversely correlated with the ability to repair AF–DNA adducts, and vice versa. For example, lower repair activity of AF–DNA adducts in mouse lung and the ability to induce repair of AF–DNA adducts in the mouse liver are consistent with the susceptibility of mice to lung carcinogenesis that is higher than that to liver carcinogenesis.[73]

Guanines in double-stranded DNA are preferred binding targets, as compared to those in single-stranded DNA.[74] Theoretical models show that GGGG sequences are major targets for covalent binding. Within this sequence, the third G residue was calculated to be the most favorable to bind AFB_1.[75] In double-stranded DNA, the flanking nucleotides greatly affect the efficiency of AFB_1 binding. For example, the Gs (in bold) in AG**A**, TG**A**, and G**C**C are poor targets; in T**G**T, C**G**C, **G**GG, and GG**C**, moderate targets; and in CC**G**, GG**G**, CC**G**G, CC**G**CC, and CG**G**CG, strong targets. Reaction rates of AFB_1 with moderate and strong targets are 2–3 and 6–10 times faster than with poor ones, respectively.[76] In vivo, not all regions of DNA are equally susceptible to binding; for example, genes coding for ribosomal RNA in the nucleolus[77] and internucleosomal DNA[78] preferentially bind AFB_1, because they are not protected by chromosomal proteins.

6.2.3 Genetic Consequences of AFB₁–DNA Binding

The AFB_1-N^7-guanine adduct, FAPY adducts, and apurinic sites are premutagenic lesions.[79] In bacteria (*Salmonella typhimurium*), approximately 60 adducts per genome are required to produce a lethal event, and 40 adducts per genome induce a frequency of 10^{-4} reversions (point mutations) to histidine prototrophy.[46] Only 0.3 adducts per genome are required to induce the same frequency of forward mutations in guanine–hypoxanthine phosphoribosyl transferase.[52]

6.2.3.1   Mutagenesis

Most of the mutations discussed above are G→T transversions, resulting from placement of a T against the AFB_1-N^7-guanine. However, apurinic (aguaninic) sites originating in AFB_1-N^7-guanine (see above) are mutagenic, in that an error-prone polymerase induced under SOS conditions has a preference to place an adenine against the abasic site, leading to a G→T transversion as well, that occurs exclusively at the abasic site.[80,81]

In vivo replication of single-stranded DNA containing this adduct yield predominantly G→T transversions targeted to the adduct site, and 13% of the mutations occur one base upstream (5′) to the adduct.[65] Less common are G→C transversions and G→A transversions,[79] and a minor fraction consists of frameshifts.[82,83]

Thus, the mutations in AFB_1-treated cells are best explained as originating mainly in AFB_1-N^7-guanine adducts rather than in abasic sites. AFB_1 is an inducer of the SOS response mutagenesis in bacteria and the latter is required for AFB_1 mutagenesis.[65,75,84–86] AFB_1 induces an SOS-like response in mammalian cells.[87]

6.2.3.2   Immunosuppression

Aflatoxin B_1 is an immunosuppressor in mice, rats, and rabbits[13, 88–90] and is immunotoxic to lectin-stimulated human peripheral blood lymphocytes in vitro[91] due to its capability to impair DNA, RNA, and protein synthesis. Actively dividing cells such as those of the immune system are more sensitive to these effects as compared to nondividing ones.

6.2.3.3   Teratogenicity of Aflatoxin B_1

Aflatoxin B_1 causes malformations in numerous organs in embryos of various species of mammals, birds, amphibians, and fish.[92–94] The exact mechanism by which AFB_1 acts as a teratogen is not clear. However, because teratogenicity is associated with mutations and gross alteration in the structure of chromosomes such as sister chromatid exchanges, chromosomal aberrations, induction of micronuclei in human cells,[95] the DNA binding property of AFB_1 may be the key reaction in teratogenicity. AFB_1 ingested by pregnant females is readily transferred via the placenta to the embryos of animals[96] and humans.[97]

6.2.3.4   Relationship between Primary Liver Cancer and the Specificity of AFB₁ in DNA Binding and Mutagenesis

One half of human tumors contain mutant (activated) forms of the tumor suppressor gene p53, making it the most frequently mutated cancer-related gene in human cancer. Its activation involves primarily point mutations that lead to amino acid substitutions. Sequence analysis of the mutations reveals that there is an association between the types of the altered DNA bases, the mutagen, and carcinogenesis in a specific tissue or organ.

For example, altered p53 in malignant skin cancers in humans contained CC→TT mutations and C→T substitutions exclusively at dipyrimidine sites. These alterations are known to result from DNA lesions induced exclusively by ultraviolet light. Alterations in p53 in internal cancers do not contain these ultraviolet-specific mutations.[98,99]

c-Ki-*ras*, c-Ha-*ras*, and c-N-*ras* protooncogenes are frequently mutated in experimental liver tumors in rats and mice. In AFB$_1$-treated mice, 75 of 76 liver tumors contained mutations in codon 12 (GGT), where all of the mutations were located in guanine residues,[100] strongly indicating that the primary lesion was the binding of AFB$_1$to guanine residues at this codon. Similar predominance of GGT→GAT, GGT→TGT, and GGT→GTT mutations in codon 12 of c-Ki-*ras* or c-N-*ras* occurs in liver tumors in rats.[101,102] Although frequently mutated in many human cancers, *ras* activation is not associated with HCC,[103] even in regions where dietary exposure to AFB$_1$ is a risk factor.[104] But, the p53 tumor suppressor is frequently mutated in many cancers in humans, including HCC. Surveys compiling numerous (>1000) individual cases of HCC in humans revealed that high levels of AFB$_1$ in the environment and in the diet in West Africa, Mozambique, southern Africa, Qidong and Tongan in China, and Mexico correlated with a high prevalence of HCC and with a high prevalence of mutations involving guanines in codon 249 of p53.[105–109] Such guanine residues are strong or moderate targets for AFB$_1$ binding.[76] In Alaska, Europe, or Japan, where exposure to AF is low or does not occur, mutations in codon 249 in HCCs are very rare.[110–112] Thus, G→T transversions in codon 249 of p53 are consistent with the mutational specificity of AFB$_1$ in vitro and in vivo. The identification of specific AFB$_1$-induced mutations in tumors of humans living in areas contaminated with AFB$_1$ makes it possible to more accurately identify the causing agent. The AFB$_1$ story is one of the best examples for molecular epidemiology in action.

6.2.3.5 Synergy between Aflatoxin B$_1$ and Hepatitis Virus in Hepatocellular Carcinoma

Aflatoxins and viral hepatitis are the most important environmental factors in HCC in humans. In order to determine the relationship between these factors, the frequency of HCC in China and in Taiwan was determined in people exposed to AFB$_1$ and to HBV.

Exposure to AFB$_1$ was estimated by the determination of the concentration of AFB$_1$ detoxification products or AF–guanine adducts in urine or by immunohistochemical detection of AFB$_1$–DNA adduct in liver tissue. These methods replaced older ones based on the determination of the concentration of AFB$_1$ in food products in homes and the daily intake of these foods. Infection with hepatitis virus was determined by the presence of HBV antigen. Four studies (Table 6.1) revealed that HBV alone was associated with relative risk of HCC of about 12; AFB$_1$ alone with a relative risk of about 6, and the combined exposure to with a relative risk of about 64,

TABLE 6.1

Synergistic Action between AFB_1 and HBV in Hepatocarcinogenesis

Location	Relative Risk of Hepatocellular Carcinoma			References
	HBV	AFB_1	HBV and AFB_1	
Shanghai	4.8	1.9	60.1	[114]
Shanghai	7.3	3.4	59.4	[115]
Taiwan	17.4	0.3	70.0	[116]
Taiwan	17.0	17.4	67.6	[117]
Mean ± S.D.	11.6 ± 6.5	5.8 ± 7.9	64 ± 5.3	

Source: From Kew, M.C., *Liver Int.*, 23, 405, 2003.

roughly the product of the risk of HBV and AFB_1. Thus, AFB_1 and HBV are synergistic in the induction of HCC. Vaccination against hepatitis viruses may have a greater impact than that of AFB_1 on the incidence of HCC in countries with endemic HCC.

6.2.4 Prevention of AFB_1-Induced Hepatocellular Carcinoma

6.2.4.1 Monitoring and Detection

The contamination of foodstuffs and feedstuffs with aflatoxins is strictly monitored throughout the world[121] using chromatographic methods and enzyme-linked immunosorbent assays (ELISAs). A very sensitive liquid chromatography/tandem mass spectrometry (LC/MS/MS) method has been recently developed for AF and other mycotoxins with a detection of 9 fg/μL (approximately 30 pM AFB_1).[122] Several formats of biosensors for the detection of aflatoxin are being developed, including surface plasmon resonance and microbead assays, and fiber optic probes.[123] A method using isotope dilution LC/MS/MS has been recently developed for the detection of AF–lysine adducts in the serum.[124]

Similar to the appearance of tumor antigens in the bloodstream, patients with solid cancers have DNA of tumor cells in their circulation. This DNA that originates probably in apoptotic or necrotic tumor cells, exhibit the same mutations and altered microsatellites contained in the solid tumor.[125] Thus, DNA from plasma of patients with HCC contained the specific mutation in codon 249 of p53.[126,127] The mutation was detected also in DNA from plasma of people from aflatoxin stricken areas 5 years before the diagnosis of HCC.[128]

The reader is referred to recent reviews of the toxicity of aflatoxins and other mycotoxins[129] and about the chemical basis for AFB_1 mutagenesis, and the synergism between AFB_1 with HBV in the induction of HCC.[130]

6.2.4.2 Dietary Supplements for Chemoprevention

HSCAS (NovaSil) is an anticaking additive in animal feeds. It adsorbs AFB_1 with astoundingly high capacity and high affinity. 110 g AFB_1/kg were bound in aqueous solution or milk containing 20 μM AFB$_1$ and 10 μg/mL HSCAS incubated at 37°C for 24 h.[131] Toxic effects were not detected in human volunteers fed 1–3 g HSCAS/day for 2 weeks.[132] This amount of clay can adsorb 330 mg AFB$_1$.[133] Note that the highest daily exposure of humans to AFB$_1$ was 15 μg/day (222 ng/kg body weight) in Mozambique (Figure 6.1).[120] Dietary HSCAS greatly decreased the bioavailability of AFB$_1$ in poultry; it mitigated the toxicity of AFB$_1$ in young pigs, lambs, chicks, turkeys, and rats, and decreased the concentration of AFB$_1$ in the milk of cows and goats (reviewed in ref. 134). HSCAS is a promising dietary additive that should prevent HCC in AF-endemic areas.

Chlorophyllin is a semisynthetic, water-soluble form of chlorophyll that contains Cu in lieu of Mg. It is a popular colorant of food and a component of many medications. Chlorophyllin form complexes with xenobiotics, including carcinogens, inhibiting their absorption by the digestive system. Chlorophyllin inhibited hepatocarcinogenesis induced by AFB$_1$ in experimental animals. In China, human volunteers in endemic AFB$_1$ areas who were administered 100 mg chlorophyllin in every meal for 4 months were tested for the appearance of AFB$_1$–guanine adducts in their urine. Chlorophyllin treatment decreased the level of the AFB$_1$ biomarker by 55%, without apparent toxicity. Thus, in humans that are inevitably exposed to AFB$_1$, chlorophyllin is an effective, safe means to decrease exposure.[135,136]

Oltipraz [4-methyl-5-(pyrazinyl)-3H-1,2-dithiole-3-thione] is a synthetic drug that is a potent inhibitor of CYP1A2, of CYP3A4 that oxidizes AFB$_1$ to AFB$_1$-8,9-oxide, and of CYP1A2 that converts AFB$_1$ to AFM$_1$. Oltipraz also induces phase II enzymes such as GSH-S-transferases that are involved in the detoxification metabolism of aflatoxin. In humans exposed to AB1, oltipraz modulated the levels of aflatoxin biomarkers.[136]

References

1. Williams, J.H. et al., Human aflatoxicosis in developing countries: A review of toxicology, exposure, potential health consequences, and interventions. *Am. J. Clin. Nutr.*, 80:1106–1122, 2004.
2. Busby, W.F. Jr., and Wogan, G.N., Aflatoxins, in *Chemical Carcinogens*, Searle, C.E., (Ed.), ACS Monograph 182, American Chemical Society, Washington, DC, 1984, pp. 946–1135.
3. Shank, R.C., *Mycotoxins and N-Nitroso Compounds: Environmental Risks*, vol. I, Shank, R.C., (Ed.), CRC Press, Boca Raton, FL, 1981, pp. 107–140.
4. Shank, R.C., Epidemiology of aflatoxin carcinogenesis, in *Environmental Cancer*, Kraybill, H.F. and Mehlman, M.A., (Eds.), John Wiley & Sons, New York, 1977, pp. 291–318.
5. van Rensburg, S.J., Role of epidemiology in causation of mycotoxin health risk, in *Mycotoxins in Human and Animal Health*, Rodricks, J.V., Hesseltine, C.W., and Mehlman, M.A., (Eds.), Pathotox, Park Forest South, IL, 1977, pp. 699–711.

6. Shank, R.C. et al., Aflatoxins in autopsy of specimens from Thai children with an acute disease of unknown etiology. *Food Cosmet. Toxicol.*, 9:501–507, 1971.
7. Nelson, D.B. et al., Aflatoxins and Reye's syndrome: A case control study. *Pediatrics*, 66:865–869, 1980.
8. van Nieuwenhuize, J.P. et al., Aflatoxinen: Epidemiologish onderzoek naar carcinogeniteit bij langdurige "low level" exposite van eon fabriekspopulatie. *T. Soc. Geneesk*, 51:754–760, 1973.
9. Sorenson, W.G. et al., Aflatoxin in respirable corn dust particles. *J. Toxicol. Environ. Health*, 7:669–672, 1981.
10. Hayes, R.B. et al., Aflatoxin exposures in the industrial setting: An epidemiological study of mortality. *Food Chem. Toxicol.*, 22:39–43, 1984.
11. Dvorackova, I., Aflatoxin inhalation and alveolar cell carcinoma. *Br. Med. J.*, 1:691, 1986.
12. Harrison, J.C. and Garner, R.C., Immunological and HPLC detection of aflatoxin adducts in human tissues after an acute poisoning incident in S.E. Asia. *Carcinogenesis*, 12:741–743, 1991.
13. Jakab, G.J. et al., Respiratory aflatoxicosis: Suppression of pulmonary and systemic host defenses in rats and mice. *Toxicol. Appl. Pharomacol.*, 125:198–205, 1994.
14. Zarba, A. et al., Aflatoxin B1-DNA adduct formation in the rat liver following exposure by aerosol inhalation. *Carcinogenesis*, 13:1031–1033, 1992.
15. Zilinskas, R.A., Iraq's biological weapons. The past as future? *J. Am. Med. Assoc.*, 278:418–424, 1997.
16. Cohen, S.M. and Ellwein, L.B., Cell proliferation in carcinogenesis. *Science*, 249:1007–1011, 1990.
17. Seitz, H.K. and Stickel, F., Risk factors and mechanisms of hepatocarcinogenesis with special emphasis on alcohol and oxidative stress. *Biol. Chem.*, 387:349–360, 2006.
18. Stark, A.A. et al., Aflatoxin B1 mutagenesis and adduct formation in *Salmonella typhimurium*. *Proc. Natl. Acad. Sci. U.S.A.*, 76:1343–1347, 1979.
19. Wogan, G.N. et al., Macromolecular binding of aflatoxin B1 and sterigmatocystin: Relationship of adduct patterns to carcinogenesis and mutagenesis, in *Naturally Occurring Carcinogens-mutagens and Modulators of Carcinogenesis*, Miller, E.C., Miller, J.A., Hirono, I., Sugimura, T., and Takayama, A., (Eds.), University Park Press, Baltimore, MD, 1979, pp. 19–33.
20. Stark, A.A., Molecular aspects of aflatoxin B1 mutagenesis and carcinogenesis, in *Mycotoxins and Phycotoxins*, Steyn, P.S. and Vleggaar, R., (Eds.), Elsevier Science, Amsterdam, 1986, pp. 435–445.
21. Crespi, C.L. et al., Human cytochrome P-450A3: Sequence, role of the enzyme in the metabolic activation of promutagens, comparison to nitrosamine activation by human cytochrome P-450IIE1. *Carcinogenesis*, 11:1293–1300, 1990.
22. Mace, K. et al., Aflatoxin B1-induced DNA adduct formation and p53 mutations in CYP-450-expressing human liver cell lines. *Carcinogenesis*, 18:1291–1297, 1997.
23. Zarba, A. et al., Aflatoxin M_1 in human breast milk from The Gambia, West Africa, quantified by combined monoclonal antibody immunoaffinity chromatography and HPLC. *Carcinogenesis*, 13:891–894, 1992.
24. Moss, E.J. et al., The mercapturic acid pathway metabolites of a glutathione conjugate of aflatoxin B1. *Chem. Biol. Interact.*, 55:139–155, 1985.
25. Scholl, P.F. et al., Synthesis and characterization of aflatoxin B1 mercapturic acids and their identification in rat urine. *Chem. Res. Toxicol.*, 10:1144–1151, 1997.

26. Roebuck, B.D. et al., *In vitro* metabolism of aflatoxin B2 by animal and human liver. *Cancer Res.*, 38:999–1002, 1978.
27. Massey, T.E., Cellular and molecular targets in pulmonary chemical carcinogenesis: Studies with aflatoxin B1. *Can. J. Physiol. Pharmacol.*, 74:621–628, 1996.
28. Daniels, J.K. et al., Biotranasformation of aflatoxin B1 in rabbit lung and liver microsomes. *Carcinogenesis*, 11:823–827, 1990.
29. Daniels, J.M. et al., DNA binding and mutagenicity of aflatoxin B1 catalyzed by isolated rabbit lung cells. *Carcinogenesis*, 14:1429–1434, 1993.
30. Coulombe, R.A. et al., Metabolism of AFB1 in the upper airways of the rabbit: Role of the nonciliated tracheal epithelial cells. *Cancer Res.*, 46:4091–4096, 1986.
31. Stewart, R.K. and Massey, T.E., Kinetic studies of glutathione-S-transferase (GST)-catalyzed conjugation of aflatoxin B1-8,9-epoxide in rabbit lung and liver. *Toxicologist*, 13:63, 1993.
32. Ball, R.W. et al., Comparative activation of aflatoxin B1 by mammalian pulmonary tissue. *Toxicol. Lett.*, 75:119–125, 1995.
33. Devereux, T.R. et al., Xenobiotic metabolism in human alveolar type II cells isolated by centrifugal elutriation and density gradient centrifugation. *Cancer Res.*, 46:5438–5443, 1986.
34. Anttila, S. et al., Smoking and peripheral types of cancer are related to high level of pulmonary cytochrome P-450IA in lung cancer patients. *Int. J. Cancer*, 47:681–685, 1991.
35. Liu, L. and Massey, T.E., Bioactivation of AFB1 by lipoxygenases, prostaglandin H synthase and cytochrome P-450 monooxygenase in Guinea-pig tissues. *Carcinogenesis*, 13:533–539, 1992.
36. Liu, L. et al., *In vitro* prostaglandin H synthase- and monooxygenase-mediated binding of AFB1 to DNA in Guinea-pig tissue microsomes. *Carcinogenesis*, 11:1915–1919, 1990.
37. Liu, L. et al., *In vitro* cytochrome P-450 monooxygenase and prostaglandin H synthase-mediated AFB1 biotransformation in Guinea-pig tissues: Effect of β-naphthoflavone treatment. *Arch. Toxicol.*, 67:379–385, 1993.
38. Kelly, J.D. et al., Aflatoxin B1 activation in the human lung. *Toxicol. Appl. Pharmacol.*, 144:88–95, 1997.
39. Donnelly, P.J. et al., Biotransformation of aflatoxin B1 in the human lung. *Carcinogenesis*, 17:2487–2494, 1996.
40. Donnelly, P.J. et al., Arachidonic acid dependent bioactivation of AFB1 in human lung. *Toxicologist*, 14:336, 1994.
41. Donnelly, P.J. et al., Bioactivation of AFB1 in human alveolar type II cells and macrophages. *Proc. Am. Assoc. Cancer Res.*, 36:153, 1995.
42. Harrison, J.C. and Garner, R.C., Immunological and HPLC detection of aflatoxin adducts in human tissues after an acute poisoning incident in S.E. Africa. *Carcinogenesis*, 12:741–743, 1991.
43. Biswas, G. et al., Comparative kinetic studies of aflatoxin B1 binding to pulmonary and hepatic DNA of rat and hamster receiving the carcinogen intratracheally. *Teratol. Carcinog. Mutagen.*, 13:259–268, 1993.
44. Coulombe, R.A. et al., Pharmacokinetics of intratracheally administered aflatoxin B1. *Toxicol. Appl. Pharmacol.*, 109:19–206, 1991.
45. Imaoka, S. et al., Rat pulmonary microsomal cytochrome P-450 enzymes involved in the activation of procarcinogens. *Mut. Res.*, 284:233–241, 1992.

46. Israel Kalinsky, H. et al., Photoactivated aflatoxins are mutagens to *Salmonella typhimurium* and bind covalently to DNA *in vitro. Carcinogenesis*, 3:423–429, 1982.
47. Israel Kalinsky, H. et al., Comparative aflatoxin B1 mutagenesis in *Salmonella typhimurium* TA100 in metabolic and photoactivation systems. *Cancer Res.*, 44:1831–1839, 1984.
48. Stark, A.A. et al., DNA strand scission and apurinic sites induced by photo-activated aflatoxins. *Cancer Res.*, 48:3070–3076, 1988.
49. Shaulsky, G. et al., Properties of aflatoxin DNA adducts formed by photoacti-vation and characterization of the major photoadduct as aflatoxin N7 guanine. *Carcinogenesis*, 11:519–527, 1990.
50. Stark, A.A. et al., Involvement of singlet oxygen in the photoactivation of aflatoxins B1 and B2 to DNA binding forms *in vitro. Carcinogenesis*, 11:529–534, 1990.
51. Stark, A.A. and Liberman, D.F., Synergism between aflatoxins in covalent binding to DNA and in mutagenesis in the photoactivation system. *Mutation Res.*, 247:77–86, 1991.
52. Stark, A.A. et al., Aflatoxin B1 mutagenesis, DNA binding, and adduct forma-tion in *Salmonella typhimurium. Proc. Natl. Acad. Sci. U.S.A.*, 76:1343–1347, 1979.
53. Stark, A.A. and Giroux, C.N., Mutagenesis in *Streptococcus pneumoniae (pneumo-coccus)* by transformation with DNA modified by the carcinogen-mutagen, aflatoxin B1. *Mut. Res.*, 107:23–32, 1983.
54. McLean, M. and Dutton, M.F., Cellular interactions and metabolism of afla-toxin: An update. *Pharmacol. Ther.*, 65:163–192, 1995.
55. Amaya-Farfan, J., Aflatoxin B1-induced hepatic steatosis: Role of carbonyl compounds and active diols on steatogenesis. *Lancet*, 353:747–748, 1999.
56. Luyendyk, J.P. et al., Augmentation of aflatoxin B1 hepatotoxicity by endotoxin: Involvement of endothelium and the coagulation system. *Toxicol Sci.*, 72:171–181, 2003.
57. Wogan, G.N., Aflatoxin carcinogenesis, *Meth. Cancer Res.*, 7:309–344, 1973.
58. McGlynn, K.A. et al., Susceptibility to aflatoxin B1-related primary hepatocel-lular carcinoma in mice and humans. *Cancer Res.*, 63:4594–4601, 2003.
59. Yu, F.L. et al., Evidence for the covalent binding of aflatoxin B1-dichloride to cytosine in DNA. *Carcinogenesis*, 12:997–1002, 1991.
60. D'Andrea, A.D. and Haseltine, W.A., Modification of DNA by aflatoxin B1 creates alkali-labile lesions in DNA at positions of guanine and adenine. *Proc. Natl. Acad. Sci. U.S.A.*, 75:4120–4124, 1978.
61. Essigmann, J.M. et al., Structural identification of the major DNA adduct formed by aflatoxin B1 *in vitro. Proc. Natl. Acad. Sci. U.S.A.*, 74:1870–1874, 1977.
62. Croy, R.G. et al., Identification of the principal aflatoxin B1-DNA adduct formed *in vivo* in rat liver. *Proc. Natl. Acad. Sci. U.S.A.*, 75:1745–1749, 1978.
63. Kobertz, W.R. et al., An intercalation inhibitor altering the target selectivity of DNA damaging agents: Synthesis of site-specific aflatoxin B1 adducts in a p53 mutational hotspot. *Proc. Natl. Acad. Sci. U.S.A.*, 94:9579–9584, 1997.
64. Heinonen, J.T. et al., Determination of aflatoxin B1 biotransformation and binding to hepatic macromolecules in human precision liver slices. *Toxicol. Appl. Pharmacol.*, 136:1–7, 1996.
65. Bailey, E.A. et al., Mutational properties of the primary aflatoxin B1-DNA adduct. *Proc. Natl. Acad. Sci. U.S.A.*, 93:1535–1539, 1996.
66. Stark, A.A. et al., DNA strand scission and apurinic sites induced by photo-activated aflatoxins. *Cancer Res.*, 48:3070–3076, 1988.

67. Mao, H. et al., An intercalated and thermally stable FAPY adduct of aflatoxin B1 in a DNA duplex: Structural refinement from 1H NMR. *Biochemistry*, 37:4374–4387, 1998.
68. Croy, R.G. and Wogan, G.N., Temporal patterns of covalent DNA adducts in rat liver after single and multiple doses of aflatoxin B1, *Cancer Res.* 41:197–203, 1981.
69. Groopman, J.D. et al., Molecular epidemiology of aflatoxin exposures: Validation of aflatoxin-N7-guanine levels in urine as a biomarker in experimental rat models and humans. *Environ. Health Perspect.*, 99:107–113, 1993.
70. Alekseyev, Y.O. et al., Aflatoxin B_1 formamidopyrimidine adducts are preferentially repaired by the nucleotide excision repair pathway in vivo. *Carcinogenesis*, 25(6):1045–1051, 2004.
71. Leadon, S.A. et al., Excision repair of aflatoxin B_1-DNA adducts in human fibroblasts, *Cancer Res.*, 41:5125–5129, 1981.
72. Takahashi, Y. et al., Enhanced spontaneous and aflatoxin-induced liver tumorigenesis in xeroderma pigmentosum group A genedeficient mice, *Carcinogenesis*, 23:627–633, 2002.
73. Bedard, L.L. et al., Susceptibility to aflatoxin B_1-induced carcinogenesis correlates with tissue specific differences in DNA repair activity in mouse and in rat, *Cancer Res.*, 65:1265–1270, 2005.
74. Jacobsen, J.S. et al., DNA replication-blocking properties of adducts formed by aflatoxin B1-2,3-dichloride and aflatoxin B1-2,3-oxide. *Mut. Res.*, 179:89–101, 1987.
75. Bonnett, M. and Taylor, E.R., The structure of aflatoxin B1-DNA adduct at N^7 of guanine. Theoretical intercalation and covalent adduct models. *J. Biochem. Structure Dynamics*, 7:127–149, 1989.
76. Muench, K.F. et al., Sequence specificity in aflatoxin B1-DNA interactions. *Proc. Natl. Acad. Sci. U.S.A.*, 80:6–10, 1983.
77. Irvin, T.R. and Wogan, G.N., Quantitation of aflatoxin B1 adduction within the ribosomal RNA gene sequences of rat liver DNA. *Proc. Natl. Acad. Sci. U.S.A.*, 81:664–668, 1984.
78. Bailey, G.S. et al., Carcinogen AFB1 is located preferentially in internucleosomal deoxyribonucleic acid following exposure *in vivo* in rainbow trout. *Biochemistry*, 19:5836–5842, 1980.
79. Prieto-Alamo, M.J. et al., Mutational specificity of aflatoxin B1: Comparison of *in vivo* host-mediated assay with *in vitro* S9 metabolic activation. *Carcinogenesis*, 17:1997–2002, 1996.
80. Schapper, R.M. et al., Infidelity of DNA synthesis associated with bypass of apurinic sites. *Proc. Natl. Acad. Sci. U.S.A.*, 80:487–491, 1984.
81. Tessman, I. and Kennedy, M.A., DNA polymerase II of *Escherichia coli* in the bypass of abasic sites in *vivo*. *Genetics*, 136:439–448, 1994.
82. Zhu, Y. et al., Aflatoxin B1, 2-aminoanthracene, and 7,12-dimethylbenz[a]anthracene-induced frameshift mutations in human APRT. *Environ. Molec. Mutagen.*, 26:234–239, 1995.
83. Bennett, C.B. et al., Frameshifts: Genetic requirements for frameshift reversion induced by bulky DNA adducts in M13 DNA. *Mut. Res.*, 249:19–27, 1991.
84. Stark, A.A. and Giroux, C.N., Mutagenicity and cytotoxicity of the carcinogen mutagen aflatoxin B1 in *Streptococcus pneumoniae* (*Pneumococcus*) and *Salmonella typhimurium*: Dependence on DNA repair functions. *Mut. Res.*, 106:195–208, 1982.

85. Sahasrabudhe, S. et al., Mutagenesis by aflatoxin in M13 DNA: Base-substitution mechanisms and the origin of strand bias. *Mol. Gen. Genet.*, 217:20–25, 1989.
86. Foster, P.L. et al., Induction of base substitution mutations by aflatoxin B1 is *mucAB* dependent in *Escherichia coli. J. Bacteriol.*, 170:3415–3420, 1988.
87. Sarasin, A.R. and Hanawalt, P.C., Carcinogens enhance survival of UV-irradiated simian virus 40 in treated monkey kidney cells: Induction of a recovery pathway?, *Proc. Natl. Acad. Sci. U.S.A.*, 75:346–350, 1978.
88. Venturini, M.C. et al., Mycotoxin T-2 and aflatoxin B1 as immunosuppressors in mice chronically infected with *Toxoplasma gondii. J. Comp. Pathol.*, 115:229–237, 1996.
89. Dimitri, R.A. and Gabal, M.A., Immunosuppressant activity of aflatoxin ingestion in rabbits measured by response to *Mycobacterium bovis* antigen. I. Cell-mediated immune response measured by skin test reaction. *Vet. Hum. Toxicol.*, 38:333–336, 1996.
90. Raisuddin, S. et al., Immunostimulating effects of protein A in immunosuppressed aflatoxin-intoxicated rats. *Int. J. Immunopharmacol.*, 16:977–984, 1994.
91. Methenitou, G. et al., Immunomodulative effects of aflatoxins and selenium on human eriperal blood lymphocytes. *Vet. Hum. Toxicol.*, 38:274–277, 1996.
92. Roll, R. et al., Embryotoxicity and mutagenicity of mycotoxins. *J. Environ. Pathol. Toxicol. Oncol.*, 10:1–7, 1990.
93. Bloom, S.E., Sister chromatid exchange studies in the chick embryo and neonate: Actions of mutagens in a developing system. *Basic Life Sci.*, 29:509–533, 1984.
94. Geissler, F. and Faustman, E.M., Developmental toxicity of aflatoxin B1 in the rodent embryo *in vitro*: Contribution of exogenous biotransformation systems to toxicity. *Teratology*, 37:101–111, 1988.
95. Miele, M. et al., Aflatoxin exposure and cytogenetic alterations in individuals from Gambia, West Africa. *Mut. Res.*, 349:209–217, 1996.
96. Autrup, H. Transplacental transfer of genotoxins and transplacental carcinogenesis. *Environ. Health perspect.*, 101:33–38, 1993.
97. Denning, D.W. et al., Transplacental transfer of aflatoxin in humans. *Carcinogenesis*, 11:1033–1035, 1990.
98. Ziegler, A. et al., Tumor suppressor gene mutations and photocarcinogenesis. *Photochem. Photobiol.*, 63:432–435, 1996.
99. Brash, D.E. et al., A role for sunlight in skin cancer: UV-induced p53 mutations in squamous cell carcinoma. *Proc. Natl. Acad. Sci. U.S.A.*, 88:10124–10128, 1991.
100. Donnelly, P.J. et al., Activation of K-ras in aflatoxin B1-induced lung tumors from AC3F1 (A/J × C3H/HeJ) mice. *Carcinogenesis*, 17:1735–1740, 1996.
101. McMahon, G. et al., Characterization of c-Ki-ras and N-ras oncogenes in aflatoxin B1-induced rat liver tumors. *Proc. Natl. Acad. Sci. U.S.A.*, 87:1104–1108, 1990.
102. Soman, N.R. and Wogan, G.N., Activation of the c-Ki-ras oncogene in aflatoxin B1-induced hepatocellular carcinoma and adenoma in the rat: Detection by denaturing gradient gel electrophoresis. *Proc. Natl. Acad. Sci. U.S.A.*, 90:2045–2099, 1993.
103. Tada, M. et al., Analysis of ras gene mutations in human hepatic malignant tumors by polymerase chain reaction and direct sequencing. *Cancer Res.*, 50:1121–1124, 1990.
104. Leon, M. and Kew, M.C., Analysis of ras gene mutations in hepatocellular carcinoma in southern African blacks. *Anticancer Res.*, 15:859–861, 1995.

105. Montesano, R. et al., Hepatocellular carcinoma: From gene to public health. *J. Natl. Cancer Inst.*, 89:1844–1851, 1997.
106. Shen, H.M. and Ong, C.N., Mutations of the p53 tumor suppressor gene and ras oncogenes in aflatoxin hepatocarcinogenesis. *Mut. Res.*, 366:23–44, 1996.
107. Yang, M. et al., Mutations at codon 249 of p53 gene in human hepatocellular carcinomas from Tongan, *China Mut. Res.*, 381:25–29, 1997.
108. Soini, Y. et al., An aflatoxin-associated mutational hotspot at codon 249 in the p53 tumor suppressor gene occurs in hepatocellular carcinomas from Mexico. *Carcinogenesis*, 17:1007–1012, 1996.
109. Aguilar, F. et al., Geographic variation of p53 mutational profile in nonmalignant human liver. *Science*, 264:1317–1319, 1994.
110. De-Benedetti, V.M. et al., p53 is not mutated in hepatocellular carcinomas from Alaska natives. *Cancer Epidemiol. Biomarkers Prev.*, 4:79–82, 1995.
111. Volkmann, M. et al., p53 overexpression is frequent in European hepatocellular carcinoma and largely independent of the codon 249 hot spot mutation. *Oncogene*, 9:195–204, 1994.
112. Hayashi, H. et al., The mutation of codon 249 in the p53 gene is not specific in Japanese hepatocellular carcinoma. *Liver*, 13:279–281, 1993.
113. Kew, M.C., Synergistic action between AFB1 and HBV in hepatocarcinogenesis. *Liver Int.*, 23:405–409, 2003.
114. Ross, R.K. et al., Urinary aflatoxin biomarkers and risk of hepatocellular carcinoma. *Lancet*, 339:943–946, 1992.
115. Qian, G.S. et al., A follow-up study of urinary markers of aflatoxin exposure and liver cancer risk in Shanghai, People's Republic of China. *Cancer Epidemiol. Biomarkers Prev.*, 3:3–10, 1994.
116. Wang, L.-Y. et al., Aflatoxin exposure and risk of hepatocellular carcinoma in Taiwan. *Int. J. Cancer*, 67:620–630, 1996.
117. Lunn, R.M. et al., p53 mutations, chronic hepatitis B virus infection, and aflatoxin exposure in hepatocellular carcinoma in Taiwan. *Cancer Res.*, 57:3471–3477, 1997.
118. Peers, F.G. et al., Dietary aflatoxins and human liver cancer: A study in Swaziland. *Int. J. Cancer*, 17:167–176, 1976.
119. Peers, F.G. and Linsel, C.A., Dietary aflatoxins and liver cancer—a population based study in Kenya. *Br. J. Cancer*, 27:473–484, 1973.
120. van Rensburg, S.J. et al., Primary liver cancer rate and aflatoxin intake in a high cancer area. *S. Afr. Med. J.*, 48:2508a–2508d, 1974.
121. Stark, A.A. and Paster, N., New information on the carcinogenic risks associated with mycotoxin contamination in the diet, in *Nutrition in a Sustainable Environment*, Wahlqvist, M.L., Truswell, A.S., Smith, R., Nestel, P.L. (Eds.), Smith-Gordon & Co., London, 1994, pp. 60–64.
122. Delmulle, B. et al., Development of a liquid chromatography/tandem mass spectrometry method for the simultaneous determination of 16 mycotoxins on cellulose filters and in fungal cultures, *Rapid Commun. Mass Spectrom.*, 20:771–775, 2006.
123. Maragos, C.M., Novel assays and sensor platforms for the detection of aflatoxins. *Adv Exp. Med. Biol.*, 504:85–93, 2005.
124. McCoy, L. et al., Analysis of aflatoxin B_1-lysine adducts in human serum by isotope dilution liquid chromatography tandem mass spectrometry. *Rapid Commun. Mass Spectrom.*, 19, 2203–2210, 2005.
125. Goebel, G. et al., Circulating nucleic acids in plasma or serum (CNAPS) as prognostic and predictive markers in patients with solid neoplasias. *Dis. Markers*, 21:105–120, 2005.

126. Kirk, G.D. et al., Ser-249 p53 mutations in plasma DNA of patients with hepatocellular carcinoma from The Gambia. *J. Natl. Cancer Inst.*, 92:148–153, 2000.
127. Jackson, P.E. et al., Specific p53 mutations detected in plasma and tumors of hepatocellular carcinoma patients by electrospray ionization mass spectrometry. *Cancer Res.*, 61:33–35, 2001.
128. Jackson, P.E., Prospective detection of codon 249 mutations in plasma of hepatocellular carcinoma patients. *Carcinogenesis*, 24:1–27, 2003.
129. Bennett, J.W. and Klich, M., Mycotoxins, *Clin. Microbiol. Rev.*, 16:497–516, 2003.
130. Smela, M.E. et al., The chemistry, biology of aflatoxin B1: From mutational spectrometry to carcinogenesis. *Carcinogenesis*, 22:535–545, 2001.
131. Grant, P.G. and Phillips, T.D., Isothermal adsorption of aflatoxin B_1 on HSCAS clay. *J. Agric. Food Chem.*, 46:599–605, 1998.
132. Wang, J.S. et al., Short-term safety evaluation of processed calcium montmorillonite clay (NovaSil) in humans. *Food Addit. Contam.*, 22:270–279, 2005.
133. Phillips, T.D., Dietary clay in the chemoprevention of aflatoxin-induced disease. *Toxicol. Sci.* 52 (Suppl. 2):118–126, 1999.
134. Egner, P.A. et al., Chlorophyllin intervention reduces aflatoxin-DNA adducts in individuals at high risk for liver cancer. *Proc. Natl. Acad. Sci. U.S.A.*, 98:14601–14606, 2001.
135. Egner, P.A. et al., Chemoprevention with chlorophyllin in individuals exposed to dietary aflatoxin. *Mut. Res.*, 523–524:209–216, 2003.
136. Kensler, T.W. et al., Chemoprevention of hepatocellular carcinoma in aflatoxin endemic areas. *Gastroenterology*, 127(5) (Suppl. 1):S310–S318, 2004.

Section II

Detecting and Monitoring Microbial Food Contamination

7

Rapid Methods for Detecting Microbial Contaminants in Foods: Past, Present, and Future

Daniel Y.C. Fung

CONTENTS

7.1 Introduction

Because of global food trades, concern of food safety and security, threat of bioterrorism, national and international public health monitoring, food spoilage potential, development and spread of new microbial agents and related issues, and the rapid and accurate determination of the numbers and kinds of microbes in our food systems are important means to help protect the general public in any society. Rapid methods and automation in microbiology is a dynamic area in applied microbiology dealing with the study of improved methods in the isolation, early detection, characterization, and enumeration of microorganisms and their products in clinical, food, industrial, and environmental samples. In the past 25 years this field has emerged into an important subdivision of the general field of applied microbiology and is gaining momentum nationally and internationally as an area of research and application to monitor the numbers, kinds, and metabolites of microorganisms related to food spoilage, food preservation, food fermentation, food safety, and foodborne pathogens. This chapter provides information and discussions on major developments in many aspects of this rapidly changing discipline. The purpose is to provide an overview of the current status of the total field and predict the developments in the near future.

7.2   History and Key Developments

Medical microbiologists started to be involved with rapid methods around mid-1960s and this started to accelerate in the 1970s, with continued developments in the 1980s, 1990s, and up to the present day. Food microbiologists were lagging about 10 years behind the medical microbiologists for about 20 years, but in the past decade they have greatly increased their activities in this field. From 1965 to 1975, it can be called the age of miniaturization and diagnostic kit developments. From 1975 to 1985, it was the age of immunological test kits developments. From 1985 to 1995, it was the age of genetic probes, molecular testing systems, and polymerase chain reaction (PCR) applications. Currently (1995–2007), we are in the biosensor, computer chip technology, and microarray system development era in response to human genome projects and the evolving field of "proteomics" and related fields. Spanning across these major areas was the development of instrumentations and automation for mechanization of these methods and technologies and in biomass monitoring. Fung (2002) made a comprehensive review of the historical development of rapid methods and automation in microbiology in the inaugural issue of *Critical Reviews of Food Science and Food Safety* published by Institute of Food Technologists. Many methods and procedures currently in use in food microbiology laboratories were developed more than 100 years ago. The "conventional" methods used by many regulatory laboratories around the world are based on these laborious, large-volume usages of liquid and solid media and reagents, and time consuming procedures both in operation and data collection. However, these methods remain as the gold standards in applied microbiology and in the books of regulatory agencies nationally and internationally to the present time.

A look into older bacteriology textbooks and laboratory manuals revealed some form of improved operations for handling large numbers of culture tubes, test tubes, plates, and inoculation procedures. The most important book dealing with automation was *Miniaturization of Microbiological Methods*, written by Paul A. Hartman in 1968. The book provided over 1200 citations of techniques for the cultivation of bacteria, fungi, protozoa, and other plants and animal cells. The purpose of the book was to describe techniques that were more rapid, convenient, or reliable than conventional laboratory methods by miniaturization. Several interesting articles appeared in the early 1970s concerning this field. Goldschmidt (1970) had a chapter entitled "Instrumentation for microbiology: Horizons unlimited" in the book *Rapid Diagnosis Methods in Medical Microbiology* by Graber (1970). Richardson (1972) had an article on "Automation in the diary laboratory" in the *Journal of Milk and Food Technology*, and Trotman (1973) on "The philosophy of the application of automatic methods to hospital diagnostic bacteriology" in *Biochemical Engineering*.

Many scientific meetings, seminars, and symposia were held to discuss rapid methods in the early 1970s. The key identifiable start of the field was the first International Symposium on Rapid Methods and Automation in Microbiology held in Stockholm, Sweden, in 1973. There were about 500–600 people at this meeting. Subsequently, symposia of this series were held in Cambridge, United Kingdom (1976), Washington, DC (1981), Berlin (1984), Florence, Italy (1987), and Helsinki, Finland (1990). The last meeting of this series was held in London, United Kingdom, in 1993. The proceedings of these meetings were published after the meetings. The most valuable ones were the two books edited by Heden and Illeni (1975a,b): *Automation in Microbiology and Immunology* and *New Approaches to the Identification of Microorganisms*. These two books, although outdated by now, contain the basic approaches and philosophies of the field of rapid methods.

In between these major meetings, many national and international conferences also were held on similar topics mostly in Europe. In the past 10 years an explosion of meetings and symposia occurred in the United States, Europe, and around the world organized by professional societies such as *Institute of Food Technologists, American Society for Microbiology, National Environmental Health Association, Biodeterioration Society, AOAC International*, etc., and by universities, governmental agencies, and industrial companies. An interesting development occurred in recent years when professional conference managing companies and trade magazine companies started to organize these meetings and attracted quite a diversified audience. Another important development was the initiation of hands-on workshops concerning these rapid methods. Some of the workshops were for one or two days, with lectures and limited demonstrations and hands-on experiences of various systems. The most comprehensive program was developed by the author in 1981 at Kansas State University, Manhattan, Kansas. The program lasted 8 days. The first workshop had 16 participants from several countries. The number of participants steadily increased through the years to about 60 participants. The total number of participants, lecturers, students, and guest speakers exceeded 3500 scientists from

60 countries and all over the United States. The workshop celebrated its 25th anniversary in 2005 and is planning for the 27th workshop in June, 2007. All these conferences, workshops, symposia, and meetings greatly heightened the interests and participation of an ever-expanding audience on a global scale.

7.3 Advances in Sample Preparation and Treatments

One of the most important steps for successful microbiological analysis of any material is sample preparation. Without proper sampling procedures, the data obtained will have limited meaning and usefulness. With the advancement of microbiological techniques and miniaturization of kits and test systems to ever smaller sizes, proper sample preparation becomes critical. The following discussions are sample preparation methods for applied microbiological analysis for foods and food plant environments. Microbiological samples can be grouped as solid samples, liquid samples, surface samples, and air samples. Each type of sample has its unique properties and concerns in sample preparation and analysis. These procedures are important for both conventional microbiological techniques as well as new and sophisticated rapid methods.

7.3.1 Solid Samples

Common laboratory procedures for solid samples include aseptic techniques to collect sample, and rapid transport (less than 24 h) to laboratory site in frozen state for frozen foods and chilled state for most other foods. The purpose is to minimize growth or death of the microorganisms in the food to be analyzed. The next step is to aseptically remove a subsample such as 5, 10, 25 g, or more for testing. Sometimes samples are obtained from different lots and composited for analysis. In food microbiology, almost always the food is diluted to 1:10 dilution (i.e., 1 part of food in 9 parts of sterile diluent) and then homogenized by a variety of methods. It should be noted that 1 g of food sample is equivalent to 1 mL of diluent (based on the specific gravity of water) for ease of calculation of dilution factors in microbiological protocol. After dilution, the sample needs to be homogenized. Traditionally, a sterile blender or osterizer is used to homogenize the food suspension for 1–2 min before further diluting the sample for microbiological analysis. The disadvantages of using a blender include (1) cleaning and re-sterilization between each use, (2) generation of aerosols contaminating the environment, and (3) mechanical generation of heat may kill some bacteria. In the past 25 years, the Stomacher invented by Anthony Sharpe has become standard equipment in food analysis laboratories. About 40,000 Stomacher units are in use worldwide. The sample is placed in a sterile plastic bag and an appropriate amount of sterile diluent is added.

The sample in the bag is then "massaged" by two paddles of the instrument for 1–2 min and then the content can be analyzed with or without further dilution. The advantages of the Stomacher include (1) no need to resterilize the instrument between samples because the sample (housed in a sterile plastic bag) does not come in contact with the instrument, (2) disposable bags allow analysis of a large number of samples efficiently, (3) no heat or aerosols will be generated, and (4) the bag with the sample can serve as a container for time-course studies. Recently, Anthony Sharpe invented the Pulsifier (Microgen Bioproducts, Surrey, United Kingdom) for dislodging microorganisms from foods without excessively breaking the food structure. The Pulsifier has an oval ring that can house a plastic bag with the sample and diluent. When the instrument is activated the ring will vibrate vigorously for a predetermined time (30–60 s). During this time microorganisms on the food surface or in the food will be dislodged into the diluent with minimum destruction of the food. Fung et al. (1998) evaluated the Pulsifier against the Stomacher with 96 food items (including beef, pork, veal, fish, shrimp, cheese, peas, a variety of vegetables, cereal, and fruits) and found that the systems gave essentially the same viable cell count in the food, but the Pulsified samples were much clearer than the Stomached samples. A more recent report by Kang et al. (2001) found that the Pulsifier and Stomacher had a correlation coefficient of 0.971 and 0.959 for total aerobic count and coliform count, respectively, with 50 samples of lean meat tissues. The Pulsified samples, however, contained much less meat debris than Stomached samples. In the case of Stomached samples, much meat debris occurred, which interfered with plating samples on agar. Wu et al. (2003) made a detailed study of the Stomacher and the Pulsifier on microbiology from 30 vegetables and obtained equivalent counts from the two instruments but the samples from the Pulsifier were far clearer. The superior quality of microbial suspensions with minimum food particles from the Pulsifier has positive implications for general analysis as well as for techniques such as adenosine triphosphate (ATP) bioluminescence tests, DNA/RNA hybridization, PCR amplifications, enzymatic assays, etc.

7.3.2   Liquid Samples

Liquid samples are easier to manipulate than solid samples. After appropriate mixing (by vigorous hand shaking or by instrument), one only needs to aseptically introduce a known volume of liquid sample into a container and then add a desired volume of sterile diluent to obtain the desired dilution ratio (1:10, 1:100, etc.). Further dilutions can be made as necessary. There are now many automated pipetting instruments available for sample dilutions. Viscous and semisolid samples need special considerations such as the use of large mouth pipettes during operation. Regardless of the consistency of the semisolid sample, 1 mL of sample is considered as 1 mL of liquid for ease of making dilution calculations.

7.3.3 Surface Samples

Sampling of surfaces of food or the environment presents a different set of concerns. The analyst needs to decide on the proper unit to report the findings, such as number of bacteria per inch square, per cm square, or other units. One can analyze different shapes of the surface such as a square, rectangle, triangle, or circle, etc. A sterile template will be useful for this purpose. Occasionally, one has to analyze unusual shapes such as the surface of an egg, apple, the entire surface of a chicken, etc. The calculations of these areas becomes quite complex. For intact meat or other soft tissues, one can excise an area of the food by using a sterile knife assuming that all the organisms are on the surface and that the meat itself is sterile. Often a sterile moist cotton swab is used to obtain microbes from the surface of a known area and then the swab is placed into a diluent of known volume (e.g., 5 mL), shaken and then plated on a general purpose agar or a selective agar. Instead of a cotton swab, one can use contact materials to sample surfaces. This includes selective and nonselective agar in Rodac plate, adhesive tape, sterile gauge, sterile sponge, etc.

The nature and characteristics of the surfaces are also very important. Obtaining microbiological samples from dry surfaces, wet surfaces, oily surfaces, slimy surfaces, meat, chicken skin, orange skin, stainless steel, concrete, rocks, hair nets, etc., are very different. A lot of microorganisms will remain on the surface even after repeatedly sampling the same area. Biofilms are very hard to completely remove from any surface. This, however, should not be a deterrent to use surface sampling techniques if one can relate the numbers obtained to another parameter such as cleanliness of the surface or quality of a food product. Lee and Fung (1986) made a comprehensive review on surface sampling techniques for bacteriology.

7.3.4 Air Samples

Air sampling in food microbiology received much less attention compared with other sample techniques already discussed. Due to recent concerns of environmental air pollution, indoor air quality, public health, and the threat of bioterrorism, there is a renewed interest in rapid techniques to monitor microbes and their toxins in the air. The most common way to estimate air quality is the use of "air plates," where the lid of an agar plate is removed and the agar surface exposed to air of the environment for a determined time such as 10 min, 30 min, or a couple of hours. The plate is then covered and incubated and later colonies are counted. If the colony numbers exceed a certain value, for example 15 per plate, the air quality may be considered unacceptable. However this simple method is passive and the information is not too quantitative. A much better way is to actively pass a known volume of air through an instrument to measure biological particles over an agar surface (impaction) to obtain viable cell numbers after incubation of the agar, or trap microorganisms with a liquid sample (impingement) and then analyze the liquid for various viable cells. There are a variety of commercially available air samplers. Some of them are quite sophisticated such as the Andersen air sampler that can separate particle sizes from the environment in six stages from large particles (more than 5 µm in diameter) to small particles (0.2 µm). The author has used the SAS sampler (PBI, Milan, Italy) for many years with good results. With this instrument, a Rodac plate or an ordinary plate with a suitable agar is clipped in place. A cover with precision pattern of holes (to direct air flow precisely) is then screwed on. After activating the instrument, a known volume of air is sucked through the holes and the particles will hit and be lodged onto the surface of the agar. After operation (e.g., 60 L of air in 20 s) the air sampler cover is removed and the lid of the agar plate is replaced and the plate is incubated. The number of colonies developed on the agar can be converted to colony forming units (CFU) per cubic meter. Al-Dagal and Fung (1993) suggested that for food processing plants 0–100 CFU/m^3 is considered clean air, 100–300 CFU/m^3 is acceptable air, and over 300 CFU/m^3 is considered not acceptable. As a comparison, more than 500 CFU/m^3 of air is unacceptable according to the standard used in Singapore for food plants.

Applied food microbiologists are constantly searching for better sample preparation methods to improve recovery of microbes from foods and the environment. This section only dealt with improvements related to solid and liquid foods, surfaces of food and food contact areas, and air samples. A great variety of physical, chemical, physicochemical, and biological sampling methods used in clinical sampling, industrial sampling, and environmental sampling can also be explored by food microbiologists to make sampling of microorganisms in foods more precise and accurate.

7.4   Advances in Total Viable Cell-Count Methodologies

One of the most important information concerning food quality, food spoilage, food safety, and potential implication of foodborne pathogens is the total viable cell count of food, water, food contact surfaces, and air of the food plants. The conventional "standard plate count" method has been in use for the past 100 years in applied microbiology. The method involves preparing the sample, diluting the sample, plating the sample with a general nonselective agar, incubating the plates at 35°C, and counting the colonies after 48 h. The operation of the conventional standard plate count method, although simple, is time-consuming both in terms of operation and data collection. Also, this method utilizes a large number of test tubes, pipettes, dilution bottles, dilution buffer, sterile plates, incubation space, and the related disposable and clean up of reusable materials and resterilizing them for further use.

Several methods have been developed, tested, and used effectively in the past 20 years as alternative methods for viable cell count. Most of these methods were first designed to perform viable cell counts and relate the counts to standard plate counts. Later coliform count, fecal coliform count, and yeast and mold counts were introduced in these systems. Further developments in these systems include differential counts, pathogen counts, and even pathogen detection after further manipulations. Many of these methods have been extensively tested in many laboratories throughout the world and went through AOAC International collaborative study approvals. The aim of these methods is to provide reliable viable cell counts of food and water in more convenient, rapid, simple, and cost-effective alternative formats compared to the cumbersome standard plate count method.

The spiral plating method is an automated system to obtain viable cell count (Spiral Biotech, Bethesda, Maryland). By use of a stylus, this instrument can spread a liquid sample on the surface of a pre-poured agar plate (selective or nonselective) in a spiral shape (the Archimedes spiral) with a concentration gradient starting from the center and decreasing as the spiral progresses outward on the rotating plate. The volume of the liquid deposited at any segment of the agar plate is known. After the liquid containing microorganisms is spread, the agar plate is incubated overnight at an appropriate temperature for the colonies to develop. The colonies appearing along the spiral pathway can be counted either manually or electronically. The time for plating a sample is only several seconds compared to minutes used in the conventional method. Also, using a laser counter, an analyst can obtain an accurate count in a few seconds as compared with a few minutes, in the tiring procedure of counting colonies by the naked eye. The system has been used extensively for the past 20 years with satisfactory microbiological results from meat, poultry, seafood, vegetable, fruits, dairy products, spices, etc. New versions of the spiral plater are introduced as Autoplater (Spiral Biotech, Maryland) and Whitley Automatic Spiral Plater (Microbiology International, Rockville, Maryland). With these automatic instruments, an analyst needs only to present the liquid sample and the instrument completely and automatically processes the sample, including re-sterilizing the unit for the next sample.

The ISOGRID system (Neogen, Inc., East Lansing, Michigan) consists of a square filter with hydrophobic grids printed on the filter to form 1600 squares for each filter. A food sample is first weighted, homogenized, diluted, enzyme treated, and then passed through the filter assisted by vacuum. Microbes are trapped on the filter and into the squares. The filter is then placed on pre-poured nonselective or selective agar and then incubated for a specific time and temperature. Since a growing microbial colony cannot migrate over the hydrophobic material, all colonies are confounded into a square shape. The analyst can then count the squares as individual colonies. Since there is a chance that more than one bacterium were trapped in one square, the system has a most probable number (MPN) conversion table to provide statistically accurate viable cell counts. Automatic instruments are also available to count these square colonies in seconds. Again, this method has been used to test a great variety of foods in the past 20 years.

Petrifilm (3M Co., St. Paul, Minnesota) is an ingenious system with appropriate rehydratable nutrients embedded in a series of films in the unit. The unit is a little larger than the size of a credit card. To obtain viable cell count the protective top layer is lifted and 1 mL of liquid sample is introduced to the center of the unit and then the cover is replaced. A plastic template is placed on the cover to make a round mold. The rehydrated medium will support the growth of microorganisms after suitable incubation time and temperature. The colonies are directly counted in the unit. This system has a shelf-life of over 1 year in cold storage. The attractiveness of this system is that it is simple to use, small in size, has a long shelf-life, preparation of agar is not needed, and easy to read results. Recently, the company also introduced a Petrifilm counter so that an analyst only needs to place the Petrifilm with colonies into the unit and the unit will automatically count and record the viable cell count in the computer. The manual form of the Petrifilm has been used for many food systems and is gaining international acceptance as an alternative method for viable cell count.

Redigel system (3M Co., St Paul, Minnesota) consists of tubes of sterile nutrient with a pectin gel in the tube but no conventional agar. This liquid system is ready for use and no heat is needed to melt the system since there is no agar in the liquid. After an analyst mixes 1 mL of liquid sample with the liquid in the tube, the resultant contents are poured into a special petri dish coated with calcium. The pectin and calcium will react and form a gel that will solidify in about 20 min. The plate is then incubated at the proper time and temperature, and the colonies will be counted the same way as the conventional standard plate count method.

The four methods described above have been in use for almost 25 years. Chain and Fung (1991) made a comprehensive evaluation of all four methods against the conventional standard plate count method on seven different foods, 20 samples each, and found that the alternative systems and the conventional method were highly comparable at an agreement of $r = 0.95$. In the same study, they also found that the alternative systems cost less than the conventional system for making viable cell counts.

The author also miniaturized the entire viable cell-count method by use of the Microtiter system for dilution and miniaturized droplets to deliver samples on agar plates (4–8 drops per agar plate) and obtained viable cell counts in a very efficient manner (Fung and Kraft, 1968; Fung and LaGrange, 1969). The counting range of each droplet is between 10 and 100 colonies per drop. This method received positive collaborative evaluation among several public health and university laboratories (Fung et al., 1976).

A newer alternative method, the SimPlate system (BioControl, Bellevue, Washington), has 84 wells imprinted in a round plastic plate. After the lid is removed, a diluted food sample (1 mL) is dispensed onto the center landing pad and 10 mL of rehydrated nutrient liquid provided by the manufacturer is poured onto the landing pad. The mixture (food and nutrient liquid) is distributed evenly into the wells by swirling the SimPlate in a gentle, circular motion. Excessive liquid is absorbed by a pad housed in the unit. After 24 h of incubation at 35°C, the plate is placed under UV light. Fluorescent-positive wells are counted and the number is converted in the MPN table to determine the number of bacteria present in the SimPlate. The method is simple to use with minimum amount of preparation. A 198 well unit is also available for samples with high counts. Using different medium, the unit can also make counts of total coliforms and *Escherichia coli* counts, as well as yeast and mold counts. The above methods are designed to count aerobic microorganisms.

To count anaerobic microorganisms, one has to introduce the sample into the melted agar; and after solidification, the plates need to be incubated in an enclosed anaerobic jar. In the anaerobic jar, oxygen is removed by the hydrogen generated by the "gas pack" in the jar to create an anaerobic environment. After incubation, the colonies can be counted and reported as anaerobic count of the food. The method is simple but requires expensive anaerobic jars and disposable gas packs. Also, it takes about 1 h before the interior of the jar becomes anaerobic. Some strict anaerobic microorganisms may die during this 1 h period of reduction of oxygen. The author developed a simple anaerobic double tube system that is easy to use and provides an instant anaerobic condition for the cultivation of anaerobes from foods (Fung and Lee, 1981). In this system, the desired agar (ca. 23 mL) is first autoclaved in a large test tube (OD 25 × 150 mm). When needed, the agar is melted and tempered at 48°C. A liquid (1 mL) or solid (1 gm) sample or a filter such as ISOGRID, which can capture microorganisms from 1, 10, or 100 mL sample, is placed into the melted agar. A smaller sterile test tube (OD 16 × 150 mm) is inserted into the large tube containing the food sample or filter in the melted agar. By doing so, a thin film is formed between the two test tubes. The unit is tightly closed by a screw cap. The entire unit is placed into an incubator for the colonies to develop. No anaerobic jar is needed for this simple anaerobic system. After incubation, the colonies developing in the agar film can be counted and provide an anaerobic count of the food being tested. This simple method has been used extensively for applied anaerobic microbiology in the author's laboratory for about 20 years (Ali and Fung, 1991; Schmidt et al., 2000).

Another effective viable cell-count method in applied microbiology is the MPN system. In a paper published in 1918, McCrady (1918) presented detailed MPN tables for making viable cell counts of water samples. McCrady effectively argued that MPN method of dilution to extinction of water and evaluate fermentation tube was more accurate than the colony counts resulted in the agar plates after incubation. Interestingly enough even in 1918 the title of the paper was "Tables for rapid interpretation of fermentation tube results!" However the MPN method (3-tube, 5-tube, or

16-tube MPN in three dilution series) is very time-consuming and involves a large number of tubes, media, and incubation space. The author is the first person to miniaturize the 3-tube MPN system in the Microtiter plate in 1969 (Fung and Kraft, 1969). In a similar vein, the author also miniaturized the MPN method in the Microtiter plate by diluting a sample in a 3-tube miniaturized series (Fung and Kraft, 1969). In one Microtiter plate, one can dilute four samples each in triplicate (3-tube MPN) to eight series of 1:10 dilution. After incubation, the turbidity of the wells is recorded and a modified 3-tube MPN table can be used to calculate the MPN of the original sample. This procedure recently received renewed interest in the scientific community.

Walser (2000) in Switzerland reported the use of an automated system for Microtiter plate assay to perform classical MPN of drinking water. He used a pipetting robot equipped with sterile pipetting tips for automatic dilution of the samples, and after incubation, placed the plate in a Microtiter plate reader and obtained MPN results with the use of a computer. The system can cope with low or high bacterial load from 0 to 20,000 colonies/mL. The system takes out the tedious and personnel influence of routine microbiological works and can be applied to determine MPN of fecal organisms in water as well as other microorganisms of interest in food microbiology.

Irwin et al. (2000) in the United States also worked on a similar system by using a modified Gauss–Newton algorithm and 96-well microtechnique for calculating MPN using Microsoft Excel spreadsheets. These improvements are possible in 2000 compared with the original work of the author in 1969 because (1) automated instruments are now available in many laboratories to dispense liquid into the Microtiter plate; automated dilution instruments are also available to facilitate rapid and aseptic dilutions of samples; (2) auto mated readers of Microtiter wells are now common place to efficiently read turbidity, color, and fluorescence of the liquid in the wells for calculation of MPN; and (3) elegant mathematical models, computer interpretations and analysis, and printout of data are now available, which the author could not have envisioned back in 1969.

At the 2006 International Association for Food Protection annual meeting in Calgary, Canada, in June 2006, bioMerieux, Inc. (Hazelwood, Missouri) officially introduced a totally automated 16-tube MPN system in a very convenient and mechanized TEMPO system, which integrates preparation, injection of sample into the miniaturized chambers (16 tube, 3 series MPN system), and incubation of the integrated clear plastic MPN unit. The analyst simply presents to the instrument the sample with suitable liquid nutrients and the instrument can automatically deliver the liquid sample (1 mL) into the 3 series of 16-tube MPN unit. The unit is then incubated overnight at the appropriate temperature. After incubation, the unit is placed in another instrument which can automatically read the fluorescence of each well and report the data as MPN/mL of water or food. This, in the opinion of the author, is a major development in automated viable cell enumeration in the field of rapid methods for food and water microbiology testing. By using different selective liquid media, indicator organisms and even potential pathogens can be effectively enumerated from food and water.

A few "real time" viable cell-count methods have been developed and tested in recent years. These methods rely on using vital stains to stain live cells or ATP detection of live cells. All these methods need careful sample preparation, filtration, careful selection of dyes and reagents, and instrumentation. Usually the entire system is quite costly. However, they can provide one shift results and can handle a large number of samples.

The direct epifluorescent filter techniques (DFET) method has been tested for many years and is in use in the United Kingdom for raw milk quality assurance programs and Nordic countries for ground beef quality assurance programs. In this method, the microorganisms are first trapped on a filter and then the filter is stained with acridine orange dye. The slide is observed under UV microscopy. Live cells usually fluoresce orange–red, orange–yellow, or orange–brown, whereas dead cells fluoresce green. The slide can be read by the eye or by an automated counting system. A viable cell count can be made in less than an hour.

The Chemunex Scan RDI system (Monmouth Junction, New Jersey) involves filtering cells on a membrane and staining cells with vital dyes (Fluorassure), and after about 90 min incubation (for bacteria), the membrane with stained cell is read in a scanning chamber that can scan and count fluorescing viable cells. This system has been used to test disinfecting solutions against such organisms as *Pseudomonas aeruginosa*, *Serratia marcescens*, *E. coli*, and *Staphylococcus aureus* with satisfactory results.

The MicroStar System developed by Millipore Corporation (Benford, Massachusetts) utilizes ATP bioluminescence technology by trapping bacteria in a specialized membrane (Milliflex). Individual live cells are trapped in the matrix of the filter and grow into microcolonies. The filter is then sprayed with permeabilizing reagent in a reaction chamber to release ATP. The bioluminescence reagent is then sprayed onto the filter. Live cells will give off light due to the presence of ATP and the light is measured by a CCD camera and fluorescent particles (live cells) are counted.

These are new developments in staining technology, ATP technology, and instrumentation for viable cell counts. The application of these methods in the food industry is still in the evaluation stage. The future looks promising.

7.5 Advances in Miniaturization and Diagnostic Kits

Identification of normal flora, spoilage organisms, foodborne pathogens, starter cultures, etc., in food microbiology is an important part of microbiological manipulations. Conventional methods, dating back to more than 100 years ago, utilize large volumes of medium (10 mL or more) to test for a particular characteristic of a bacterium (e.g., lactose broth for lactose fermentation by *E. coli*). Inoculating a test culture into these individual tubes one at a time is also very cumbersome. Through the years, many microbiologists have devised vessels and smaller tubes to reduce the volumes used for these tests (Hartman, 1968). This author has systematically developed many miniaturized methods to reduce the volume of reagents and media (from 5–10 mL to about 0.2 mL) for microbiological testing in a convenient Microtiter plate, which has 96 wells arranged in an 8×12 format. The basic components of the miniaturized system are the commercially sterilized Microtiter plates for housing the test cultures, a multiple inoculation device, and containers to house solid media (large petri dishes) and liquid media (in another series of Microtiter plates with 0.2 mL of liquid per well). The procedure involves placing liquid cultures (pure cultures) to be studied into sterile wells of a Microtiter plate (approximately 0.2 mL for each well) to form a master plate. Each Microtiter plate can hold up to 96 different cultures, 48 duplicate cultures, or various combinations as desired. The cultures are then transferred by a sterile multipoint inoculator (96 pins protruding from a template) to solid or liquid media. Sterilization of the inoculator is by alcohol flaming. Each transfer represents 96 separate inoculations in the conventional method. After incubation at an appropriate temperature, the growth of cultures on solid media or liquid media can be observed and recorded, and the data can be analyzed. These methods are ideal for studying large numbers of isolates or for research involving challenging large numbers of microbes against a host of test compounds. Through the years, using the miniaturized systems the author has characterized thousands of bacterial cultures isolated from meat and other foods, studied the effect of organic dyes against bacteria and yeasts, and performed challenging studies of various compounds against microbes with excellent results. Many useful microbiological media were discovered through this line of research. For example, an aniline blue *Candida albicans* medium was developed and marketed by DIFCO under the name of Candida Isolation Agar. The sensitivity and specificity were 98.0% and 99.5%, respectively, with a predictive value of 99.1% (Goldschmidt et al., 1991).

Other scientists also have miniaturized many systems and developed them into diagnostic kits around late 1960s to 1970s. Currently, API systems, Enterotube, Minitek, Crystal ID system, MicroID, RapID systems, Biolog, and Vitek systems are available. Most of these systems were first developed for identification of enterics (*Salmonella, Shigella, Proteus, Enterobacter,* etc.). Later, many of the companies expanded the capacity to identify nonfermentors, anaerobes, gram-positive organisms, and even yeast and molds. Most of the early comparative analyses centered around evaluation of these kits for clinical specimens. Comparative analysis of diagnostic kits and selection criteria for miniaturized systems were made by Cox et al. (1984) and Fung et al. (1989). They concluded that miniaturized systems are accurate, efficient, labor saving, space saving, and cheaper than the conventional methods. Originally, an analyst needs to read the color reaction of each well in the diagnostic kit and then use a manual identification code to "key" out the organisms. Recently, diagnostic companies have developed automatic readers phasing in with computers to provide rapid and accurate identification of the unknown cultures.

The most successful and sophisticated miniaturized automated identification system is the Vitek system (bioMerieux, Hazelwood, Missouri), which utilizes a plastic card that contains 30 tiny wells in which each has a different reagent. The unknown culture in a liquid form is "pressurized" into the wells in a vacuum chamber and then the cards are placed in an incubator for a period of time ranging from 4 to 12 h. The instrument periodically scans each card and compares the color changes or gas production of each tiny well with the database of known cultures. Vitek can identify a typical *E. coli* culture in 2–4 h. Each Vitek unit can handle 120 cards or more automatically. There are a few thousand Vitek units in use currently in the world. The database is especially good for clinical isolates. A new generation of Vitek instrument (Vitek 2) will be launched in 2007.

Biolog system (Hayward, California) is also a miniaturized system using the Microtiter format for growth and reaction information similar to the original ideas of the author. Pure cultures are first isolated on agar and then suspended in a liquid to the appropriate density (approximately 6 log cell/mL). The culture is then dispensed into a Microtiter plate containing different carbon sources in 95 wells and 1 nutrient control well. The plate with the pure cultures is then incubated overnight after which the Microtiter plate is evaluated and the color pattern of the wells with carbon utilization is observed and compared with profiles of typical patterns of microbes. This manual evaluation is too tedious to perform and the company developed a software system for the users to enter the data in a computer and then receive the identification. A more convenient mode is to put the Microtiter plate in an instrument that can scan the pattern of the positive wells and conduct a match with known cultures to make an identification. This system is easy to operate, and with the use of the automatic data analysis, the system is a useful tool to characterize and identify unknown cultures. This system is very ambitious and tries to identify more than 1400 genera and species of environmental, food, and medical isolates from major groups of gram-positive, gram-negative, and other organisms. The data base of many cultures is still limited and it needs further development to identify cultures from food and the environment. Nevertheless this system provides a simple operational format with good identification for typical isolates.

There is no question that miniaturization of microbiological methods has saved much materials and operational time and has provided the required efficiency and convenience in diagnostic microbiology. The flexible systems developed by the author and others can be used in many research and development laboratories for studying a large number of cultures. The commercial systems have played key roles in diagnostic microbiology and have saved many lives due to rapid and accurate characterization of pathogenic bacteria. These miniaturized systems and diagnostic kits will continue to be very useful and important in the medical and food microbiology arenas.

7.6   Advances in Immunological Testings

Antigen and antibody reaction has been used for decades for detecting and characterizing microorganisms and their components in medical and diagnostic microbiology. Antibodies are produced in animal systems when a foreign particle (antigen) is injected into the system. By collecting the antibodies and purifying the antibodies one can use these antibodies to detect the corresponding antigens. Thus when a *Salmonella* or a component of *Salmonella* is injected into a rabbit the animal will produce antibodies against *Salmonella* or the component (e.g., somatic antigen). By collecting and purifying these antibodies, one can use these antisera to react with a culture of suspected *Salmonella*. When a positive reaction commences, agglutination of antigens (*Salmonella*) and antibodies (antibodies against *Salmonella*) will occur and can be observed on a slide by a trained technician. This is the basis for serotyping bacteria such as *Salmonella, E. coli* O157:H7, *Listeria monocytogenes*, etc. These antibodies can be polyclonal (a mixture of several antibodies in the antisera, which can react with different sites of the antigens) or monoclonal (there is only one pure antibody in the antiserum, which will react with only one epitope of the antigens). Both polyclonal antibodies and monoclonal antibodies have been used extensively in applied food microbiology. There are many ways to perform antigen–antibody reactions but the most popular format in recent years is the "sandwiched" enzyme linked immunosorbent assay or popularly known as the ELISA test.

Briefly, antibodies (e.g., anti-*Salmonella* antibody) are fixed on a solid support (e.g., wells of a Microtiter plate). A solution containing a suspect target antigen (e.g. *Salmonella*) is introduced into the Microtiter well. If the solution has *Salmonella* the antibodies will capture the *Salmonella*.

After washing away food debris and excess materials another anti-*Salmonella* antibody complex is added into the solution. The second anti-*Salmonella* antibody will react with another part of the trapped *Salmonella*. This second antibody is linked with an enzyme such as horseradish peroxidase. After another washing to remove debris, a chromagen complex such as tetramethylbenzidine and hydrogen peroxide is added. The enzyme will react with the chromagen and will produce a color-compound, which will indicate that the first antibody has captured *Salmonella*. If all the reaction procedures are done properly and the liquid in a Microtiter well exhibits a color reaction then the sample is considered positive for *Salmonella*.

This procedure is simple to operate and has been used for decades with excellent results. It should be mentioned that these ELISA tests need about 1 million cells to be reactive and therefore before performing the ELISA tests the food sample has to go through an overnight incubation so that the target organism has reached a detectable level. The total time to detect a pathogen by these systems should include the enrichment time of the target pathogens.

Many diagnostic companies (such as BioControl, Organon Teknika, Tecra, etc.) have marketed ELISA test kits for foodborne pathogens and toxins such as *Salmonella, E. coli,* staphylococcal enterotoxins, etc. However, the time involved in samples addition, incubating, washing and discarding of liquids, adding of another antibody complex, washing, and finally adding of reagents for color reaction all contribute to inconvenience of the manual operation of the ELISA test. Recently some companies have completely automated the entire ELISA procedure.

The VIDAS system (bioMerieux, Hazelwood, Missouri) is an automated system that can perform the entire ELISA procedure automatically and can complete an assay from 45 min to 2 h depending on the test kit. Since VIDAS utilizes a more sensitive fluorescent immunoassay for reporting the results, their system is named ELFA. All the analyst needs to do is to present to the reagent strip a liquid sample of an overnight enriched sample. The reagent strip contains all the necessary reagents in a ready-to-use format. The instrument will automatically transfer the sample into a plastic tube called the SPR (solid-phase receptacle), which contains antibodies to capture the target pathogen or toxin. The SPR will be automatically transferred to a series of wells in succession to perform the ELFA test. After the final reaction, the result can be read and the interpretation of positive or negative test will be automatically determined by the instrument. Presently, VIDAS can detect *Listeria, L. monocytogenes, Salmonella, E. coli* O157, staphylococcal enterotoxin, and *Campylobacter.* They also market an immuno-concentration kit for *Salmonella* and *E. coli* O157. More than 10,000 units of VIDAS units were in use in 2001.

BioControl (Bellevue, Washington) markets an Assurance EIA system that can be adapted to automation for high-volume testing. Assurance EIA is available for *Salmonella, Listeria, E. coli* O157:H7, and *Campylobacter.*

The message of the above discussion is that many ELISA test kits are now highly standardized and can be performed automatically to increase efficiency and reduce human errors.

Another exciting development in immunology is the use of lateral flow technology to perform antigen–antibody tests. In this system, the unit has three reaction regions. The first well contains antibodies to react with target antigens. These antibodies have color particles attached to them. A liquid sample (after overnight enrichment) is added to this well, and if the target organism (e.g. *E. coli* O157:H7) is present it will react with the antibodies. The complex will migrate laterally by capillary action to the second region, which contains a second antibody designed to capture the target organism. If the target organism is present, the complex will be captured and a blue line will form due to the color particles attached to the first antibody.

Excess antibodies will continue to migrate to the third region, which contains another antibody that can react with the first antibody (which has now become an antigen), to the third antibody and will form a blue color band. This is a "control" band indicating that the system is functioning properly. The entire procedure takes only about 10 min. This is truly a rapid test!

Reveal system (Neogen, Lansing, Michigan) and VIP system (BioControl, Bellevue, Washington) are the two main companies marketing this type of system for *E. coli* O157, *Salmonella*, and *Listeria*. The newest entry to this field is Eichrom Technologies, which markets a similar lateral migration system called Eclipse for the detection of *E. coli* O157:H7. Merck KgaA (Darmstadt, Germany) is also working on a similar lateral migration system for many common foodborne pathogens using a more sensitive gold particle system to report the reactions.

A number of interesting methods utilizing growth of the target pathogen are also available to detect antigen–antibody reactions.

The BioControl 1–2 test (BioControl, Bellevue, Washington) is designed to detect motile *Salmonella* from foods. In this system, the food sample is first pre-enriched for 24 h in a broth and then 0.1 mL is inoculated into one of the chambers in an L-shaped system. The chamber contains selective enrichment liquid medium for *Salmonella*. There is a small hole connecting the liquid chamber with a soft agar chamber through which *Salmonella* can migrate. An opening on the top of the soft agar chamber allows the analyst to deposit a drop of polyvalent anti-H antibodies against flagella of *Salmonella*. The antibodies move downward in the soft agar due to gravity and diffusion. If *Salmonella* is present, it will migrate throughout the soft agar. As the *Salmonella* and the anti-H antibodies meet, they will react and form a visible V-shaped "immunoband." The presence of the immunoband indicates the presumptive positive for *Salmonella* in the food sample. This reaction occurs after overnight incubation of the unit. This system is easy to use and interpret, and has gained popularity because of its simplicity.

Tecra (Roseville, Australia) developed a unique *Salmonella* detection system that combines immunocapturing and growth of the target pathogen and ELISA test in a simple to use self-contained unit. The food is first pre-enriched in a liquid medium overnight and an aliquot is added into the first tube of the unit. Into this tube a dipstick coated with *Salmonella* antibodies is introduced and left in place for 20 min at which time the antibodies will capture the *Salmonella*, if present. The dip-stick with *Salmonella* attached will then be washed and placed into a tube containing growth medium. The dipstick is left in this tube for 4 h. During this time, if *Salmonella* is present, it will start to replicate and the newly produced *Salmonella* will automatically be trapped by the coated antibodies. Thus, after 4 h of replication, the dipstick will be saturated with trapped *Salmonella*. The dipstick will be transferred to another tube containing a second antibody conjugated to enzyme and allowed to react for 20 min. After this second antigen–antibody reaction, the dipstick is washed in the fifth tube and then placed into the last tube for color development similar to other ELISA tests. A purple color developed on the dipstick indicates the presence of *Salmonella* in the food. The entire process from incubation of food sample to reading of the test results is about 22 h making it an attractive system for detection of *Salmonella*. The system can now also detect *Listeria*.

The BioControl 1–2 test and the unique *Salmonella* test are designed for laboratories with a low volume of tests. Thus, both the automatic systems and the hands-on unit systems have their place in different food testing laboratory situations.

A truly innovative development in applied microbiology is the immuno-magnetic separation system. Vicam (Somerville, Massachusetts) pioneered this concept by coating antibodies against *Listeria* on metallic particles. Large numbers of these particles (in the millions) are added into a liquid suspected to contain *Listeria* cells. The antibodies on the particles will capture the *Listeria* cells after rotating the mixture for about an hour. After the reaction, the tube is placed next to a powerful magnet, which will immobilize all the metallic particles to the side of the glass test tube regardless of whether the particles have or have not captured the *Listeria* cells. The rest of the liquid will be decanted. By removing the magnet from the tube, the metallic particles can again be suspended in a liquid. At this point, the only cells in the solution will be the captured *Listeria*. By introducing a smaller volume of liquid (e.g., 10% of the original volume), the cells are now concentrated by a factor of 10. Cells from this liquid can be detected by direct plating on selective agar, ELISA tests, PCR reaction, or other microbiological procedures in almost pure culture state. Immunomagnetic capture can save at least one day in the total protocol of pre-enrichment and enrichment steps of pathogen detection in food.

Dynal (Oslo, Norway) developed this concept further by use of very homogenized paramagnetic beads that can carry a variety of molecules such as antibodies, antigens, DNA, etc. Dynal has developed beads to capture *E. coli* O157, *Listeria*, *Cryptosporidium*, *Giardia*, etc. Furthermore, the beads can be supplied without any coating materials and scientists can tailor to their needs by coating the necessary antibodies or other capturing molecules for detection of target organisms. Currently, many diagnostic systems (ELISA test, PCR, etc.) are combining immunomagnetic capture steps to reduce incubation and increase sensitivity of the entire protocol.

Fluorescent antibody techniques have been used for decades for the detection of *Salmonella* and other pathogens. Similar to the DEFT test designed for viable cell count, fluorescent antibodies can be used to detect a great variety of target microorganisms. Tortorello and Gendel (1993) used this technique to detect *E. coli* O157:H7 in milk and juice.

Antigen–antibody reactions are a powerful system for rapid detection of all kinds of pathogens and molecules. This section describes some of the more useful methods developed for applied food microbiology. Some systems are highly automated and some systems are exceedingly simple to operate. It should be emphasized that many of the immunological tests described in this section provide "presumptive-positive" or "presumptive-negative" screening-test results. For negative screening results, the food in question is allowed to be shipped for commerce. For presumptive-positive test results, the food will not be allowed for shipment until confirmation of the positive is done by the conventional microbiological methods.

This field of immunological testing will continue to evolve as detection methodologies are being explored.

7.7   Advances in Instrumentation and Biomass Measurements

As the field of rapid methods and automation develops, the boundaries between instrumentation and diagnostic tests begin to merge. As mentioned in Section 7.6, instrumentation is now playing an important function in diagnostic kit systems and the trend will continue. The following discussions are mainly on instrumentation related to signal measurements of microbial growth.

Instruments are needed to monitor changes in a population such as ATP levels, specific enzymes, pH, electrical impedance, conductance and capacitance, generation of heat, radioactive carbon dioxide, etc. It is important to note that for the information to be useful, these parameters must be related to viable cell count of the same sample series. In general, the larger the number of viable cells in the sample, the shorter the detection time of these systems. A scattergram is then plotted and used for further comparison of unknown samples. The assumption is that as the number of microorganisms increases in the sample, these physical, biophysical, and biochemical events will also increase accordingly. When a sample has 5 log or 6 log organisms/mL, detection time can be achieved in about 4 h.

All living things utilize ATP. In the presence of a firefly enzyme system (luciferase and luciferin system), oxygen, and magnesium ions, ATP will facilitate the reaction to generate light. The amount of light generated by this reaction is proportional to the amount of ATP in the sample. Thus, the light units can be used to estimate the biomass of cells in a sample. The light emitted by this process can be monitored by a sensitive and automated fluorimeter. Some of the instruments can detect as little as 100–1000 femtogram (1 femtogram, fg, is –15 log in gram). The amount of ATP in one colony-forming unit has been reported as 0.47 fg with a range of 0.22–1.03 fg. Using this principle, many researchers have used ATP to estimate microbial cells in solid and liquid foods.

At the beginning, scientists attempted to use ATP to estimate the total number of viable cell counts in foods. The results are inconsistent because

1. Different microorganisms have different amounts of ATP per cell. For example, a yeast cell can have 100 times more ATP than a bacterial cell.

2. Even for the same organism the amount of ATP per cell is different at different growth stages.

3. Background ATP from other biomass such as blood and biological fluids in the foods interferes with the target bacterial ATP.

Only after much research and development, scientists can separate nonmicrobial ATP from microbial ATP and obtain reasonable accuracy in relating ATP to viable cell counts in foods. Since obtaining an ATP reading takes only a few minutes, the potential of further exploring this method exists. To date, not much routine work has been applied using ATP to estimate viable cell counts in food microbiology laboratories.

From another viewpoint, the presence of ATP in certain food such as wine is undesirable regardless of the source. Thus, monitoring ATP can be a useful tool for quality assurance in the winery.

There is a paradigm shift in the field of ATP detection in recent years. Instead of detecting ATP of microorganisms, the systems are now designed to detect ATP from any source for hygiene monitoring. The idea is that a dirty food-processing environment will have a high ATP level and a properly cleansed environment will have a low ATP level regardless of what contributed to the ATP in these environments. Once this concept is accepted by the food industry, there will be an explosion of ATP systems on the market.

In all of these systems, the key is to be able to obtain an ATP reading in the form of relative light units (RLUs) and relate these units to cleanliness of the food-processing surfaces. Most systems design an acceptable RLU, unacceptable RLU, and a marginal RLU for different surfaces in food plants. Since there is no standard in what constitutes an absolute acceptable ATP level on any given environment, these RLUs are quite arbitrary. In general, a dirty environment will have high RLUs and after proper cleaning the RLUs will decrease. Besides the sensitivity of the instruments, for an analyst to select a particular system the following attributes are considered: simplicity of operation, compactness of the unit, computer adaptability, cost of the units, support from the company, and documentation of usefulness of the system.

Besides the above mentioned issues, Dreibelbis (1999) in a study of five ATP instruments for hygiene monitoring of a food plant considered the following attributes to be important as selection criteria of the systems: the ability of the technicians in the microbiological laboratory to use the ATP bioluminescence hygiene monitoring system without supervision, the reputation of the ATP system in the industry, and the quality of services received from the manufacturer during the evaluation of the product.

Currently the following ATP instruments are available: Lumac (Landgraaf, the Netherlands), BioTrace (Plainsboro, New Jersey), Ligthning

(BioControl, Bellevue, Washington), Hy-Lite (EM Science, Darmstadt, Germany), Charm 4000 (Charm Sciences, Malden, Massachusetts), Celsis system SURE (Cambridge, United Kingdom), Zylux (Maryville, Tennessee), Profile 1 (New Horizon, Columbia, Maryland), and others. As microorganisms grow and metabolize nutrients, large molecules change to smaller molecules in a liquid system and cause a change in electrical conductivity and resistance in the liquid as well as at the interphase of electrodes. These changes can be expressed as impedance, conductance, and capacitance changes. When a population of cells reaches about 5 log/mL it will cause a change of these parameters. Thus, when a food has a large initial population, the time to make this change will be shorter than a food that has a smaller initial population. The time for the curve to change from the baseline and accelerate upward is the detection time of the test sample, which is inversely proportional to the initial concentration of microorganisms in the food. In order to use these methods, a series of standard curves must be constructed by making viable cell counts of a series of food with different initial concentration of cells and then measuring the resultant detection time. A scattergram can then be plotted. Thereafter, in the same food system, the number of the initial population of the food can be estimated by the detection time on the scattergram.

The Bactometer (bioMerieux, Hazelwood, Missouri) has been in use for many years to measure impedance changes in foods, water, cosmetics, etc. by microorganisms. Samples are placed in the wells of a 16-well module that is then plugged into the incubator to start the monitoring sequence. As the cells reach the critical number (5–6 log/mL), the change in impedance increases sharply and the monitor screen shows a slope similar to the log phase of a growth curve. The detection time can then be obtained to determine the initial population of the sample. If one sets a cut-off point of 6 log organisms/g of food for acceptance or rejection of the product and the detection time is 4 h ± 15 min, then one can use the detection time as a criterion for quality assurance of the product. Foods that exhibit no change of impedance curve more than 4 h 15 min in the instrument are acceptable while foods that exhibit a change of impedance curve before 3 h 45 min will not be acceptable. For convenience, the instrument is designed such that the sample bar for a food on the screen will flash red for unacceptable sample, green for acceptable sample, and yellow for marginally acceptable sample. A similar system called RABIT (rapid automated bacterial impedance technique), marketed by Bioscience International (Bethesda, Maryland) is available for monitoring microbial activities in food and beverages. Instead of a 16-well module used in the Bactometer, individual tubes containing electrodes are used to house the food samples.

The Malthus system (Crawley, United Kingdom) uses conductance changes of the fluid to indicate microbial growth. It generates conductance curves similar to impedance curves used in the Bactometer. It uses individual tubes for food samples. Water heated to the desirable temperature (e.g., 35°C) is used as the temperature control instead of heated air in the previous two systems. All these systems have been evaluated by various scientists in the past 10–15 years with satisfactory results. All have their advantages and disadvantages depending on the type of food being analyzed. These systems can also be used to monitor target organisms such as coliform, yeast, and mold by specially designed culture media. In fact, the Mathlus system has a *Salmonella* detection protocol that has AOAC International approval.

BacT/Alert Microbiolial Detection System (Organon Tecknika, Durham, North Carolina) utilizes colorimetric detection of carbon dioxide production by microorganisms in a liquid system using sophisticated computer algorithms and instrumentation. Food samples are diluted and placed in special bottles with appropriate nutrients for growth of microorganisms and production of carbon dioxide. At the bottom of the bottle there is a sensor that is responsive to the amount of carbon dioxide in the liquid. When a critical amount of the gas is produced, the sensor changes from dark green to yellow and this change is automatically detected by reflectance colorimetry. The units can accommodate 120 or 240 culture bottles. Detection time of a typical culture of *E. coli* is about 6–8 h.

BioSys (BioSys, Inc., Ann Arbor, Michigan) utilizes color changes of media during the growth of cultures to detect and estimate organisms in foods and liquid systems. The uniqueness of the system is that the color compounds developed during microbial growth are diffused into an agar column in the unit and the changes are measured automatically without the interference of food particles. Depending on the initial microbial load in the food, same shift microbial information can be obtained. The system is easy to use and can accommodate 32 samples for one incubation temperature or 128 samples for four independent incubation temperatures in different models. The system is designed for bioburden testing and HACCP control and can test for indirect total viable cell, coliform, *E. coli*, yeast, mold, lactic acid bacteria counts, swab samples, and environmental samples.

Basically, any type of instrument that can continuously and automatically monitor turbidity and color changes of a liquid in the presence of microbial growth can be used for rapid detection of the presence of microorganisms. There will definitely be more systems of this nature in the market in years to come.

7.8 Advances in Genetic Testings

Up to this point, all the rapid tests discussed for detection and characterization of microorganisms were based on phenotypic expression of genotypic characteristics of microorganisms. Phenotypic expression of cells is subject to growth conditions such as temperature, pH, nutrient availability, oxidation–reduction potentials, environmental and chemical stresses, toxins, water activities, etc.

Even immunological tests depend on phenotypic expression of cells to produce the target antigens to be detected by the available antibodies or vice versa. The conventional gold standards of diagnostic microbiology rely on phenotypic expression of cells and are inherently subject to variation.

Genotypic characteristics of a cell are far more stable. Natural mutation rate of a bacterial culture is about 1 in 100 million cells. Thus, there is a push in recent years to make genetic test results as the confirmative and definitive identification step in diagnostic microbiology. The debate is still continuing and the final decision has not been reached by governmental and regulatory bodies for microbiological testing. Genetic based diagnostic and identification systems are discussed in this section.

Hybridization of the DNA sequence of an unknown bacterium by a known DNA probe is the first stage of genetic testings. Genetrak system (Framingham, Massachusetts) is a sensitive method and convenient system to detect pathogens such as *Salmonella, Listeria, Campylobacter,* and *E. coli* O157 in foods. At the beginning, the system utilized radioactive compounds bound to DNA probes to detect DNA of unknown cultures. The drawbacks of the first generation of this type of probes are (1) most food laboratories are not eager to work with radioactive materials in routine analysis and (2) there are limited copies of DNA in a cell. The second generation of probes uses enzymatic reactions to detect the presence of the pathogens and uses RNA as the target molecule. In a cell, there is only one complete copy of DNA; however, there may be 1,000–10,000 copies of ribosomal RNA. Thus, the new generation of probes is designed to probe target RNA using color reactions. After enrichment of cells (e.g., *Salmonella*) in a food sample for about 18 h, the cells (target cells as well as other microbes) are lysed by a detergent to release cellular materials (DNA, RNA, and other molecules) into the enrichment solution. Two RNA probes (designed to react with one piece of target *Salmonella* RNA) are added into the solution. The capture probe with a long tail of a nucleotide (e.g., adenine, AAAAA) is designed to capture the RNA onto a dipstick with a long tail of thymine (TTTTT). The reporter probe with an enzyme attached will react with any part of the RNA fragment. If *Salmonella* RNA molecules are present, the capture probes will attach to one end of the RNA and the report probes will attach to the other end. A dipstick coated with many copies of a chain of complementary nucleotide (e.g., thymine, TTTTT) will be placed into the solution. Since adenine (A) will hybridize with thymine (T), the chain (TTTTT) on the dipstick will react with the AAAAA and thus capture the target RNA complex onto the stick. After washing away debris and other molecules in the liquid, a chromagen is added. If the target RNA is captured then the enzyme present in the second probe will react with the chromagen and will produce a color reaction indicating the presence of the pathogen in the food. In this case, the food is positive for *Salmonella*. The Genetrak has been evaluated and tested for many years and has AOAC International approval of the procedure for many food types. More recently, Genetrak has adapted a Microtiter format for more efficient and automated operation of the system.

Polymerase chain reaction (PCR) is now an accepted method to detect pathogens by amplification of the target DNA and detecting the target PCR products. Basically, a DNA molecule (double helix) of a target pathogen (e.g., *Salmonella*) is first denatured at about 95°C to form single strands; then the temperature is lowered to about 55°C for two primers (small oligonucleotides specific for *Salmonella*) to anneal to specific regions of the single-stranded DNA. The temperature is increased to about 70°C for a special heat stable polymerase, the TAQ enzyme from *Thermus aquaticus*, to add complementary bases (A, T, G, or C) to the single-stranded DNA and complete the extension to form a new double strand of DNA. This is called a thermal cycle. After this cycle, the tube will be heated to 95°C again for the next cycle. After one thermal cycle one copy of DNA will become two copies. After about 21 cycles and 31 cycles, one million and one billion copies of the DNA will be formed, respectively. This entire process can be accomplished in less than an hour in an automatic thermal cycler. Theoretically, if a food contains one copy of *Salmonella* DNA, the PCR method can detect the presence of this pathogen in a very short time. After PCR reactions, one still needs to detect the presence of the PCR products to indicate the presence of the pathogen. The following are brief discussions of four commercial kits for PCR reactions and detection of PCR products.

The BAX for Screening family of PCR assays for foodborne pathogens (Qualicon, Inc., Wilmington, Delaware) combines DNA amplification and automated homogeneous detection to determine the presence or absence of a specific target. All primers, polymerase, and deoxynucleotides necessary for PCR as well as a positive control and an intercalating dye are incorporated into a single tablet. The system works directly from an overnight enrichment of the target organisms. No DNA extraction is required. Assays are available for *Salmonella* (Mrozinski et al., 1998), *E. coli* O157:H7 (Johnson et al., 1998; Hochberg et al., 2000), *Listeria* genus, and *L. monocytogenes* (Steward and Gendel, 1998; Norton et al., 2000, 2001). The system uses an array of 96 blue LEDs as the excitation source and a photomultiplier tube to detect the emitted fluorescent signal. This integrated system improves the ease-of-use of the assay. In addition to simplifying the detection process, the new method converts the system to a homogeneous PCR test. The homogenous detection process monitors the decrease in fluorescence of a double-stranded DNA (dsDNA), intercalating dye in solution with dsDNA as a function of temperature. Following amplification, melting curves are generated by slowly ramping up the temperature of the sample to a denaturing level (95°C). As the dsDNA denatures, the dye becomes unbound from the DNA duplex, and the fluorescent signal decreases. This change in fluorescence can be plotted against temperature to yield a melting curve waveform. This assay thus eliminates the need for gel-based detection and yields data amenable to storage and retrieval in an electronic database. In addition, this method reduces the hands-on time of the assay and reduces the subjectivity of the reported results. Further, melting curve analysis makes possible the ability to detect multiple PCR products in a single tube. The inclusivity and exclusivity of the BAX system assays reach almost 100%, meaning that false-positive and false-negative rates are almost zero. Additionally, the automated BAX system can now be used with assays for the detection of *Cryptosporidium parvum* and *Campylobacter jejuni/coli* and for the quantitative and qualitative detection of genetically modified organisms in soy and corn.

The new BAX system is far more convenient than the old system in which a gel electrophoresis step was required to detect PCR products after thermal cycling. Recently Qualican announced that the BAX system is able to detect yeast and mold by PCR method.

The following two methods have been developed also to bypass the electrophoresis step to detect PCR products and can provide real-time PCR information.

TaqMan system of Applied Biosystems (Foster City, California) also amplifies DNA by PCR protocol. However, during the amplification step a special molecule is annealed to the single-stranded DNA to report the liner amplification. The molecule has the appropriate sequence for the target DNA. It also has two attached particles. One is a fluorescent particle and the other is a quencher particle. When the two particles are close to each other no fluorescence occurs. However, when the TAQ polymerase is adding bases to the liner single strand of DNA, it will break this molecule away from the strand (like the PacMan in computer games). As this occurs, the two particles will separate from each other and fluorescence will occur. By measuring fluorescence in the tube, a successful PCR reaction can be determined. Note that the reaction and reporting of a successful PCR protocol occur in the same tube, thus eliminating the need to detect PCR products by electrophoresis in the old BAX system.

A new system called molecular beacon technology (Stratagene, La Jolla, California) has been developed and can be used for food microbiology in the future (Robinson et al., 2000). In this technology, all reactions are again in the same tube. A molecular beacon is a tailor-made hairpin-shaped hybridization probe. The probe is used to attach to target PCR products. On one end of the probe there is attached a fluorophore and on the other end a quencher of the fluorophore. In the absence of the target PCR products the beacon is in a hairpin shape and there is no fluorescence. However, during PCR reactions and the generation of target PCR products, the beacons will attach to the PCR products and cause the hairpin molecule to unfold. As the quencher moves away from the fluorophore, fluorescence will occur and this can be measured. The measurement can be done as the PCR reaction is in progression, thus allowing real-time detection of target PCR products and thus the presence of the target pathogen in the sample. This system has the same efficiency as the TaqMan system but the difference is that the beacons detect the PCR products themselves, while in the TaqMan system, it only reports the occurrence of a liner PCR reaction and not the presence of the

PCR product directly. By using molecular beacons containing different fluorophores, one can detect different PCR products in the same reaction tubes, and thus can be able to perform multiplex tests of several target pathogens or molecules. The use of this technology is very new and not well known in food microbiology areas. The aforementioned methods utilize fluorescence to report PCR reactions. When there are more target DNAs in the system, detection time will be shorter as compared to less target DNAs; thus these systems are termed "real-time" PCR systems.

Theoretically, the PCR system can detect one copy of target pathogen from a food sample (e.g., *Salmonella* DNA). In practice, about 200 cells are needed to be detected by current PCR methods. Thus, even in a PCR protocol the food must be enriched for a period of time, e.g., overnight or at least 8 h incubation of food in a suitable enrichment liquid so that there are enough cells for the PCR process to be reliable. Besides the technical manipulations of the systems, which can be complicated for many food microbiology laboratories, two major problems need to be addressed: inhibitors of PCR reactions and the question of live and dead cells. In food, there are many enzymes, proteins, and other compounds that can interfere with the PCR reaction and result in false negatives. These inhibitors must be removed or diluted. Since PCR reaction amplifies target DNA molecules, even DNA from dead cells can be amplified and thus food with dead *Salmonella* can be declared as *Salmonella* positive by PCR results. Thus, food properly cooked but containing DNA of dead cells may be unnecessarily destroyed because of a positive PCR test.

PCR can be a powerful tool for food microbiology once all the problems are solved and analysts are convinced of the applicability in routine analysis of foods.

The aforementioned genetic methods are for detection of target pathogens in foods and other samples. They do not provide identification of the cultures to the species and subspecies level so critical in epidemiological investigations of outbreaks or routine monitoring of occurrence of microorganisms in the environment. The following discussions will center around the developments in genetic characterization of bacterial cultures.

The RiboPrinter Microbial Characterization System (Du Pont Qualicon, Wilmington, Delaware) characterizes and identifies organisms to genus, species, and subspecies levels automatically. To obtain a RiboPrint of an organism, the following steps are followed:

1. A pure colony of bacteria suspected to be the target organism (e.g., *Salmonella*) is picked from an agar plate by a sterile plastic stick.
2. Cells from the stick are suspended in a buffer solution by mechanical agitation.
3. An aliquot of the cell suspension is loaded into the sample carrier to be placed into the instrument. Each sample carrier has space for eight individual colony picks.

4. The instrument will automatically prepare the DNA for analysis by restriction enzyme and lysis buffer to open the bacteria, and release and cut DNA molecules. The DNA fragments will go through an electrophoresis gel to separate DNA fragments into discrete bands. Lastly, the DNA probes, conjugate, and substrate will react with the separated DNA fragments and light emission from the hybridized fragments is then photographed. The data are stored and compared with known patterns of the particular organism.

The entire process takes 8 h for eight samples. However, at 2 h intervals, another eight samples can be loaded for analysis.

Different bacteria will exhibit different patterns (e.g., *Salmonella* versus *E. coli*) and even the same species can exhibit different patterns (e.g., *L. monocytogenes* has 49 distinct patterns). Some examples of numbers of RiboPrint Patterns for some important food pathogens are: *Salmonella*, 145; *Listeria*, 89; *E. coli*, 134; *Staphylococcus*, 406; and *Vibrio*, 63. Additionally, the database includes 300 *Lactobacillus*, 43 *Lactococcus*, 11 *Leuconostoc*, and 34 *Pediococcus*. The current identification database provides 3267 RiboPrint patterns representing 98 genera and 695 species.

One of the values of this information is that in the case of a foodborne outbreak, scientists not only can identify the etiological agent (e.g., *L. monocytogenes*) but can also pinpoint the source of the responsible subspecies. For example, in the investigation concerning an outbreak of *L. monocytogenes*, cultures were isolated from the slicer of the product and also from the drains of the plant. The question is which source is responsible fo the outbreak. By matching RiboPrint patterns of the two sources of *L. monocytogenes* against the foodborne outbreak culture, it was found that the isolate from the slicer matched the outbreak culture, and thus determined the true source of the problem. The RiboPrinter system is a very powerful tool for electronic data sharing worldwide.

These links can monitor the occurrence of foodborne pathogens and other important organisms as long as different laboratories utilize the same system for obtaining the RiboPrint Patterns.

Another important system is the pulsed-field gel electrophoresis patterns of pathogens. In this system, pure cultures of pathogens are isolated and digested with restriction enzymes and the DNA fragments are subjected to a system known as pulsed-field gel electrophoresis, which effectively separates DNA fragments on the gel (DNA fingerprinting). For example, in a foodborne outbreak of *E. coli* O157:H7, biochemically identical *E. coli* O157:H7 cultures can exhibit different patterns. By comparing the gel patterns from different sources one can trace the origin of the infection or search for the spread of the disease and thereby control the problem.

In order to compare data from various laboratories across the country the PulseNet system is established under the National Molecular Subtyping Network for Foodborne Disease Surveillance at the Centers for Disease

Control and Prevention (CDC). An extensive training program has been established so that all the collaborating laboratories use the same protocol and are electronically linked to share DNA fingerprinting patterns of major pathogens. As soon as a suspect culture is noted as a possible source of an outbreak, all the collaborating laboratories are alerted to search for the occurrence of the same pattern to determine the scope of the problem and share information in real time.

There are many other genetic base methods but they are not directly related to food microbiology and are beyond the scope of this review. It is safe to say that many genetic base methods are slowly but surely finding their ways into food microbiology laboratories and they will provide valuable information for quality assurance, quality control, and food safety programs in the future.

7.9   Advances in Biosensors

Biosensor is an exciting field in applied microbiology. The basic idea is simple but the actual operation is quite complex and involves much instrumentation. Basically, a biosensor is a molecule or a group of molecules of biological origin attached to a signal recognition material.

When an analyte comes in contact with the biosensor, the interaction will initiate a recognition signal that can be reported in an instrument.

Many types of biosensors have been developed such as enzymes (a great variety of enzymes have been used), antibodies (polyclonal and monoclonal), nucleic acids, cellular materials, etc.

Sometime whole cells can also be used as biosensors. Analytes detected include toxin (staphylococcal enterotoxins, tetrodotoxins, saxitoxin, botulinum toxin, etc.), specific pathogens (e.g., *Salmonella, Staphylococcus, E. coli* O157:H7, etc.), carbohydrates (e.g., fructose, lactose, galactose, etc.), insecticides and herbicides, ATP, antibiotics (e.g., penicillins), and others. The recognition signals used include electrochemical (e.g., potentiometry, voltage changes, conductance and impedance, light addressable, etc.), optical (such as UV, bioluminescence and chemiluminescence, fluorescence, laser scattering, reflection and refraction of light, surface plasmon resonance, polarized light, etc.) and miscellaneous transducers (such as piezoelectric crystals, thermistor, acoustic waves, quartz crystal, etc.).

An example of a simple enzyme biosensor is sensor for glucose. The reaction involves the oxidation of glucose (the analyte) by glucose oxidase (the biosensor) with the end-products of gluconic acid and hydrogen peroxide. The reaction was reported by a Clark oxygen electrode which monitors the decrease in oxygen concentration amperometrically. The range of measurement is from 1 to 30 mM, and response time of 1–1.5 min and the recovery time of 30 s. Lifetime of the unit is several months. Some of the advantages of enzyme biosensors are binding to the subject, highly selective, and rapid acting. Some of the disadvantages are expensive loss of activity when they are immobilized on a transducer, and loss of activities due to deactivation. Other enzymes used include galactosidase, glucoamlyase, acetylcholinesterase, invertase, lactate oxidase, etc. Excellent review articles and books on biosensors are presented by Eggins (1997), Cunningham (1998), Goldschmidt (1999), and others.

Recently, much attention has been directed to the field of "biochips" and "microchips" development to detect a great variety of molecules including foodborne pathogens.

Due to the advancement in miniaturization technology as many as 50,000 individual spots (e.g., DNA microarrays) with each spot containing millions of copies of a specific DNA probe can be immobilized on a specialized microscope slide. Fluorescent-labeled targets can be hybridized to these spots and be detected. An excellent article by Deyholos et al. (2001) described the application of microarrays to discover genes associated with a particular biological process such as the response of the plant (*Arabidopsis*) to NaCl-stress and detailed analysis of a specific biological pathway such as one-carbon metabolism in maize.

Biochips can also be designed to detect all kinds of foodborne pathogens by imprinting a variety of antibodies or DNA molecules against specific pathogens on the chip for the simultaneous detection of pathogens such as *Salmonella, Listeria, E. coli, S. aureus*, etc., on the same chip. According to Elaine Heron of Applied Biosystems of Foster City, California (Heron, 2000), biochips are an exceedingly important technology in life sciences and the market value is estimated to be as high as $5 billion by the middle of this decade. This technology is especially important in the rapidly developing field of proteomics, which requires massive amount of data that generate valuable information.

Certainly, the developments of these biochips and microarray chips are impressive for obtaining a large amount of information for biological sciences. As for foodborne pathogen detection, there are several important issues to consider. These biochips are designed to detect minute quantities of target molecule. The target molecules must be free from contaminants before being applied to the biochips. In food microbiology, the minimum requirement for pathogen detection is 1 and viable target cell in 25 g of a food such as ground beef. A biochip will not be able to seek out such a cell from the food matrix without extensive cell amplification (either by growth or PCR) or sample preparation by filtration, separation, absorption, centrifugation, etc., as described in this article. Any food particle in the sample will easily clot the channels used in biochips. These preparations will not allow the biochips to provide "real-time" detection of pathogens in foods.

Another concern is the viability of the pathogens to be detected by biochips. Monitoring the presence of some target molecule will only provide the presence or absence of the target pathogen and will not provide viability of the pathogen in question. Some form of culture enrichment to ensure growth is still needed in order to obtain meaningful results. It is conceivable that the biomass of microbes can be monitored by biochips, but instantaneous detection of specific pathogens such as *Salmonella, Listeria, Campylobacter,* etc., in food matrix during food processing operation is still not possible. The potential of biochip and microarrays for food pathogen detection is great but at this moment much more research is needed to make this technology a reality in applied food microbiology.

7.10   United States and World Market and Testing Trends (1999–2008)

There is no question that many microbiological tests are being conducted nationally and internationally in food, pharmaceutical products, environmental samples, and water. The most popular tests are total viable cell count, coliform/*E. coli* count, and yeast and mold counts. A large number of tests are also performed on pathogens such as *Salmonella, Listeria* and *L. monocytogenes, E. coli* O157:H7, *S. aureus, Campylobacter,* and other organisms.

Applied microbiologists working in medical, food, environmental, and industrial settings in government, industries, academia, and the private sector are interested in the numbers and kinds of microbiological tests being done annually at local, regional, national, and international scales.

However, there are no real statistics on these numbers and only estimates are available from various groups in the past couple of decades. The author at Kansas State University has been conducting a workshop on rapid methods and automation in microbiology since 1981 and has been collecting statistics on the number of tests performed by participants in their work environment. Summary of data from 1981 to 1991 indicated that the average food microbiology laboratory performed about 20,000 total viable cell count, 13,000 coliform count, and about 2,000 specific pathogens (*Salmonella, Listeria,* etc.) tests per year. An average laboratory serving a medium-size food company would therefore perform about 35,000 tests per year. Assuming that there are 20,000 reasonably large microbiological laboratories worldwide (a conservative estimate) the number of tests per year would be a staggering 700 million tests! Even at a modest estimated cost of $2 per test, the market will be $1.4 billion per year.

Informal estimation for *Salmonella* testing from food samples per year for United States and Europe was 6–8.4 million, and for *Listeria* 3–4.2 million in 1989. More recent estimates for United States alone in 1996 was 6–7.5 million for *Salmonella* and 2.5–3.5 million for *Listeria.* The latest estimate for total viable cell count was 60 million; coliform, 50 million; yeast and mold, 10 million; *Salmonella,* 8 million; *Listeria,* 5 million; *E. coli* O157:H7, 1 million; generic *E. coli* 3–5 million; and *Campylobacter* and Staphylococcal enterotoxin, less than 1 million each (Bailey, 2000; Fung, 2000). The aforementioned numbers were pure estimation by observers of the development in this field.

Strategic Consulting, Inc. (Woodstock, Vermont) produced five major reports on the market of microbiological testing: *Industrial Microbiology Market Review* I and II (Strategic Consulting, Inc., 1998, 2004) and *Pathogen Testing in the US Food Industry* (Strategic Consulting, Inc., 2000), *Food Diagnostics: Global Review of Microbiological and Residue Testing in the Food Processing Industry* (Strategic Consulting, Inc., 2002), and *Global Review of Microbiology Testing in the Food Processing Market* (Strategic Consulting, Inc., 2005) This author received permissions to use these data in publications. This group researched diagnostic testing companies through public records and interviews of hundreds of practitioners of applied microbiology by phone or other means to obtain estimated data to compile the reports. Readers are advised to contact Strategic Consulting, Inc. for details of these reports. Below is information that the author received permission to use for this article.

In 1998, the worldwide industrial microbiological tests were estimated to be 755 million tests, quite similar to the estimation of the author mentioned above. The total market value was $1.1 billion assuming the average price per test to be $1.47. They also estimated that 56% of the tests were for food; 30% for pharmaceutical; 10% for beverages; and 4% for environmental water tests (Strategic Consulting, Inc., 1998). Of these tests, 420 millions tests were done in food laboratories with 360 million for routine tests (total viable cell counts, coliform counts and yeast and mold counts) and 60 million for specific pathogen tests (*Salmonella*, *Listeria*, *S. aureus*, and *E. coli* O157:H7 tests). Approximately one-third of all the tests were done in United States, another third in Europe, and the rest were performed by the rest of the world.

They projected that from 1998 to 2003 there will be a 24.6% increase in number of tests; 17% increase in price per test, and 45.8% increase in total revenue of the testing market by 2003. Of the 50 or so diagnostic companies reviewed, there seems to be no absolute dominance of the field by any one company although there are clear leaders in the area (Strategic Consulting, Inc., 1998). The situation is quite fluid since some companies are constantly acquiring products from other companies. Many new companies are also emerging in this area as new technologies are developed.

The 2000 U.S. Food Industry Market study indicated that the total per-year microbiological tests were 144.3 million, total pathogens were 23.5 million, with a market value of pathogen tests valued at $53.4 million and the average selling price per test $2.27. These data were obtained by surveying 5979 food processing plants with an average of 464 tests per plant per week and 24,128 tests per plant per year. Processed food constituted 36.2%; dairy, 31.8%; meat, 22.3%; and fruit and vegetable, 9.7%. The number of tests to be done in the future for fruits and vegetables will certainly increase due to recent foodborne outbreaks related to these food commodities.

Another valuable set of data is the proportion of routine tests versus pathogen tests, which is 83.7% versus 16.3%. Further breakdown of the routine versus pathogen test revealed the total viable count consisted 37.2% of all tests, coliform/*E. coli*, 30.8%; yeast and mold, 15.7%; and pathogens,

16.3%. This is an increase from 15% of pathogen tests reported in the 1998 IMMR I (Strategic Consulting, Inc., 1998). It is projected that this number will increase further in the years to come.

There is a question on the location where the pathogen samples are analyzed due to considerations of possible contamination of the food plant environments. In meat plants about 45% of the samples were analyzed in the plant; about 25% from outside laboratories and 30% in corporate and central laboratories. In the dairy industry, about 75% of the samples were analyzed by outside laboratories probably due to safety considerations and the lack of trained microbiologists in the plants. Microbial samples analyzed locally in plant and analyzed in central laboratories were 15% and 10%, respectively. For fruit and vegetable samples about 55% were analyzed by outside laboratories and 43% analyzed in plant. Very few samples were analyzed by corporate and central laboratories. This is probably because many corporations, until recently, were not aware of the problems of food-borne pathogens in these products and do not have corporate laboratory facilities. This may change as the demand for safer fruit and vegetable products increases in the coming years. For processed food, more than 60% were analyzed in plant, 35% in outside laboratories, and less than 10% in corporate laboratories. The reason for this food sector to perform its own in-plant testing is probably because processed food has relatively low microbial contamination and thus easier to handle the procedures. As a whole for all food sector, about 40% was done in plant, 40% was in outside laboratories, and 20% done in corporate central laboratories.

Estimation of the use of "rapid methods" versus "conventional method" is even harder to obtain. From the author's experiences, at this moment, about 70% of the microbial tests are done using manual or conventional methods and 30% using rapid methods. By 2008, for total test, about 50% will be using conventional methods and 50 will be using rapid tests. However, for pathogen tests 60%–70% of the tests will be in some form of rapid tests and 30%–40% will be using the conventional tests. This is because of the great improvement of rapid methods that are under development and will accelerate in the near future.

More recent information provided by Strategic Consulting, Inc. indicated that 78.7% of "routine microbiology testing" is done by traditional method and 21.3% is done by some sort of "convenience methods." For pathogen testing, 63.5% is by traditional methods, 33.7% by immunoassay methods, and 2.8% by PCR methods. The dynamics will shift toward rapid methods in the years to come. As far as microbiological testings in the world are concerned, about one-third is now done in North America, another third in Europe, and the last third in the rest of the world. This author predicts that in the next 15 years one-fourth will be done in North America, one-fourth will be done in Europe, and one-half will be done in the rest of the world due to heightened interests in the field of microbial testings around the globe. The number of microbiological tests on food, beverages, pharmaceuticals, personal-care products, environment, and processing has increased steadily from approximately 500 million tests per year in 1993 to approximately 1.2 billion in 2001, and projected to be 1.5 billion tests in 2008. The dollar value of microbiological tests has increased from $1.8 billion in 1993, to $2.3 billion in 1998, to $3.2 billion in 2003, and projected to $5 billion in 2008. Thus, the field of microbial testing is receiving healthy growth in terms of number of tests and dollar value in the world in the near and far future.

In conclusion, it is safe to say that the field of rapid methods and automation in microbiology will continue to grow in number and kinds of tests to be done in the future due to the increasing concern on food safety.

7.11 Future Predictions

It is always difficult to predict the future development in any field of endeavor. In 1995, the author was honored to present a lecture at the annual meeting of the American Society of Microbiology in Washington, D.C., as the Food Microbiology Divisional Lecturer concerning the current status and the future outlook of the field of rapid methods and automation in microbiology. The following are synopses of the 10 predictions with a look into the future made in 1995. A more detailed description of the predictions can be found in the paper by Fung in 1999.

1. *Viable cell counts will still be used.* It is the firm belief of the author that viable cell counts (total aerobic count, anaerobic count, coliform/*E. coli* count, differential count, and pathogenic count) will remain an important parameter to assess the potential safety and hygiene quality of food supplies. Although the current methods are cumbersome and labor-intensive, many improvements have been made and will continue to be made to improve the viable cell count procedure as described in Section 7.4. Special developments in early sensing of viable colonies on agar, electronic sensing of viable cells under the microscope, improvements of vital stains to count living cells, and more effective sensing of MPN of samples will greatly improve the viable cell count procedure.

2. *Real-time monitoring of hygiene will be in place.* Several exciting developments in this area have occurred such as ATP bioluminescence, catalase measurement, and instant protein detection kits. In the past several years, many ATP systems have been marketed and used. These kits are easy to use and provide useful information in a few minutes. Catalase is a very reactive enzyme. The author has worked on this enzyme for a number of years to monitor hygiene of surfaces, microbial spoilage potential of aerobic cold stored food, and end-point temperature monitoring of cooked foods. The test is simple, inexpensive, and rapid (a few seconds to minutes). This system deserves more research and

development. Monitoring of the presence of protein fat, carbohydrate, etc., on food contact surfaces can also provide rapid and
meaningful information concerning the hygiene quality of the
surfaces. Recently, BioControl (Bellevue, Washington) introduced
a protein testing kit called FLASH, which can detect the presence
of protein level on food contact surfaces almost instantaneously.
Positive surfaces change the color of the swab from yellow to
green or blue color in 5 to 10 s. This type of real-time monitoring
systems will be developed for other compounds in the future.

3. *Polymerase chain reaction (PCR), ribotyping, and genetic tests will
become reality in food laboratories.* This was a bold prediction in
1995 but now there are food companies, pharmaceutical companies, and related industries routinely using this advanced technology to monitor the presence of normal flora, spoilage flora, and
pathogens in food and other materials. This trend will advance
rapidly in the near and far future.

4. *Enzyme-linked immunosorbent assay (ELISA) and immunological tests
will be completely automated and widely used.* This prediction certainly came true. After pre-enrichment of food samples (overnight
incubation or 8 h incubation) an analyst can place the sample into
an automated system and monitor the presence of the target
pathogen in a matter of 1–2 h. Automated systems will continue
to be developed and used in the future.

5. *Dipstick technology will provide rapid answers.* Many forms of dipsticks
are available for screening of pathogens by "lateral" migration of
antigen–antibody complex. These kits can detect target organisms in
about 10 min after enrichment of the cultures overnight. This type of
technology will continue to be developed and used in the future.

6. *Biosensors will be in place for HACCP programs.* This prediction is
still for the future. A variety of biosensors are now available on the
market to monitor microbes but they are not yet suitable for use in
routine monitoring of pathogens in the food industry. More
research and development will be needed to have this technology
in use for the food industry.

7. *Instant detection of target pathogens will be possible by computer-
generated matrix in response to particular characteristics of pathogens
(biosensors, microarrays, microchips, etc.).* This prediction depends on
the development of a much more in-depth understanding of the
microbial cells and the pathogenic traits of pathogens before it can
become a reality. By the completion of the mapping of the human
genome and the development of proteomics (identification and
quantitation of proteins and elucidation of their functions) this
field is rapidly moving into practical use in the near future for
food microbiology.

8. *Effective separation, concentration of target cells will greatly assist in rapid identification.* A variety of approaches have been mentioned in this chapter. These developments have been and will continue to improve detection sensitivity and increase speed of detection of target pathogens.

9. *A microbiological alert system will be in food packages.* This prediction is certainly within the reach of modern technology. During growth and spoilage, microbial cells will generate a variety of compounds that can be detected by ingenious devices such as gas and pH indicators. It is conceivable that a series of reagents in the form of "bar codes" be placed inside the packaging materials and will change color due to the development of gas (ammonia, hydrogen sulfide, hydrogen, carbon dioxides, etc.) or acid or due to temperature abuse to indicate a potential spoilage problem.

10. *Consumers will have rapid alert kits for pathogens at home.* Nowadays there are urine tests, blood glucose test, pregnancy test, and even AIDS test kits available for the consumer to use at home. It is possible that rapid alert kits for food spoilage and even food pathogen detection available for home use will be developed. More development in this area is needed and a lot of consumer education will have to come along with these kits to make them useful and meaningful. Along with the prediction of the future of rapid method testings, it is useful to describe the 10 attributes for an ideal automated microbiology assay system as follows:

    i. Accuracy for the intended purposes: Sensitivity, minimal detectable limits, specificity of test system, versatility, potential applications, and comparison to reference methods.

    ii. Speed in productivity: Time in obtaining results, number of samples processed per run, per hour, per day.

    iii. Cost: Initial, per test, reagents, labor

    iv. Acceptability by scientific community and regulatory agencies

    v. Simplicity of operation: Sample preparation, operation of test equipment, computer versatility

    vi. Training: On site, length of time, qualification of operator.

    vii. Reagents: Preparation, stability, availability, and consistency

    viii. Company reputation

    ix. Technical services: Speed, availability, cost, and scope

    x. Utility and space requirement.

The future looks very bright for the field of rapid methods and automation in microbiology. The potential is great and many exciting developments will certainly unfold in the near and far future.

References

Al-Dagal, M.M. and D.Y.C. Fung. 1993. Aeromicrobiology: An assessment of a new meat research complex. *J. Environ. Health.* 56(1):7–14.

Ali, M.S. and D.Y.C. Fung. 1991. Occurrence of *Clostridium perfringens* in ground beef and turkey evaluated by three methods. *J. Food Protect.* 11:197–203.

Bailey, J.S. 2000. Development of a successful pathogen detection test. In Fung, D.Y.C., *Handbook of Rapid Methods and Automation in Microbiology,* Supplement 1. Kansas State University, Manhattan, Kansas.

Chain, V.S. and D.Y.C. Fung. 1991. Comparison of redigel, petrifilm, spiral plate system, isogrid, and aerobic plate count for determining the numbers of aerobic bacteria in selected food. *J. Food Protect.* 54:208–211.

Cox, N.A., D.Y.C. Fung, M.C. Goldschmidt, and J.S. Bailey. 1984. Selecting a miniaturized system for identification of *Enterobacteriaceae. J. Food Protect.* 47:74–77.

Cunningham, A.J. 1998. *Bioanalytical Sensors.* John Wiley and Sons, Inc., New York.

Deyholos, M., H. Wang, and D. Galbraith. 2001. Microarrays for gene discovery and metabolic pathway analysis in plants. *Life Science* 2(1):2–4.

Dreibelbis, S.B. 1999. Evaluation of five ATP bioluminescence hygiene monitoring systems in a commercial food processing facility. Master's Thesis. Kansas State University Library, Manhattan, Kansas.

Eggins, B. 1997. *Biosensors: An Introduction.* John Wiley and Sons, New York.

Fung, D.Y.C. 1999. Prediction in the future of rapid methods and microbiology. *Food Testing and Analysis* 5(3):18–21.

Fung, D.Y.C. 2000. *Handbook for Rapid Methods and Automation in Microbiology Workshop.* Kansas State University, Manhattan, Kansas, pp. 750.

Fung, D.Y.C. 2002. Rapid methods and automation in microbiology. Comprehensive reviews on food science and food safety. *Electron. J. Inst. Food Technol.* 1(1):3–21.

Fung, D.Y.C., R. Donahue, J.P. Jensen, W.W. Ulmann, W.J. Hausler, Jr., and W.S. LaGrange. 1976. A collaborative study of the microtiter count method and standard plate count method on viable cell count of raw milk. *J. Milk Food Technol.* 39:24–26.

Fung, D.Y.C. and A.A. Kraft. 1968. Microtiter method for the evacuation of viable cells in bacterial cultures. *Appl. Microbiol.* 16:1036–1039.

Fung, D.Y.C. and A.A. Kraft. 1969. Rapid evaluation of viable cell counts using the microtiter system and MPN technique. *J. Milk Food Technol.* 322:408–409.

Fung, D.Y.C. and W.S. LaGrange. 1969. Microtiter method for bacterial evaluation of milk. *J. Milk Food Technol.* 32:144–146.

Fung, D.Y.C. and C.M. Lee. 1981. Double-tube anaerobic bacteria cultivation system. *Food Science* 7:209–213.

Fung, D.Y.C., N.A. Cox, M.C. Goldschmidt, and J.S. Bailey. 1989. Rapid methods and automation in microbiology: A survey of professional microbiologists. *J. Food Protect.* 52:65–68.

Fung, D.Y.C., A.N. Sharpe, B.C. Hart, and Y. Liu. 1998. The Pulsifier: A new instrument for preparing food suspensions for microbiological analysis. *J. Rapid Methods Automat. Microbiol.* 6:43–49.

Graber, C.D. 1970. *Rapid Diagnosis Methods in Medical Microbiology.* Williams and Wilkins, Co., Baltimore, MD.

Goldschmidt, M.C. 1970. Instrumentation of microbiology: Horizons unlimited. In Graber, C.D., ed. *Rapid Diagnostic Methods in Medical Microbiology*. Williams and Wilkins, Co., Baltimore, MD.

Goldschmidt, M.C. 1999. Biosensors: Scope in microbiological analysis. In Robinson, R., C. Batt, and P. Patel., eds. *Encyclopedia of Food Microbiology*. Academic Press, New York, pp. 268–278.

Goldschmidt, M.C., D.Y.C. Fung, R. Grant, J. White, and T. Brown. 1991. New aniline blue dyes medium for rapid identification and isolation of *Candida albicans*. *J. Clinical Microbiol*. 29(6):1095–1099.

Hartman, P.A. 1968. *Miniaturized Microbiological Methods*. Academic Press, New York.

Heden, C.G. and T. Illeni. 1975a. *Automation in Microbiology and Immunology*. John Wiley and Sons, New York.

Heden, C.G. and T. Illeni. 1975b. *New Approaches to the Identification of Microorganisms*. John Wiley and Sons, New York.

Heron, E. 2000. Applied biosystem: Innovative technology for the life sciences. *Am. Lab* 32(24):35–38.

Hochberg, A.M., P.N. Gerhardt, T.K. Cao, W. Ocasio, W.M. Barbour, and P.M. Morinski. 2000. Sensitivity and specificity of the test kit BAX for screening/ *E. coli* O157:H7 in ground beef: Independent laboratory study. *J. AOAC Int.* 83(6):1349–1356.

Irwin, P., S. Tu, W. Damert, and J. Phillips. 2000. A modified Gauss–Newton algorithm and ninety-six well micro-technique for calculating MPN using EXCEL spread sheets. *J. Rapid Methods Automat*. 8(3):171–192.

Johnson, J.l., C.L. Brooke, and S.J. Fritschel. 1998. Comparison of BAX for screening/ *E. coli* O157:H7 vs. conventional methods for detection of extremely low levels of *Escherichia coli* O157:H7 in ground beef. *Appl. Environ. Microbiol.* 64: 4390–4395.

Kang, D.H., R.H. Doughtery, and D.Y.C. Fung. 2001. Comparison of Pulsifier and Stomacher to detach microorganisms from lean meat tissues. *J. Rapid Methods Automat. Microbiol*. 9(1):27–32.

Lee, J.Y. and D.Y.C. Fung. 1986. Surface sampling technique for bacteriology. *J. Environ. Health* 48:200–205.

McCrady, M.H. 1918. Tables for rapid interpretation of fermentation tube results. *Canadian Public Health Journal* 9:201–219.

Mrozinski, P.M., R.P. Betts, and S. Coates. 1998. Performance tested methods: Certification process for BAX for screening/*Salmonella*: A case study. *J. AOAC Intl.* 81:1147–1154.

Norton, D.M., M. McCamey, K.J. Boor, and M. Wiedmann. 2000. Application of the BAX for screening/genus *Listeria* polymerase chain reaction system for monitoring *Listeria* species in cold-smoked fish and in the smoked fish processing environment. *J. Food Prot*. 63:343–346.

Norton, D.M., M. McCamey, K.L. Gall, J.M. Scarlett, K.J. Boor, and M. Wiedmann. 2001. Molecular studies on the ecology of *Listeria monocytogenes* in the smoked fish processing industry. *App. Environ. Microbiol*. 67:198–205.

Richardson, G.H. 1972. Automation in dairy laboratory. *J. Milk Food Technol*. 35(5):279–287.

Robinson, J.K., R. Mueller, and L. Filippone. 2000. New molecular beacon technology. *Am. Lab*. 32(24):30–34.

Schmidt, K.A., R.H. Thakur, G. Jiang, and D.Y.C. Fung. 2000. Application of a double tube system for the enervation of *Clostridium tyrobutyricum*. *J. Rapid Methods Automat. Microbiol*. 8(1):21–30.

Steward, D. and S.M. Gendel. 1998. Specificity of the BAX polymerase chain reaction system for detection of the foodborne pathogen *Listeria monocytogenes*. *J. AOAC Intl.* 81:817–822.

Strategic Consulting, Inc. 1998. *Industrial Microbiology Market Review I.* Strategic Consulting Inc., Woodstock, VT.

Strategic Consulting, Inc. 2000. *Pathogen Testing in the US Food Industry.* Strategic Consulting Inc., Woodstock, VT.

Strategic Consulting, Inc. 2002. *Food Diagnostics: Global Review of Microbiological and Residue Testing in the Food Processing Industry.* Strategic Consulting Inc., Woodstock, VT.

Strategic Consulting, Inc. 2004. *Industrial Microbiology Market Review II.* Strategic Consulting Inc., Woodstock, VT.

Strategic Consulting, Inc. 2005. *Food Micro-2005. Global Review of Microbiology Testing in the Food Processing Market.* Strategic Consulting Inc., Woodstock, VT.

Trotman, R.E. 1973. Philosophy of the application of automation methods to hospital diagnostic bacteriology. *Biomed. Eng.* 8(12):519–521.

Tortorello, M. and S.M. Gendel. 1993. Fluorescent antibodies applied to direct epifluorescent filter techniques for microscopic enumeration of *Escherichia coli* O157:H7 in milk and juice. *J. Food Protect.* 56:672.

Walser, P.E. 2000. Using conventional microtiter plate technology for the automation of microbiology testing of drinking water. *J. Rapid Methods Automat. Microbiol.* 8(3):193–208.

Wu, V.C.H., P. Jitareerat, and D.Y.C. Fung. 2003. Comparison of the Pulsifier and the Stomacher for recovery of microorganisms in vegetable. *J. Rapid Methods Automation Microbiol.* 11(2):145–152.

8

Rapid Electrochemical Biosensors for the Identification and Quantification of Bacteria

Judith Rishpon and Tova Neufeld

CONTENTS

8.1 Introduction

Food-borne infections are a worldwide major health problem, which cause million illness cases each year. Variable microorganisms and toxic agents might be transmitted to humans through nutritive products and cause severe health damages. The most common food contaminates are bacteria. Many kinds of bacteria might damage food quality, thus causing infectious diseases, especially but not exclusively, of the digestion system. Not every edible compound can be pasteurized hence it is important to certify the purity of certain products before their arrival to the market. Consequently, the field of food safety requires the rapid detection of bacterial pathogens that cause severe infectious diseases and poisonings.

Although culturing methodology remains the gold standard for detection of food-borne pathogens, the technique is time consuming (24–48 h of enrichment before analysis).[1,2] Moreover, the identification of certain types of pathogens by culturing often results in false negatives due to a high background level of competing microorganisms. Another conventional method for detecting a bacterial pathogen involves the use of antibodies against the microorganisms.[3,4] This method has some drawbacks as well: the sensitivity is inadequate and the bacteria must be purified, a process requiring many hours.[5,6] The polymerase chain reaction (PCR) has been used extensively in the last few years to detect bacteria and viruses. Although the sensitivity is improved, the technique is laborious and expensive.[7,8]

Direct online monitoring of bacterial contamination will result in improved food quality and safety as well as greater efficiency of food production. In order to achieve these goals, analytical devices allowing rapid "on the spot" performances must be used. Not only should these devices provide fast and sensitive measurements but also they must be simple to operate and inexpensive as well. In this respect, biosensors offer an attractive opportunity.

Biosensors are measuring devices which combine the high sensitivity and specificity of a "biological unit" with a physical signal-converting and processing unit. They are used normally, in applications in which electronic signals provide proportional information on the concentration of some specific substance in the analyzed medium. In bioelectrochemical sensors, a biological element (enzyme, antibody etc.) is placed in proximity with an electrode. A bioelectrochemical sensor is an analytical device, which uses biologically sensitive material to detect chemical or biochemical species directly (Figure 8.1). During the biochemical reaction, ions or electroactive substances may be produced.[9] By using well-established electrochemical techniques, the biochemical response is converted into an amplified quantifiable electrical signal. Amperometric and potentiometric enzyme electrodes are well known in characterization of bioactive surfaces, and have

Electric signal

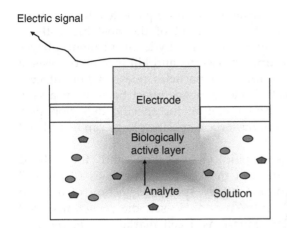

FIGURE 8.1
A bioelectrochemical sensor.

been commercialized. Their use in diagnostic devices has been an active research area in the past few years. Thus, bioelectrochemical sensors combine the selectivity of biological recognition with the high sensitivity and relative simplicity of modern electroanalytical techniques. Normally, they are utilized in applications in which electronic signals provide quantitative information on the concentration of selected substances in an analyzed medium. Since the first enzyme-based sensor for glucose, which was introduced by Clark in 1962,[10] there has been extensive use of enzyme-based biosensors involving a wide variety of substrates.

Enzyme biosensors in general and enzyme immunoassays (EIA) in particular play an important role in clinical diagnostics, veterinary medicine, environmental control, and bioprocess analysis. Due to high selectivity and sensitivity, EIA enable us the detection of a broad-spectrum of analytes in complex samples. Decentralizing quantitative immunoassays from hospital laboratories, where complex instrumentation as well as highly qualified technical staff is required, can be achieved by combining immunoenzymatic systems with electrodes to create immunoelectrochemical sensors that provide immediate results. We have developed an enzyme immunosensor, made of two enzymes and two antibodies, which can detect bacteria in food samples.

It is possible to take advantage of the intrinsic enzymatic activity of a bacterium for analytical purposes. The ubiquitous enzyme β-D-galactosidase is often used as a general marker for total coliforms. The β-D-galactosidase activity of noncoliforms is at least 2 log units below that of induced coliforms, affecting the results only when the bacteria are present in high concentrations.[11] We developed a sensitive, inexpensive amperometric enzyme biosensor based on the electrochemical detection of β-galactosidase activity, using *p*-amino-phenyl-β-D-galactopyranoside (PAPG) as substrate, for determining the density of coliforms, represented by *Escherichia coli* and *Klebsiella pneumoniae.*

Bacteriophages (phages) are obligate intracellular parasites that multiply inside bacteria by making use of some or all of the host biosynthetic machinery (i.e., viruses that infect bacteria.). Lytic or virulent phages are phages, which can only multiply in bacteria and kill the cell by lysis at the end of the life cycle. The number of particles released per infected bacteria may be as high as 1000. Bacteriophages infect bacteria in a very selective manner and can be used therefore for specific detection purposes.[12,13] For any strain or type of bacteria, a specific phage can be utilized for identification.

The combination of phage-specific identification and the related release of an intrinsic enzymatic cell marker following lysis of the cell provides a powerful means for the highly specific detection of a given bacterial strain. Blasco et al.[14] and Wu et al.[15] used the phage-mediated release of the enzyme adenylate kinase as a cell marker for *E. coli* and Salmonella. The enzymatic conversion of ADP to ATP is followed by the appearance of bioluminescence using an external firefly luciferase. A method reported by Goodridge et al.[16,17] involves a fluorescent bacteriophage assay for detecting *E. coli* O157:H7 in ground beef and raw milk. This method, based on staining the bacteriophages with a fluorescent dye, enables the detection of 100 colony-forming units (cfu)/mL of target bacteria in artificially contaminated milk after a 10 h enrichment step.

A phagemid is a modified phage that contains a bacterial extrachromosomal, autonomously replicating circular DNA molecule called a plasmid. This phagemid has the ability to infect bacteria but cannot replicate as an intact phage. Under most conditions, the phagemid propagates autonomously like a normal plasmid and replicates along with the bacterial cell cycle, but it can be released from the bacteria (rescue) only by coinfection with a second helper phage to lyse the bacteria.[18] The plasmid pFLAG-ATS-BAP carries a "reporter" gene coding for the detectable bacterial enzyme, alkaline phosphatase, as well as a genetically selective marker, Amp[r], which confers resistance to ampicillin. Filamentous phages like M13 infect hosts by injecting their DNA through a protein fiber structure of the bacteria called the sex pilus. To initiate infection, the phage binds to the minor coat protein, pIII, present only on the tip of the F pilus on male bacteria, *E. coli* F+.[19] The binding induces retraction of the pilus, resulting in the injection of the single-stranded DNA of the phage into the bacterial cell. A specific peptide in the phagemid then genetically directs the reporter enzyme, bacterial alkaline phosphatase, to the periplasmic space between the outer plasma membrane and the cell wall of the bacteria. The cell wall is porous, allowing the substrate, *p*-amino phenyl phosphate, to enter easily into the periplasmic space. Hence, the activity of the reporter enzyme can be directly measured in the electrochemical cell without further treatment of the sample. The product of the reaction, *p*-aminophenol (*p*-AP), diffused out is the same as in the previous bacteria.

8.2 Experimental

8.2.1 General

The biosensors used were based on amperometric measurement system with three electrodes: A working electrode, a reference electrode, and a counter electrode. The electrochemical measurements used here were made with disposable screen-printed electrodes (Figure 8.2). Graphite ink was used as the working and counter electrodes and Ag/AgCl ink was used for the reference electrode. The electrochemical cells were made of polystyrene tubes (volume of 0.3 mL). The electrochemical apparatus consisted eight-channeled potentiostat that allowed the simultaneous measurement of eight bacteria samples with efficient mixing. Figure 8.3 describes schematically the computerized system, the electrochemical cells connected to the multipotentiostat and mixing device.

8.2.2 Amperometric Enzyme-Channeling Immunosensor

To detect bacteria in a pure culture, we developed a novel, rapid, one step, separation-free immunosensor that is based on an enzyme-channeling immunoassay (ECIA).[20,21] The principle of the method is shown in Figure 8.4. According to this method, the product of one enzyme reaction is the substrate for a second enzyme reaction. The binding interaction brings the two enzymes to proximity and catalyzes the conversion of the initial substrate to a final detectable electroactive product. Cyclic regeneration of the substrate, accumulation of a redox mediator, and control of the hydrodynamic conditions at the sensor/solution interface enable the direct preferential measurement of a surface-bound enzyme label with high sensitivity. The method does not require a separation step to remove excess free label from the bulk solution. This type of biosensor not only measures separate components but also determines the concentration of bacteria.

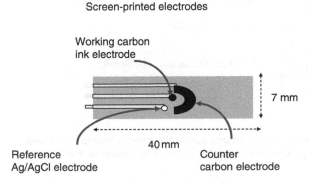

Screen-printed electrodes

Working carbon
ink electrode

7 mm

40 mm

Reference
Ag/AgCl electrode

Counter
carbon electrode

FIGURE 8.2
A screen-print electrode.

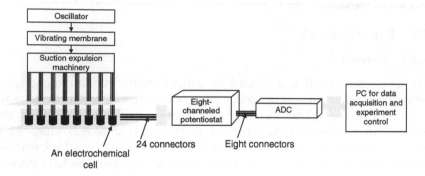

FIGURE 8.3
Scheme of the apparatus for eight simultaneous measurements.

We used a sandwich immunoassay. Protein A, the major cell wall component of *Staphylococcus aureus*, can be detected by binding the bacteria to an electrode surface that has been modified by immunoglobulin G from rabbit (RbIgG). Graphite electrodes (pencil leads) were coated by a polyethylenimine (0.5%) film with the coimmobilized capture antibody, RbIgG, and glucose oxidase (GOD), (all from Sigma, St. Louis, Missouri). The remaining unbound sites were blocked with 0.1 M glycine, (Fluka). Standard solutions of *S. aureus* (10^2–10^6 cells/mL) (Sigma, St. Louis, Missouri) were prepared in phosphate-buffered saline. The electrode was placed in buffer solutions

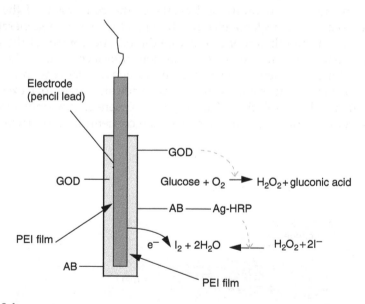

FIGURE 8.4
Schematic illustration of the separation-free, amperometric enzyme-channeling immunoassay with immobilized antibody and glucose oxidase on the PEI-modified electrode surface.

and an aliquot (10 μL) of *S. aureus* standard solution was added, and the RbIgG–GOD electrode was rotated for 10 min at 1000 rpm. at room temperature to enhance the kinetics of immunobinding between the cells and the antibody. Then, the electrode was washed and transferred to the electrochemical cell containing 0.1 M acetate buffer, 0.1 M NaCl, 3 mM KI, and 0.01% BSA. Aliquot (10 μL) of RbIgG–HRP (4 μg/mL) was added to the cell, thus placing the bacterial cells between two antibodies. After 10 min of incubation, an aliquot (10 μL) of glucose (0.1 M) was added to the cell, and the response to glucose was recorded. On the electrode surface, the GOD had catalyzed the oxidation of glucose to H_2O_2, and the iodine produced in the peroxidase-catalyzed H_2O_2/iodide redox system was monitored amperometrically by the electrochemical reduction of iodine back to iodide. As the GOD and the horseradish peroxidase (HRP) were in proximity, one could follow the labeled peroxidase activity, which was related to the GOD activity.

We have used a similar assay for the detection of *Salmonella*. Heat-killed *Salmonella typhimurium* cells (positive control), affinity-purified antibodies to *Salmonella*, and peroxidase-labeled affinity purified antibody to *Salmonella* were obtained from Kirkegaard & Perry Laboratories Inc., Gaithersburg, Maryland.

Electron microscopy of *S. aureus* cells on the electrode surface was performed with a JEOL-840a scanning electron microscope with an acceleration voltage of 25 kV, a magnification of 10,000, and an objective aperture of 1 mm.

8.2.3   Detection of Coliforms

We used three bacterial concentration ranges: high (10^3–10^7 CFU/mL), medium (60 CFU/mL), and very low (~1 CFU/mL). Two wild-type bacterial strains were used: *E. coli* and *K. pneumoniae*. Both strains were obtained from the strain collection of our laboratory.

Bacterial cultures were inoculated into flasks containing 10 mL of LB medium; isopropyl-β-D-thiogalactopyranoside (IPTG) was added, to a final concentration of 0.5 mM, to induce β-D-galactosidase activity. For the high concentration, the cultures were then grown for 2–3 h at 37°C with vigorous shaking until they reached the logarithmic phase (~2 × 10^8 CFU/mL). The log–phase cultures were then diluted to concentrations of 10^3–10^7 CFU/mL in 1 L of sterile water. The next step, permeabilization was performed in 10 mL of LB medium containing polymyxin B sulfate (10 μg/mL) and lysozyme (25 μg/mL) by vigorous shaking for 45 min at 30°C, followed by filtration (0.45 μm) and then the activity of β-D-galactosidase was electrochemically determined.

For the medium and very low concentrations, a preincubation step was required. Bacterial suspensions were incubated in 10 mL of LB medium and 0.5 mM of IPTG, and aerated by shaking at 37°C. Samples were withdrawn at 1 h intervals for permeabilization and the determination of β-D-galactosidase activity.

For specific detection of *E. coli*, we coated the immunosensor with a polyclonal anti-*E. coli* antibody to bind the bacteria to the electrode. The antibody-modified electrodes were immersed in the bacterial suspension (after incubation), washed, and checked for ~β-D-galactosidase activity.

8.2.4 Utilization of Phages

Experimental procedure for high bacterial concentration 10^5–10^9 cfu/mL: 100 μL of stationary–phase cultures were incubated in a 15 mL sterile tube with 2 μL of 10^{10} pfu/mL lambda vir phage in the presence of 10 mM $MgSO_4$, 0.2% maltose and 0.5 mM IPTG, in a total volume of 220 μL, for 15 min at 37°C without shaking. Control mixtures did not contain phage lambda. After 15 min, LB was added and completed to 4 mL total volume, and the mixture was further incubated for 3 h as before. The 4 mL cultures were filtered through a 0.22 μm filter to separate the medium from intact cells and cell debris. The filtrates were used for the electrochemical measurements

For medium–low bacterial concentration (10^2–10^5 cfu/mL) the bacterial cells were first preincubated for 2, 3, or 4 h with vigorous shaking at 37°C. Afterward, 1 mL of phage solution with different concentration, 10^5–10^4 pfu/mL, was added to the bacterial mixture and the procedure above was applied.

For very low bacterial concentration 1 cfu/100 mL–10^2 cfu/mL, a preconcentration step was used. High volumes (100–2000 mL) samples were first filtered through 0.22 μm filter. The filters were then preincubated for 4 h. Next, the procedure for low–medium concentration was used.

8.2.5 Utilization of a Phagemid

We have used a commercial plasmid, pFLAG-ATS-BAP, carrying the reporter gene coding for alkaline phosphatase and the genetic marker Amp^r conferring ampicillin resistance that was purchased from Sigma Chemicals Co., St. Louis, Missouri.

An aliquot (100 μL) of a logarithmic *E. coli* TG1 culture was centrifuged for 5 min at 7000 rpm. The pellet was diluted with 10 mL of 100 mM $MgCl_2$ solution and incubated for 30 min on ice. The cells were centrifuged for 5 min at 7000 rpm, diluted with 10 mL of 100 mM $CaCl_2$ solution, and placed for 30 min on ice. The cells were then centrifuged for 5 min at 7000 rpm, and the pellet was diluted with 1 mL of 10 mM $CaCl_2$ solution containing 10% glycerol. Aliquots of 200 μL were kept at 70°C.

Competent TG1 bacterial cells (200 μL, as prepared above) were allowed to thaw slowly for 30 min on ice. The plasmid pFLAG-ATS-BAP (100 ng) was added to the tube and incubated for 30 min on ice. The *E. coli* tube was moved to heat shock for 3 min at 42°C and cooled for 5 min on ice. LB medium (1 mL) was added to the *E. coli* tube and incubated for 1 h at 37°C. An aliquot of 100 μL of the transformed cells was plated onto an LB-ampicillin (100 μg/mL) agar plate. An overnight culture of transformed *E. coli* cells, 3 mL, was centrifuged for 1 min at 13,000 rpm. The plasmid was purified using a Gen Elute Miniprep Kit, according to the manufacturer's protocol, and stored at ~20°C. The transformed *E. coli* cells bearing the plasmid pFLAG-ATS-BAP in LB liquid medium containing ampicillin were then grown overnight with shaking at 20°C. An aliquot (100 μL) of the overnight *E. coli* culture was inoculated into 3 mL 2YT medium containing 100 μg/mL ampicillin and 1% glucose and grown until reaching the logarithmic phase. For infection, 15 μL of 4×10^{10} pfu/mL M13KO7 helper phage was added and incubated for 30 min at 37°C without shaking. A pfu (plaque forming unit) arises from a single infectious phage. The culture was further incubated for 30 min at the same temperature with shaking. The cells were centrifuged for 5 min at 13,000 rpm, and the pellet was diluted with 100 mL 2YT medium containing ampicillin (100 μg/mL) and kanamycin (50 μg/mL) for overnight incubation with mild shaking at 30°C. After the overnight incubation, the culture was centrifuged for 20 min at 5000 rpm at 4°C and the supernatant collected. A sterile solution of 20% polyethylene glycol (PEG) containing 2.5 M NaCl was added gently to the supernatant at a ratio related to one-fifth of the supernatant volume. The solution was incubated for at least 2.5 h on ice, without stirring. The solution was then centrifuged for 30 min at 3000 rpm, 4°C, and the pellet was diluted with 1 mL sterile PBS buffer. After recentrifugation for 5 min at 13,000 rpm, the supernatant was purified by filtering through a 0.45 μm sterile filter membrane and stored at 20°C.

8.2.5.1 Titration of Phagemid Concentration

A mid-logarithmic phase *E. coli* TG1 culture and a decimal dilution of the purified phagemid solution were used for titration. An aliquot (10 μL) of each dilution was added to 90 μL bacteria. All samples were incubated for 1 h at 37°C without shaking. A 10 μL drop of each sample was plated on a TYE-Amp plate and dried for 10 min in a sterile hood. The plate was incubated overnight at 37°C and the titer determined according to the number of pfu. The titer used for this work was 4×10^{10} pfu/mL.

8.2.5.2 Phagemid Infection of 10^5–10^8 Cells/mL E. coli TG1 Samples

Liquid bacterial cultures were grown in 2YT medium at 37°C until O.D$_{600}$ = 0.5 was reached. Decimal serial bacterial dilutions, ranging from 10^5 to 10^8 cells/mL, were used for the experiments. An aliquot (1 mL) of each bacterial dilution was infected with 20 μL M13KO7 phagemid (4×10^{10} pfu/mL). Control mixtures did not contain phagemid. The mixtures were incubated for 1 h at 37°C without shaking to allow the phagemid to attach to its receptor. Ampicillin and IPTG (for bacterial alkaline phosphatase induction under *TAC* promoter) were then added to the bacterial mixtures at the respective concentrations of 100 µg/mL and 0.5 mM. The samples were incubated at 37°C with shaking for different times, ranging from 30 min to 3–4 h.

8.2.5.3   *Phagemid Infection of 1–10⁴ Cells/mL* E. coli *TG1 Samples*

Bacterial cultures were grown on 2YT medium at 37°C until O.D$_{600}$ = 0.5 was reached. Fifty milliliters of each dilution of bacteria, ranging from 1 to 10^4 cells/mL, was filtered and the cells collected on a 0.22 µm sterile filter. The filters were transferred to 2 mL 2YT medium; the bacteria were released by shaking for 10 min at 37°C. The content of each tube was divided and placed into two separate tubes: one tube was infected with 20 µL of phagemid (4×10^{10} pfu/mL), and the other, into which the phagemid was not introduced, served as a control for the collection filter. All samples were incubated for 30 min at 37°C without shaking for phagemid attachment. Ampicillin and IPTG were added to the bacterial mixtures at the respective concentrations of 100 µg/mL and 0.5 mM and incubated for 90 min at 37°C.

8.2.5.4   *Lysis of Phagemid-Infected* E. coli *TG1 Samples*

Bacterial samples, infected with phagemid as described in the former section, were incubated for 1 h with polymixin B and lysozyme at the respective concentrations of 10 µg/mL and 25 µg/mL at 37°C to lyse the bacteria.

8.2.5.5   *Phagemid Infection of Other Bacterial Strains*

Different bacterial strains, *Salmonella typhimurium, Bacillus cereus, Staphylococcus aureus*, and *Escherichia coli* TG1 cultures, were used for this experiment. Infection was performed as described above for the high concentration samples.

8.2.5.6   *Phagemid Infection in the Presence of Other Bacterial Strains*

Different bacterial strains, *B. cereus, Klebsiella pneumoniae*, and *E. coli* TG1 cultures, were grown on 2YT medium at 37°C until O.D$_{600}$ = 0.5 was reached. Dilutions of 1–10⁴ *E. coli* TG1 cells/mL were used for these experiments. Different dilutions of *E. coli* were introduced to a constant high concentration (10^5 cells/mL) of other strains of bacteria (*B. cereus, K. pneumoniae*) in 2YT medium. Infection was performed as described above.

8.3   Results and Discussion

8.3.1   Amperometric Enzyme-Channeling Immunosensor

Figure 8.5 shows an electron microscopy picture of two electrodes exposed to *S. aureus*: one with captured antibody immobilized on it and the other one

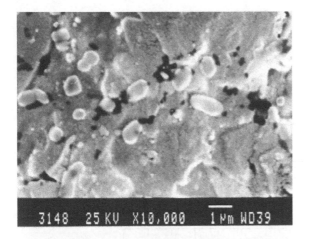

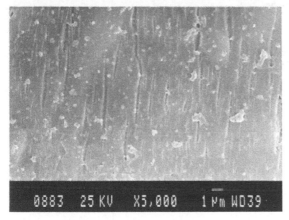

FIGURE 8.5
Electron microscopy of bacteria-modified electrode. (Top) Electrode bearing an immobilized antibody on it surface. (Bottom) Electrode without antibody captured on its surface.

without antibody. It is clearly seen that the electrode without antibody does not bear any bacteria on it. Evidently, this control experiment confirms the absence of nonspecific adsorption of bacteria to the electrodes.

Current changes caused by HRP activity were related to the variations in cell concentrations, ranging from 0 to 4×10^4 cells/mL. The measurements results are presented in Figure 8.6A. Similar results were obtained with *Salmonella*.

The immunoassay represented here is performed with an amperometric immunosensor, using a disposable cell and electrodes. The sensor enables preferential measurement of surface-bound conjugate relative to the excess, enzyme-labeled reagent in the bulk sample solution.

8.3.2 Detection and Enumeration of Coliforms

Figure 8.7 shows an example of the amperometric response of *E. coli* cultures (10^7 and 10^8 CFU/mL). We used the slope (Δcurrent/Δtime) within the

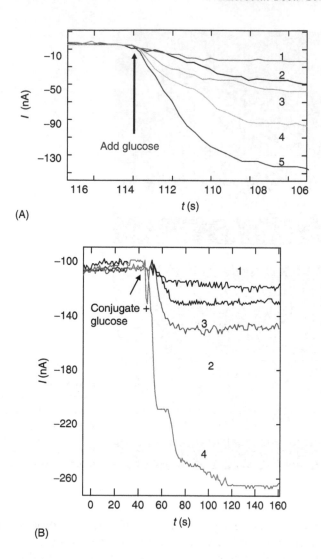

(A)

(B)

FIGURE 8.6
The response curves generated by amperometric immunosensor to specific bacteria at various concentrations. (A) *Staphylococcus aureus* (1) 0 cells/mL; (2) 1000 cells/mL; (3) 2000 cells/mL; (4) 20,000 cells/mL; (5) 40,000 cells/mL. (B) In the presence of *Salmonella* (1) 0 cells/mL; (2) 10^3 cells/mL; (3) 10^4 cells/mL; (4) 10^6 cells/mL.

linear range (the first 10 min) as the index for β-galactosidase activity. The results presented in Figure 8.8 show that a detectable signal could be measured for both coliform types in concentrations ranging between approximately 10^3 and 10^7 CFU/mL.

A good linear correlation was found between the number of bacteria measured by the plate counting method and the electrochemical response

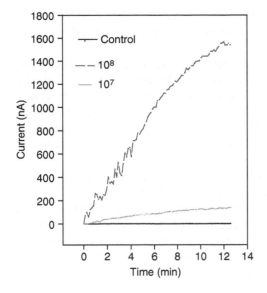

FIGURE 8.7
The amperometric response of *E. coli* cultures (10^8, 10^7 CFU/mL), with *p*-aminophenyl-β-D-galactopyranoside (PAPG) as substrate (0.8 mg/mL in LB medium). The control was without bacteria. (From Schwartz-Mittelmann, A., Ron, E.Z., and Rishpon, J., *Anal. Chem.*, 74, 903, 2002. With permission.)

measured as—Δcurrent/Δtime, with a correlation coefficient (R^2) of 0.9641 for *E. coli* and 0.932 for *K. pneumoniae*. The results are better than those reported for fluorimetric detection, where correlation coefficients of 0.8 and 0.83 were found[7,15]. The detection limit for both coliform types was ~10^3 CFU/mL. This sensitivity is comparable with the results obtained with fluorimetric and chemiluminometric methods (~10^3 CFU/mL) and

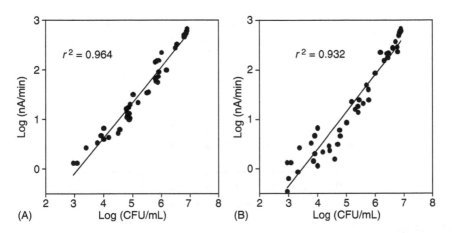

FIGURE 8.8
Quantification of (A) *E. coli* and (B) *K. pneumoniae* after filtering 1 L of water containing bacterial concentrations ranging from ~10^3 to 10^7 CFU/mL. The filter was placed in 10 mL of LB medium and permeabilization. (From Schwartz-Mittelmann, A., Ron, E.Z., and Rishpon, J., *Anal. Chem.*, 74, 903, 2002. With permission.)

better than the sensitivity of the colorimetric method ($\sim 10^6$ CFU/mL)[10,23]. For lower bacterial concentrations, however, further modifications were required.

We checked the feasibility of detecting medium concentrations (60 CFU/mL) and very small concentrations of bacteria (~ 1 CFU/mL) by filtering 1 L of water inoculated with bacteria and incubation in LB medium. At hourly intervals, samples were withdrawn, permeabilized, and analyzed. The results presented in Figure 8.9 show that *E. coli* at a concentration of 60 CFU/mL could be detected after 3 h of incubation, whereas *K. pneumoniae* at a similar concentration was detectable after 4 h of incubation.

E. coli at the very low concentration of 1.2 CFU/mL was detectable after 5 h of incubation and *K. pneumoniae* at a concentration of 1.3 CFU/mL after 6 h of incubation indicate that even very small concentrations of bacteria can be detected within a single working day. Although other rapid methods for detecting small concentrations of coliforms, based on fluorescent and chemiluminescent substrates, require similar incubation periods, they are dependent on the availability of an extremely sensitive detection apparatus, such as a CCD camera.[22]

The use of immunoassays is one of the presently available approaches to the specific identification of a target protein. For specific detection of *E. coli*,

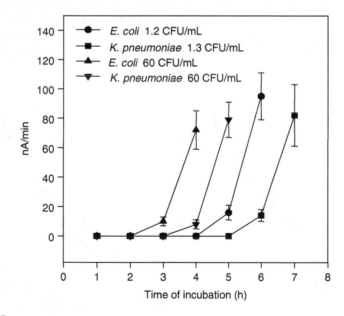

FIGURE 8.9
Detection of *E. coli*, at concentrations of 60 CFU/mL and 1.2 CFU/mL, and *K. pneumoniae*, at concentrations of 60 CFU/mL and 1.3 CFU/mL, in 1 L of water after filtration, incubation in LB medium at 37°C, and permeabilization. Each point represents the mean of three measurements ± standard deviation. (From Schwartz-Mittelmann, A., Ron, E.Z., and Rishpon, J., *Anal. Chem.*, 74, 903, 2002. With permission.)

we coated the working electrode with a polyclonal anti-*E. coli* antibody to bind the bacteria to an electrode. The antibody-modified electrodes were immersed in the bacterial suspension (after incubation), washed, and checked for β-D-galactosidase activity. After an incubation period of 6 h, we could detect *E. coli* at a concentration of 1.2 CFU/mL. *K. pneumoniae*, also β-D-galactosidase positive, was not detected by this method (Figure 8.10).

8.3.3 Enumeration and Identification of Specific Bacteria

Detection and measurements of various *E. coli* concentrations was performed with three main different techniques depending on the initial concentration of the bacterial sample. At first, we measured *E. coli* concentrations, ranging between 10^5 and -10^9 cfu/mL (cfu, colony forming unit), a small portion of 100 μL of the selected sample was infected with the phage, and transferred to 4 mL test tube for further incubation. Bacterial source was always at the stationary phase, after an overnight incubation, in order to simulate a typical environmental sample that usually do not represent a bacteria in the logarithmic stage. The initial concentration of the bacteria, in the test tube, is actually 40 times lower. However, as explained above, we were interested to detect and measure the real concentration of the bacterial sample, and not the initial concentration inside the tube. After 3 h incubation and immediately before the electrochemical measurement, the tests tubes were filtered in order to measure only the β-galactosidase

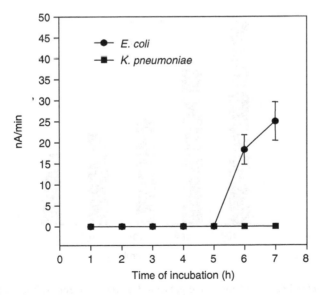

FIGURE 8.10
Specific detection by antibody-coated electrodes of 1.2 CFU/mL of *E. coli* in 1 L of water after filtration, incubation in LB medium at 37°C, and permeabilization. Each point represents the mean of three measurements ± standard deviation. (From Schwartz-Mittelmann, A., Ron, E.Z., and Rishpon, J., *Anal. Chem.*, 74, 903, 2002. With permission.)

released to the medium due to the specific lysis of *E. coli* by lambda vir phage. Thus, we avoid measuring the activity of the enzyme in the remaining intact *E. coli* cells or other β-galactosidase-producing bacteria[23] The results obtained are shown in Figure 8.11. There is a very good correlation

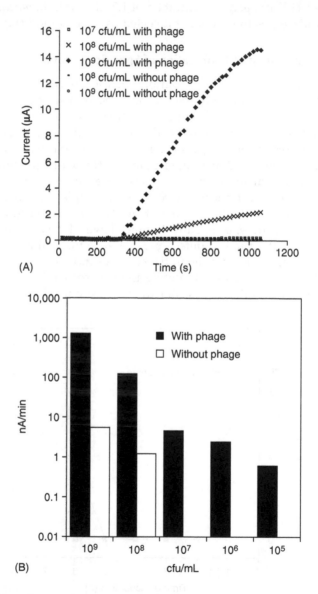

FIGURE 8.11
(A) Typical electrochemical response of β-galactosidase released from 100 μL stationary *E. coli* samples, after infection and incubation for 3 h at 37°C, with 2 μL of 10^8 pfu/mL lambda vir, in a total volume of 4 mL LB medium containing 0.2% lactose and 0.5 mM IPTG. (B) Results obtained by measuring the activity of released β-galactosidase from 100 μL *E. coli* samples ranging between 10^5 and 10^9 cfu/mL. The results are shown in nA/min, the rate of reaction measured. *Y* axis is in the logarithmic scale. (From Neufeld, T., Schwartz-Mittelmann, A., Biran, D., Ron, E.Z., and Rishpon, J., *Anal. Chem.*, 75, 580, 2003. With permission.)

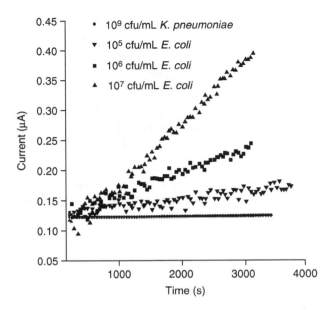

FIGURE 8.12
The electrochemical β-galactosidase activity measured from 100 μL stationary *Klebsiella pneumoniae* samples, after infection and incubation for 3 h at 37°C, with 2 μL of 10^8 pfu/mL lambda vir phage, in a total volume of 4 mL LB medium containing 0.2% lactose and 0.5 mM IPTG. (From Neufeld, T., Schwartz-Mittelmann, A., Biran, D., Ron, E.Z., and Rishpon, J., *Anal. Chem.*, 75, 580, 2003. With permission.)

between the initial concentrations of *E. coli* infected by the virulent phage lambda and the electrochemical response generated by the activity of the enzyme β-galactosidase.[24]

The action of the phage is very specific to *E. coli* as the samples containing *K. pneumoniae*, (10^9 cfu/mL) which is β-D-galactosidase positive, did not show any activity (Figure 8.12). The β-D-galactosidase activity of full lysed high concentration of *E. coli* samples was three orders of magnitude higher than the samples of *K. pneumoniae* since, there was no phage-mediated release of the enzyme to the medium. Our results are well correlated with the data shown previously by Schwartz et al[24] and Tryland et al[26] that nontarget β-D-galactosidase positive bacteria, is low, as the β-D-galactosidase activity of *K. pneumoniae* bacteria is at least 2 log units below that of *E. coli* bacteria.

Experiments for determination of multiplicity of infection (MOI), the ratio of the number of infectious virions to the number of susceptible cells in the tested culture are very important to establish an optimized mode of operation. The results are shown in Figure 8.13. *E. coli* culture, at constant initial concentration of 2.5×10^4 cfu/mL was infected with different suspensions of phage lambda vir and the electrochemical activity of the enzyme was measured. We show that best MOI ratio is in the low range, between 0.05 and 0.005. Application of such a low MOI value enables the bacterial

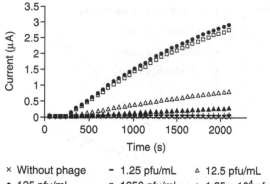

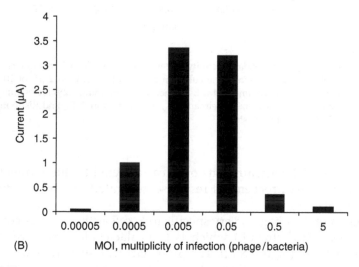

FIGURE 8.13

(A) Electrochemical response of β-D-galactosidase activity generated by *E. coli* cultures, at constant initial concentration of 2.5×10^4 cfu/mL, infected with different concentrations of phage lambda vir. (B) Determination of the optimal MOI value, phage/bacteria ratio. 100 μL of stationary phase *E. coli* samples, were infected and incubated for 3 h at 37°C, with 2 μL of lambda vir phage in different concentrations, in a total volume of 4 mL LB medium containing 0.2% lactose and 0.5 mM IPTG. The electrochemical measurements were performed in 0.3 mL cell volume with 0.8 mg/mL PAPG, β-D-galactosidase substrate, with $E = 0.3$ V applied potential. (From Neufeld, T., Schwartz-Mittelmann, A., Biran, D., Ron, E.Z., and Rishpon, J., *Anal. Chem.*, 75, 580, 2003. With permission.)

culture, to grow initially and produce enough β-galactosidase before full lysis occurs. A large number of virulent phage progeny are produced during the 3 h incubation time leading to release of the enzyme to the medium through cell lysis.

Our next step was to increase the sensitivity of the method. For that purpose, we had to change the mode of infection with the phage. Preincubation of the bacterial cultures (before adding the phage) was needed. In this way we could achieve higher enzyme activity in a relatively short time, compared to the mode used above. Furthermore, preincubation will allow us to use a relatively high phage concentration, instead of low concentration (as calculated in the former section), that means, using higher than 0.05–0.005 MOI ratios. In addition, according to the mode of infection used in the first part, detection of lower bacterial concentration will require an extremely low concentration of phage lambda, which, may result in a very long incubation time. In order to emphasize this claim, an *E.coli* culture was preincubated for 2 h, infected with two different concentration of the phage, and further incubated until lysis occurred (2 h). Figure 8.13 shows that increasing the phage concentration from 2.5×10^4 to 2.5×10^5 pfu/mL leads to increase in the enzyme activity and thus, in the same detection time (overall of 4 h) we can detect a 100 μL sample of 10^5 cfu/mL (final concentration was 2.5×10^3 cfu/mL).

Detection of lower concentrations of bacteria ($<2.5 \times 10^3$ cfu/mL) became possible by extending the preincubation time. As a result, the growing culture that was not in the logarithmic stage could, possibly, enter this stage and produce higher quantities of β-galactosidase (Figure 8.14). We can measure different sample concentrations ranging from the relatively high 10^5 cfu/mL to even as low as 10^2 cfu/mL within 3 or 4 h preincubation, respectively, followed by 2 h incubation with the phage. It should be emphasized that we took only 100 μL sample of the aforementioned concentrations diluted in 4 mL medium, which means, that the bacterial culture started with only 2.5 cfu/mL when the source concentration was 10^2 cfu/mL. In this way there is no need to make any pretreatment, e.g., concentrating or filtering large volumes of water samples besides taking only 100 μL volume. We could determine the bacterial concentration according to the incubation time employed.

Although, we could detect as low as 100 cfu/mL of *E. coli* sample using the preincubation method, we anticipated that measuring very low concentration of bacteria such as 1 cfu/mL or even 1 cfu/100 mL may be time consuming. Our goal was to develop a detection method that will take within a standard working day, in other words, no more than 8 h. For that purpose, we used the procedure described in the experimental part for very low concentration. We could detect and distinguish between 10 cfu/mL, 1 cfu/mL, and particularly, 1 cfu/100 mL, with high accuracy according to the results shown in Figure 8.14. The results are demonstrated by measuring three different samples of each bacterial concentration in the presence or absence of phage lambda. Cells collected on the filter in the absence of the phage did not generate any electrochemical signal, given that there was no nonspecific lysis.

The results obtained are exhibited as the total cfu collected from 100, 10, 1 cfu/mL, and 1 cfu/100 mL samples, vs. the electrochemical signal measured

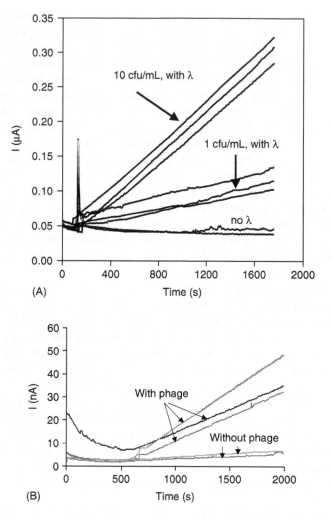

FIGURE 8.14

Detection of low concentration of *E. coli* of 10 cfu/mL, (A) 1 cfu/mL and (B) 1 cfu/100 mL. Each represents triplicates of the measured sample. (From Neufeld, T., Schwartz-Mittelmann, A., Biran, D., Ron, E.Z., and Rishpon, J., *Anal. Chem.*, 75, 580, 2003. With permission.)

(Figure 8.15). We can measure as low as 1 cfu/100 mL within less than 8 h with no need to grow the bacterial samples overnight on culture plates. Moreover, we could identify specifically the bacterial type present in the sample, since the phage binds to specific receptors on the bacterial surface.

8.3.4 Utilization of a Phagemid

Bacterial cultures of *E. coli* TG1 were grown to mid-log stage at 37°C in order to induce pilus formation, and diluted to samples ranging from 10^9 to

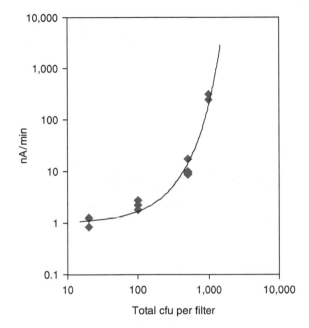

FIGURE 8.15
Total cfu collected on the filter and the relative enzyme activity generated at the electrochemical electrode in the presence of phage lambda vir. The results are exhibited on the logarithmic scale. (From Neufeld, T., Schwartz-Mittelmann, A., Biran, D., Ron, E.Z., and Rishpon, J., *Anal. Chem.*, 75, 580, 2003. With permission.)

10^5 cfu/mL. Each sample was infected with the phagemid at high and constant concentration of 4×10^{10} pfu/mL following 1 h incubation period. The samples were measured immediately without any additional treatment such as filtration, chemical permeabilization, or lysis. By introducing the M13KO7 phagemid into other strains of bacteria, we examined whether the phagemid infection is specific for *E. coli* TG1. The strains tested were *B. cereus*, *S. typhimurium*, and *S. aureus*. Figure 8.16 shows the results of infection at very high bacterial concentrations of 10^8 and 10^9 cells/mL. The infection was specific because only the *E. coli* TG1 culture showed alkaline phosphatase activity. A minor signal, from 15- to 20-fold less than that for *E. coli* TG1, detected in *B. cereus* at 10^9 cells/mL, was probably due to the innate alkaline phosphatase enzyme activity typical for *Bacillus* spp.[27,28] Such activity, which disappeared almost completely in *B. cereus*, is not considered a problem because polluted water samples contain about 4–5 orders of magnitude lower bacterial concentrations than those tested in this experiment. *S. typhimurium* and *S. aureus*, showed no activity at all.

At low *E. coli* concentrations, prolonged incubation with the phagemid was required to obtain a signal. To test the effect of the incubation time on the amperometric signal, we withdrew samples at 30 min intervals for electrochemical measurement. As low as 10^4 cfu/mL were detectable after 4 h incubation without any prefiltration, preincubation, or further lysis-aided treatment, all of which are required in other methods.[29] The time-dependence of enzymatic activity is shown in Figure 8.17. Low bacterial concentrations required additional treatment like prefiltration and a preincubation period before phage infection.

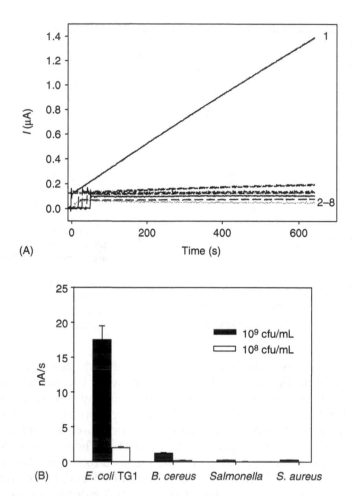

FIGURE 8.16

Bacterial strain specificity tested at high concentrations of *Bacillus cereus*, *S. typhimurium*, and *S. aureus* and compared with *E. coli* TG1 (A) Amperometric response of infected bacterial cultures. (1) *E. coli* TG1 infected with the M13K07 phagemid, (2)–(8) other bacterial responses to the phagemid infection. (B) Comparison of infected *E. coli* TG1 shown in (A) with the other cultures tested. Results are represented as Δcurrent/Δtime (with error bars [$n = 6$]). (From Neufeld, T., Mittelmann, A.S., Buchner, V., and Rishpon, J., *Anal. Chem.*, 77, 652, 2005. With permission.)

To measure very low concentrations of *E. coli*, we collected on a filter 50 mL of bacteria, ranging from 680 to 1 cfu/mL, which were shaken for 10 min to release the bacteria into the liquid medium. The samples were divided into two tubes for the 30 min infection step and the 90 min incubation period in the presence or absence of the phagemid. The duration of the whole procedure was 130 min. The results of the electrochemical measurements are shown in Figure 8.18. We found a good correlation between the sample concentration and the electrochemical signal. No signal was

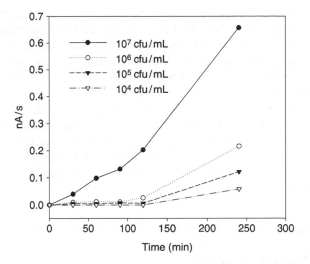

FIGURE 8.17
Effect of incubation time on the amperometric signal generated by different *E. coli* TG1 samples ranging between 10^7 and 10^4 cfu/mL infected with the phagemid. (From Neufeld, T., Mittelmann, A.S., Buchner, V., and Rishpon, J., *Anal. Chem.*, 77, 652, 2005. With permission.)

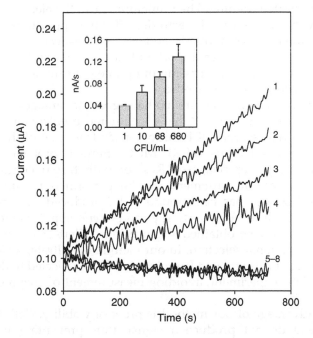

FIGURE 8.18
Amperometric response to alkaline phosphatase activity expressed at low concentrations of *E. coli* TG1 infected with the phagemid at (1) 1000 cfu/mL, (2) 100 cfu/mL, (3) 10 cfu/mL, (4) 1 cfu/mL, and in noninfected bacterial samples (5)–(8). The results in the insert are represented as Δcurrent/Δtime ($n = 6$). (From Neufeld, T., Mittelmann, A.S., Buchner, V., and Rishpon, J., *Anal. Chem.*, 77, 652, 2005. With permission.)

obtained from control experiments in the absence of the phagemid because the low concentration of the natural bacterial alkaline phosphatase activity is under the detection limit of the system, and noninfected bacteria were excluded by ampicillin selection. This procedure can be manipulated for measuring even lower concentrations of bacteria (1 cfu/100 mL) by filtering between 2 and 5 L of the test water sample.

We tested the ability of the phagemid assay to identify *E. coli* TG1 in a mixture containing two other strains of bacteria. *E. coli* TG1 cultures in the range of $1-10^3$ cfu/mL were mixed with 10^5 cells/mL of *B. cereus* and 10^5 cells/mL of *K. pneumoniae*. We found that that even at the lowest concentration of 1 cfu/mL a measurable signal was detected in the phagemid-infected *E. coli* samples.

8.4 Concluding Remarks

In this chapter, we described rapid and sensitive amperometric techniques for the quantification of total bacteria and identification of specific bacteria. The techniques are simple to operate, and does not require any particular skills or complicated training. The miniature size of the electrochemical cell, combined with screen-printed electrodes offer the opportunity of working with low volumes of compounds and reagents, especially when dealing with hazardous materials. An important feature of our system is the possibility of the simultaneous processing of up to eight samples and the use of disposable screen-printed electrodes.

The electrochemical measurements have great advantages in contrast to fluorescence measurements[31–33] that encountered problems in distinguishing the natural fluorescence of Pseudomonads from that of the commonly used fluorescent substrate called MUG. Similar problems can arise with luciferase reporter phages (LRPs) or with turbid culture samples. The electrochemical measurement can be performed in turbid culture. β-D-galactosidase also has been found to be produced by some noncoliform bacteria, such as *Aeronomas* spp. and *Vibrio* spp.[34] Therefore, false-positive results may be obtained when using colilert-18 or any other test without any additional selection. In our method the filtrate, which contains the released enzyme originated from lysed cells, is subjected to the substrate in the end of the experiment, avoiding measurement of enzyme present in intact cells.

Another advantage of our method is proof of viability. Cells that cannot grow or dead do not produce a signal, thus preventing false results. Methods using antibodies have more probability to have such problems.

Finally, the biosensors described are potentially useful tools in improving food quality by allowing careful examination of edible materials before spreading them to the markets, or checking food components before their use in commercial products.

References

1. Baeumner, A.J., Leonard, B., McElwee, J., and Montagna, R.A., A rapid biosensor for viable B. anthracis spores, *Anal. Bioanal. Chem.*, 380, 15–23, 2004.
2. Turnbough, C.L., Discovery of phage display peptide ligands for species-specific detection of *Bacillus* spores, *J. Microb. Met.*, 53, 263–271, 2003.
3. Diaz-Gonzalez, M., Gonzalez-Garcia, M.B., and Costa-Garcia, A., Immunosensor for Mycobacterium tuberculosis on screen-printed carbon electrodes, *Biosens. Bioelect.*, 20 2035–2043, 2005.
4. Petrenko, V.A. and Sorokulova, I.B., Detection of biological threats. A challenge for directed molecular evolution, *J. Microbl. Met.*, 58, 147–168, 2004.
5. Rubina, A.Y., Dyukova, V.I., Dementieva, E.I., Stomakhin, A.A., Nesmeyanov, V.A., Grishin, E.V., and Zasedatelev, A.S., Quantitative immunoassay of biotoxins on hydrogel-based protein microchips, *Anal. Biochem.*, 340, 317–329, 2005.
6. Zhou, B., Wirsching, P., and Janda, K.D., Human antibodies against Bacillus: A model study for detection of an protection against anthrax and the bioterrorist threat, *Proc. Natl Acad. Sci. U.S.A.*, 99, 5241–5246, 2002.
7. de Viedma, D.G., Rapid detection of resistance in Mycobacterium tuberculosis: A review discussing molecular approaches, *Clin. Microbiol. Infect.*, 9, 349–359, 2003.
8. Iqbal, S.S., Mayo, M.W., Bruno, J.G., Bronk, B.V., Batt, C.A., and Chambers, J.P., A review of molecular recognition technologies for detection of biological threat agents, *Biosens. Bioelect.*, 15, 549–578, 2000.
9. Bard, A.J. and Faulkner, L.R., in *Electrochemical Methods: Fundamental and Applications*, John Wiley & Sons, Inc., 1980, pp. 136–249.
10. Clark, L.C. and Lyons, C., Electrode systems for continuous monitoring in cardiovascular surgery, *N.Y. Acad. Sci.*, 102, 29, 1962.
11. Tryland, I. and Fiksdal, L., Enzyme characteristics of beta-D-galactosidase- and beta-D-glucuronidase-positive bacteria and their interference in rapid methods for detection of waterborne coliforms and *Escherichia coli*, *A. Environ. Microb.*, 64, 1018–1023, 1998.
12. McNerney, R., T.B.: The return of the phage. A review of fifty years of mycobacteriophage research, *Int. J. Tuberc. Lung Dis.*, 3 (3), 179–184, 1999.
13. Ronner, A.B. and Cliver, D.O., Isolation and characterization of a coliphage specific for *Escherichia coli*-0157-H7, *J. Food Protect.*, 53, 944–947, 1990.
14. Blasco, R., Murphy, M.J., Sanders, M.F., and Squirrell, D.J., Specific assays for bacteria using phage mediated release of adenylate kinase, *J. Appl. Microbiol.*, 84 (4), 661–666, 1998.
15. Wu, Y., Brovko, L., and Griffiths, M.W., Influence of phage population on the phage-mediated bioluminescent adenylate kinase (AK) assay for detection of bacteria, *Lett. Appl. Microbiol.*, 33 (4), 311–315, 2001.
16. Goodridge, L., Chen, J.R., and Griffiths, M., The use of a fluorescent bacteriophage assay for detection of *Escherichia coli* O157:H7 in inoculated ground beef and raw milk, *Internl. J. Food Microbiol.*, 47 (1–2), 43–50, 1999.
17. Goodridge, L., Chen, J.R., and Griffiths, M., Development and characterization of a fluorescent-bacteriophage assay for detection of *Escherichia coli* O157:H7, *Appl. Environ. Microbiol.*, 65 (4), 1397–1404, 1999.
18. Kramer, R.A., Cox, F., van der Horst, M., van den Oudenrijn, S., Res, P.C.M., Bia, J., Logtenberg, T., and de Kruif, J., A novel helper phage that improves

phage display selection efficiency by preventing the amplification of phages without recombinant protein, *Nucl. Acid. Res.*, 31 (11), 2003.

19. Brock, T.D. and Madigan, M.T., *Biology of Microorganisms*, 6th ed., Prentice Hall Engelwood Cliffs, NJ, 1991, 263–265.

20. Rishpon, J. and Ivnitski, D., Amperometric enzyme-channeling immunosensor, *Enz. Eng. XIII*, 799, 508–513, 1996.

21. Ivnitski, D. and Rishpon, J., A one-step, separation-free amperometric enzyme immunosensor, *Biosens. Bioelect.*, 11 (4), 409–417, 1996.

22. Vanpoucke, S.O. and Nelis, H.J., Development of a sensitive chemiluminometric assay for the detection of beta-galactosidase in permeabilized coliform bacteria and comparison with fluorometry and colorimetry, *Appl. Environ. Microbiol.*, 4505–4509, 1995.

23. Leclerc, H., Mossel, D.A.A., Edberg, S.C., and Struijk, C.B., Advances in the bacteriology of the coliform group: Their suitability as markers of microbial water safety, *Annu. Rev. Microbiol.*, 55, 201–234, 2001.

24. Schwartz-Mittelmann, A., Ron, E.Z., and Rishpon, J., Amperometric quantification of total coliforms and specific detection of Escherichia coli, *Anal. Chem.*, 74 (4), 903–907, 2002.

25. Neufeld, T., Schwartz-Mittelmann, A., Biran, D., Ron, E.Z., and Rishpon, J., Combined phage typing and amperometric detection of released enzymatic activity for the specific identification and quantification of bacteria, *Anal. Chem.*, 75 (3), 580–585, 2003.

26. Tryland, I. and Fiksdal, L., Enzyme characteristics of beta-D-galactosidase- and beta-D-glucuronidase-positive bacteria and their interference in rapid methods for detection of waterborne coliforms and *Escherichia coli*, *Appl. Environ. Microbiol.*, 64 (3), 1018–1023, 1998.

27. Bursik, M. and Nemec, M., Alkaline phosphatase production during sporulation of *Bacillus cereus*, *Folia Microbiol.*, 44 (1), 90–92, 1999.

28. Vinter, V. and Smid, F., Content of alkaline-phosphatase (Ec3.1.3.1) in spores of *Bacillus cereus* and *Bacillus megaterium* depends on the presence of inorganic-phosphate in the medium during sporulation, *Folia Microbiol.*, 29 (5), 389–389, 1984.

29. van Poucke, S.O. and Nelis, H.J., Rapid detection of fluorescent and chemiluminescent total coliforms and *Escherichia coli* on membrane filters, *J. Microbiol. Methods*, 42 (3), 233–244, 2000.

30. Neufeld, T., Mittelmann, A.S., Buchner, V., and Rishpon, J., Electrochemical phagemid assay for the specific detection of bacteria using Escherichia coli TG-1 and the M13KO7 phagemid in a model system, *Anal. Chem.*, 77 (2), 652–657, 2005.

31. Bloemberg, G.V., Otoole, G.A., Lugtenberg, B.J.J., et al., Green fluorescent protein as a marker for *Pseudomonas* spp., *Appl. Environ. Microbiol.*, 63, 4543–4551, 1997.

32. Hartman, P.A., Petzel, J.P., and Kaspar, C.W., New methods for indicator organisms, *Food Technol.*, 39, 53–53, 1985.

33. Timms-Wilson, T.M., Bryant, B.K., and Bailey, M.J., Strain characterization and 16S–23S probe development for differentiating geographically dispersed isolates of the phytopathogen *Ralstonia solanacearum*, *Environ. Microbiol.*, 3, 785–797, 2001.

34. Geissler, K., Manafi, M., Amoros, I., and Alonso, J.L., Quantitative determination of total coliforms and *Escherichia coli* in marine waters with chromogenic and fluorogenic media, *J. Appl. Microbiol.*, 88, 280–285, 2000.

9

Applications of the Polymerase Chain Reaction for Detection, Identification, and Typing of Food-Borne Microorganisms

Pina M. Fratamico and Susumu Kawasaki

CONTENTS

Mention of trade names or commercial products is solely for the purpose of providing specific information and does not imply recommendation or endorsement by the U.S. Department of Agriculture.

9.1 Detection of Food-Borne Pathogens

Public awareness of microorganisms transmitted by food which pose a severe threat to human health has increased dramatically in recent years. Food-borne pathogenic microorganisms include bacterial pathogens, such as *Salmonella* and *Campylobacter* spp., *Listeria monocytogenes*, *Escherichia coli* O157:H7 and other Shiga toxin-producing *E. coli*, *Yersinia enterocolitica*, and *Clostridium perfringens*, protozoan parasites, including *Giardia*, *Cryptosporidium*, and *Cyclospora*, and enteric viruses including hepatitis A and noroviruses. In a report from the Centers for Disease Control and Prevention, it was estimated that there are approximately 76 million cases of food-borne illnesses each year in the United States with 325,000 hospitalizations, and 5000 deaths.[1] The Council for Agricultural Science and Technology Task Force Report estimated that the annual incidence of microbial food-borne disease cases in the United States ranges from 6.5 to 33 million, with as many as 9000 deaths annually.[2] Thus, there is a need for rapid, sensitive, and reliable methods for detection of food-borne pathogens and for investigating cases and outbreaks of illness caused by these agents. Furthermore, development of rapid diagnostic systems that have the capability to link sample processing, preparation, and simultaneous detection of multiple pathogens and new threats, including potential biothreat agents, is important for food safety.

9.1.1 Conventional Methods

Conventional methods for detection, isolation, and identification of food-borne bacteria require enrichment culturing of food samples for various lengths of time to allow growth of target organisms followed by subculturing on a medium that contains selective agents or which allows for different-iation of targeted bacterial colonies from among the background microflora. Presumptive colonies are ultimately identified by performing a series of bio-chemical and serological tests. Additionally, tests for the presence of toxins produced by the targeted organism, as well as for other virulence character-istics, may also be performed. Although traditional cultural methods are relatively sensitive, such methods are often laborious and time consuming, requiring up to 4–7 days or longer to obtain definitive results.

9.1.2 Rapid Methods

Advancements in technology have resulted in the development of various types of rapid methods for detection, identification, and enumeration of food-borne pathogens. In addition to providing results in a shorter length of time than conventional methods, rapid assays are often more sensitive, specific, and more accurate than classical methods. Rapid methods include miniaturized biochemical kits and antibody- and nucleic acid-based assays.

9.1.2.1 Immunoassays

Immunologic methods depend on the binding specificity of an antibody to an antigen, usually displayed on the surface of a microorganism, or to a secreted toxin. Immunoassays, such as enzyme-linked immunosorbent assays (ELISA), latex agglutination, immunodiffusion assays, nanoparticle-labeled microfluidic immunoassays, and antibody-based biosensors,[3,4] which employ polyclonal or monoclonal antibodies directed against specific antigens of microorganisms, have found application in food testing. A variety of immunoassay kits are available commercially. However, there are limitations with the use of immunoassays, and these include: (1) cross-reactivity of the antibody with antigenically similar organisms giving rise to false positive results, (2) quantitative differences in expression of the target antigen related to growth parameters, (3) enzyme inhibitors present in foods, and (4) limited availability of antibodies against specific pathogens or specificity only at the species level or below. Generally, immunoassays yield presumptive results which must be confirmed by biochemical and serological testing of isolates.

9.1.2.2 Nucleic Acid-Based Methods

Nucleic acid hybridization techniques employing labeled gene probes for the detection and identification of specific microorganisms, including food-borne pathogens have been described.[5,6] Generally, probes are labeled nucleotide sequences ranging in length from 15 to 20 to several thousand base pairs, which under specific conditions hybridize to complementary target sequences. The resulting nucleic acid hybrids can then be detected in a number of ways, including using isotopic, chemiluminescent, chromogenic, or fluorescent techniques. The sensitivity of gene probe hybridization assays are in the range of 10^4–10^6 target gene copies. Commercially prepared colorimetric gene probe kits employing specific DNA probes in a dipstick hybridization format are available from GENE-TRAK (Hopkinton, Massachusetts) for detection of *Listeria*, *E. coli*, *Salmonella*, *Staphylococcus*, *Campylobacter*, and *Y. enterocolitica*, and a gene probe assay for detection of *Listeria.* is available from Gen-Probe (San Diego, California). Sensitivity of the assays is about 10^6 colony-forming units (CFU)/mL. The GeneGen Test Systems (SY-LAB Geraete GmbH., Purkersdorf, Austria) combine DNA amplification followed by detection of the amplified product by hybridization. Kits are available for detection of enterohemorrhagic *E. coli* (EHEC), *Salmonella*, *Listeria* spp. and *L. monocytogenes*, and *Campylobacter*. It is possible to detect less than 10 CFU/25 g of food within 24 h after enrichment.

The PCR is a nucleic acid amplification technique, which has found wide application and has simplified and enhanced procedures such as DNA cloning, sequencing, and mutating and genetic fingerprinting. The PCR has also become increasingly popular as a diagnostic tool to rapidly and reliably detect pathogenic microorganisms both in the clinical setting and in food and environmental microbiology laboratories. The PCR technique allows in vitro amplification of a specific fragment of DNA using a pair of oligonucleotide primers (used to initiate replication) that hybridize to opposite strands of the targeted DNA and "bracket" the section of the DNA that is to be repeatedly copied. Commonly, a target gene sequence unique to the species of interest is selected, and it is frequently a virulence gene. Following the PCR, the amplified product (also referred to as an amplicon), which is of defined length and contains the oligonucleotide primer sequences at its ends, can be detected in a number of ways (see below). The significant feature of the PCR is that a unique template sequence of the target organisms can be repeatedly replicated against a background of a large number of contaminating DNA sequences, for example, in the presence of DNA from nontarget microorganisms found in food samples.

9.2 Conventional PCR

To perform the PCR, a master mixture is usually prepared (to ensure uniformity of reagent concentrations among the PCR reactions) consisting of PCR buffer containing Tris-HCl, pH 8.3, KCl, and $MgCl_2$, the four deoxynucleotide triphosphates (dNTPs), a pair of DNA primers (typically 15–30 bases long), *Taq* DNA polymerase, template DNA (i.e., sequence which is to be amplified by the PCR), and water. The simplest method for preparation of template DNA from bacterial cells is to boil intact cells in a water bath or to lyse them using a thermal cycler set at 99°C for 10 min, for example. The master mixture and template DNA released from lysed bacteria are mixed in individual PCR reaction tubes. Gelatin, bovine serum albumin, or non-ionic detergents such as Triton X-100 are often included in PCR reactions to help stabilize *Taq* DNA polymerase and prevent the formation of secondary structures. The inclusion of low concentrations of nonionic detergents also may reverse the inhibitory effects of ionic detergents such as SDS which may be used in sample processing, and they also help to inhibit the activity of proteolytic enzymes which may be present. The sequence and concentration of the primers are very important for overall assay success. The primer/template ratio influences the specificity of the PCR, and thus, it should be optimized to prevent formation of nonspecific products and to obtain good product yield.

For total reaction volumes of 50 μL (25 or 100 μL volumes can also be used), 1–10 μL of template DNA from the material to be analyzed is added to 49–40 μL of reaction mixture, respectively, (i.e., master mixture) in 0.2 mL volume reaction tubes. The tubes are placed in a thermal cycling instrument, which is programed to go through cycles of high temperature DNA denaturation to separate the DNA strands, followed by lower temperatures for primer annealing and primer extension (i.e., template copying). The amount of template DNA approximately doubles with each cycle, thus theoretically, after 30 cycles, the DNA can be amplified 10^9-fold assuming 100% efficiency during each cycle. However, in practice, since the amount and activity of the enzyme become limiting and because of other factors, approximately 10^6-fold amplification of the target sequence is achieved. Typically, after an initial high temperature denaturation step, the PCR cycling parameters are 94°C–95°C for 1 min, 50°C–65°C annealing temperature for 1 min (depending on melting temperature $[T_m]$ of primers), and 72°C for 1 min for primer extension. To promote completion of partially extended products and annealing of single-stranded complementary products, a final extension step at 72°C for 5–15 min is frequently included after the last cycle. Unwanted, nonspecific sequences may be amplified if the annealing temperature is too low, and expected amplicons may not be detectable if the temperature is too high. Several annealing temperatures should be tested, starting at 5°C below the calculated T_m of the primers. The various reagents, kits, and equipment required to perform the PCR are available from many commercial suppliers and oligonucleotide primers can be synthesized in the laboratory, but generally, are custom synthesized by a number of commercial companies.

9.2.1 Detection of PCR Products

A number of techniques can be employed to detect and confirm the identity of PCR amplification products. The most commonly used procedure is agarose gel electrophoresis with ethidium bromide staining, which allows visualization of products due to the ability of the stain to intercalate into the DNA. Accurate size determination of the amplicons is accomplished by comparison to a set of size markers that are applied to adjacent wells of the same gel. Other nucleic acid stains such as SYBR Green (Molecular Probes, Inc., Eugene, Oregon) or EvaGreen (Biotium, Inc., Hayward, California), which may be more sensitive than ethidium bromide, are commercially available. Amplicons can also be stained by a silver-staining technique which does not require UV transillumination for visualization of the DNA. Hybridization techniques in which products are transferred to membranes followed by detection using radioactive- or nonradioactive-labeled specific probes are more sensitive than gel electrophoresis, allowing a 10^2- to 10^3-fold increase in detection sensitivity.[7] Alternatively, specific oligonucleotides can be covalently bound to membranes, then hybridized to amplification products that were biotinylated during the PCR. Streptavidin–horseradish peroxidase binds to the biotinylated DNA which then permits colorimetric detection.[8]

Numerous ELISA formats have been developed for detection of amplicons. For example, PCR amplification can be performed with a digoxigenin-labeled primer and a biotinylated probe. The biotin–digoxigenin hybrids can then be quantified by an ELISA through binding to streptavidin-coated microtiter plates followed by detection using a peroxidase-labeled antidigoxigenin antibody.[9] Detection of a *L. monocytogenes*-specific *hlyA* gene product was achieved using an antibody directed to RNA–DNA hybrids formed upon hybridization with a probe bound to a microtiter plate.[10]

With electrochemiluminescence detection systems, PCR products are labeled with biotin and ruthenium (II) trisbipyridyl ($Ru(bpy)_3^{2+}$) and then captured by streptavidin-coated magnetic beads before electrochemiluminescent detection.[11] Detection of DNA using this technique was more sensitive than visualization of the product by ethidium bromide staining. The PCR products can also be sized, detected, and purified using HPLC, and HPLC systems have been described for quantification of specific nucleic acid sequences.[12] Reversed-phase HPLC with UV detection at 254 nm was used for quantitative and qualitative analysis of RT-PCR products.[13] However, HPLC systems are not routinely used because the equipment is costly and not practical for analysis of large numbers of samples. In recent years, conventional PCR has advanced from end point detection of products to detection while the reaction is occurring. Amplification and detection of the amplicon occurs in a "real-time" mode in the same reaction vessel, and the PCR is referred to as real-time PCR (see below).

9.3 Real-Time PCR

9.3.1 Real-Time Detection Chemistries

There are a number of advantages of real-time compared with conventional PCR. They are: (1) the closed-tube detection format lowers the potential for carryover contamination and false-positive results; (2) there is a shorter analytical turnaround time; (3) probe-based real-time PCR product detection results in higher assay sensitivity and specificity; (4) there is no need for post-PCR processing steps to detect the products; and (5) there is a quantitative detection range spanning about 7–8 orders of magnitude with real-time PCR assays compared to 2–3 logs for traditional PCR.

Real-time PCR systems rely upon detection and quantitation of signal generated from a fluorescent reporter, which increases in direct proportion to the amount of PCR product. The cycle threshold (C_t) is defined as the first cycle in which there is a significant increase in fluorescence above a specified threshold, and plotting fluorescence against cycle number yields a curve that represents the accumulation of PCR product over the duration of the PCR reaction. A standard curve can be generated from C_t values for a series of reactions using dilutions containing known quantities of target DNA. The amount of target in unknown samples can be derived by measuring the C_t and using the standard curve to determine starting copy number. Alternatively, quantitation can be "relative," where the C_t values are compared to those of an internal standard, which is usually a housekeeping gene.

A number of fluorescence systems have been employed for real-time PCR, and among the various chemistries available, intercalating dyes, such as SYBR Green I or SYTO 9 are the most economical and convenient to use. SYBR Green I, the first commercially available dye for real-time PCR, is a thermostable intercalating cyanine dye that binds to double-stranded DNA, and emits a fluorescent signal that increases proportionately with the amount of PCR product. However, one drawback is that the dye is nonspecific; thus any nonspecific product that is obtained will result in an incorrect increase in the fluorescent signal. To overcome this drawback, an additional time–temperature program after the PCR reaction is used to generate a melting curve to determine the quality and accuracy of the real-time PCR data. Fluorescence is monitored as the sample is slowly heated from a temperature below the melting point to above the melting point of the products. A drop in fluorescence is observed at the point where the double-stranded DNA melts and the dye dissociates. Melt curves can distinguish between specific and nonspecific products based on the melting temperature (T_m) of the amplicons, since each amplification product melts at different temperatures based on the length and GC content.

Holland et al.[14] developed a detection system that makes use of the 5′ to 3′ exonuclease activity of *Taq* DNA polymerase to cleave a labeled hybridization probe during the extension phase of the PCR. TaqMan probes (proprietary name) are short oligonucleotides that contain a 5′ reporter dye and a 3′ quenching dye. When intact, the fluorescence of the reporter dye is suppressed by the quencher. During the PCR reaction, the TaqMan probe hybridizes to a complementary sequence on the template between the two primer-binding sites. When *Taq* polymerase encounters the bound probe during extension from the primer, it cleaves the probe, separating the reporter dye from the quencher. The fluorescence increases in proportion to the quantity of amplicons generated. TaqMan-based real-time PCR assays have been used for detection of food-borne pathogens.[15–18]

Molecular beacons are similar to TaqMan probes, having 5′ fluorescent and 3′ quencher dyes, but they are not designed to be cleaved during the PCR reaction. They are stem-and-loop shaped probes, consisting of a PCR product-specific portion (loop, 20–24 nucleotides) and complementary stem sequences (4–6 nucleotides) that hold the probes in a hairpin configuration at low temperatures. At high temperatures, the PCR product and probe are single stranded, and as the temperature is lowered the molecular beacon hybridizes to the PCR product resulting in a conformational change that spatially separates the quencher from the reporter dye and a light signal from the reporter dye can be detected.[19–22]

A third hybridization probe detection system, relying on the fluorescence resonance energy transfer (FRET) principle was initially developed for use with the LightCycler instrument (Roche). The FRET system employs two probes, one labeled with a donor fluorochrome (fluorescein) at the 3′ end and the other labeled with an acceptor dye at the 5′ end. The probes are designed to hybridize to the template during the annealing phase of the PCR in a head-to-tail arrangement. When both are hybridized so that they are in proximity to one another, the energy emitted from the donor excites the acceptor fluorophore, which then emits red fluorescent light at a different wavelength that can be detected.[23,24]

Scorpion probes or Scorpion primers consist of a primer and probe linked to each other. When not hybridized, the Scorpion probe maintains a stem–loop configuration. The 3′ portion of the stem contains a sequence linked to the 5′ end of the primer via a nonamplifiable monomer that is complementary to a region in the PCR product. The probe binds to its target after extension of the Scorpion primer, producing an increase in fluorescence due to separation of the reporter from the quencher dyes.[25] Light upon extension (LUX) primers are labeled with a single fluorophore and are self quenched until they are incorporated into the PCR product. After annealing, fluorescence is generated due to a change in their secondary structure.[26] Additional real-time PCR fluorescence systems include amplifluors, which include primer and probe in one molecule[27] and MGB Eclipse probes, which have a minor groove binder (MGB) ligand at the 5′ end and a fluorophore at the 3′ end. PCR specificity is higher with the use of shorter, more specific probe sequences.[28]

Instruments currently available for performing real-time PCR include the LightCycler (Roche Diagnostics Corp.), the RAPID and the RAZOR (Idaho Technologies), a hand-portable instrument that was codeveloped with the Department of Defense, the MyiQ and the iCycler iQ (Bio-Rad), the ABI Prism 7000, 7300, 7500, and 7900HT (Applied Biosystems), the Quantica (Techne), the M × 4000 and M × 3000p (Stratagene), the Rotor Gene (Corbett Research), the Chromo 4, Opticon, and Opticon 2 (MJ Research), the SynChron (Genetic Discovery Technology), and the Smart Cycler systems

(Cepheid). The Smart Cycler is unique in that each processing block contains 16 independently controlled, programmable I-CORE (intelligent cooling/heating optical reaction) modules, such that 16 different PCR protocols can be run simultaneously, facilitating optimization of PCR assays. Furthermore, up to six processing blocks can be linked together allowing simultaneous analysis of 96 discrete samples. Automated nucleic acid extraction instruments, such as the MagNa Pure LC and the ABI Prism 6700 or 6100, can be coupled with the Light Cycler and ABI real-time PCR instruments, respectively. The GeneXpert System (Cepheid) combines cartridge-based sample preparation with amplification and product detection in a fully integrated instrument.

9.4 Advantages of PCR-Based Methods

There are a number of advantages of PCR-based methods over other types of assays for detection of food-borne pathogens. The PCR is a rapid technique, with both high sensitivity and specificity. With the choice of appropriate oligonucleotide primers targeting unique genetic markers, PCR assays can be designed to be very specific for the target organism. This contrasts with cross-reactions of the antisera that can occur with immunoassays. Due to the relatively high sensitivity of PCR assays, preenrichment and enrichment steps could potentially be eliminated completely or shortened considerably. Instead of plating and performing biochemical and serological tests, the PCR may be performed directly on food samples after a short enrichment step.[29]

Because of the lack of rapid and sensitive assays for detection of food-borne viruses and parasites, the extent of cases and outbreaks of diseases caused by these microorganisms may be grossly underestimated.[2] Viruses and parasites are more difficult to be recovered from foods, and enrichment culturing in liquid medium, as is performed to increase the levels of bacteria, is not possible with food-borne viruses and parasites. Nucleic acid-based amplification systems are a promising alternative to cumbersome, time-consuming, and less sensitive traditional methods used for detection and identification of viruses and parasites.

The PCR is also a functional tool for detection and identification of bacteria that cannot be identified by culture techniques. For example, a PCR-based 16S rRNA technique was used to identify *Tropheryma whippelii*, a nonculturable, possibly food-borne bacterium responsible for Whipple's disease.[30] As another example, there is no appropriate cultural method which can distinguish strains of enterotoxigenic *E. coli* (ETEC) from nonpathogenic strains. Several PCR-based assays have been developed for detection of these organisms in foods, targeting genes involved in virulence of ETEC, allowing identification of pathogenic strains among a majority of nonpathogenic isolates.[31,32] The PCR also has the ability to detect bacteria that are viable but nonculturable by traditional procedures. An additional advantage is that PCR-based methods are amenable to automation, leading potentially to more cost-effective, high-throughput testing of foods for the presence of undesirable microorganisms.

9.5 Concerns with the Use of PCR-Based Methods

To an unaccustomed laboratory analyst, the successful implementation of the PCR for detection of pathogens in foods and other complex samples such as blood or fecal specimens can be fraught with some problems and setbacks. The usefulness of the PCR for detection of microorganisms in these types of samples is limited by the presence of substances such as bilirubin, bile salts, hemoglobin degradation products, polyphenolic compounds, proteinases, complex polysaccharides and fat, which inhibit the DNA polymerase, bind magnesium, or denature the DNA.[33,34] Sensitivity is dramatically decreased if the PCR is performed on crude samples containing inhibitors; therefore, sample preparation steps and DNA extraction are often required before performing the PCR. Several methods that have been used for this purpose include aqueous polymer two-phase systems, immunomagnetic separation, centrifugation, or filtration. Furthermore, many DNA extraction kits and reagents such as PrepMan Ultra (Applied Biosystems), the DNeasy Tissue Kit (Qiagen), and the UltraClean Fecal DNA Kit (Mo Bio Laboratories, Inc.) are commercially available. Appropriate controls should be performed in each assay to assess if negative results could be due to the presence of PCR inhibitors in the sample. Also, since there may be very low numbers of the target organisms in foods, either a concentration step or enrichment culturing of samples is usually required to increase the relative number of target microorganisms and achieve adequate PCR sensitivity.

The PCR can detect DNA from nonviable, as well as from live target cells. With enrichment culturing, however, only live cells multiply, thus diluting out the presence of dead cells. Nevertheless, the PCR may not be suitable for testing pasteurized, cooked, or irradiated samples, which may contain considerable numbers of dead microorganisms.[35,36] Yet, it may be important to know if organisms such as *Staphylococcus aureus* or *Clostridium botulinum* were present in such samples, since this signals the possibility that toxins produced by these organisms, which can survive irradiation and heat processing steps, may be present. Detection of only viable cells can be accomplished by detecting bacterial mRNA using reverse transcription PCR. However, the instability of mRNA and reproducibility are problems encountered with the use of RT-PCR on food samples. Another technique used to discriminate DNA from live and dead cells is referred to as ethidium monoazide (EMA)-PCR. The EMA penetrates only dead cells with compromised cell membranes and covalently binds to the DNA, preventing its amplification by the PCR.[37]

Various parameters determine the overall efficiency, reproducibility, and specificity of PCR assays and these require optimization. Several important parameters affecting the PCR include the quality of the DNA template, magnesium ion concentration, primer design and concentration, pH, PCR temperature cycling profile (i.e., annealing, extension and denaturation temperatures and duration times, number of cycles), dNTP concentration, and size of amplicons. With each new PCR assay for different target organisms and for different foods, protocol optimization is required.

Carryover of DNA from one reaction, which contaminates subsequent reactions or cross contamination between samples can cause false-positive results. However, implementation of adequate quality control measures can help to minimize amplicon carryover and contamination in PCR assays. Plugged pipette tips or positive displacement pipettes should be used to avoid sample and reagent contamination. It is advisable to have separate workstations for each of these four tasks: reagent mixture preparation, sample preparation, template addition, and post-PCR detection. A benchtop hood equipped with UV lights is useful for decontamination. At each workstation there should be dedicated equipment and supplies, and in addition, 10%–20% bleach solutions should be used to regularly clean workbenches, pipettors, and other equipment and supplies. To control carryover contamination, an enzymatic method can be used, which is based on uracil N-glycosylase (UNG) that preferentially degrades uracil-containing DNA synthesized in the presence of dUTP.[38] Another method involves the addition of isopsoralen derivatives to the PCR mixture and following amplification, the reaction tube is irradiated with UV light resulting in the formation of cyclobutane monoadducts with pyrimidine bases in the DNA.[39] The modified DNA cannot serve as template in subsequent PCR reactions. Other chemical inactivation techniques, such as use of hydroxylamine for postamplification inactivation of PCR products, have also been described.[40]

9.6 PCR Troubleshooting

A number of strategies have been employed to overcome PCR problems associated with interference from food or other types of complex samples.[41,42] These include centrifugation of samples followed by washing of the target bacteria to remove residual inhibiting substances before the PCR,[43] recovery of bacteria by filtration,[44,45] purification of crude DNA extracts by gel chromatography[34,46] and by DNA affinity columns,[47] and removal of inhibitors and concentration of bacteria in food samples by buoyant density centrifugation.[48] Food and other complex samples can be diluted to decrease the concentration of inhibitors; however, sensitivity of PCR detection is reduced correspondingly with the dilution factor.

Most commonly, sample preparation methods consist of cell lysis to release the DNA, followed by purification and concentration of the DNA. Extraction using phenol–chloroform followed by precipitation of the DNA using ethanol has commonly been used; however, numerous commercially prepared template purification kits and reagents that allow release of DNA from the cells and separation from PCR inhibitory components are also available. Some of the protocols may involve lysis of cells, followed by binding to solid-phase matrices and elution of the DNA which is then suitable for the PCR. Other protocols consist of concentration of bacteria by centrifugation, cell lysis, and use of commercially available extraction reagents to sequester PCR inhibitors from food or other complex matrices.

Another technique, referred to as immunomagnetic separation (IMS), involves the use of magnetic beads coated with antibodies against the target organism to sequester the bacteria from a large part of the contaminating microflora and from interfering food components. The IMS technique also results in concentration of target bacteria in the sample, and thus assay sensitivity is enhanced. This technique has been employed to remove inhibiting components from enrichment samples of ground beef and bovine feces before performing the PCR.[49]

One common problem with the PCR is the amplification of nonspecific target sequences. Nonspecific amplification can be reduced using hot start PCR techniques, where the polymerase activity is inhibited during reaction preparation. Hot start PCR is commonly performed using a DNA polymerase that is supplied in an inactive form, requiring a few minutes of heating at 94°C–96°C for activation or using wax-barrier methods. Nested PCR, which involves the use of two pairs of PCR primers for a single locus can overcome problems associated with low copy numbers, for example, a low number of target organisms in the presence of high levels of nontarget bacteria and PCR inhibitors. Nested PCR involves a first round of amplification for 20–30 cycles followed by a second run using the product of the first PCR. PCR enhancers, such as formamide, DMSO, glycerol, betaine, and others, lower the template melting temperature, aiding primer annealing and extension of the template through regions of secondary structure. In addition, the magnesium concentration in the reaction can alter product yield by affecting polymerase activity; if it is too low, little or no product may be produced. If the concentration is too high, artifactual products can result from nonspecific priming of template DNA. The optimal magnesium concentration, which is generally between 1.5 and –5 mM, should be determined for each primer pair and template DNA combination.

9.7 Conventional and Real-Time Multiplex PCR

Multiplex PCR assays enable simultaneous amplification of multiple targets of interest in a single reaction using two or more primer pairs, resulting in savings in time, labor, and cost. However, compared to PCR assays in which one sequence is amplified, multiplex assays require more extensive optimization of annealing conditions and reagent concentrations for maximal amplification efficiency and to avoid the formation of spurious amplification products and uneven amplification of target sequences. For optimization of PCR conditions, it is preferable to keep the primer concentrations low, since high quantities of product may cause interference.[50] Primers with nearly identical annealing temperatures and which do not display homology either internally or to one another should be used. Multiplex PCR assays have been used to detect and identify one organism by amplification of more than one gene or multiple organisms can be detected simultaneously by targeting unique sequences from each organism.[49,51,52]

In real-time multiplex PCR assays, probes that bind to their respective PCR products are labeled with different fluorophores that have unique emission spectra or using a fluorescent dye such as SYBR Green I followed by melting curve analysis. Josefsen et al.[53] compared real-time PCR using the ABI-PRISM 7700 and the Rotor-Gene 3000 instruments for detection of thermotolerant *Campylobacter* spp., *C. jejuni*, *C. coli*, and *C. lari*, in naturally contaminated chicken rinse samples. There was good agreement between PCR assays performed using both instruments and with an International Standard Organization (ISO)-based culture method. Bellin et al.[54] developed a real-time multiplex PCR assay targeting the Shiga toxin 1 (stx_1) and Shiga toxin 2 (stx_2) genes in enterohemorrhagic *E. coli* using FRET hybridization probes and the LightCycler instrument. The assay was carried out in a single reaction capillary and completed within 45 min. A melting curve analysis could discriminate between stx_2 and stx_{2e}, which is the gene variant associated with pig edema disease. A multiplex real-time RT-PCR assay was used for the simultaneous detection of noroviruses of genogroups I and II, human astroviruses, and enteroviruses using the LightCycler and the SYBR Green dye.[55] The real-time PCR was 10 times more sensitive than conventional end point PCR.

9.8 Detection and Identification of Microorganisms by the PCR

9.8.1 Bacteria

Numerous reports have appeared on the use of the PCR for detection of bacterial pathogens either found as natural contaminants or seeded in foods. Some of these include detection of *Yersinia* and Shiga toxin-producing *E. coli* in culture and in artificially inoculated foods[56] *Campylobacter* in water, sewage, and food samples,[57] stressed *Salmonella* in dairy and egg products,[58] and *L. monocytogenes* in food products (Table 9.1).[59,60]

A multiplex PCR method was developed for *E. coli* O157:H7 by employing primers specific for the *eaeA* gene, conserved sequences of Shiga

TABLE 9.1

PCR-Based Methods for Detection of Food-Borne Microorganisms

Microorganisms	Target Genes	Type of Sample	Sensitivity	Reference
Bacteria				
Vibrio parahaemolyticus	*tlh* OR8, *tdh*, *trh*	Oysters	1 CFU/g	[18]
Salmonella spp.	*iagA*	Alfalfa sprouts, cilantro, cantaloupes mixed salad	4 CFU/25 g	[22]
Salmonella spp., *Escherichia coli* O157:H7	*invA*, *eaeA*, *stx₁*, *stx₂*, hemolysin	Apple cider, carcass wash water, ground beef, bovine feces	≤1 CFU/g or mL	[49]
Yersinia enterocolitica	*virF*, *ail*	Pork, cheese, zucchini	0.5 CFU/cm²	[52]
Yersinia, Shiga toxin-producing *E. coli*	*virF*, *yadA*, *stx₁*, *stx₂*	Tofu, chocolate milk	Not given	[56]
Campylobacter jejuni, Campylobacter coli	Intergenic sequence between *flaA* and *flab*	Water, sewage, beef, chicken, pork	≤3 CFU/g	[57]
Salmonella spp.	Random genomic fragment	Eggs, ice cream, cheese	5.9 cells/25 g	[58]
Listeria monocytogenes	*prfA*	Salmon	94 CFU/g	[59]
L. monocytogenes	*iap*	Catfish fillets, milk	1–2 CFU/g, 20 CFU/mL	[60]
L. monocytogenes	*hly*	Raw pork, fermented sausage, cooked ham, frankfurter sausage, raw and cold-smoked salmon	8 genome equivalents	[58]
Yeast and Molds				
Dekkera-Brettanomyces Strains	*Dekkera* genomic DNA DNA fragment	Sherry	Fewer than 10 cells	[63]
Bacteria, yeasts, molds	Elongation factor	Milk	10 cells/mL	[64]
Aflatoxigenic molds	*ver-1*, *omt-1*, *apa-2*	Corn	10² spores/g	[65]
Fusarium culmorum	472-bp RAPD fragment	Cereal	5–50 fg of *F. culmorum* DNA	[66]

	Target gene/region	Sample	Detection limit	Ref.
Saccharomyces Cerevisiae	Cloned random amplified PCR product	Wine	3.8 CFU/mL (sweet wine) 5.0 CFU/mL (red wine)	[67]
Viruses				
Hepatitis A virus	C-terminus of capsid protein VP3 and A-terminus of protein VP1	Oyster	10 PFU/20 g	[68]
Enteroviruses	Conserved 5' noncoding region	Sewage effluent, groundwater	0.028 PFU/mL	[69]
Hepatitis A virus	C-terminus of capsid protein VP3 and A-terminus of protein VP1	Liquid waste, shellfish	Four virus particles	[70]
Small round-structured viruses, enteroviruses	5' UTR, VP7 gene, 3D, capsid, RNA polymerase	Human stool, seafood	3–30 $TCID_{50}$/1.25 g	[71]
Genogroup I and II noroviruses	RNA-dependent RNA polymerase	Human stool	Not given	[72]
Hepatitis A	5' noncoding region	Shellfish, human stool, and serum	0.05 infection units, 10 ssRNA molecules, 1 viral RNA molecule	[73]
Parasites				
Toxoplasma gondii	B1 gene, 529-bp DNA repeat element	Clinical samples	200 fg, 20 fg	[24]
Cryptosporidium spp.	18S rRNA gene	Human stool	$<10^3$ CFU/200 mg stool	[25]
C. parvum	18S rRNA gene	Water	1–10 oocytes	[74]
C. parvum	CpR1, *C. parvum* specific genomic fragment	Raw milk	1–10 oocytes/20 mL	[75]
T. gondii	P30 gene	Cured meats	5×10^3 trophozoites/g	[76]
Cyclospora sp., *Eimeria* spp.	18S rRNA gene	Raspberry wash sediments	10–19 oocytes/PCR	[77]

toxin 1 and 2 genes (stx_1, stx_2), and for a hemolysin gene found on a 60 MDa plasmid. Amplification products of 1087 (*eaeA*), 227/224 (stx_1/stx_2), and 166 (hemolysin) base pairs were successfully amplified simultaneously in a single reaction.[51] This multiplex PCR method was used to specifically identify EHEC displaying serotype O157. Since *E. coli* O157:H7 and *Salmonella* can contaminate similar types of food and other samples, a multiplex PCR was designed to allow simultaneous detection of both *E. coli* O157:H7 and *Salmonella* spp. in sample enrichment cultures.[49] Apple cider, beef carcass wash water, ground beef, and bovine feces were inoculated with approximately 1–250 CFU/g or mL of both *E. coli* O157:H7 and *S. typhimurium*, and following enrichment culturing, the samples were subjected to a DNA extraction technique or to immuno-magnetic separation and then tested by the multiplex PCR assay. Four pairs of primers were employed in the PCR: three primers for amplification of *E. coli* O157:H7 *eaeA*, both stx_1 and stx_2, and plasmid sequences, and one primer for the amplification of a portion of the *Salmonella invA* gene. Four fragments of the expected sizes were amplified in a single reaction and visualized following agarose gel electrophoresis in all of the samples inoculated with ≤ 1 CFU of *E. coli* O157:H7 and *Salmonella* per gram or milliliter. Results could be obtained in approximately 30 h from inoculation of the sample.

There have been numerous reports describing real-time PCR assays for detection of food-borne bacterial pathogens. A multiplex real-time Taq-Man PCR targeting four genomic loci was used to detect *Vibrio parahae-molyticus* in seeded and naturally contaminated oysters.[18] The sensitivity of the assay was 200 pg of purified DNA, and *V. parahaemolyticus* was detectable at an initial inoculum level of 1 CFU/g of oyster tissue after overnight enrichment. *Salmonella* spp. were detected in whole and fresh-cut fruit and vegetable samples using a molecular beacon-based real-time PCR assay, the iQ-Check kit, targeting the *Salmonella iagA* gene (invasion associated gene).[22] The sensitivity of the assay was 4 CFU/25 g of produce after 16 h of enrichment in buffered peptone water. A quantitative TaqMan real-time PCR assay targeting the *L. monocytogenes hly* (listerioly-sin) gene was used to detect the pathogen in various foods, including raw pork meat, fermented pork sausage, cooked ham, frankfurter sausage, and raw and cold-smoked salmon.[61] An internal amplification control (IAC) consisting of DNA containing a fragment of the rapeseed *BnACCg8* gene flanked by the *hly*-specific target was used to assess PCR inhibition due to food matrix components. Two TaqMan probes, one targeting the *hly* gene and the other targeting the IAC, enabled simultaneous detection of both signals. Inclusion of a quantitative internal control in real-time PCR assays allows detection of false–negative results due to operator error or the presence of PCR inhibitory compounds and can also be used to correct quantitative data when partial inhibition or enhancement of the reaction occurs.

9.8.2 Yeasts and Molds

The PCR has also found application for rapid detection of molds and yeasts involved in food spoilage. By a multiplex PCR assay, Pearson and McKee[62] were able to simultaneously detect three strains of yeast which cause food spoilage. Other reports described PCR-based assays to detect spoilage yeasts in red wine,[63] viable bacteria, molds, and yeasts in milk,[64] and aflatoxigenic molds in grains such as corn.[65] The phytopathogenic fungus, *Fusarium culmorum*, was detected in cereal samples using a nested PCR method performed in a single tube.[66] Using different concentrations of primers for the first and second PCR and different annealing temperatures, the nested PCR could be performed in the same tube. The assay had a detection limit of 5–50 fg of DNA, and gave positive results with samples from seed mixtures in which 1% of the seeds was contaminated with *F. culmorum*. A real-time PCR assay using the SYBR Green I dye was used to detect *Saccharomyces cerevisae* in sweet and red wines, with detection limits of 3.8 CFU/mL and 5 CFU/mL, respectively.[67]

9.8.3 Viruses

In the past decade, the expanding information on the sequences of viral genomes has allowed the development of PCR-based assays to ascertain the presence of viruses in food, environmental, and other samples. Several techniques for virus detection include magnetic immunoseparation PCR,[68] an integrated cell culture-reverse transcriptase PCR (RT-PCR) method for detection of enteroviruses,[69] antigen capture PCR for detection of hepatitis A virus in environmental samples,[70] and a seminested RT-PCR for viruses in seafoods.[71] A concern with PCR methods for detection of enteric viruses in foods is the inability to differentiate infectious from noninfectious (inactivated) viruses. This limitation can be overcome if the PCR is preceded by propagation of infectious virus particles in cell or tissue culture. Richards et al.[72] designed two sets of degenerate primers, which were used in a real-time PCR assay with SYBR Green I to detect 13 different genetic clusters of genogroups I and II noroviruses. A real-time TaqMan reverse transcriptase PCR was used to detect and quantify all hepatitis A genotypes in clinical and shellfish samples targeting a conserved 5' noncoding region.[73]

9.8.4 Parasites

A number of PCR assays have been designed for detection of protozoan parasites in food and environmental samples and in fecal specimens. The PCR is rapid, sensitive, and specific and is an attractive alternative to tedious techniques involving microscopy, which are less amenable to batch processing of samples. Johnson et al.[74] found that sensitivity of the PCR was similar to that obtained by immunofluorescence for the detection of *Cryptosporidium* oocysts in wastewater concentrates. The PCR combined with digoxigenin-labeled probe hybridization was used for detection of *C. parvum* in raw milk,[75] for detection of *Toxoplasma gondii* in cured meats,[76] and for detection and identification of *Cyclospora* spp. and *Eimeria* spp. in raspberries.[77] Detailed reviews on the use of the PCR for detection of food-borne pathogens have been published by Hill[78] and Olsen et al.[6] A real-time PCR assay using Scorpion probes targeting the 18S rRNA gene was used to detect all human pathogenic *Cryptosporidium* spp.[25] Reischl et al.[24] compared two PCR assays using the LightCycler, one targeting the *T. gondii* B1 gene and the other targeting a 529-bp repeat element. The detection limit of the B1-specific LightCycler PCR assay was 200 fg after 35 cycles of amplification, and with the 529-bp element-specific PCR the limit of detection was 20 fg. Quantitative PCR showed that the 529-bp repeat element of *T. gondii* was repeated more than 300-fold in the genome, and sequencing of PCR amplicons demonstrated that the sequence was highly conserved. Thus the 529-bp target sequence was preferred to a less repeated and more divergent target sequence to improve the sensitivity and specificity of the PCR.

9.9 Commercially Available PCR Kits and Related Materials

The BAX pathogen detection systems, manufactured by Qualicon are fluorogenic PCR-based assays available for detection of several food-borne pathogens, including of *E. coli* O157:H7, *Salmonella*, and *Listeria*, and for differentiating *C. jejuni*, *C.coli*, and *C. lari*. After enrichment and a short pretreatment of the sample, a simplified PCR assay is performed using tableted, prepackaged reagents. Several reports have indicated that the BAX systems were considerably faster, simpler, and more sensitive than cultural methods and demonstrated comparable results.[79–82] TaqMan-based real-time PCR kits for detection of a number of food-borne pathogens are available from Applied Biosystems.[83–85] Krause et al.[86] compared the TaqMan *C. jejuni* PCR kit to two reference culture methods for detection of the pathogen in chicken and environmental samples and found that the PCR method complied with NordVal (the Nordic validation organization) criteria for validation of alternative microbiological methods. It was approved as an alternative method for detection of *Campylobacter* in chicken samples. Other kits employing real-time detection include the LightCycler foolproof kits for *Salmonella*, *L. monocytogenes*, *E. coli* O157, and *Campylobacter* (Roche), the RealArt *L. monocytogenes*, *Campoylobacter*, and *Salmonella* PCR kits (Qiagen), the SureFood pathogen *Salmonella*, *Campylobacter*, and *Listeria* kits (Congen), the Artus *L. monocytogenes*, *Salmonella*, and *Campylobacter* kits (Artus), and the Warnex Rapid Pathogen Detection System kits, which use molecular beacon technology.

Various materials are available to optimize and improve PCR performance. Modified DNA polymerases such as Amplitaq Gold (PE Applied Bioystems), HotStarTaq and HotStar HiFidelity DNA Polymerase (Qiagen),

SureStart *Taq* DNA Polymerase (Stratagene), JumpStart *Taq* DNA Polymerase (Sigma-Aldrich), HotMaster *Taq* DNA Polymerase (Eppendorf), or Platinum *Taq* DNA polymerase (Invitrogen) are available for "hot start" PCR. Also available are PCR optimization kits, such as SureBrand PCR Optimization Kit (Bioline), and MasterAmp PCR Optimization Kit (Epicentre Biotechnologies), PCR Optimizer Kit (Invitrogen), and others that simplify determination of optimal PCR conditions for individual assays. The MasterAmp PCR Enhancer (with betaine), the Perfect Match PCR Enhancer (Stratagene) and other similar products improve product yield and specificity for target sequences, especially those containing a high GC content or secondary structure. Ready to use PCR mixes, tablets, or lyophilized reagents to which only template and primers need to be added by the user, such as Omnimix HS reagents (Takara Bio Inc.) and FailSafe PCR PreMix Selection Kit (Epicentre BioTechnologies) are available. Long-range PCR systems, including the TripleMaster PCR System (Eppendorf), the MasterAmp Extra-Long PCR Kit (Epicentre Biotechnologies), and the Expand Long Template PCR System (Roche Applied Science) are used for amplification of very large (up to 30–40 kb) templates. These systems provide unique enzyme combinations: a nonproofreading polymerase with 5′ to 3′ polymerase activity, and an enzyme with 3′ to 5′ proofreading ability to provide high fidelity and the capability to amplify very long sequences.

9.10 Quantitative PCR

Since the PCR involves the exponential amplification of target nucleic acid sequences, it is commonly assumed that quantitation of the number of input target molecules cannot easily be achieved. Although there have not been many reports on the use of PCR-based techniques for quantitating pathogens in foods, several approaches for determining the level of input copy number have been described.[60,87,88]

Competitive PCR involves the addition of varying amounts of a DNA sequence bearing the same primer annealing sites as the template. The degree to which the added DNA competes will depend on its initial concentration relative to that of the test sequence. The amount of initial target sequence can be obtained from the point on the curve where target and standard values are equal.

The endogenous standard assay utilizes an endogenous sequence, which is expressed at a relatively constant level in all of the samples. The level of amplification of the target sequence is then compared to that of the standard. Drawbacks with this method are that it is generally only a comparative technique and the actual copy number cannot easily be determined, and that the endogenous standard may be expressed at levels far higher than the target sequence, making dilutions of the sample necessary.

The synthetic internal standard method involves the addition of synthetic standards designed to carry very slight sequence variations, which make them readily distinguishable from the sequences of interest. Usually, a unique restriction site is created in the synthetic standard, such that after amplification and restriction enzyme digestion, only the standard will yield two small digestion products. Several ELISA systems employing biotinylated primers with the PCR or involving hybridization of product to capture oligonucleotides have also been described for quantifying PCR products.[89]

Takahashi et al.[90] developed a quantitative real-time PCR-based assay targeting the *toxR* gene of *Vibrio vulnificus* and used it to detect and quantify the pathogen in seawater and oyster samples. A standard curve was constructed from samples containing known concentrations of *V. vulnificus*, and this curve was then used as a reference standard for extrapolating quantitative information from seawater and oyster samples. The assay could detect as few as 10 cells/mL of seawater and oyster homogenate. Furthermore, real-time reverse transcriptase PCR (see below) has become a useful tool to quantify gene expression and has been used to evaluate the effects of environmental conditions on expression of bacterial virulence genes.[91,92]

9.11   Reverse Transcription PCR

Reverse transcription PCR (RT-PCR) is a sensitive technique for RNA detection and quantitation. Since RNA cannot serve as a template for the PCR, reverse transcription is combined with the PCR to make RNA into a complementary DNA (cDNA) molecule suitable for PCR amplification. Thus, the combination of reverse transcription and PCR is referred to as RT-PCR. As discussed above, food or other types of samples containing high numbers of nonviable cells may give positive results with conventional PCR. The RT-PCR permits differentiation between viable and nonviable cells if mRNA serves as the target of amplification. Bacterial mRNA has a very short half-life and is rapidly degraded with processes that render the cells nonviable. Klein and Juneja[93] used RT-PCR for detection of viable *L. monocytogenes*. The RT-PCR assay, based on amplification of *L. monocytogenes* mRNA (the *iap* gene), was used to detect only viable cells. A PCR product was detected in cooked meat samples initially inoculated with 3 CFU/g. A 2-h enrichment was necessary to increase the sensitivity of the RT-PCR, and their results showed that nonviable cells would have been detected following short enrichment periods if PCR had been used. Sheridan et al.[94] studied the relationship between viability and detection of specific *E. coli* mRNAs. They found that the type of cell inactivation treatment and subsequent holding conditions influenced the ability to detect mRNA targets; however, the presence of 16S rRNA was detected in samples containing dead cells, and it persisted for long periods. A number of RT-PCR assays for detection of RNA viruses, such as hepatitis A virus, have also been reported.[68,70,95,96] As an example, real-time RT-PCR was used to identify oysters contaminated with noroviruses as the cause of an international outbreak and to quantify the level of viruses in the oysters.[96]

9.12   Other Nucleic Acid Amplification Methods

9.12.1   Ligase Chain Reaction

A procedure called the Ligase chain reaction (LCR) involves the formation of new target DNA molecules through the joining, by a thermostable DNA ligase, of probe molecules which anneal to the target DNA such that they are immediately adjacent to each other. If there is a mismatch at the ligation site, the primers are not ligated by the enzyme. The LCR is cyclic, with ligated product serving as template for the next reaction; product is formed without DNA replication. LCR is useful for discriminating between DNA sequences differing in a single base pair. Wiedmann et al.[97] used a PCR-coupled LCR assay to distinguish *L. monocytogenes* from other *Listeria* spp. by targeting a single base pair difference in the *Listeria* 16S rRNA gene. A similar approach was used to distinguish between the food spoilage yeasts *Zygosaccharomyces bisporus* and *Z. bailii*, and to differentiate these species from other related species.[98] However, the ligase chain reaction has been used more widely for clinical diagnostics than for detection of pathogens in food.

9.12.2   Strand Displacement Amplification

The isothermal strand displacement amplification (SDA) technique can result in about 10^8-fold amplification of the target after 2 h at ca. 40°C. A restriction enzyme is used to nick a hemimodified recognition site, and a DNA polymerase initiates synthesis of a new DNA strand at the nick, while displacing the existing strand. The modified target sequences are amplified exponentially by repeated nicking, strand displacement, and priming of displaced strands. A multiplex SDA procedure was used to amplify DNA from *Mycobacterium* spp., and the amplified target molecules were detected by DNA polymerase-catalyzed extension of ^{32}P-labeled probes hybridized to the different targets.[99] Ge et al.[100] combined strand displacement amplification of the *hlyA* gene of EHEC O157:H7 and other EHEC serotypes with detection of product by fluorescence polarization for detection of the pathogen within 35 min of reaction initiation. The assay was used to detect *E. coli* O157:H7 in drinking and recreational water and in bovine drinking trough water, and the sensitivity was 4.3 bacteria.

9.12.3 Nucleic Acid Sequence-Based Amplification

Nucleic acid sequence-based amplification (NASBA) involves isothermal (37°–42°C) amplification usually of an RNA template. The reaction consists of continuous cycles of reverse transcriptase-mediated synthesis of cDNA from an RNA target sequence, followed by in vitro transcription by RNA polymerase from the double-stranded cDNA template. The NASBA method requires two primers, one that bears a bacteriophage T7 promoter sequence at the 3′ end and which binds to the 3′ end of the target sequence and another that is derived from the 5′ end of the target sequence. The coordination of three enzymes are required: reverse transcriptase to synthesize the cDNA, RNase H to digest the RNA strand of RNA:DNA heteroduplexes, and T7 RNA polymerase to synthesize as many as 100 copies of RNA used as substrate in the next cycle. Using a NASBA-based method, Uyttendaele and coworkers[101] were able to detect *C. jejuni* in foods inoculated with as few as 3 CFU/10 g after 18 h of selective enrichment. NASBA targeting mRNA of *L. monocytogenes* inoculated into dairy and egg products successfully detected the organism at an initial inoculum level of less than 10 CFU/g.[102] NASBA has been employed for detection of *Campylobacter* spp., *L. monocytogenes*, *Salmonella* spp., *Cryptosporidium parvum*, and foodborne viruses using 16S rRNA and mRNA as target molecules.[103] The technique was used to detect viable *S. enterica* in fresh meats, poultry, and other foods targeting mRNA transcribed from the *Salmonella dnaK* gene using the NucliSens kit (BioMerieux), which is a NASBA assay with electrochemiluminesence detection of product.[104,105] Rodríguez-Lázaro et al.[106] developed a molecular beacon-based real-time NASBA targeting the *dnaA* gene for detection of *Mycobacterium avium* subspecies *Paratuberculosis* in water and milk. The assay had a sensitivity of 150–200 cells per reaction, and was able to detect 10^3 target bacteria in artificially contaminated drinking water. A multiplex NASBA method for simultaneous detection of hepatitis A and genogroup I and II noroviruses in ready-to-eat foods has been described.[107]

9.12.4 Rolling Circle Amplification and Ramification Amplification

Rolling circle amplification (RCA) employs processes similar to those used by viruses to replicate their genomes. RCA uses restriction digestion and exonuclease digestion to produce single-stranded DNA targets, which can then hybridize to specific oligonucleotides called padlock probes. The padlock probes circularize following hybridization to target DNA or RNA sequences and are then ligated to provide a template for rolling circle amplification employing a DNA polymerase with strand displacement activity. The padlock probe contains a specific target sequence that is detected using a fluorescent complementary probe. RCA was used to detect and enumerate microorganisms[108,109] If a second strand displacement primer is encoded in the circular probe, the process grows exponentially and the technique is referred to as ramification amplification. Ramification amplification (RAM) results in a large branching or ramified DNA complex. Using a circular probe specific for the Shiga toxin 2 gene, Li et al.[110] could detect as few as 10 *E. coli* O157:H7 cells per reaction, and this was accomplished using a real-time RAM assay (using the SYBR Green I dye), as well.

9.12.5 Qβ Replicase

The Qβ replicase amplification method was named after the enzyme which replicates the RNA genome of bacteriophage Qβ and is used for amplification of RNA probe molecules. A section of the Qβ genome is replaced with an RNA probe specific for the target sequence such that the unique folded structure of the genome is not altered. Probe molecules, which specifically anneal to the target sequence are enzymatically replicated then detected.[111] The level of amplification can approach 10^9-fold for 30-min incubation; however, nonspecific amplification is a limitation of Qβ replicase assays.

9.12.6 Loop-Mediated Isothermal Amplification

In 2000, Notomi et al.[112] described a method referred to as loop-mediated isothermal amplification (LAMP) for DNA amplification under isothermal conditions with high specificity, efficiency, and rapidity. This reaction uses DNA polymerase with strand displacement activity (*Bca*BEST DNA polymerase) and four primers to amplify the target gene, with recognition of six distinct sequences. There are two specially designed inner primers and two outer primers that are used in the initial steps, and only the inner primers are then used for strand displacement DNA synthesis. The LAMP procedure is illustrated in Figure 9.1. In the first step, DNA synthesis from the two sets of inner primers and outer primers results in the formation of a dumbbell like DNA structure. Later, one inner primer hybridizes to the loop on the product and initiates strand displacement synthesis, yielding the original stem–loop structure and another with a longer stem. The amplification products are stem–loop DNA structures with several inverted repeats of the target and cauliflower-like structures with multiple loops. The cycling reaction, performed under a single temperature of 60°C–65°C results in the accumulation of 10^9 copies in less than 1 h. Moreover, DNA amplification by the LAMP reaction can be correlated with precipitation of magnesium pyrophosphate, which is a by-product of the reaction, leading to turbidity. Alternatively, DNA intercalating dyes can be used to measure fluorescence generated with the LAMP reaction.

Ohtsuka et al.[113] used a LAMP assay to detect *Salmonella* in naturally contaminated liquid egg samples. *Salmonella* was detected in a higher number of samples using the LAMP assay compared to a conventional PCR assay. Parida et al.[114] used a reverse transcription LAMP assay with six specially designed primers that recognized eight distinct sequences of the target (envelope gene) to detect the West Nile virus. The RT-LAMP

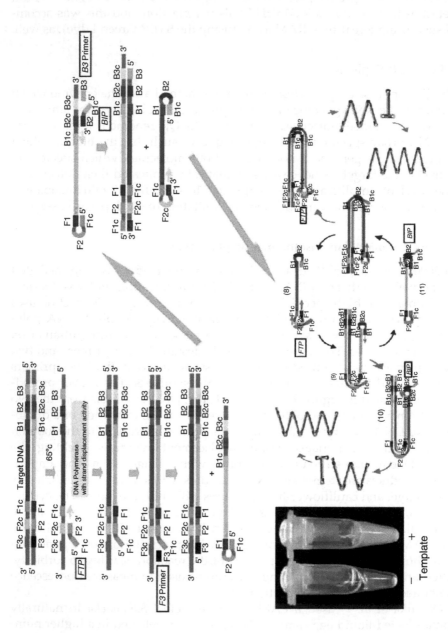

FIGURE 9.1
Illustration of the LAMP procedure.

assay demonstrated 10-fold higher sensitivity compared to an RT-PCR assay, with a detection limit of 0.1 PFU of virus.

9.12.7 Isothermal and Chimeric Primer-Initiated Amplification of Nucleic Acids

Isothermal and chimeric primer-initiated amplification of nucleic acids (ICAN) is an isothermal amplification method that employs chimera-primers composed of RNA at the 3′ end and DNA at the 5′ end, RNase H, and DNA polymerase. Firstly, the primers hybridize to the target gene, and nucleotide replication is initiated by the DNA polymerase that has strand displacement activity (*Bca*BEST DNA polymerase) (Figure 9.2) An intermediate product is formed after a template exchange reaction. RNase H then cuts out RNA portions derived from the chimeric primers. This is followed by an elongation reaction beginning from the site at which the RNA portions were cut out and is accompanied by strand displacement and template switching. This chain reaction is repeated, amplifying genes of interest with high specificity and efficiency. The amount of product is generally 10-fold higher by ICAN than by the PCR.

Isogai et al.[115] described the detection of *Salmonella* spp. from chicken carcasses, egg yolk, and cattle fecal samples targeting the *invA* gene by the PCR and by the ICAN method combined with detection by ELISA. The number of bacteria detectable by the ICAN technique was less than 50 CFU/mL of chicken rinse solution. Twelve out of fourteen chicken rinse samples were positive using the ICAN technique; however, only 7 of the 14 samples were positive by the standard PCR assay. ICAN was performed using the TaKaRa ICAN—*Salmonella* Detection Kit-ELISA (Takara Bio Co. Ltd., Kyoto, Japan).

9.13 DNA Microarrays

DNA microarrays combine nucleic acid amplification strategies for parallel high throughput detection, and represent a potential solution to the challenge of multiplexed pathogen detection. DNA arrays employed for pathogen detection consist of large numbers of probes (oligonucleotides or PCR products) immobilized on specially treated glass slides. DNA samples for analysis are chemically labeled with fluorescent dyes or are labeled during PCR amplification and are then hybridized with their complementary sequences on the chip. Following hybridization and washing steps, the arrays are examined using a high-resolution scanner. Microarrays can be used to detect labeled PCR products by hybridization to an array composed of pathogen-specific probes. Sergeev et al.[116] used degenerate primers to amplify variable regions of *Staphylococcus aureus* enterotoxin genes and hybridized chemically labeled ssDNA (derived from PCR reactions specific

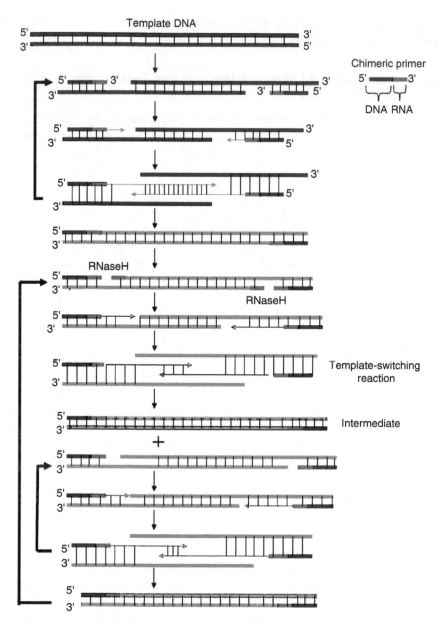

FIGURE 9.2
Illustration of the ICAN procedure.

for enterotoxin genes) to microarrays onto which probes specific for each of the different enterotoxin genes were bound. Call et al.[117] were able to detect 55 CFU of *E. coli* O157:H7 per milliliter of chicken rinsate without an enrichment step using immunomagnetic capture followed by PCR amplification and hybridization of the products onto a microarray containing oligonucleotide probes (25–30 mer) complementary for four virulence genes of *E. coli* O157:H7. The microarray assay was 32-fold more sensitive than gel electrophoresis for PCR product detection. Chizhikov et al.[118] detected microbial virulence factors (*eaeA, slt-I, slt-II, fliC, rfbE,* and *ipaH*) of multiple pathogens by hybridizing Cy5-labeled fluorescent PCR products to the gene-specific oligonucleotides spotted on microarrays. A similar approach was used by Keramas et al.[119] to detect *Campylobacter* spp. directly from fecal cloacal swabs targeting the 16S rRNA, the 16S-23S rRNA intergenic region, and specific *Campylobacter* genes. Other investigators have also reported on the use of DNA microarrays combined with the PCR to detect pathogens, including *Yersinia enterocolitica* and *Enterobacter sakazakii* in food and for speciating pathogens.[120–123]

9.14 PCR-Based Techniques for Typing Microorganisms

Many outbreaks of food-borne disease are due to exposure to a common source of the etiologic agent. Isolates are usually clonal, meaning they are derived from a common ancestor, and are found to be indistinguishable from one another by a variety of subtyping methods. Molecular typing methods targeting bacterial lipopolysaccharides, fatty acids, proteins, or nucleic acids are gradually replacing phenotype-based subtyping methods such as serotyping, phage typing, biotyping, or bacteriocin typing. The relatively high discriminatory ability, ease of performance, and reproducibility of many nucleic acid-based typing techniques that have been developed in recent years have led to their application to study the relatedness of bacterial isolates and have allowed epidemiological investigations to be conducted more rapidly and thoroughly.[124]

Plasmid typing involves analysis of the sizes of plasmids (i.e., extrachromosomal, circular pieces of supercoiled double-stranded DNA) possessed by microorganisms. Pulsed field gel electrophoresis (PFGE) is a commonly used genotypic typing method which involves the generation of large fragments of chromosomal DNA through the use of restriction enzymes that cut genomic DNA infrequently. The fragments are then separated by electrophoretic procedures that allow resolution of DNA molecules ranging in size from 100 to 200,000 base pairs. The technique of PFGE is very discriminating and reproducible, and has been found to be very useful for epidemiological investigations.[125] Ribotyping involves restriction digestion of chromosomal DNA and agarose gel electrophoresis to separate the fragments, followed by transfer of the fragments onto a nylon or nitrocellulose membrane. The DNA is then probed with either labeled rRNA sequences, cDNA made from the rRNA, a recombinant plasmid in which the *rrn* operon of *E. coli* is inserted, or synthetic oligonucleotides made from 16S or 16S plus 23S gene sequences.[124] A "fingerprint" pattern of up to 15 bands is generated from binding of the probes to DNA fragments containing ribosomal genes. An automated ribotyping system, known as the RiboPrinter Microbial Characterization System (Qualicon) is commercially available.[126] Compared to PFGE analysis, PCR-based typing techniques offer the advantages of rapidity, simplicity, the need for smaller amounts of DNA, and often, lower cost.

9.14.1   Random-Amplified Polymorphic DNA

One PCR-based typing technique known as random-amplified polymorphic DNA (RAPD) or also known as arbitrarily primed PCR (AP-PCR) involves the use of a single primer that has no known homology to the target DNA. The reaction occurs with low annealing temperatures allowing the primer to bind to DNA at sites where the match is imperfect, thus at multiple locations on the two DNA strands. The sequences between the primer annealing sites are amplified and fragments, which form a fingerprint of the genomic DNA, are visualized on ethidium bromide-stained agarose gels. The RAPD assays have been successfully applied for molecular typing of a number of organisms including *L. monocytogenes* and *Bacillus cereus*.[127,128] Andrade et al.[129] were able to differentiate yeasts found in dry-cured meat products at the species and strain level; however, the level of discrimination was dependent on the specific primers used.

9.14.2   Amplified Restriction Fragment Length Polymorphism

Amplified restriction fragment length polymorphism (AFLP) is based on detection of DNA restriction fragments by PCR amplification. The DNA is subjected to restriction enzyme digestion followed by amplification of the fragments by ligation of adapter sequences to the ends of the restriction fragments which serve as sites for primer annealing. To reduce the number of fragments generated, the primers can have a number of selective bases at their 3' ends extending into the restriction fragments allowing amplification of only those fragments in which the nucleotides flanking the restriction sites match the 3' primer extensions.[130] Analysis of *L. monocytogenes* food isolates by PCR-RFLP and AFLP techniques demonstrated that although the AFLP method was more complex than PCR-RFLP, it had a higher discriminatory power and was very reproducible.[131]

9.14.3   PCR-Restriction Fragment Length Polymorphism

PCR-restriction fragment length polymorphism (PCR-RFLP) analysis involves PCR amplification of a known DNA sequence such as a virulence region, followed by cutting the amplification product with a restriction enzyme. Analysis of the DNA fingerprint is performed by agarose gel electrophoresis. Fields et al.[132] used PCR-RFLP analysis of the *E. coli fliC* gene to differentiate flagellar antigen groups, and found that in conjunction with serotyping, PCR-RFLP allowed identification of *E. coli* O157:H7 and related strains. Petersen and Newell (2001)[133] compared two PCR-RFLP techniques based on the *C. jejuni flaA* and *flaB* genes and found that higher discrimination of strains was achieved using separately amplified PCR fragments of both *fla* genes.

9.14.4   Rep-PCR

A typing technique referred to as rep-PCR entails the use of primers complementary to highly conserved, repetitive sequences present in multiple copies on the genome. Since the distance between the repetitive elements varies among strains, PCR amplification of the DNA sequences found between them results in generation of a distinct fingerprint. As is true for other genomic typing methods, the resulting fingerprint is analogous to UPC codes used in supermarkets. Families of repetitive sequences that have been identified in bacteria include repetitive extragenic palindromic (REP) sequences, enterobacterial repetitive intergenic consensus (ERIC) sequences, and BOX elements. The rep-PCR typing protocols employing these sequences are referred to as REP-PCR, ERIC-PCR, and BOX-PCR, respectively. Rep-PCR was used to type *L. monocytogenes* strains isolated form humans, animals, and foods,[134] and to determine the genetic relatedness of *Bacillus sphaericus* strains.[135] Rep-PCR was useful for genotyping *Bacillus* spp. and for screening dry food products for typical DNA banding profiles consistent with profiles for enterotoxigenic *Bacillus* spp.[136]

9.14.5   PCR-Ribotyping

The PCR amplification of the intergenic spacer regions between genes coding for 16S and 23S rRNA is known as PCR-ribotyping. In addition to variations in the sequences of the spacer regions, many bacteria possess multiple rRNA alleles, each differing in the length of the spacer regions. A variable number of amplified fragments can be generated allowing differentiation of bacterial isolates based on the pattern of the fragments.[137] Hrstka et al.[138] used PFGE, PCR ribotyping, and enterobacterial repetitive intergenic consensus motif-PCR techniques to genotype toxic shock syndrome toxin-1-positive *Staphylococcus aureus* strains to determine the prevalence of particular genotypes. A predominant genotype, T1, was identified using the three methods.

9.14.6   Sau-PCR

A technique called Sau-PCR involves digestion of genomic DNA using the restriction enzyme *Sau*3A, which is a 4-bp (GATC) cutter, followed by amplification of the DNA using a primer that has the *Sau*3A recognition site as part of its sequence.[139] Profiles of products generated are used to perform cluster analysis. Cocolin et al.[140] employed Sau-PCR to differentiate strains of *L. monocytogenes* isolated from different sources in Italy.

9.14.7   Denaturing Gradient Gel Electrophoresis and Temperature Gradient Gel Electrophoresis

The denaturing gradient gel electrophoresis (DGGE)[141] and temperature gradient gel electrophoresis (TGGE)[142] techniques are used to separate PCR products based on sequence differences that result in different melting characteristics. DGGE separates PCR products of similar size but with sequence differences that result in differential denaturing characteristics. DGGE electrophoresis is performed using a polyacrylamide gel with a relatively broad denaturing gradient (20%–80%) under a constant temperature. As the DNA migrates through the gel, it encounters increasingly higher concentrations of denaturant. The separation of the fragments is based on the decreased electrophoretic mobility of partially melted double-stranded DNA in the linear gradient in the gel formed by a mixture of urea and formamide. Sequence variation in the "melting domain" results in different melting temperatures, and molecules with different sequences stop migrating at different positions in the gel. As little as a single base pair can cause a mobility shift. Cocolin et al.[143] used DGGE for direct identification of *Listeria* spp. isolated from various sources and in food samples after enrichment. A fragment of the *iap* gene from different *Listeria* spp. was amplified, followed by analysis of the PCR products by DGGE. The method could distinguish different *Listeria* spp. and could partially differentiate different serotypes within *L. monocytogenes*. The TGGE technique is similar to DGGE; however, it uses a temperature gradient instead of a chemical gradient to denature the DNA. Manzano et al.[144] used primers designed to the ITS2 DNA region of *S. cerevisiae* and PCR-TGGE to distinguish *S. cerevisiae* and *S. paradoxus*, and the technique could distinguish between strains of *S. cerevisiae*. Population shifts and the ecology of *S. cerevisiae* during wine fermentation were monitored at the strain level. With both PCR-TGGE and PCR-DGGE, a sequence of guanines and cytosines (GC clamp) can be added to the 5′ end of one of the PCR primers, resulting in a PCR product with a GC-rich sequence. Due to the high melting domain of the GC clamp, the complete dissociation of the two DNA strands is prevented, increasing the separation of the different sequences.

9.14.8   PCR-Single-Strand Conformation Polymorphisms

The basis of the PCR-single-strand conformation polymorphisms (PCR-SSCP) technique is that the electrophoretic mobility of a single-stranded DNA molecule depends on both its size, as well as its secondary structure determined by the nucleotide sequence. The technique is relatively simple and does not require the use of costly instruments. The DNA region of interest is amplified by the PCR, heat denatured, and separated on non-denaturing polyacrylamide gels. Mutations or polymorphisms are detected as shifts in mobility. PCR-SSCP[145] was used to detect point mutations in human genomic DNA, and a mobility shift was observed due to a single base substitution in cloned DNA fragments, as well as in fragments of total genomic DNA. Based on nucleotide variation in the heat shock protein gene, *groEL*, Nair et al.[146] described the possibility of using PCR-SSCP to differentiate *Salmonella* strains at the serovar level and for differentiation of strains within a serovar. Since GC clamp primers, gradient gels, or specific equipment is not required, SSCP is more simple and straightforward than DGGE or TGGE.

9.14.9   16S rDNA Sequencing (Homology Search)

For microbial identification, 16S rRNA gene sequencing is widely used as DNA sequencing instruments are now readily available in many laboratories. The 16S rRNA gene contains regions that are highly conserved and common among all previously studied bacteria, and these regions are interspersed with variable or divergent sequences that can differentiate one species from another. Universal primers targeting conserved sequences of the 16S rRNA gene and that flank the variable regions can be used to amplify a portion of this gene. The PCR product can then be sequenced, and the bacterial species is identified by performing homology searches against DNA sequence databases. This technique is useful for the identification of new bacterial species, and results are obtained relatively rapidly since it is not necessary to culture the bacteria to perform biochemical profile testing or other types of tests for identification. The MicroSeq 500 16S Ribosomal DNA-Based Bacterial Identification System (Applied Biosystems) is a commercially available sequence-based system.

9.15   Nanotechnology: On-Chip PCR

Nanotechnology, as it applies to diagnostics, is a rapidly developing new analysis technology that is driving the development of nanochip, nanoarray, and lab-on-a-chip systems. Procedures involving on-chip PCR amplification and detection of products have been described.[147–149] The PCR described by Nickisch-Rosenegk et al.[149] involved PCR amplification with primers immobilized on a chip, and the products were visualized through the use of intercalating dyes or by confocal microarray scanning or fluorescence microscopy using Cy5-dye fluorescence of the modified free primer. Moreover, microchip devices are being developed that integrate cell lysis, multiplex PCR amplification, electrophoretic separation of PCR products, and product detection.[150–152] An integrated plastic microfluidic device combined DNA amplification, injection of amplicons through a gel valve, followed by on-chip electrophoretic separation and detection of labeled PCR products using laser-induced fluorescence.[153] The system was used to detect *E. coli* O157 and *S. typhimurium*, and the limit of detection was six copies of target DNA. Liu et al.[154] described a completely self-contained integrated biochip device that was used to perform sample preparation, followed by PCR and product detection. *E. coli* was inoculated into whole-blood samples, and after immunomagnetic separation and cell lysis, target sequences were detected following PCR and DNA-microarray detection. Westin et al.[155] developed a microchip array with primers anchored to the surface, which were used to perform multiplex SDA-based amplification and detection in situ on the chip. Research groups are considering the use of small portable on-chip PCR systems for detection of a number of bioterrorism agents in a single test sample. Microminiaturization of nucleic acid-based techniques will have a significant impact on diagnostic and food testing, potentially enabling the assays to be performed by relatively unskilled operators in nonlaboratory settings.

References

1. Mead, P.S., Slutsker, L., Dietz, V., McCraig, L.F., Bresee, J.S., Shapiro, C., Griffin, P.M., and Tauxe, R.V., Food-related illness and death in the United States. *Emerg. Infect. Dis.*, 5, 607, 1999.
2. Council for Agricultural Science and Technology Task Force Report, Foodborne pathogens: Review of recommendations, No. 122. Council for Agricultural Science and Technology, 1998.
3. Gracias, K.S. and McKillip, J.L., A review of conventional detection and enumeration methods for pathogenic bacteria in food. *Can. J. Microbiol.*, 50, 883, 2004.
4. Lin, F.Y.H., Sabri, M. Alirezaie, J., Li, D., and Sherman, P.M., Development of a nanoparticle-labeled microfluidic immunoassay for detection of pathogenic microorganisms. *Clin. Diagn. Lab. Immunol.*, 12, 418, 2005.
5. Dooley, J.S.G., Nucleic acid probes for the food industry, *Biotech. Adv.*, 12, 669, 1994.
6. Olsen, J.E., Aabo, S., Hill, W., Notermans, S., Wernar, K., Granum, P.E., Popovic, T., Rasmussen, H.N., and Olsvik, Ø., Probes and polymerase chain reaction for detection of food-borne bacterial pathogens, *Int. J. Food Microbiol.*, 28, 1, 1995.
7. Deng, M.Y. and Fratamico, P.M., A multiplex PCR for rapid identification of Shiga-like toxin-producing *Escherichia coli* O157:H7 isolated from foods, *J. Food Prot.*, 59, 570, 1996.
8. Saiki, R.K., Walsh, P.S., Levenson, C.H., and Erlich, H.A., Genetic analysis of amplified DNA with immobilized sequence-specific oligonucleotide probes, *Proc. Natl. Acad. Sci. USA*, 86, 6230, 1989.
9. Gutierrez, R., Garcia, T., Gonzalez, I., Sanz, B., Hernandez, P.E., and Martin, R., Quantitative detection of meat spoilage bacteria by using the polymerase chain reaction (PCR) and an enzyme linked immunosorbent assay (ELISA), *Lett. Appl. Microbiol.*, 26, 372, 1998.
10. Blais, B.W., Transcriptional enhancement of the *Listeria monocytogenes* PCR and simple immunoenzymatic assay of the product using anti-RNA:DNA antibodies, *Appl. Environ. Microbiol.*, 60, 348, 1994.

11. Yu, H., Bruno, J.G., Cheng, T.C., Calomiris, J.J., Goode, M.T., and Gatto-Menking, D.L., A comparative study of PCR product detection and quantitation by electro-chemiluminescence and fluorescence, *J. Biolumin. Chemilumin.*, 10, 239, 1995.

12. Hayward-Lester, A., Chilton, B.S., Underhill, P.A., Oefner, P.J., and Doris, P.A., Quantification of specific nucleic acids, regulated RNA processing, and genomic polymorphisms using reversed-phase HPLC, in *Gene Quantification*, Ferré, F., (Ed.), Birkhäuser, Boston, MA, 1997, 45.

13. Bachmair, F., Huber, C., and Daxenbichler, G. Quantitation of gene expression by means of HPLC analysis of RT-PCR products, *Clin. Chem. Acta.*, 279, 25, 1999.

14. Holland, P.M., Abramson, R.D., Watson, R., and Gelfand, D.H. Detection of specific polymerase chain reaction product utilizing the 5′→3′ exonuclease activity of *Thermus aquaticus* DNA polymerase, *Proc. Natl. Acad. Sci. U.S.A.*, 88, 7276, 1991.

15. Vishnubhatla, A., Fung, D.Y.C., Oberst, R.D., Hays, M.P., Nagaraja, T.G., and Flood, S.J.A., Rapid 5′ nuclease (TaqMan) assay for detection of virulent strains of *Yersinia enterocolitica*, *Appl. Environ. Microbiol.*, 66, 4131, 2000.

16. Sharma, V.K., Detection and quantitation of enterohemorrhagic *Escherichia coli* O157, O111, and O26 in beef and bovine feces by real-time polymerase chain reaction, *J. Food Prot.*, 65, 1371, 2002.

17. Cheung, P.W., Chan, C.W., Wong, W., Cheung, T.L., and Kam, K.M., Evaluation of two real-time polymerase chain reaction pathogen detection kits for *Salmonella* spp. in food, *Lett. Appl. Microbiol.*, 39, 509, 2004.

18. Ward, L.N. and Bej, A.K., Detection of *Vibrio parahaemolyticus* in shellfish by use of multiplexed real-time PCR with TaqMan fluorescent probes, *Appl. Environ. Microbiol.*, 72, 2031, 2006.

19. Vet, J.A.M., Majthia, A.R., Marras, S.A.E., Tyagi, S., Dube, S., Poiesz, B.J., and Kramer, F.R., Multiplex detection of four pathogenic retroviruses using molecular beacons, *Proc. Natl. Acad. Sci. U.S.A.*, 96, 6394, 1999.

20. Chen, W., Martinez, G., and Mulchandani, A., Molecular beacons: A real-time polymerase chain reaction assay for detecting *Salmonella*, *Anal. Biochem.*, 280, 166, 2000.

21. Fortin, N.Y., Mulchandani, A., and Chen, W., Use of real-time polymerase chain reaction and molecular beacons for the detection of *Escherichia coli* O157:H7, *Anal. Biochem.*, 289, 281, 2001.

22. Liming, S.H. and Bhagwat, A.A., Application of a molecular beacon—real-time PCR technology to detect *Salmonella* species contaminating fruits and vegetables, *Int. J. Food Microbiol.*, 95, 177, 2004.

23. Palladino, S., Kay, I.D., Costa, A.M., Lambert, E.J., and Flexman, J.P., Real-time PCR for the rapid detection of *vanA* and *vanB* genes, *Diagn. Microbiol. Infect. Dis.*, 45, 81, 2003.

24. Reischl, U., Bretagne, S., Krüger, D., Frnault, P., and Costa, R.J.-M., Comparison of two DNA targets for the diagnosis of toxoplasmosis by real-time PCR using fluorescence resonance energy transfer hybridization probes, *BMC Infect. Dis.*, 3, 7, 2003.

25. Stroup, S.E., Roy, S., Mchele, J., Maro, V., Ntabaguzi, S., Siddique, A., Kang, G., Guerrant, R.L., Kirkpatrick, B.D., Fayer, R., Herbein, J., Ward, H., Haque, R., and Houpt, E.R., Real-time PCR detection and speciation of *Cryptosporidium* infection using Scorpion probes, *J. Med. Microbiol.*, 55, 1217, 2006.

26. Gilmour, M.W., Tracz, D.M., Andrysiak, A.K., Clark, C.G., Tyson, S., Severini, A., and Ng, L.-K., Use of the *espZ* gene encoded in the locus of enterocyte

effacement for molecular typing of Shiga toxin-producing *Escherichia coli*, *J. Clin. Microbiol.*, 44, 449, 2006.

27. Rodríguez-Lázaro, D., Hernández, M., Scortti, M. Esteve, T., Vásquez-Boland, J.A., and Pla, M., Quantitative detection of *Listeria monocytogenes* and *Listeria innocua* by real-time PCR: Assessment of *hly*, *iap*, and *lin02483* targets and AmpliFluor technology, *Appl. Environ. Microbiol.*, 70, 1366, 2004.

28. Afonina, I.A., Reed, M.W., Lusby, E., Shiskina, L.G., and Belousov, Y.S., Minor groove binder-conjugated DNA probes for quantitative DNA detection by hybridization-triggered fluorescence, *Biotoechniques*, 32, 940, 2002.

29. Koch, W.H., Payne, W.L., Wentz, B.A., and Cebula, T.A., Rapid polymerase chain reaction method for detection of *Vibrio cholerae* in foods, *Appl. Environ. Microbiol.*, 59, 556, 1993.

30. Relman, D.A., Schmidt, T.M., MacDermott, R.P., and Falkow, S., Identification of the uncultured bacillus of Whipple's disease, *N. Engl. J. Med.*, 327, 293, 1992.

31. Deng, M.Y., Cliver, D.O., Day, S.P., and Fratamico, P.M., Enterotoxigenic *Escherichia coli* detected in foods by PCR and an enzyme-linked oligonucleotide probe, *Int. J. Food Microbiol.*, 30, 217, 1996.

32. Tsen, H.Y., Jian, L.Z., and Chi, W.R., Use of a multiplex PCR system for the simultaneous detection of heat labile toxin I and heat stable toxin II genes of enterotoxigenic *Escherichia coli* in skim milk and porcine stool, *J. Food Prot.*, 61, 141, 1998.

33. Rossen, L., Nørskov, P., Holmstrøm, K., and Rasmussen, O.F., Inhibition of PCR by components of food samples, microbial diagnostic assays and DNA-extraction solutions, *Int. J. Food Microbiol.*, 17, 37, 1992.

34. Monteiro, L., Bonnemaison, D., Vekris, A., Petry, K.G., Bonnet, J., Vidal, R., Cabrita, J., and Mégraud, F., Complex polysaccharides as PCR inhibitors in feces: *Helicobacter pylori* model, *J. Clin. Microbiol.*, 35, 995, 1997.

35. Josephson, K.L., Gerba, C.P., and Pepper, I.L., Polymerase chain reaction detection of nonviable bacterial pathogens, *Appl. Environ. Microbiol.*, 59, 3513, 1993.

36. Arnal, C., Crance, J.M., Gantzer, G., Schwartzbrod, L., Deloince, R., and Billaudel, S., Persistence of infectious hepatitis A virus and its genome in artificial seawater, *Zentralbl. Hyg. Umweltmed.*, 201, 279, 1998.

37. Lee, J.-L. and Levin, R.E., Use of ethidium monoazide for quantification of viable and dead mixed bacterial flora from fish fillets by polymerase chain reaction, *J. Microbiol. Methods*, 67, 456, 2006.

38. Longo, M.C., Berninger, M.S., and Hartley, J.L., Use of uracil DNA glycosylase to control carry-over contamination in polymerase chain reactions, *Gene*, 93, 2847, 1990.

39. Cimino, G.D., Metchette, K.C., Tessman, J.W., Hearst, J.E., and Isaacs, S.T., Post-PCR sterilization: A method to control carryover contamination for the polymerase chain reaction, *Nucl. Acids Res.*, 19, 99, 1991.

40. Persing, D.H. and Cimino, G.D., Amplification product inactivation methods, in *Diagnostic Molecular Microbiology, Principles and Applications*, Persing, D.H., Smith, T.F., Tenover, F.C., and White, T.J., (Eds.), American Society for Microbiology, Washington, DC, 1993, 105.

41. Greenfield, L. and White, T.J., Sample preparation methods, in *Diagnostic Molecular Microbiology, Principles and Applications*, Persing, D.H., Smith, T.F., Tenover, F.C., and White, T.J., (Eds.), American Society for Microbiology, Washington, DC, 1993, 122.

42. Lantz, P., Hahn-Hägerdal, B., and Rådström, P., Sample preparation methods and PCR-based detection of food pathogens, *Trends Food Sci. Technol.*, 5, 384, 1994.

43. Jinneman, K.C., Trost, P.A., Hill, W.E., Weagant, S.D., Bryant, J.L., Kaysner, C.A., and Wekell, M.M., Comparison of template preparation methods from foods for amplification of *Escherichia coli* O157 Shiga-like toxins type I and II by multiplex polymerase chain reaction, *J. Food Prot.*, 58, 722, 1995.

44. Starbuck, M.A.B., Hill, P.J., and Stewart, G.S.A.B., Ultra sensitive detection of *Listeria monocytogenes* in milk by the polymerase chain reaction (PCR), *Lett. Appl. Microbiol.*, 15, 248, 1992.

45. Oyofo, R.A. and Rollins, D.M., Efficacy of filter types for detecting *Campylobacter jejuni* and *Campylobacter coli* in environmental water samples by polymerase chain reaction, *Appl. Environ. Microbiol.*, 59, 4090, 1993.

46. Tsai, Y-L. and Olson, B.H., Rapid method for separation of bacterial DNA from humic substances in sediments for polymerase chain reaction, *Appl. Environ. Microbiol.*, 58, 2292, 1992.

47. Anderson, M.R. and Omiecinski, C.J., Direct extraction of bacterial plasmids from food for polymerase chain reaction, *Appl. Environ. Microbiol.*, 58, 4080, 1992.

48. Lindqvist, R., Preparation of PCR samples from food by a rapid and simple centrifugation technique evaluated by detection of *Escherichia coli* O157:H7, *Int. J. Food Microbiol.*, 37, 73, 1997.

49. Fratamico, P.M. and Strobaugh, T.P., Simultaneous detection of *Salmonella* spp. and *Escherichia coli* O157:H7 by multiplex PCR, *J. Indust. Microbiol. Biotechnol.*, 21, 92, 1998.

50. Kawasaki, S., Horikoshi, N., Takeshita, K., Sameshima, T., and Kawamoto, S., Development of a multiplex PCR protocol for detection of Salmonella spp., Listeria monocytogenes, and Escherichia coli O157:H7 from meat samples, *J. Food Prot.*, 68, 551, 2005.

51. Fratamico, P.M., Sackitey, S.K., Wiedmann, M., and Deng, M.Y., Detection of *Escherichia coli* O157:H7 by multiplex PCR, *J. Clin. Microbiol.*, 33, 2188, 1995.

52. Bhaduri, S. and Cottrell, B., Direct detection and isolation of plasmid-bearing virulent serotypes of *Yersinia enterocolitica* from various foods, *Appl. Environ. Microbiol.*, 63, 4952, 1997.

53. Josefsen, M.H., Jacobsen, N.R., and Hoorfar, J., Enrichment followed by quantitative PCR both for rapid detection and as a tool for quantitative risk assessment of foodborne thermotolerant campylobacters, *Appl. Environ. Microbiol.*, 70, 3588, 2004.

54. Bellin, T., Pulz, M., Matussek, A., Hempen, H., and Gunzer, F., Rapid detection of enterohemorrhagic *Escherichia coli* by real-time PCR with fluorescent hybridization probes., *J. Clin. Microbiol.*, 39, 370, 2001.

55. Beuret, C., Simultaneous detection of enteric viruses by multiplex real-time RT-PCR, *J. Virol. Methods*, 115, 1, 2004.

56. Weagant, S.D., Jagow, J.A., Jinneman, K.C., Omiecinski, C.J., Kaysner, C.A., and Hill, W.E., Development of digoxigenin-labeled PCR amplicon probes for use in the detection and identification of enteropathogenic *Yersinia* and Shiga toxin-producing *Escherichia coli* from foods, *J. Food Prot.*, 62, 438, 1999.

57. Waage, A.S., Vardund, T., Lund, V., and Kapperud, G., Detection of small numbers of *Campylobacter jejuni* and *Campylobacter coli* cells in environmental water, sewage, and food samples by a seminested PCR assay, *Appl. Environ. Microbiol.*, 65, 1636, 1999.

58. Rijpens, N., Herman, L., Vereecken, F., Jannes, G., DeSmedt, J., and DeZutter, L., Rapid detection of stressed *Salmonella* spp. in dairy and egg products using immunomagnetic separation and PCR, *Int. J. Food Microbiol.*, 46, 37, 1999.

59. Simon, M.C., Gray, D.I., and Cook, H., DNA extraction and PCR methods for the detection of *Listeria monocytogenes* in cold smoked salmon, *Appl. Envrion. Microbiol.*, 62, 822, 1996.

60. Wang, C. and Hong, C., Quantitative PCR for *Listeria monocytogenes* with colorimetric detection, *J. Food Prot.*, 62, 35, 1999.

61. Rodríguez-Lázaro, D., Pla, M., Scortti, M., Monzó, Vásquez-Boland, J.A., A novel real-time PCR for *Listeria monocytogenes* that monitors analytical performance via an internal amplification control, *Appl. Environ. Microbiol.*, 71, 9008, 2005.

62. Pearson, B. and McKee, R., Rapid identification of *Saccharomyces cerevisiae*, *Zygosaccharomyces bailii* and *Zygosaccharomyces rouxii*, *Int. J. Food Microbiol.*, 16, 63, 1992.

63. Ibeas, J.I., Lozano, I., Perdigones, F., and Jimenez, J., Detection of *Dekkera-Brettanomyces* strains in sherry by a nested PCR method, *Appl. Environ. Microbiol.*, 62, 998, 1996.

64. Vaitilingom, M., Gendre, F., and Brignon, P., Direct detection of viable bacteria, molds, and yeasts by reverse transcriptase PCR in contaminated milk samples after heat treatment, *Appl. Environ. Microbiol.*, 64, 1157, 1998.

65. Shapira, R., Paster, N., Eyal, O., Menasherov, M., Mett, A., and Salomon, R., Detection of aflatoxigenic molds in grains by PCR, *Appl. Environ. Microbiol.*, 62, 3270, 1996.

66. Klemsdal, S.S. and Elen, O., Development of a highly sensitive nested-PCR method using a single closed tube for detection of *Fusarium culmorum* in cereal samples, *Lett. Appl. Microbiol.*, 42, 544, 2006.

67. Martorell, P., Querol, A., and Fernández-Espinar, M.T., Rapid identification and enumeration of *Saccharomyces cerevisiae* cells in wine by real-time PCR. *Appl. Environ. Microbiol.*, 71, 6823, 2005.

68. Lopez-Sabater, E.L., Deng, M.Y., and Cliver, D.O., Magnetic immunoseparation PCR assay (MIPA) for detection of hepatitis A virus (HAV) in American oyster (*Crassostrera virginica*), *Lett. Appl. Microbiol.*, 24, 101, 1997.

69. Reynolds, K.A., Gerba, C.P., and Pepper, I.L., Detection of infectious enteroviruses by an integrated cell culture-PCR procedure, *Appl. Environ. Microbiol.*, 62, 1424, 1996.

70. Deng, M.Y., Day, S.P., and Cliver, D.O., Detection of hepatitis A virus in environmental samples by antigen-capture PCR, *Appl. Environ. Microbiol.*, 60, 1927, 1994.

71. Hafliger, D., Gilgen, M., Luthy, J., and Hubner, P., Seminested RT-PCR systems for small round structured viruses and detection of enteric viruses in seafoods, *Int. J. Food Microbiol.*, 37, 27, 1997.

72. Richards, G.P., Watson, M.A., Fankhauser, R.L., and Monroe, S.S., Genogroup I and II noroviruses detected in stool samples by real-time reverse transcription-PCR using highly degenerate universal primers, *Appl. Environ. Microbiol.*, 70, 7179, 2004.

73. Costafreda, M.I., Bosch, A., and Pintó, R.M., Development, evaluation, and standardization of a real-time TaqMan reverse transcription-PCR assay for quantification of hepatitis A virus in clinical and shellfish samples, *Appl. Environ. Microbiol.*, 72, 3846, 2006.

74. Johnson, D.W., Pieniazek, N.J., Griffin, D.W., Misener, L., and Rose, J.B., Development of a PCR protocol for sensitive detection of *Cryptosporidium* oocysts in water samples, *Appl. Environ. Microbiol.*, 61, 3849, 1995.

75. Laberge, I., Ibrahim, A., Barta, J.R., and Griffiths, M.W., Detection of *Cryptosporidium parvum* in raw milk by PCR and oligonucleotide probe hybridization, *Appl. Environ. Microbiol.*, 62, 3259, 1996.

76. Warnekulasuriya, M.R., Johnson, J.D., and Holliman, R.E., Detection of *Toxoplasma gondii* in cured meats, *Int. J. Food Microbiol.*, 45, 211, 1998.

77. Jinneman, K.C., Wetherington, J.H., Hill, W.E., Adams, A.M., Johnson, J.M., Tenge, B.J., Dang, N.L., Manger, R.L., and Wekell, M.M., Template preparation for PCR and RFLP of amplification products for the detection and identification of *Cyclospora* spp. and *Eimeria* spp. oocysts directly from raspberries, *J. Food Prot.*, 61, 1497, 1998.

78. Hill, W.E., The polymerase chain reaction: Applications for the detection of foodborne pathogens, *Crit. Rev. Food Sci. Nutr.*, 36, 123, 1996.

79. Johnson, J.L., Brooke, C.L., and Fritschel, S.J., Comparison of the BAX for Screening/*E. coli* O157:H7 method with conventional methods for detection of extremely low levels of *Escherichia coli* O157:H7 in ground beef, *Appl. Environ. Microbiol.*, 64, 4390, 1998.

80. Bailey, J.S., Detection of *Salmonella* cells within 24 to 26 hours in poultry samples with the polymerase chain reaction BAX system, *J. Food Prot.*, 61, 792, 1998.

81. Bennett, A.R., Greenwood, D., Tennant, C., Banks, J.G., and Betts, R.P., Rapid and definitive detection of *Salmonella* in foods by PCR, *Lett. Appl. Microbiol.*, 26, 437, 1998.

82. Silbernagel, K., Jechorek, R., and Carver, C., Evaluation of the BAX system for detection of *Salmonella* in selected foods: Collaborative study, *J. AOAC Int.*, 86, 1149, 2003.

83. Bassler, H.A., Flood, S.J.A., Livak, K.J., Marmaro, J., Knorr, R., and Batt, C.A., Use of a fluorogenic probe in a PCR-based assay for the detection of *Listeria monocytogenes*. *Appl. Environ. Microbiol.*, 61, 3724, 1995.

84. Chen, S., Yee, A., Griffiths, M., Larkin, C., Yamashiro, C.T., Behari, R., Paszko-Kolva, C., Rahn, K., and Grandis, S.A., The evaluation of a fluorogenic polymerase chain reaction assay for the detection of *Salmonella* species in food commodities, *Int. J. Food Microbiol.*, 35, 239, 1997.

85. Oberst, R.D., Hays, M.P., Bohra, L.K., Phebus, R.K., Yamashiro, C.T., Paszko-Kolva, C., Flood, S.J.A., Sargeant, J.M., and Gillespie, J.R., PCR-based DNA amplification and presumptive detection of *Escherichia coli* O157:H7 with an internal fluorogenic probe and the 5' nuclease (TaqMan) assay, *Appl. Environ. Microbiol.*, 64, 3389, 1998.

86. Krause, M., Josefsen, M.H., Lund, M., Jacobsen, N.R., Brorsen, L., Moos, M., Stockmarr, A., and Hoorfar, J., Comparative, collaborative, and on-site validation of a TaqMan PCR method as a tool for certified production of fresh, *Campylobacter*-free chickens. *Appl. Environ. Microbiol.*, 72, 5463, 2006.

87. Atmar, R.L., Neill, F.H., Romalde, J.L., LeGuyader, F., Woodley, C.M., Metcalf, T.G., and Estes, M.K., Detection of Norwalk virus and hepatitis A virus in shellfish tissues with the PCR, *Appl. Environ. Microbiol.*, 61, 3014, 1995.

88. Arnal, C., Ferre-Aubineau, V., Migotte, B., Imbert-Marcille, B.M., and Billaudel, S., Quantification of hepatitis A virus in shellfish by competitive reverse transcription-PCR with coextraction of standard RNA, *Appl. Environ. Microbiol.*, 65, 322, 1999.

89. Lantz, O., Bonney, E., Umlauf, S., and Taoufik, Y., Kinetic ELISA-PCR: A versatile quantitative PCR method, in *Gene Quantification*, Ferré, F., (Ed.), Birkhäuser, Boston, MA, 1997, 145.

90. Takahashi, H., Hara-Kudo, Y., Miyasaka, J., Kumagai, S., and Konuma, H., Development of a quantitative real-time polymerase chain reaction targeted to the *toxR* for detection of *Vibrio vulnificus, J. Microbiol. Methods*, 61, 77, 2005.

91. Duport, C., Zigha, A., Rosenfeld, E., and Schmitt, P., Control of enterotoxin gene expression in *Bacillus cereus* F4430/73 involves the redox-sensitive ResDE signal transduction system, *J. Bacteriol.*, 188, 6640, 2006.

92. Hanna, S.E. and Wang, H.H., Assessment of environmental factors on *Listeria monocytogenes* Scott A *inlA* gene expression by relative quantitative Taqman real-time reverse transcriptase PCR, *J. Food Prot.*, 69, 2754, 2006.

93. Klein, P.G. and Juneja, V.K., Sensitive detection of viable *Listeria monocytogenes* by reverse transcription-PCR, *Appl. Environ. Microbiol.*, 63, 4441, 1997.

94. Sheridan, G.E.C., Masters, C.I., Shallcross, J.A., and Mackey, B.M., Detection of mRNA by reverse transcription-PCR as an indicator of viability in *Escherichia coli* cells, *Appl. Environ. Microbiol.*, 64, 1313, 1998.

95. Goswami, B.B., Koch, W.H., and Cebula, T.A., Detection of hepatitis A virus in *Mercenaria mercenaria* by coupled reverse transcription and polymerase chain reaction, *Appl. Environ. Microbiol.*, 59, 2765, 1993.

96. Le Guyader, F.S., Bon, F., DeMedici, D., Parnaudeau, S., Bertone, A., Crudeli, S., Doyle, A., Zidane, M., Suffredini, E., Kohli, E., Maddalo, F., Monini, M., Gallay, A., Pommepuy, M., Pothier, P., and Ruggeri, F.M., Detection of multiple noroviruses associated with an international gastroenteritis outbreak linked to oyster consumption, *J. Clin. Microbiol.*, 44, 3878, 2006.

97. Wiedmann, M., Czajka, J., Barany, F., and Batt, C.A., Discrimination of *Listeria monocytogenes* from other *Listeria* species by ligase chain reaction, *Appl. Environ. Microbiol.*, 58, 3443, 1992.

98. Stubbs, S., Hutson, R., James, S., and Collins, M.D., Differentiation of the spoilage yeast *Zygosaccharomyces bailii* from other *Zygosaccharomyces* species using 18S rDNA as target for a non-radioactive ligase detection reaction, *Lett. Appl. Microbiol.*, 19, 268, 1994.

99. Walker, G.T., Nadeau, J.G., Spears, P.A., Schram, J.L., Nycz, C.M., and Shank, D.D., Multiplex strand displacement amplification (SDA) and detection of DNA sequences from *Mycobacterium tuberculosis* and other mycobacteria, *Nucl. Acids Res.*, 22, 2670, 1994.

100. Ge, B., Larkin, C., Ahn, S., Jolley, M., Nasir, M., Meng, J., and Hall, R.H., Identification of *Escherichia coli* O157:H7 and other enterohemorrhagic serotypes by EHEC–*hlyA* targeting, strand displacement amplification, and fluorescence polarization, *Mol. Cell Probes*, 16, 85, 2002.

101. Uyttendaele, M., Schukkink, R., VanGemen, B., and Debevere, J., Detection of *Campylobacter jejuni* added to foods by using a combined selective enrichment and nucleic acid sequence-based amplification (NASBA), *Appl. Environ. Microbiol.*, 61, 1341, 1995.

102. Blais, B.W., Turner, G., Sooknanan, R., and Malek, L.T., A nucleic acid sequence-based amplification system for detection of *Listeria monocytogenes hlyA* sequences, *Appl. Environ. Microbiol.*, 63, 310, 1997.

103. Cook, N., The use of NASBA for the detection of microbial pathogens in food and environmental samples, *J. Microbiol. Methods*, 53, 165, 2003.

104. Simpkins, S.A., Chan, A.B., Hays, J., Pöpping, B., and Cook, N., A RNA transcription-based amplification technique (NASBA) for the detection of viable *Salmonella enterica*, *Lett. Appl. Microbiol.*, 20, 75, 2000.

105. D'Souza, D.H. and Jaykus, L.-A., Nucleic acid sequence based amplification for the rapid and sensitive detection of *Salmonella enterica* from foods. *J. Appl. Microbiol.*, 95, 1343, 2003.

106. Rodríguez-Lázaro, D., Lloyd, J., Herrewegh, A., Ikonomopoulos, J., D'Agostino, M., Pla, M., and Cook, N., A molecular beacon-based real-time NASBA assay for detection of *Mycobacterium avium* subsp. *paratuberculosis* in water and milk. *FEMS Microbiol. Lett.*, 237, 119, 2004.

107. Jean, J., D'Souza, D.H., and Jaykus, L.A., Multiplex nucleic acid sequence-based amplification for simultaneous detection of several enteric viruses in model ready-to-eat foods, *Appl. Environ. Microbiol.*, 70, 6603, 2004.

108. Maruyama, F., Kenzaka, T., Yamaguchi, N., Tani, K., and Nasu, M., Visualization and enumeration of bacteria carrying a specific gene sequence by in situ rolling circle amplification, *Appl. Environ. Microbiol.*, 71, 7933, 2005.

109. Wang, B., Potter, S.J., Lin, Y., Cunningham, A.L., Dwyer, D.E., Su, Y., Ma, X., Hou, Y., and Saksena, N.K., Rapid and sensitive detection of severe acute respiratory syndrome coronavirus by rolling circle amplification, *J. Clin. Microbiol.*, 43, 2339, 2005.

110. Li, F., Zhao, C., Zhang, W., Cui, S., Meng, J., Wu, J., and Zhang, D.Y., Use of ramification amplification assay for detection of *Escherichia coli* O157:H7 and other *E. coli* Shiga toxin-producing strains, *J. Clin. Microbiol.*, 43, 6086, 2005.

111. Wolcott, M.J., Advances in nucleic acid-based detection methods, *Clin. Microbiol. Rev.*, 5, 370, 1992.

112. Notomi, T., Okayama, H., Masubuchi, H., Yonekawa, T., Watanabe, K., Amino, N., and Hase, T., Loop-mediated isothermal amplification of DNA. *Nucl. Acids Res.*, 28 (12), E63, 2000.

113. Ohtsuka, K., Yanagawa, K., Takatori, K., and Kudo, Y.H., Detection of *Salmonella enterica* in naturally contaminated liquid eggs by loop-mediated isothermal amplification, and characterization of *Salmonella* isolate, *Appl. Environ. Microbiol.*, 6730, 71, 2005.

114. Parida, M., Posadas, G., Inoue, S., Hasebe, F., and Morita, K., Real-time reverse transcription loop-mediated isothermal amplification for rapid detection of West Nile Virus, *J. Clin. Microbiol.*, 257, 42, 2004.

115. Isogai, E., Makungu, C., Yabe, J., Sinkala, P., Nambota, A., Isogai, H., Fukushi, H., Silungwe, M., Mubita, C., Syakalima, M., Hang'ombe, B.M., Kozaki, S., and Yasuda, J., Detection of *Salmonella invA* by isothermal and chimeric primer-initiated amplification of nucleic acids (ICAN) in Zambia, *Comp. Immunol. Microbiol. Infect. Dis.*, 363, 28, 2005.

116. Sergeev, N., Volokhov, D., Chizhikov, V., and Rasooly, A., Simultaneous analysis of multiple staphylococcal enterotoxin genes by an oligonucleotide microarray assay, *J. Clin. Microbiol.*, 42, 2134, 2004.

117. Call, D.R., Brockman, F.J., and Chandler, D.P., Detecting and genotyping *Escherichia coli* O157:H7 using multiplexed PCR and nucleic acid microarrays, *Int. J. Food Microbiol.*, 67, 71, 2001.

118. Chizhikov, V., Rasooly, A., Chumakov, K., and Levy, D.D., Microarray analysis of microbioal virulence factors, *Appl. Environ. Microbiol.*, 67, 3258, 2001.

119. Keramas, G., Bang, D.D., Lund, M., Madsen, M., Bunkenborg, H., Telleman, P., and Christensen, C.B.V., Use of culture, PCR analysis, and DNA microarrays

for detection of *Campylobacter jejuni* and *Campylobacter coli* from chicken feces, *J. Clin. Microbiol.*, 42, 3985, 2004.

120. Volokov, D., Rasooly, A., Chumakov, K., and Chizhikov, V., Identification of *Listeria* species by microarray-based assay, *J. Clin. Microbiol.*, 40, 4720, 2002.

121. Volokov, D., Chizhikov, V., Chumakov, K., and Rasooly, A., Microarray-based identification of thermophilic *Campylobacter jejuni*, *C. coli*, *C. lari*, and *C. upsaliensis*, *J. Clin. Microbiol.*, 41, 4071, 2003.

122. Myers, K.M., Gaba, J., and Al-Khaldi, S.F., Molecular identification of *Yersinia enterocolitica* isolated from pasteurized whole milk using DNA microarray chip hybridization. *Mol. Cell. Probes*, 20, 71, 2006.

123. Liu, Y., Gao, Q., Zhang, X., Hou, Y., Yang, J., and Huang X., PCR and oligonucleotide array for detection of *Enterobacter sakazakii* in infant formula, *Mol. Cell. Probes*, 20, 11, 2006.

124. Farber, J.M., An introduction to the hows and whys of molecular typing, *J. Food Prot.*, 59, 1091, 1996.

125. Barrett, T.J., Lior, H., Green, J.H., Khakhria, R., Wells, J.G., Bell, B.P., Greene, K.D, Lewis, J., and Griffin, P.M., Laboratory investigation of a multistate food-borne outbreak of *Escherichia coli* O157:H7 by using pulsed field-gel electrophoresis and phage typing, *J. Clin. Microbiol.*, 32, 3013, 1994.

126. Oscar, T.P., Identification and characterization of *Salmonella* isolates by automated ribotyping, *J. Food Prot.*, 61, 519, 1998.

127. Czajka, J. and Batt, C.A., Verification of causal relationships between *Listeria monocytogenes* isolates implicated in food-borne outbreaks of listeriosis by randomly-amplified polymorphic DNA patterns, *J. Clin. Microbiol.*, 32, 1280, 1994.

128. Nilsson, J., Svensson, B., Ekelund, K., and Christiansson, A., A RAPD-PCR method for large-scale typing of *Bacillus cereus*, *Lett. Appl. Microbiol.*, 27, 168, 1998.

129. Andrade, M.J., Rodríguez, M., Sánchez, B., Aranda, E., and Córdoba, J.J., DNA typing methods for differentiation of yeasts related to dry-cured meat products, *Int. J. Food Microbiol.*, 107, 48, 2006.

130. Restrepo, R., Duque, M., Tohme, J., and Verdier, V., AFLP fingerprinting: An efficient technique for detecting genetic variation of *Xanthomonas axonopodis* pv. *manihotis*, *Microbiology*, 145, 107, 1999.

131. Mikasova, E., Oravcova, K., Kaclikova, E., Kuchta, T., and Krahovska, H., Typing of food-borne *Listeria monocytogenes* by polymerase chain reaction-restriction enzyme analysis and amplified fragment length polymorphism, *New Microbiol.*, 28, 265, 2005.

132. Fields, P.I., Blom, K., Hughes, H.J., Helsel, L.O., Feng, P., and Swaminathan, B., Molecular characterization of the gene encoding H antigen in *Escherichia coli* and development of a PCR-restriction fragment length polymorphism test for identification of *E. coli* O157:H7 and O157:NM, *J. Clin. Microbiol.*, 35, 1066, 1997.

133. Petersen, L. and Newell, D.G., The ability of Fla-typing schemes to discriminate between strains of *Campylobacter jejuni*, *J. Appl. Microbiol.*, 91, 217, 2001.

134. Jeršek, B., Gilot, P., Gubina, M., Klun, N., Mehle, J., Tcherneva, E., Rijpens, N., and Herman, L., Typing of *Listeria monocytogenes* strains by repetitive element sequence-based PCR, *J. Clin. Microbiol.*, 37, 103, 1999.

135. Miteva, V., Selenska-Pobell, S., and Mitev, V., Random and repetitive primer amplified polymorphic DNA analysis of *Bacillus sphaericus*, *J. Appl. Microbiol.*, 86, 928, 1999.

136. Cooper, R.M. and McKillip, J.L., Enterotoxigenic *Bacillus* spp. DNA fingerprint revealed in naturally contaminated nonfat dry milk powder using rep-PCR, *J. Basic Microbiol.*, 46, 358, 2006.

137. Cartwright, C.P., Stock, F., Beekmann, S.E., Williams, E.C., and Gill, V.J., PCR amplification of rRNA intergenic spacer regions as a method for epidemiologic typing of *Clostridium difficile*, *J. Clin. Microbiol.*, 33, 184, 1995.

138. Hrstka, R., Růžičková, Petráš, P., Pantšček, R., Rosypal, S., and Doškař, J., Genotypic characterization of toxic shock syndrome toxin-1-producing strains of *Staphylococcus aureus* isolated in the Czech Republic, *Int. J. Med. Microbiol.*, 296, 49, 2006.

139. Corich, V., Mattiazzi, A., Soldati, E., Carraro, A., and Giacomini, A., Sau-PCR, a novel amplification technique for genetic fingerprinting of microorganisms, *Appl. Environ. Microbiol.*, 71, 6401, 2005.

140. Cocolin, L., Stella, S., Nappi, R., Bozzetta, E., Cantoni, C., and Comi G., Analysis of PCR-based methods for characterization of *Listeria monocytogenes* strains isolated from different sources, *Int. J. Food Microbiol.*,103, 167, 2005.

141. Theophilus, B.D.M., Latham, T., Grabowski, G.A., and Smith, F.I., Comparison of RNase A, a chemical cleavage and GC-clamped denaturing gradient gel electrophoresis for the detection of mutations in exon 9 of the human acid B-glucosidase gene, *Nucl. Acids Res.*, 7707, 17, 1989.

142. Henco, K. and Heibey, M., Quantitative PCR: The determination of template copy numbers by temperature gradient gel electrophoresis (TGGE). *Nucl. Acids Res.*, 6733, 18, 1990.

143. Cocolin, L., Rantsiou, K., Iacumin, L., Cantoni, C., and Comi, G., Direct identification in food samples of *Listeria* spp. and *Listeria monocytogenes* by molecular methods, *Appl. Environ. Microbiol.*, 6273, 68, 2002.

144. Manzano, M., Cocolin, L., Iacumun, L., Cantoni, C., and Comi, G., A PCR-TGGE (temperature gradient gel electrophoresis) technique to assess differentiation among enological *Saccharomyces cerevisiae* strains. *Int. J. Food Microbiol.*, 333, 101, 2005.

145. Orita, M., Iwahana, H., Kanazawa, H., Hayashi, K., and Sekiya, T., Detection of polymorphisms of human DNA by gel electrophoresis as single-strand conformation polymorphisms. *Proc. Natl. Acad. Sci. U.S.A.*, 2766, 86, 1989.

146. Nair, S., Lin, T.K., Pang, T., and Altwegg, M., Characterization of *Salmonella* serovars by PCR-single-strand conformation polymorphism analysis, *J. Clin. Microbiol.*, 2346, 40, 2002.

147. Kricka, L.J., Miniaturization of analytical system, *Clin. Chem.*, 44, 2008, 1998.

148. Kricka, L.J., Microchips, microarrays, biochips and nanochips: Personal laboratories for the 21st century, *Clin. Chem. Acta.*, 307, 219, 2001.

149. Nickisch-Rosenegk, M., Marschan, X., Andresen, D., Abraham, A., Heise, C., and Bier, F.F., On-chip PCR amplification of very long templates using immobilized primers on glassy surfaces, *Biosens. Bioelectron.*, 20, 1491, 2005.

150. Cheng, J., Shoffner, M.A., Hvichia, G.E., Kricka, L.J., and Wilding, P., Chip PCR. II. Investigation of different PCR amplification systems in microfabricated silicon-glass chips, *Nucl. Acids Res.*, 24, 380, 1996.

151. Woolley, A.T., Hadley, D., Landre, P., deMello, A.J., Mathies, R.A., and Northrup, M.A., Functional integration of PCR amplification and capillary electrophoresis in a microfabricated DNA analysis device, *Anal. Chem.*, 68, 4081, 1996.

152. Waters, L.C., Jacobson, S.C., Kroutchinina, N., Khandurina, J., Foote, R.S., and Ramsey, J.M., Multiple sample PCR amplification and electrophoretic analysis on a microchip, *Anal. Chem.*, 70, 158, 1998.

153. Koh, C.G., Tan, W., Zhao, M.-Q., Ricco, A.J., and Fan, Z.H., Integrating polymerase chain reaction, valving, and electrophoresis in a plastic device for bacterial detection, *Anal. Chem.*, 75, 4591, 2003.
154. Liu, R.H., Yang, J., Lenigk, R., Bonanno, J., and Grodzinski, P., Self-contained, fully integrated biochip for sample preparation, polymerase chain reaction amplification, and DNA microarray detection, *Anal. Chem.*, 76, 1824, 2004.
155. Westin, L., Xu, X., Miller, C., Wang, L., Edman, C.F., and Nerenberg, M., Anchored multiplex amplification on a microelectronic chip array, *Nature Biotechnol.*, 18, 199, 2000.

10

Advances in Prion Detection

Rodrigo Morales, Dennisse González, Claudio Soto,
and Joaquín Castilla

CONTENTS

10.1   Introduction

Prion diseases or transmissible spongiform encephalopathies (TSEs) are a group of fatal, transmissible neurodegenerative diseases affecting humans and animals (Table 10.1). They are usually characterized by the presence of protease-resistant prion protein (PrP^{res}), an abnormal, protease-resistant isoform of the normal host cell surface protein[1] denoted PrP^C. No amino acid sequence or posttranslational differences have been detected between PrP^C and its pathological form, PrP^{Sc}. The conversion of PrP^C into PrP^{Sc} involves a conformational change, whereby the α-helical content diminishes and the amount of β-sheet increases.[2] Depending on how they arise, TSEs can be classified as sporadic, hereditary, or infectious; most have been experimentally transmitted and, with some exceptions, the presence of PrP^{res} is related to their infectivity.[1,3–5] The etiology of spontaneous and familial TSE has been only described in humans and includes the Creutzfeldt–Jakob disease (CJD), the Gertsmann–Straüssler–Scheinker syndrome, and fatal familial insomnia.[6–12] It is generally accepted that misfolding of the cellular prion protein (PrP^C) leads to the build up in the brain of an insoluble, pathologic PrP isoform (PrP^{Sc}). PrP^{Sc} aggregation and accumulation in the brain produce spongiform brain degeneration (vacuolization), neuronal death, astrocytosis, and microglial proliferation.[2] Clinically, the disease is manifested mainly by rapidly progressive dementia, visual and motor impairments, and inexorable death.

TABLE 10.1

Prion Diseases, Hosts, and Mechanism of Infection

Disease	Host	Mechanism of Infection	Reference
Sporadic CJD	Human	Unknown	[128]
Sporadic fatal insomnia	Human	Unknown	[129]
Fatal familial insomnia	Human	Mutations in the *prnp* gene	[130]
Familial CJD	Human	Mutations in the *prnp* gene	[131]
Gerstmann–Straussler–Scheinker syndrome	Human	Mutations in the *prnp* gene	[132]
Iatrogenic CJD	Human	Acquired from human sources (growth hormone, corneal grafts, others).	[133]
Kuru	Human	Cannibalism	[134]
Variant CJD	Human	Ingestion of BSE-contaminated food	[45]
Scrapie	Sheep and goat	Unknown	[135]
Transmissible mink encephalopathy	Mink	Probably ingestion of TSE-contaminated food	[136]
Chronic wasting disease	Cervids	Unknown	[47]
Bovine spongiform encephalopathy (BSE) or mad cow disease	Cattle	Ingestion of TSE-contaminated food	[137]
Feline spongiform encephalopathy	Cats	Ingestion of BSE-contaminated food	[138]

Although prion diseases are rare in humans, the established link between a new variant form of CJD (vCJD) and the consumption of cattle meat contaminated by BSE have raised concern about a possible outbreak of a large epidemic in the human population.[13–16] Over the past few years, BSE has become a significant health problem affecting many countries, and it seems now apparent that vCJD can be iatrogenically transmitted from human to human by blood transfusion.[17–19] Exacerbating this state of affairs is the lack of a reliable test to identify individuals incubating the disease during the long and silent period from the onset of infection to the appearance of clinical symptoms.[20,21]

At the molecular level, the main difference between vCJD and other human prion diseases such as sporadic CJD (sCJD) is the accumulation of PrP^{Sc} in the lymphoreticular system.[22] Furthermore, 100% of the vCJD patients are methionine homozygous at codon 129 in the PrP gene (*prnp*), while this genotype represents only 48%–52% of the Caucasian population.[23,24] This distribution is not shared with other human prion diseases. Although it has been recently demonstrated that the other M129V and V129V genotypes could be infected by vCJD, at this moment, homozygosis at codon 129 seems one of the most important risk factors associated to developing prion diseases by the host.[25]

10.1.1 How Is a Normal Protein Converted to a TSE Agent?

The prion protein is a glycoprotein of around 210 amino acids coded by one unique gene (*prnp*) that appears attached to the outer plasmatic membrane by a glycosylphosphatidylinositol (GPI) anchor.[2] The protein is expressed in most of the mammalian cells including CNS, lymphoreticular tissues, and muscle.[2,26] Although its function is still unknown, some studies suggest that it could be participating in copper uptake, protection against oxidative stress, cell adhesion, modulation of apoptotic process, and modulation of neuronal excitability, among others.[27–31]

In spite of PrP^{C} and PrP^{Sc} sharing the same amino acid sequence, their biochemical and physiological properties differ. While the secondary structure of PrP^{C} is composed mainly of α-helix, PrP^{Sc} is highly enriched in β-sheet structure, resulting in the formation of a protein core resistant to proteases digestion, chemical agents, radiation, high temperature, and non-denaturing detergents.[2]

Aggregates of PrP^{Sc} form fibrilar structures.[32] The kinetics follows a nucleation–polymerization model with presumably two stages. The first step is a nucleation phase, which is rate limiting to form stable polymerization nucleus or seeds composed of monomeric PrP (Figure 10.1). Then, a fast elongation phase occurs in which the PrP^{C} interacts with PrP^{Sc} changing its conformation to a β-sheet rich structure. In TSE diseases the rate limiting phase could be bypassed for the addition of seeds from the environment (as PrP^{Sc} is contained in food, surgical procedures, blood transfusions, etc.), increasing the kinetics of the PrP^{Sc} formation.[33]

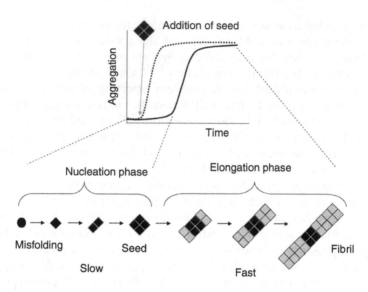

FIGURE 10.1
Nucleation-polymerization model for PrP^{Sc} formation. PrP^{Sc} fibrils formation follows a kinetics characteristic of polymerization-crystallization process. The first step is the limiting-rate reaction in which monomers of PrP^{C} are misfolded into a β-sheet rich structure and form a polymerization nucleus or seed (nucleation phase). This slow step can be accelerated for addition of preformed seed (dashed line). The second step is the elongation phase in which fibrils grow at the ends of preformed fibrils by recruitment of PrP^{C}.

10.1.2 From Food to Brain

How a protein maintains its infective properties across the digestive tract is astonishing. It is known experimentally that PrP^{Sc} is resistant to degradation by standard digestive enzymes. The result of its digestion is a protease-resistant fragment that remains infectious even at low pH characteristic of the stomach.[34] However, how prions can cross the intestinal epithelium is still unclear. Some evidence indicates that post-digested infectious fragments are complexed with ferritin (a protein highly present in meat) and is basolaterally translocated across epithelial cells.[35] Another plausible explanation would be that the infectious agent crosses the barrier through microfold (M) cells (specialized cells for transepithelial transport of macromolecules and particles) in an intact misfolded conformation.[36] These cells are part of Peyer's patches (lymphoid follicles localized in the epithelial layer of the small intestine). Then, the TSE agent is transported to the lymphoid tissue, where reside follicular dendritic cells (FDC) that maintain PrP^{Sc} and other proteins attached in the plasmatic membrane for long periods.[37] These properties of FDC and other immune cells are crucial for replication of the infectious agent.[38] Supporting evidence indicates that PrP^{C} binds to C1q (a complement protein) creating a complex capable of binding to the FDC membrane and other migratory immune cells as dendritic cells or phagocytic cells such as macrophages. For this, C1q might participate in TSE agent uptake and spread along different and distant targets.[39]

Data from TSE-inoculated rodents indicate that the transfer from lymphoid tissue to CNS is through the enteric nervous system, both by sympathetic and parasympathetic nerves, i.e., splenic nerve and vagus nerve, respectively. This process is denominated neuroinvasion, where the TSE agent moves retrogradely until it reaches the brain, where it replicates and aggregates producing cellular damage and, as a consequence, typical clinical signs and death.[40]

10.1.3 Species Barrier Phenomenon

The species barrier phenomenon is defined as the difficulty associated with a specific prion to infect other species.[41] Although the molecular mechanisms involved in this intriguing phenomenon are not completely known, the conformational similarity between both host PrP^C and the TSE-causing agent (PrP^{Sc}) determines the strength of the barrier. Unfortunately, the conformation of PrP^{Sc} and PrP^C is not determined entirely by the PrP amino acid sequence. Thus, it has been described by many different PrP^{Sc} conformations, named prion strains, in the same host, and therefore with the same PrP amino acid sequence.[42] In other words, the same PrP^C could yield different PrP^{Sc} with many different conformations depending on which prion has been used to convert it. Interestingly, different prion strains might result in distinctive infective capabilities expressed by the incubation time of the TSE agent, brain lesion profile, and other biochemical parameters. The following examples could resume the importance of this phenomenon for public heath: (1) A natural scrapie agent from sheep does not infect humans but efficiently infects cattle, developing a bovine encephalopathy spongiform that is able to infect humans[43] and (2) while scrapie is a noninfectious disease for humans, the infectivity of the new ovine prion generated as a result of BSE inoculation in sheep remains still unknown. Recent experiments have revealed that both ovine prions show a non-distinguishable pathology in sheep, but they show differential biochemical characteristics.[44] Biological studies related to infectivity in humans are addressed. However, these studies will take several years; thus it is a priority to improve current prion detection tests in order to increase their sensitivity and also to differentiate between these two ovine prion strains, in order to avoid BSE-contamination food for human consumption.

10.1.4 Animal TSEs as Zoonoses

The most important outbreak of TSE for human public health arose in the late 1980s and early 1990s. The United Kingdom population was exposed to BSE-contaminated food and as a consequence more than 150 human deaths have been reported.[45]

Another TSE affecting animals for human consumption is currently in the spotlight. Chronic wasting disease (CWD), a prion disease that naturally affects deer (*Odocoileus* spp.) and Rocky Mountain elk (*Cervus elaphus nelsoni*) has been detected in the United States and Canada since late 1960s, both in free-ranging and captive animals.[46,47] In 2005, a first case of CWD in moose (*Alces alces*) was reported (unpublished data) and recently it has been published that infective prions can be found in preparations from semitendinosus/semimembranous muscles of CWD-affected mule deer[26], raising the question if venison-consuming people are at risk of developing some prion diseases, repeating the BSE episode in the United Kingdom. Nevertheless, there are no epidemiological links between CWD outbreak and vCJD or other sCJDs in United States. To address this question, several experimental approaches have been taken. Mice expressing human PrP inoculated with CWD-brain extract failed to develop prion diseases.[48] Furthermore, in vitro studies evidence a strong species barrier between cervid and human PrP.[49] However, two squirrel monkeys challenged intracerebrally with brain tissue from CWD-infected deer died due to prion disease after 31 and 34 months.[50] Unfortunately, the previous evidence data do not clarify if CWD-venison is an infectious source for humans, and more experiments should be done to clarify it.

One of the most intriguing features of prion diseases is the large incubation time, which depends on the prion strain and species, inoculation route, host, and dose of the TSE agent. This variability and the uncertain presence of prions in accessible fluids (blood, CSF, saliva, and urine) make an early clinical diagnosis of the disease difficult. In the present chapter, we review the latest advances in prion detection. These are principally focused on the improvement of high-throughput screening and sensitivity, trying to detect prions in preclinical phases and in more accessible tissues.

10.2   Current Methods in Prion Detection

10.2.1   Needs for an Ultra-Sensitive Method for Prion Detection

Currently no commercial assays available are accurate enough or highly sensitive for prion detection. However, five recent events in the prion field have increased the need for developing methods capable of detecting minute amounts of the prion infectious agent: (1) the diagnosis of three new cases of vCJD contracted by blood transfusion in the United Kingdom[18] and consequently the uncertainty about the real incidence of vCJD in the asymptomatic United Kingdom population, (2) the first case of BSE in sheep and its unknown ability to infect humans, (3) the detection of infectious prion agent in muscle from sheep[51] and cervid,[26,50] (4) the transmission of the CWD agent to nonhuman primates,[50] and (5) the detection of prions in other tissues and fluids, e.g., urine.[52] Although these new incidents are demanding more accurate and more sensitive detection methods, at present, postmortem analysis must be performed in order to faithfully diagnose prion-related disorders. It is a priority in this field to improve the actual detection methods mainly to avoid TSE outbreak similar to the one in Europe. In other words, highly sensitive and pre-symptomatic detection methods are required to prevent TSE-contaminated food from entering the human food chain again.

The food industry has been seriously affected after the most recent and extensive outbreak of BSE in cattle, which occurred in Europe in the 1980s.[53] BSE has important implications for human health, and the consumption of BSE-contaminated meat or meat products has been linked to the advent of a new human TSE disease, the variant Creutzfeldt–Jakob disease.[13–16] The potential spread of BSE to other domestic animals such as sheep, cervids, and pigs has consequences for human health, and these populations of animals need to be monitored for signs of BSE infection. On the other hand, the high incidence of CWD in wild-ranging cervids in U.S. territory[54] and the actual data about the infectivity of these prions in primates are demanding the use of a more accurate detection method in edible samples.[55,56]

Both, strain and species barrier phenomena are complicating the investigations about prion infectivity in humans due to the singularity of its outstanding features as infectious proteins. These phenomena are responsible for what most of investigators in the field think: while scrapie is not infectious at all in the human being, a scrapie prion coming from the inoculation with the BSE agent may be infectious in spite of being pathologically indistinguishable from a natural case of scrapie. This concern is having a huge repercussion in the ovine food industry, as it happened in the past with cattle. Since the memory of prions after crossing species barriers is unpredictable we have to rule out infectivity in humans using animal models as bioassays. Hundreds of different prions have been tested for several years in animal models, principally in hamsters and mice. At present, other more sophisticated animal models have been generated to answer these questions. Unfortunately, there is not a way to predict how hazardous to humans a prion strain could be. However, as it will be described later, some detection techniques could be adapted in order to address this question.

Different strategies have been developed that focus on the improvement of sensitivity, specificity, and suitability for high throughput of current prion detection methods. They include (1) increasing the sensitivity by improving the affinity of the antibody to bind the PrP molecule, (2) increasing the concentration of the infectious material, (3) selective recognition of disease associated isoform of PrP, and (4) amplification of the infectious agent, among others. In the present chapter, we describe several detection methods for prions that are currently in use but also others, the most promising, which may probably be in use in a short-term future. Most of them will be used for the screening of "packaged" products, but also directly in presymptomatic livestock.

10.2.2 In Vitro Assays for Prion Detection

10.2.2.1 Histopathological Study

In spite of using an assay with a low sensitivity, histopathological studies are still an essential method for confirmatory studies and it was the first method used for prion diagnosis.[57] In fact, the name of TSE comes from the histopathological analysis of brain samples, where spongiform degeneration of the brain is observed. The current histopathological procedure does not differ very much from other histopathological studies used in other infectious diseases. The pathognomonic depositions of PrP^{Sc} (prion agent) in CNS and other lymphoreticular tissues and the spongiosis specific to CNS make this method highly precise. However, the limitations of this method are clear and the negative results obtained should be cautiously analyzed. For example, (1) samples obtained from carcasses after a long postmortem period are not useful for this assay, (2) it is frequent that positive cases are denoted negatives using this technique because not all brain areas show the same TSE characteristics, i.e., differential histopathological patterns of BSE and BASE (atypical BSE),[58] (3) other tissues different from CNS result in negatives most of the time depending on the prion strain evaluated, and (4) in asymptomatic phases the amount of prions and the lesions are undetectable. In addition, since this assay is time consuming and is not suitable for high-throughput studies, it is not useful in the food industry and is only appropriate for suspected livestock analysis.

10.2.2.2 Western Blot-Based Tests

10.2.2.2.1 Prionics-Check Western Test

This Western blot-based test takes advantage of the protease-resistant feature of PrP^{Sc}. The sample is treated by proteinase K digestion and is resolved in a SDS-PAGE gel. The PrP^{res} fragment (27–30 kDa for the diglycosylated band versus ~36 kDa of PrP^{C}) is detected using the 6H4 monoclonal antibody. The principal advantage of this technique is the possibility to see the pathognomonic sign unique to these diseases, i.e., the PrP^{res} signal, after PK digestion, making this method highly specific.[59] Meanwhile, this assay is less time consuming compared to other assays; it is also easy to perform and many samples can be analyzed in a relatively short period of time. The main disadvantage of this assay is its low sensitivity, an indispensable characteristic needed in the food industry.

10.2.2.3 ELISA-Based Tests

10.2.2.3.1 Enfer Test

This standard ELISA-based assay is one of the first methods for BSE prion detection approved by the European Union.[59] Although it was selected because of its sensitivity, which is higher than that of the Western blot, and the possibility to use it in a high throughput manner, the number of false positives is still high. For this reason, the positive cases are usually confirmed using another Western blot-based assay.

10.2.2.3.2 CEA/BioRad Test

Although the false positives remain high in this assay, the principal advantage of this procedure is its sensitivity, much higher than other standard ELISA-based assays.[59] Thus, this DAS (double antibody sandwich) ELISA is capable of detecting brain samples to a dilution of up to $10^{-2.5}$, making it suitable for pre-diagnostic analysis. The immunoassay is based on the detection of the PK resistant core of PrP^{Sc} after denaturation and concentration processes, and is also used in high throughput procedures.

10.2.2.3.3 Prionics-Check LIA Test

This is one of the fastest assays for BSE prion detection.[60] However, this test does not show any other advantage in sensitivity or specificity when compared to Western blot assay or other ELISA-based assays. The method uses two monoclonal antibodies to bind the PrP^{Sc}. In the first step, the samples are incubated with one of the monoclonal antibodies and the mixture is transferred to another microtitre plate coated with the other monoclonal antibody. As in other ELISA-based tests, the high number of false positives is its main disadvantage.

10.2.2.3.4 Prionics PrioSTRIP System

This recent test based on the same principles as other STRIP-based immunoassays (a primary antibody is conjugated with blue latex beads that allow the recognition after the migration of the samples in the kit's strips) makes the BSE detection a very simple and friendly procedure. The principal advantage is its simplicity (more than 400 samples can be analyzed by one person in around 2 h), and high sensitivity and specificity close to 100%.[61] Unfortunately, its incomparable characteristics are restricted by the use of specific samples based on brain homogenates from obex.

10.2.2.4 BSE and Scrapie Discriminatory Test

As mentioned above, species barrier and prion strain phenomena could lead to the generation of many different infectious proteins. Each one could be a potential hazardous agent for humans. For this reason, the BSE transmission to sheep and the consequent generation of a new scrapie strain able to infect humans[62] is currently one of the most important concerns in the prion field. In addition, this concern is extended to the food industry since ovine and goat products are one of the most popular meat-products after cow, chicken, and pork.

Natural and experimental transmissions of BSE in sheep have revealed that the new sheep infected BSE (sBSE) strain presents several biochemical differences compared to natural or experimental cases of scrapie.[62,63] The most important feature is its *sui generis* electrophoretical motility in

SDS-PAGE gels compared with scrapie and BSE.[64] Thus, the electrophoretical motility of the unglycosylated form after PK digestion in scrapie is 18.1 kDa, whereas in sBSE it is 16.5 kDa.[64] Based on these differences, several discriminatory tests have been developed. The principal method is a standard Western blot using two very well-known antibodies: 6H4 and P4.[65] While the 6H4 monoclonal antibody is able to recognize PrP^{Sc} after PK digestion from both scrapie and sBSE cases, P4 is only able to detect PrP^{Sc} from scrapie but not sBSE.[63–65] This is possible due to the specific epitopes that each antibody is recognizing: the 6H4 epitope is located between the amino acids 148–156 of ovine PrP, while the P4 epitope is located in positions 94–99, critical in terms of PK digestion, and therefore, recognition.[64] Unfortunately, false positives could appear in the case of CH1641 sheep prion strain, due principally to its unique conformation compared to the rest of scrapie agents.[65]

The European Union guidelines command the use of primary molecular testing with a discriminatory immuno-blotting to all samples from clinical suspect cases. In case the presence of BSE cannot be excluded in ovine samples, the Community Reference Laboratory should carry out at least a second discriminatory immuno-blotting, a discriminatory immunocytochemistry, and a discriminatory ELISA. Finally, samples indicative for BSE by the three different methods and samples inconclusive should be further analyzed by a mouse bioassay for final confirmation.

10.2.2.5   Conformational Assays

10.2.2.5.1   Conformational-Dependent Immunoassay Test

The conformational-dependent immunoassay (CDI) is an original immunoassay that is based on the specific antibody binding to an epitope that is always available in PrP^C in standard conditions and becomes available in PrP^{Sc} only after denaturation.[66,67] The procedure requires splitting the sample into two aliquots that are treated or not with a denaturant agent. The rest of the procedure is standard for an ELISA-based technique. Although the first immunoassay based on these conformational-dependent properties was accepted in the United States for CWD prion detection, recently a new assay for BSE prion detection has been accepted by the European Union. Although the sensitivity of this assay is higher than other regular ELISAs, the general procedure is more complicated and requires more time than usual. Probably, the principal advantage of this method is its use in all kinds of atypical BSE and scrapie strains. Since the method is based on the conformational differences between PrP^C and PrP^{Sc}, we cannot rule out that noninfectious PrP^C, misfolded as a consequence of mutations in its amino acid sequence, causes false positives.

10.2.2.5.2   Multimer Detection System

The multimer detection system is a promising assay still under development and is based on the property of the misfolded proteins to generate aggregates, as it happens with the PrP^{Sc} in prion diseases.[68] The method is based on a DAS-ELISA where two antibodies recognizing the same epitope are used. The fact that the antibodies used recognize the same epitope in any PrP yield a positive result when two or more PrP molecules are together, as in the case of aggregates of PrP^{Sc}. The proof of concept of this assay has been successfully established using recombinant protein, brain from infected hamsters, and blood from different sources. However, this procedure has an important disadvantage because other kinds of non-pathological aggregations are sources of false positives. On the other hand, the principle of this method could be applied to other protein aggregates as Aβ in Alzheimer disease or huntingtin in Huntington disease.

10.2.2.5.3 Misfolded Protein Diagnostic Assay

The misfolded protein diagnostic assay (MPD) technology developed by Adlyfe, and performed originally for prion blood detection, is based on the PrP misfolded isoform recognition by fluorescent peptides instead of standard antibodies.[69] When conformational changes occur in the fluorescent peptides after the binding to a misfolded PrP, slight differences in the fluorescence are detectable. This technique has been experimentally tested in blood from different animal models in preclinical and clinical cases from endemic and experimental prion diseases, including human, cattle, and sheep. However, more data about the specificity and sensitivity are needed.

10.2.2.5.4 Prionics Conformational Assay

In 1997, B. Oerch and coworkers developed the first antibody able to recognize specifically PrP^{Sc} but not PrP^{C}.[70] The principal advantage of this antibody, called 15B3, is the possibility to be used in immunoprecipitation and concentration procedures. Since it is specific for misfolded PrPs, it is also able to recognize mutant isoforms that have been described as non-pathological.[71] Currently, Prionics has developed a new assay based on this IgM monoclonal antibody that combines its specific characteristic with a regular ELISA test.[70] Although this system is still under development it would be necessary to know more details about its sensitivity and specificity, especially in other non-pathological forms of prion related diseases. However, this antibody is a great tool in prion studies where a pathological process is involved but PrP^{Sc} (as a protease resistant isoform) is not present.

10.2.2.5.5 Other Conformational Antibodies

Although still under development, other conformational antibodies have shown interesting results in the detection of specific prionopathies as the V5B2 monoclonal antibody, which is able to recognize specifically PrP^{Sc} in CJD.[72]

Another example also under development is the monoclonal antibody OCD4 that recognizes specifically DNA or DNA binding proteins, and is able to capture PrP from brains affected by prion diseases in both humans and animals but not from unaffected controls.[73]

10.2.2.6 Spectroscopic Techniques: Multispectral Ultraviolet Fluoroscopy

Conceptually, multispectral ultraviolet fluoroscopy (MUFS) is a smart method that uses the conformational differences between PrP^C and PrP^{Sc} to detect them differentially by fluorescent emission after ultraviolet excitation.[74] The advantage of this assay is that no treatment to the sample is necessary and, in addition, it could allow distinguishing between diverse structures of PrP^{Sc} (prion strains). However, this technology shows a poor sensitivity and is completely impractical in current diagnosis systems.

10.2.2.6.1 Confocal Dual-Color Fluorescence Correlation Spectroscopy

In confocal dual-color fluorescence correlation spectroscopy (FCS), a sophisticated method, the sample is mixed with PrP specific fluorescent antibodies. Based on the assumption that the polymeric PrP^{Sc} shows more antibody binding sites versus the monomeric PrP^C, these slight differences of fluorescence after the antibody binding are detected using excitation by laser beams and a confocal microscope equipped with a single photon counter.[75] Although the technique is more sensitive than any Western blot or ELISA, it is not suitable for high-throughput approaches, being an excellent technique for dedicated laboratory studies.

10.2.2.6.2 Fourier-Transformed Infrared Spectroscopy

The Fourier-transformed infrared (FTIR) spectroscopy assay was used initially for the detection of PrP^{Sc} in blood samples.[76] The method is based on the differences in the infrared spectra shown by the different isoforms of PrP. The test shows very good and promising results in terms of sensitivity and specificity. However, its principal problem is the high experience required to interpret the result obtained. On the other hand, it seems to be difficult to perform as a large-scale diagnostic method.

10.2.2.7 Prion Concentration and Specific Ligands

10.2.2.7.1 Sodium Phosphotungstic Acid

After the discovery of sodium phosphotungstic acid (NaPTA) as a molecule able to precipitate PrP^{Sc} predominantly over PrP^C, many laboratories have included this technique as a standard procedure in prion detection.[66,67,77] However, although this procedure increases the sensitivity about 10 times when coupled to other techniques such as Western blot or ELISA, it is not a very practical technique for high-throughput screening. The method has been applied satisfactorily for prion detection in several tissues with very interesting results.[67,78,79] This technique can also be applied to big samples, including food, where the amount of prion can be undetectable using other techniques. In general, this technique is a great alternative as pretreatment when an increase in sensitivity is required.

10.2.2.7.2 PrP^{Sc} Binding Peptides

It has been described how some peptides and proteins are able to bind specifically PrP^{Sc} but not PrP^{C}. Although plasminogen was one of the first examples published, likely due to its not total specificity for PrP^{Sc} binding, no tests have been developed at this moment using this approach.[80] However, further investigations have given way to the design of other synthetic peptides with similar properties.[81] The main advantage in the use of synthetic peptides is the possibility for modifications: fluorescent dye linked, enzyme activity linked, and coated by magnetic beads, among others. The biotechnology company Chiron is working in this direction, using a peptide that specifically binds PrP^{Sc} and is coated to magnetic beads.[82] This approach allows the concentration of PrP^{Sc}, which can then be used for further analysis using PrP specific antibodies. In unpublished results, the company has showed detection up to a 10^{-5} dilution of BSE infected brain homogenates, 1000-fold the standard limit for a regular Western blot or ELISA.[83]

This system is also suitable for high throughput, but more data are required about its specificity to be approved.

10.2.2.7.3 Seprion Ligand Platform

Polyanionic molecules are intriguing molecules able to bind PrP^{Sc} and disrupt the infectivity in cell cultures,[83] or even enhance amplification of infectious particles in vitro.[84] Microsense Biotechnologies has developed a system using these kinds of polyanionic polymers that are able to specifically capture rogue prion protein and avoid the need of proteinase K. This allows accelerating the detection process compared to conventional Western blot or ELISA. The analysis proposed by Microsense Biotechnologies takes around 4 h and is suitable for high throughput.[85] This system has been tested in spiked plasma using PrP^{CJD} from brain and spleen, and the detection level obtained was 330 infectious units (IU)/mL in brain spiked plasma and 10^2 IU/mL of spleen spiked plasma. Although the studies are not completed and more evidence are necessary for it to be approved as a regular assay, the preliminary results are very promising compared with other techniques on development.

10.2.2.7.4 Other Specific Ligands

A recent discovery has showed that the antibiotic streptomycin is able to bind specifically oligomeric PrP^{Sc}.[86] This property has been used in the study of 150 (52 negative controls and 98 CJD cases) CJD infected brain samples demonstrating 100% specificity and 100% sensitivity.[87] Since the streptomycin-PrP^{Sc} complex cannot be retained on an antibody coated microplate, it is necessary that its previous denaturalization be attached to the microplate coupled to chemical ligands (calyx-arenes). The company Biomérieux has successfully developed this diagnostic assay in a high throughput manner.[87] Although this new approach is highly promising, more studies of specificity and sensitivity will have to be carried out using the final assay.

10.2.3 Amplification Assays for Prion Detection

In the methods described above for prion detection, different approaches based on the direct detection of PrP^{Sc} as the only validated surrogate marker for the disease have been shown. In all cases, the sensitivity and specificity were limited by the affinity of the ligand (antibody, peptide, polyanions, or other molecules) for the PrP^{Sc}. Most of them, in spite of presenting sufficient sensitivity for postmortem diagnosis are not sensitive enough for presymptomatic samples and, needless to say, to detect prions in other less infectious tissues that, unfortunately, are the most probable food contaminants. For this reason, other approaches are necessary to overcome the problem that most of the assays showed. In the same manner that PCR based on DNA amplification is the most used technique for infectious agents' detection, the amplification of prion proteins might be likely the unique way to increase the sensitivity enough to avoid TSE contaminated tissues from entering the human food chain. In this section, we review four different approaches based on in vitro or in vivo prion amplification and replication as methods for detection.

10.2.3.1   In Vitro Amplification

10.2.3.1.1   Cell-Free Conversion

Nucleation of the misfolded form of PrP and polymerization of the recruiting isoforms resulting from conversion are the responsible processes in the development of prion diseases. Misfolded protein nuclei formation is the key step of amyloid formation. As shown in Figure 10.1, the lag phase is usually long, but after nuclei formation, an exponential recruitment of misfolded protein occurs, triggering the disease. Cell-free conversion is based on this kind of kinetics, where PrP^{Sc} acts as a seed accelerating the misfolding conversion process.

As it happens in vivo, the cell-free conversion technique uses the PrP^{C} as the source for the generation of new PrP^{Sc}.[49,88,89] The PrP^{C} produced in the cells is radiolabeled using ^{35}S-methionine and separated by immunoprecipitation. The PrP^{Sc} acting as seed is purified by conventional methods and both highly purified components are mixed and incubated in the absence of any other component. To evaluate the amplification of the infectious material, radioactivity of the new PK resistant PrP is measured. To avoid detection of non-converted PrP, the observations are made using Western blot, where the shift in the electrophoretical motility between non-PK treated PrP^{C} and PK treated PrP^{Sc} is observed. Since the principle of this method is based on the in vivo prion replication, the efficiency of the conversion occurring in vitro is very low and cannot be applied as a feasible detection method. In order to detect prion amplification, a dilution ratio of 50 parts of PrP^{Sc} versus one of PrP^{C} must be done. However, this in vitro procedure was the first technique able to mimic the prion replication and it has been an essential system for developing other more feasible approaches for prion diagnosis.

10.2.3.1.2 Protein Misfolding Cyclic Amplification

On the basis of the principle that it is better to imitate the nature than invent anything, the protein misfolding cyclic amplification (PMCA) technique was devised. In this technique, it is possible to simulate prion replication in the test tube in an accelerated mode.[90] PMCA is a cyclic process leading to accelerated prion replication.[90,91] Each cycle is composed of two steps (Figure 10.2A). During the first step, the sample, containing minute amounts

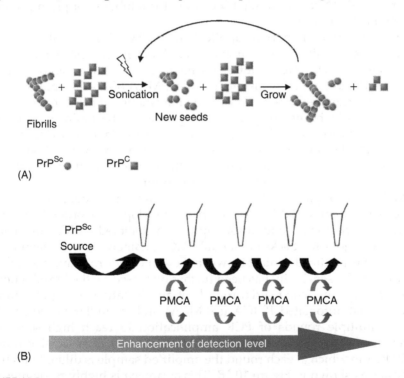

FIGURE 10.2
Protein misfolding cyclic amplification (PMCA) system. PMCA was developed to increase the total amount of PrP^{Sc} in a sample at the expense of PrP^{C}. (A) Samples are submitted to sonication in order to disrupt the PrP^{Sc} fibrils forming new seeds. Then the samples are submitted to incubation at 37°C allowing the conversion of PrP^{C} into PrP^{Sc}. Samples undergo multiple sonication–incubation cycles. (B) Serial passages of PMCA generated samples. PrP^{Sc}-containing material is diluted in normal brain homogenate as source of PrP^{C} and submitted to incubation–sonication cycles. Then the PMCA generated material is diluted in new aliquots of normal brain homogenate in order to "refresh" the source of PrP^{C}.

of PrP^{Sc} and a large excess of PrP^{C}, is incubated to induce formation of PrP^{Sc} aggregates. In the second step, the sample is sonicated in order to break down the aggregates, thus multiplying the number of growth sites for subsequent conversion. With each successive cycle, there is an exponential increase in the number of "seeds" and thus the conversion process is dramatically accelerated (Figure 10.2A).[90] The cyclic nature of the system permits the use of as many cycles as required to reach the amplification state needed for the detection of PrP^{Sc} in a given sample.

Reproduction of the process of prion conversion using PMCA represents a novel platform technology, which is likely to have a sustained impact in the field of prion biology. The ability to simulate this process in accelerated mode under controlled conditions in vitro provides an opportunity to examine many aspects of prion biology, which hitherto have been inaccessible to experimentation, i.e., (a) the molecular mechanism of species barrier and prion strains phenomena, (b) investigation of factors involved in the PrP^{C} to PrP^{Sc} conversion, (c) screening for inhibitors of prion propagation, and (d) diagnosis.

One of the most important applications of PMCA is in TSE diagnosis. As stated before, the biggest problem that biochemical tests have to overcome to detect PrP^{Sc} pre-symptomatically in tissues other than brain is the very low amount of PrP^{Sc} existing in them. PMCA offers the opportunity to enhance existing methods by amplifying the amount of PrP^{Sc} in the sample. The aim would be not only to detect prions in the brain in early pre-symptomatic cases, but also to generate a test to diagnose living animals and humans. For this purpose, a tissue other than brain is required and, in order to have an easier noninvasive method, detection of prions in body fluids such as urine or blood are the best options.

PMCA in its original mode was done by manual operation,[90] but recently an automated mode (aPMCA) has been developed in order to increase sensitivity, specificity, and throughput.[92] Automated PMCA overcomes one of the major drawbacks of manual PMCA, namely cross-contamination, since there is no direct contact between the sonicator probe and the sample. In addition, the sensitivity has been further increased by the introduction of a new concept involving serial rounds of amplification. This procedure is named serial automated PMCA (saPMCA) and is similar to the application of multiple rounds of PCR amplification to reach high sensitivity detection of DNA. Serial automated PMCA consists of successive rounds of aPMCA in which at each round the amplified sample is diluted into fresh substrate, as shown in Figure 10.2B. This approach is highly recommended when elevated levels of amplification are required, especially when working with samples containing minute initial amounts of PrP^{Sc}, such as blood, CSF, muscle, or peripheral non-lymphoid tissues. The rounds of saPMCA can be repeated as many times as needed to reach the detection threshold of Western blotting. Samples remaining negative after 10 rounds of saPMCA can be considered negative, because according to our experience, around 6–8 rounds of saPMCA can amplify the minimum amount of material required for amplification (approximately 100 molecules of PrP^{Sc} monomers) (unpublished data).

Since the replication of prions from different species is based on the same phenomenon, this technique is applicable to all of them independent of the prion strain or species trying to be detected. This advantage permits using the same procedure for any TSE-contaminated sample. Another great advantage of this amplification-based technique is the possibility to couple it to other high-sensitive biochemical detection techniques. Combining the strategy of reproducing prions in vitro with any of the high-sensitive detection methods, the early diagnosis of TSE may be achieved.

10.2.3.2 *In Vivo Amplification*

10.2.3.2.1 *Cell Infectivity Assay*

Like in a prion infectious process in animals, culture cells have been used trying to mimic the in vivo prion replication phenomenon. Although, this assay may be used theoretically as a prion detection method, there are a lot of pitfalls that make the system not suitable for the detection of the most important prions. The principal problem is that the culture cells selectively replicate prions from just a few species.[93,94] This specificity can even be extended to just a few prion strains from the same species.[95] Thus, most of the neural cells used for mouse prion replication are able to replicate only RML or RML-like prion strains but not others.[96] Unfortunately, the in vitro replication using cells has only been described for some mouse prion strains, CWD (from mule deer),[97] and some scrapie prion strains from sheep;[98] but it is impossible at this moment to mimic the same phenomenon with BSE from cattle or other human prions, making this cell-based system inadequate to be used for practical prion detection. Why a good number of the cells used for this purpose are resistant to the infection with most prions remains still unknown. In fact, the susceptible cells have been usually generated after a dedicated clonation process, since most of the cells from a standard culture are resistant for prion replication. In spite of all the problems related to this system, the sensitivity obtained using these cells replicating some mouse prions has been as high as that of the most sensitive bioassay, being possible to detect dilution up to 1000 infectious units. In this case, the great advantage of this system in comparison to other bioassays is the possibility for robotization. In other words, if in the future the intriguing phenomenon of why just certain prions are able to be replicated in cell cultures is solved, and if the system works with the rest of the prions as CJD, BSE, and scrapie, among others, this method could be converted to one of the most interesting techniques for prion detection. And at that moment it might also be useful not only for research but also for routinary food screening.

10.2.3.2.2 *Bioassays*

Bioassay is defined as any assay that uses animals to detect an infectious agent. In the 1960s, although still unknown that the agent causing TSEs was an infectious protein, the natural bioassays were crucial to study the transmissible character of the disease. Thus, samples from scrapie infected sheep were inoculated in different rodents (mouse, rat, hamster, guinea pig, gerbil, and bank vole) confirming its transmissibility.[99] In spite of the low efficiency of these first in vivo assays due to the species barrier between the ovine PrP^{Sc} and the PrP^C from rodent, they were essential tools for developing investigations in the prion field. Years later, other manageable animals (minks, raccoons, marmosets, and other primates) were used as bioassays in the detection of CWD, TME, Kuru, and CJD prions.[100-111] However, we had to wait until the British BSE-outbreak in order to see a tremendous progress in this field. The undutiful relationship between BSE in cattle and vCJD in human explained the concept of species barrier and triggered the developing of new bioassays based on transgenic (Tg) animals. As a consequence, in the last 15 years PrP Tg mice overexpressing PrP^C from different species (human,[112-115] bovine,[115-118] ovine,[119] porcine,[120] cervid,[121] and murine,[122] etc.) have been generated. The development of Tg mouse models carrying the PrP gene of species naturally affected by the TSE agents has provided the best way to overcome the difficulties in transmitting TSEs from their natural host species to laboratory animals. The incubation time in the mouse bioassay for a BSE isolate varies between 250 and 550 days depending on the mouse genetic background.[115-118] However, the bioassay based on transgenic mice expressing bovine PrP reduces the time to less than 200 days.[117]

Bioassays are playing an important role in the food industry, especially in the detection of prions from edible samples that give negative results using conventional immunological techniques. Hence, Tg mice expressing bovine PrP^C were challenged with various tissues from cattle with end-stage clinical BSE, and infectivity was found only in the central and peripheral nervous system and not in lymphatic tissues; the only exception was the Peyer's patches of the distal ileum, which most likely are the site of entry for BSE infectivity.[123] Another recent study based on transgenic mice expressing cervid PrP^C revealed the presence of infectious prions in skeletal muscles of CWD-infected deer, demonstrating that humans consuming or handling meat from CWD-infected deer are at risk of prion exposure.[26]

Other studies difficult to address in farm animals have been realized using more practical bioassays. Thus, the mother-to-offspring transmissibility study was done using transgenic mice expressing bovine PrP experimentally infected by intracerebral administration of BSE prions. In this assay, PrP^{Sc} was detected in brains of newborns from infected mothers only when mating had been allowed near to the clinical stage of the disease, when brain PrP^{Sc} deposition could be detected by Western blot analysis.[124] However, attempts to detect infectivity in milk after intracerebral inoculation in these Tg mice were unsuccessful, suggesting the involvement of other tissues as carriers of prion dissemination.

In the same manner that cattle were infected by TSE contaminated food, other species, principally captive animals in zoos, were also infected with the same source of contamination. However, natural cases of TSE in swine have not been reported in spite of this species also being exposed to the same TSE contaminated food. Castilla et al. examined the barrier from cows to pigs using a new bioassay based on transgenic mice expressing the porcine prion protein gene (poTg).[120] Intracerebral inoculation with a high-titer BSE inoculum, but not low-titer BSE inoculum, caused clinical signs of BSE, consistent with a strong species-barrier. However, second passage with brain homogenates from low-titer inoculated mice produced detectable prion protein in new poTg mice. These results suggest that the barrier is not absolute and that pigs are also susceptible to develop a TSE with unpredictable infectivity for humans.

Although the transgenic mice described above are considered the best bioassays for TSE detection, recently, a new bioassay based on a wild rodent, the bank vole (*Clethrionomys glareolus*), is showing promising results in the detection of natural scrapie (unpublished results). The results obtained in the primary transmission with some strains of scrapie indicate that the bank vole is a species much more susceptible to the scrapie agent than wild-type mice and even more susceptible than bioassays based on ovine PrP Tg mice.

At this moment, it is a priority to develop efficient bioassays that help in the risk evaluation and control of scrapie and BSE in sheep. This will provide the European agro industry with an opportunity to discard products that might contain TSE-causing agents and would guarantee the production of safer sheep and beef products.

10.3 Concluding Remarks

In the present review we have summarized the principal advances in prion detection based on methods currently in use in diagnostic laboratories and also others that should be considered, since they are showing interesting characteristics or are promising techniques under development. In Table 10.2 are represented the most reliable techniques for prion detection ordered by sensitivity. With the exception of the PMCA method, still not commercially available, no method is accurate enough to ensure that prion contaminated edible samples are not entering the human food-chain daily. However, many other aspects should be taken into account in order to evaluate the true risk for humans. Prions are unconventional infectious agents with extraordinary physicochemical features that confer on them the property to resist the most common food treatments in use. Even though the amount of prions in the current edible tissues is very low, it is able to experimentally infect the animals used in some of the available bioassays via intracerebral inoculation. Still, most of the samples able to infect by intracerebral route would not be infectious by oral ingestion. But we cannot underestimate the accumulation effect until conclusive experiments have

TABLE 10.2

Comparison of the Sensitivity of Several Methods to Detect PrP^{Sc}

Assay	Maximum Dilution Detected[a]	Minimum PrP Quantity Detected[b]	Increase in Sensitivity[c]
Standard Western blot	3.0×10^3	4.0 ng	1
ELISA	2.5×10^4	0.5 ng	8
Phosphotungstic acid precipitation	1.5×10^5	80 pg	50
Conformation-dependent immunoassay[d]	2.0×10^5	150 pg	27
Animal assay	1.0×10^5	12 fg	330,000
Single PMCA[e]	7.0×10^5	1.6 pg	2,500
Double PMCA[e]	2.0×10^{10}	0.6 fg	6,500,000
Seven rounds PMCA[e]	1.0×10^{12}	1.3 ag	3,300,000,000

[a] The maximum dilution detected corresponds to the last dilution of 263 K scrapie brain in which PrP^{Sc} is detectable.
[b] The minimum quantity of PrP^{Sc} detected in a brain sample volume of 20 μL.
[c] The increase of sensitivity is expressed in relation to the standard western blot assay using 3F4 antibody.
[d] The data for the conformation-dependent immunoassay was taken from the literature, whereas all the others were experimentally calculated.
[e] The data for single and double PMCA correspond to the average obtained in three different experiments using 100 cycles in both first and second PMCA.

been done. Thus, it would be necessary to perform experiments that mimic more accurately an actual real scenario, especially now when we dispose off the bioassays and other techniques necessary to accomplish them. For example, it would be necessary to study in primate or human PrP Tg mice if a repetitive oral dose of BSE-contaminated muscle or other common edible BSE-contaminated tissues from cattle or sheep are able to infect. In other words, even if we can guarantee that prion from different species are entering the human food-chain we cannot assure that they should be considered a risk for humans.

On the other hand, the detection of prions in blood, as one of the most accessible tissue, in a pre-symptomatic phase of the disease would be the goal that all the assays have to reach. At this moment, the PMCA is the only technique that has shown positive results at that level,[125] but only in experimental models. The extrapolation of these results to cattle, sheep, cervid, and human might be one of the most important achievements in the prion field. Fortunately, other promising techniques under development are close to having enough sensitivity for pre-symptomatic studies in accessible fluids. The combination of amplification-based techniques as PMCA or cell-infectivity assays and other detection methods will be likely the most appropriate system in the future of prion detection.

In the meantime, the prion detection methods are being improved; the food industry should apply the established guidelines in order to diminish the prion contamination in the edible tissues. These guidelines have been established according to the results obtained using the current bioassays and they determine the industrial procedures for food control. Thus, the guiding principles determine which animals should be analyzed in the abattoir and which products should be excluded from human consumption. Recently, three discoveries have substantially changed these guidelines: (1) the first natural case of BSE in goat,[126] (2) the detection of prion in muscle of CWD-infected cervid[26], and (3) the ectopic accumulation of PrP^{Sc} in organs subjected to an inflammation process.[127] The emergent scrapie strain in caprine that could be infectious for humans, the existence of the infectious agent in the most edible tissue (muscle) and the ectopic accumulation of prions in excretory organs as kidney and mammary gland that could unleash their presence in milk and urine are the new dares that the prion-detection methods should confront.

Acknowledgments

This work is partially supported by NIH grants AG0224642 and NS049173. We thank Arancha Desojo for helpful discussion of this manuscript.

References

1. Prusiner, S.B., Molecular biology of prion diseases, *Science*, 252, 1515–1522, 1991.
2. Prusiner, S.B., Prions, *Proc. Natl. Acad. Sci. U. S. A.*, 95, 13363–13383, 1998.
3. Cohen, F.E. and Prusiner, S.B., Pathologic conformations of prion proteins, *Annu. Rev. Biochem.*, 67, 793–819, 1998.
4. McKinley, M.P., Bolton, D.C., and Prusiner, S.B., A protease-resistant protein is a structural component of the scrapie prion, *Cell*, 35, 57–62, 1983.
5. Prusiner, S.B., Novel proteinaceous infectious particles cause scrapie, *Science*, 216, 136–144, 1982.
6. Beck, E., Daniel, P.M., Matthews, W.B., et al., Creutzfeldt–Jakob disease. The neuropathology of a transmission experiment, *Brain*, 92, 699–716, 1969.
7. Bendheim, P.E., The human spongiform encephalopathies, *Neurol. Clin.*, 2, 281298, 1984.
8. Collinge, J., Harding, A.E., Owen, F., et al., Diagnosis of Gerstmann-Straussler syndrome in familial dementia with prion protein gene analysis, *Lancet*, 2, 15–17, 1989.
9. Goldfarb, L.G., Petersen, R.B., Tabaton, M., et al., Fatal familial insomnia and familial Creutzfeldt–Jakob disease: Disease phenotype determined by a DNA polymorphism, *Science*, 258, 806–808, 1992.
10. Manetto, V., Medori, R., Cortelli, P., et al., Fatal familial insomnia: Clinical and pathologic study of five new cases, *Neurology*, 42, 312–319, 1992.
11. Medori, R., Tritschler, H.J., LeBlanc, A., et al., Fatal familial insomnia, a prion disease with a mutation at codon 178 of the prion protein gene, *N. Engl. J. Med.*, 326, 444–449, 1992.

12. Dormont, D., Unconventional transmissible agents or prions, *Rev. Prat.*, 44, 882–887, 1994.
13. Collinge, J., Sidle, K.C., Meads, J., et al., Molecular analysis of prion strain variation and the aetiology of 'new variant' CJD, *Nature*, 383, 685–690, 1996.
14. Collinge, J. and Rossor, M., A new variant of prion disease, *Lancet*, 347, 916–917, 1996.
15. Will, R. and Zeidler, M., Diagnosing Creutzfeldt–Jakob disease, *BMJ*, 313, 833–834, 1996.
16. Scott, M.R., Will, R., Ironside, J., et al., Compelling transgenetic evidence for transmission of bovine spongiform encephalopathy prions to humans, *Proc. Natl. Acad. Sci. U. S. A.*, 96, 15137–15142, 1999.
17. Bradley, R. and Liberski, P.P., Bovine spongiform encephalopathy (BSE): The end of the beginning or the beginning of the end?, *Folia Neuropathol.*, 42 Suppl A, 55–68, 2004.
18. Llewelyn, C.A., Hewitt, P.E., Knight, R.S., et al., Possible transmission of variant Creutzfeldt–Jakob disease by blood transfusion, *Lancet*, 363, 417–421, 2004.
19. Peden, A.H., Head, M.W., Ritchie, D.L., et al., Preclinical vCJD after blood transfusion in a *PRNP* codon 129 heterozygous patient, *Lancet*, 264, 527–529, 2004.
20. Schiermeier, Q., Testing times for BSE, *Nature*, 409, 658–659, 2001.
21. Soto, C., Diagnosing prion diseases: Needs, challenges and hopes, *Nat. Rev. Microbiol.*, 2, 809–819, 2004.
22. Ironside, J.W., McCardle, L., Horsburgh, A., et al., Pathological diagnosis of variant Creutzfeldt–Jakob disease, *APMIS*, 110, 79–87, 2002.
23. Collinge, J., Beck, J., Campbell, T., et al., Prion protein gene analysis in new variant cases of Creutzfeldt–Jakob disease, *Lancet*, 348, 56, 1996.
24. Mitrova, E., Mayer, V., Jovankovicova, V., et al., Creutzfeldt–Jakob disease risk and PRNP codon 129 polymorphism: Necessity to revalue current data, *Eur. J. Neurol.*, 12, 998–1001, 2005.
25. Ironside, J.W., Variant Creutzfeldt–Jakob disease: Risk of transmission by blood transfusion and blood therapies, *Haemophilia.*, 12 Suppl 1, 8–15, 2006.
26. Angers, R.C., Browning, S.R., Seward, T.S., et al., Prions in skeletal muscles of deer with chronic wasting disease, *Science*, 317, 1117, 2006.
27. Lasmezas, C.I., Putative functions of PrP(C), *Br. Med. Bull.*, 66, 61–70, 2003.
28. Klamt, F., Dal Pizzol, F., Conte da Frota, M.L., Jr, et al., Imbalance of antioxidant defense in mice lacking cellular prion protein, *Free Radic. Biol. Med.*, 30, 1137–1144, 2001.
29. Graner, E., Mercadante, A.F., Zanata, S.M., et al., Cellular prion protein binds laminin and mediates neuritogenesis, *Brain Res. Mol. Brain Res.*, 76, 85–92, 2000.
30. Chiarini, L.B., Freitas, A.R., Zanata, S.M., et al., Cellular prion protein transduces neuroprotective signals, *EMBO J.*, 21, 3317–3326, 2002.
31. Mallucci, G.R., Ratte, S., Asante, E.A., et al., Post-natal knockout of prion protein alters hippocampal CA1 properties, but does not result in neurodegeneration, *EMBO J.*, 21, 202–210, 2002.
32. Jones, E.M. and Surewicz, W.K., Fibril conformation as the basis of species- and strain-dependent seeding specificity of mammalian prion amyloids, *Cell*, 121, 6372, 2005.
33. Caughey, B., Prion protein conversions: Insight into mechanisms, TSE transmission barriers and strains, *Br. Med. Bull.*, 66, 109–120, 2003.

34. Martinsen, T.C., Taylor, D.M., Johnsen, R., et al., Gastric acidity protects mice against prion infection?, *Scand. J. Gastroenterol.*, 37, 497–500, 2002.
35. Mishra, R.S., Basu, S., Gu, Y., et al., Protease-resistant human prion protein and ferritin are cotransported across Caco-2 epithelial cells: Implications for species barrier in prion uptake from the intestine, *J. Neurosci.*, 24, 11280–11290, 2004.
36. Heppner, F.L., Christ, A.D., Klein, M.A., et al., Transepithelial prion transport by M cells, *Nat. Med.*, 7, 976–977, 2001.
37. Yoshida, K., van den Berg, T.K., and Dijkstra, C.D., Two functionally different follicular dendritic cells in secondary lymphoid follicles of mouse spleen, as revealed by CR1/2 and FcR gamma II-mediated immune-complex trapping, *Immunology*, 80, 34–39, 1993.
38. Oldstone, M.B., Race, R., Thomas, D., et al., Lymphotoxin-alpha- and lympho-toxin-beta-deficient mice differ in susceptibility to scrapie: Evidence against dendritic cell involvement in neuroinvasion, *J. Virol.*, 76, 4357–4363, 2002.
39. Blanquet-Grossard, F., Thielens, N.M., Vendrely, C., et al., Complement protein C1q recognizes a conformationally modified form of the prion protein, *Biochemistry*, 44, 4349–4356, 2005.
40. Mabbott, N.A. and MacPherson, G.G., Prions and their lethal journey to the brain, *Nat. Rev. Microbiol.*, 4, 201–211, 2006.
41. Moore, R.A., Vorberg, I., and Priola, S.A., Species barriers in prion diseases—Brief review, *Arch. Virol. Suppl*, 187–202, 2005.
42. Chen, S.G. and Gambetti, P., A journey through the species barrier, *Neuron*, 34, 854–856, 2002.
43. Houston, E.F. and Gravenor, M.B., Clinical signs in sheep experimentally infected with scrapie and BSE, *Vet. Rec.*, 152, 333–334, 2003.
44. Baron, T.G., Madec, J.Y., Calavas, D., et al., Comparison of French natural scrapie isolates with bovine spongiform encephalopathy and experimental scrapie infected sheep, *Neurosci. Lett.*, 284, 175–178, 2000.
45. Hilton, D.A., Pathogenesis and prevalence of variant Creutzfeldt–Jakob disease, *J. Pathol.*, 208, 134–141, 2006.
46. Williams, E.S., Chronic wasting disease, *Vet. Pathol.*, 42, 530–549, 2005.
47. Belay, E.D., Maddox, R.A., Williams, E.S., et al., Chronic wasting disease and potential transmission to humans, *Emerg. Infect. Dis.*, 10, 977–984, 2004.
48. Kong, Q., Huang, S., Zou, W., et al., Chronic wasting disease of elk: Transmissibility to humans examined by transgenic mouse models, *J. Neurosci.*, 25, 7944–7949, 2005.
49. Raymond, G.J., Bossers, A., Raymond, L.D., et al., Evidence of a molecular barrier limiting susceptibility of humans, cattle and sheep to chronic wasting disease, *EMBO J.*, 19, 4425–4430, 2000.
50. Marsh, R.F., Kincaid, A.E., Bessen, R.A., et al., Interspecies transmission of chronic wasting disease prions to squirrel monkeys (*Saimiri sciureus*), *J. Virol.*, 79, 13794–13796, 2005.
51. Andreoletti, O., Simon, S., Lacroux, C., et al., PrPSc accumulation in myocytes from sheep incubating natural scrapie, *Nat. Med.*, 10, 591–593, 2004.
52. Seeger, H., Heikenwalder, M., Zeller, N., et al., Coincident scrapie infection and nephritis lead to urinary prion excretion, *Science*, 310, 324–326, 2005.
53. Ammendrup, S., Summary review of the chronology of the major measures in relation to bovine spongiform encephalopathy (BSE) in the United Kingdom and the European Union, *Acta Vet. Scand. Suppl.*, 91, 19–20, 1999.

54. Miller, M.W. and Conner, M.M., Epidemiology of chronic wasting disease in free-ranging mule deer: Spatial, temporal, and demographic influences on observed prevalence patterns, *J. Wildl. Dis.*, 41, 275–290, 2005.
55. Belay, E.D., Gambetti, P., Schonberger, L.B., et al., Creutzfeldt–Jakob disease in unusually young patients who consumed venison, *Arch. Neurol.*, 58, 1673–1678, 2001.
56. Xie, Z., O'Rourke, K.I., Dong, Z., et al., Chronic wasting disease of elk and deer and Creutzfeldt–Jakob disease: Comparative analysis of the scrapie prion protein, *J. Biol. Chem.*, 2005.
57. Beck, E., Daniel, P.M., and Parry, H.B., Degeneration of the cerebellar and hypothalamoneurohypophysial systems in sheep with scrapie; and its relationship to human system degenerations, *Brain*, 87, 153–176, 1964.
58. Casalone, C., Zanusso, G., Acutis, P., et al., Identification of a second bovine amyloidotic spongiform encephalopathy: Molecular similarities with sporadic Creutzfeldt–Jakob disease, *Proc. Natl. Acad. Sci. U. S. A.*, 101, 3065–3070, 2004.
59. Moynagh, J. and Schimmel, H., Tests for BSE evaluated. Bovine spongiform encephalopathy, *Nature*, 400, 105, 1999.
60. Biffiger, K., Zwald, D., Kaufmann, L., et al., Validation of a luminescence immunoassay for the detection of PrP(Sc) in brain homogenate, *J. Virol. Methods*, 101, 79–84, 2002.
61. http://www.prionics.ch/prionics-e-diagnostics-priostrip-applicationlit.pdf
62. Foster, J.D., Hope, J., and Fraser, H., Transmission of bovine spongiform encephalopathy to sheep and goats, *Vet. Rec.*, 133, 339–341, 1993.
63. Stack, M.J., Balachandran, A., Chaplin, M., et al., The first Canadian indigenous case of bovine spongiform encephalopathy (BSE) has molecular characteristics for prion protein that are similar to those of BSE in the United Kingdom but differ from those of chronic wasting disease in captive elk and deer, *Can. Vet. J.*, 45, 825–830, 2004.
64. Thuring, C.M., Erkens, J.H., Jacobs, J.G., et al., Discrimination between scrapie and bovine spongiform encephalopathy in sheep by molecular size, immunoreactivity, and glycoprofile of prion protein, *J. Clin. Microbiol.*, 42, 972–980, 2004.
65. Stack, M.J., Chaplin, M.J., and Clark, J., Differentiation of prion protein glycoforms from naturally occurring sheep scrapie, sheep-passaged scrapie strains (CH1641 and SSBP1), bovine spongiform encephalopathy (BSE) cases and Romney and Cheviot breed sheep experimentally inoculated with BSE using two monoclonal antibodies, *Acta Neuropathol. (Berl)*, 104, 279–286, 2002.
66. Safar, J., Wille, H., Itri, V., et al., Eight prion strains have PrP(Sc) molecules with different conformations, *Nat. Med.*, 4, 1157–1165, 1998.
67. Safar, J.G., Scott, M., Monaghan, J., et al., Measuring prions causing bovine spongiform encephalopathy or chronic wasting disease by immunoassays and transgenic mice, *Nat. Biotechnol.*, 20, 1147–1150, 2002.
68. Seong, An., Detection of PrP^{Sc} in blood using newly developed multimer detection system, Presented in the "*10th International Transmissible Spongiform Encephalopathies meeting.*" March 7–9 2006, Baltimore, MD, 2006.
69. Orser, C., The Misfolded Protein Diagnostic (MPD) Blood Assay. In "*10th Transmissible Spongiform Encephalopathies Meeting.*" March 7–9, 2006. Baltimore, MD, 2006.
70. Korth, C., Stierli, B., Streit, P., et al., Prion (PrPSc)-specific epitope defined by a monoclonal antibody, *Nature*, 390, 74–77, 1997.

71. Nazor, K.E., Kuhn, F., Seward, T., et al., Immunodetection of disease-associated mutant PrP, which accelerates disease in GSS transgenic mice, *EMBO J.*, 24, 2472–2480, 2005.

72. Šerbec, V.Č., V, Bresjanac, M., Popović, M., Hartman, K.P., Galvani, V., Rupreht, R., Černilec, M., Vranac, T., Hafner, I., and Jerala, R., Monoclonal antibody against a peptide of human prion protein discriminates between Creutzfeldt–Jacob's disease-affected and normal brain tissue, *J. Biol. Chem.*, 279, 3694–3698, 2004.

73. Zou, W.Q., Zheng, J., Gray, D.M., et al., Antibody to DNA detects scrapie but not normal prion protein, *Proc. Natl. Acad. Sci. U. S. A.*, 101, 1380–1385, 2004.

74. Rubenstein, R., Gray, P.C., Wehlburg, C.M., et al., Detection and discrimination of PrPSc by multi-spectral ultraviolet fluorescence, *Biochem. Biophys. Res. Commun.*, 246, 100–106, 1998.

75. Bieschke, J., Giese, A., Schulz-Schaeffer, W., et al., Ultrasensitive detection of pathological prion protein aggregates by dual-color scanning for intensely fluorescent targets, *Proc. Natl. Acad. Sci. U. S. A.*, 97, 5468–5473, 2000.

76. Lasch, P., Schmitt, J., Beekes, M., et al., Antemortem identification of bovine spongiform encephalopathy from serum using infrared spectroscopy, *Anal. Chem.*, 75, 6673–6678, 2003.

77. Wadsworth, J.D., Joiner, S., Hill, A.F., et al., Tissue distribution of protease resistant prion protein in variant Creutzfeldt–Jakob disease using a highly sensitive immunoblotting assay, *Lancet*, 358, 171–180, 2001.

78. Collins, S.J., Lewis, V., Brazier, M.W., et al., Extended period of asymptomatic prion disease after low dose inoculation: Assessment of detection methods and implications for infection control, *Neurobiol. Dis.*, 20, 336–346, 2005.

79. Birkmann, E., Schafer, O., Weinmann, N., et al., Detection of prion particles in samples of BSE and scrapie by fluorescence correlation spectroscopy without proteinase K digestion, *Biol. Chem.*, 387, 95–102, 2006.

80. Fischer, M.B., Roeckl, C., Parizek, P., et al., Binding of disease-associated prion protein to plasminogen, *Nature*, 408, 479–483, 2000.

81. Rhie, A., Kirby, L., Sayer, N., et al., Characterization of 2'-fluoro-RNA aptamers that bind preferentially to disease-associated conformations of prion protein and inhibit conversion, *J. Biol. Chem.*, 278, 39697–39705, 2003.

82. Peretz, D., Towards development of a prion blood test, In *"10th Annual Transmissible Spongiform Encephalopathies Meeting"*. March 7–9, 2006. Baltimore, MD.

83. Caughey, B. and Raymond, G.J., Sulfated polyanion inhibition of scrapie-associated PrP accumulation in cultured cells, *J. Virol.*, 67, 643–650, 1993.

84. Deleault, N.R., Geoghegan, J.C., Nishina, K., et al., Protease-resistant prion protein amplification reconstituted with partially purified substrates and synthetic polyanions, *J. Biol. Chem.*, 280, 26873–26879, 2005.

85. Wilson, S., An animal model evaluation and assay protocol for screening blood for vCJD, In *"10th Annual Transmissible Spongiform Encephalopathies Meeting."* March 7–9, 2006. Baltimore, MD, USA, 2006.

86. Moussa, A., Coleman, A.W., Bencsik, A., et al., Use of streptomycin for precipitation and detection of proteinase K resistant prion protein (PrPsc) in biological samples, *Chem. Commun. (Camb.)*, 973–975, 2006.

87. Perron, H., Immunoassay for the detection of resistant prion protein (prpres) in human plasma using an original combination of chemical ligands, In *"10th Annual Transmissible Spongiform Encephalopathies Meeting"*. March 7–9, 2006. Baltimore, MD, U. S. A., 2006.

88. Kocisko, D.A., Come, J.H., Priola, S.A., et al., Cell-free formation of protease-resistant prion protein, *Nature*, 370, 471–474, 1994.
89. Bessen, R.A., Kocisko, D.A., Raymond, G.J., et al., Non-genetic propagation of strain-specific properties of scrapie prion protein, *Nature*, 375, 698–700, 1995.
90. Saborio, G.P., Permanne, B., and Soto, C., Sensitive detection of pathological prion protein by cyclic amplification of protein misfolding, *Nature*, 411, 810–813, 2001.
91. Soto, C., Saborio, G.P., and Anderes, L., Cyclic amplification of protein misfolding: Application to prion-related disorders and beyond, *Trends Neurosci.*, 25, 390–394, 2002.
92. Castilla, J., Saá, P., Hetz, C., et al., In vitro generation of infectious scrapie prions, *Cell*, 121, 195–206, 2005.
93. Enari, M., Flechsig, E., and Weissmann, C., Scrapie prion protein accumulation by scrapie-infected neuroblastoma cells abrogated by exposure to a prion protein antibody, *Proc. Natl. Acad. Sci. U. S. A.*, 98, 9295–9299, 2001.
94. Bosque, P.J. and Prusiner, S.B., Cultured cell sublines highly susceptible to prion infection, *J. Virol.*, 74, 4377–4386, 2000.
95. Arima, K., Nishida, N., Sakaguchi, S., et al., Biological and biochemical characteristics of prion strains conserved in persistently infected cell cultures, *J. Virol.*, 79, 7104–7112, 2005.
96. Klohn, P.C., Stoltze, L., Flechsig, E., et al., A quantitative, highly sensitive cell-based infectivity assay for mouse scrapie prions, *Proc. Natl. Acad. Sci. U. S. A.*, 100, 11666–11671, 2003.
97. Raymond, G.J., Olsen, E.A., Lee, K.S., et al., Inhibition of protease-resistant prion protein formation in a transformed deer cell line infected with chronic wasting disease, *J. Virol.*, 80, 596–604, 2006.
98. Archer, F., Bachelin, C., Andreoletti, O., et al., Cultured peripheral neuroglial cells are highly permissive to sheep prion infection, *J. Virol.*, 78, 482–490, 2004.
99. Chandler, R.L. and Turfrey, B.A., Inoculation of voles, Chinese hamsters, gerbils and guinea-pigs with scrapie brain material, *Res. Vet. Sci.*, 13, 219–224, 1972.
100. Gibbs, C.J., Jr., Amyx, H.L., Bacote, A., et al., Oral transmission of kuru, Creutzfeldt-Jakob disease, and scrapie to nonhuman primates, *J. Infect. Dis.*, 142, 205–208, 1980.
101. Tateishi, J., Ohta, M., Koga, M., et al., Transmission of chronic spongiform encephalopathy with kuru plaques from humans to small rodents, *Ann. Neurol.*, 5, 581–584, 1979.
102. Peterson, D.A., Wolfe, L.G., Deinhardt, F., et al., Transmission of kuru and Creutzfeldt–Jakob disease to marmoset monkeys, *Intervirology*, 2, 14–19, 1974.
103. Field, E.J., Transmission of kuru to mice, *Lancet*, 1, 981–982, 1968.
104. Gajdusek, D.C., Gibbs, C.J., and Alpers, M., Experimental transmission of a Kuru-like syndrome to chimpanzees, *Nature*, 209, 794–796, 1966.
105. Taylor, D.M., Dickinson, A.G., Fraser, H., et al., Evidence that transmissible mink encephalopathy agent is biologically inactive in mice, *Neuropathol. Appl. Neurobiol.*, 12, 207–215, 1986.
106. Kimberlin, R.H., Cole, S., and Walker, C.A., Transmissible mink encephalopathy (TME) in Chinese hamsters: Identification of two strains of TME and comparisons with scrapie, *Neuropathol. Appl. Neurobiol.*, 12, 197–206, 1986.
107. Miller, M.W. and Williams, E.S., Chronic wasting disease of cervids, *Curr. Top. Microbiol. Immunol.*, 284, 193–214, 2004.

108. Espana, C., Gajdusek, D.C., Gibbs, C.J., Jr., et al., Transmission of Creutzfeldt-Jakob disease to the stumptail macaque (Macaca arctoides), *Proc. Soc. Exp. Biol. Med.*, 149, 723–724, 1975.
109. Espana, C., Gajdusek, D.C., Gibbs, C.J., Jr., et al., Transmission of Creutzfeldt-Jakob disease to the patas monkey (Erythrocebus patas) with cytopathological changes in in vitro cultivated brain cells, *Intervirology*, 6, 150–155, 1975.
110. Tateishi, J., Koga, M., and Mori, R., Experimental transmission of Creutzfeldt-Jakob disease, *Acta Pathol. Jpn.*, 31, 943–951, 1981.
111. Tateishi, J., Doi, H., Sato, Y., et al., Experimental transmission of human subacute spongiform encephalopathy to small rodents. III. Further transmission from three patients and distribution patterns of lesions in mice, *Acta Neuropathol. (Berl)*, 53, 161–163, 1981.
112. Asante, E.A., Linehan, J.M., Desbruslais, M., et al., BSE prions propagate as either variant CJD-like or sporadic CJD-like prion strains in transgenic mice expressing human prion protein, *EMBO J.*, 21, 6358–6366, 2002.
113. Collinge, J., Palmer, M.S., Sidle, K.C., et al., Unaltered susceptibility to BSE in transgenic mice expressing human prion protein, *Nature*, 378, 779–783, 1995.
114. Telling, G.C., Scott, M., Hsiao, K.K., et al., Transmission of Creutzfeldt-Jakob disease from humans to transgenic mice expressing chimeric human-mouse prion protein, *Proc. Natl. Acad. Sci. U. S. A.*, 91, 9936–9940, 1994.
115. Scott, M.R., Peretz, D., Nguyen, H.O., et al., Transmission barriers for bovine, ovine, and human prions in transgenic mice, *J. Virol.*, 79, 5259–5271, 2005.
116. Scott, M.R., Safar, J., Telling, G., et al., Identification of a prion protein epitope modulating transmission of bovine spongiform encephalopathy prions to transgenic mice, *Proc. Natl. Acad. Sci. U. S. A.*, 94, 14279–14284, 1997.
117. Castilla, J., Gutierrez, A.A., Brun, A., et al., Early detection of PrPres in BSE-infected bovine PrP transgenic mice, *Arch. Virol.*, 148, 677–691, 2003.
118. Buschmann, A., Pfaff, E., Reifenberg, K., et al., Detection of cattle-derived BSE prions using transgenic mice overexpressing bovine PrP(C), *Arch. Virol.* (Suppl.) 75–86, 2000.
119. Vilotte, J.L., Soulier, S., Essalmani, R., et al., Markedly increased susceptibility to natural sheep scrapie of transgenic mice expressing ovine PrP, *J. Virol.*, 75, 5977–5984, 2001.
120. Castilla, J., Gutierrez-Adan, A., Brun, A., et al., Subclinical bovine spongiform encephalopathy infection in transgenic mice expressing porcine prion protein, *J. Neurosci.*, 24, 5063–5069, 2004.
121. Browning, S.R., Mason, G.L., Seward, T., et al., Transmission of prions from mule deer and elk with chronic wasting disease to transgenic mice expressing cervid PrP, *J. Virol.*, 78, 13345–13350, 2004.
122. Fischer, M., Rulicke, T., Raeber, A., et al., Prion protein (PrP) with amino-proximal deletions restoring susceptibility of PrP knockout mice to scrapie, *EMBO J.*, 15, 1255–1264, 1996.
123. Buschmann, A. and Groschup, M.H., Highly bovine spongiform encephalopathy-sensitive transgenic mice confirm the essential restriction of infectivity to the nervous system in clinically diseased cattle, *J. Infect. Dis.*, 192, 934–942, 2005.
124. Castilla, J., Brun, A., Diaz-San Segundo, F., et al., Vertical transmission of bovine spongiform encephalopathy prions evaluated in a transgenic mouse model, *J. Virol.*, 79, 8665–8668, 2005.
125. Saá, P., Castilla, J., and Soto, C., Pre-symptomatic detection of prions in blood, *Science*, 313, 92–94, 2006.

126. Eloit, M., Adjou, K., Coulpier, M., et al., BSE agent signatures in a goat, *Vet. Rec.*, 156, 523–524, 2005.
127. Heikenwalder, M., Zeller, N., Seeger, H., et al., Chronic lymphocytic inflammation specifies the organ tropism of prions, *Science*, 307, 1107–1110, 2005.
128. Linsell, L., Cousens, S.N., Smith, P.G., et al., A case-control study of sporadic Creutzfeldt–Jakob disease in the United Kingdom: Analysis of clustering, *Neurology*, 63, 2077–2083, 2004.
129. Montagna, P., Gambetti, P., Cortelli, P., et al., Familial and sporadic fatal insomnia, *Lancet Neurol.*, 2, 167–176, 2003.
130. Sundstrom, D.G. and Dreher, H.M., A deadly prion disease: Fatal familial insomnia, *J. Neurosci. Nurs.*, 35, 300–305, 2003.
131. Gambetti, P., Kong, Q., Zou, W., et al., Sporadic and familial CJD: Classification and characterisation, *Br. Med. Bull.*, 66, 213–239, 2003.
132. Salmona, M., Morbin, M., Massignan, T., et al., Structural properties of Gerstmann-Straussler-Scheinker disease amyloid protein, *J. Biol. Chem.*, 278, 48146–48153, 2003.
133. Brown, P., Transmission of spongiform encephalopathy through biological products, *Dev. Biol. Stand.*, 93, 73–78, 1998.
134. Klatzo, I., Gajdusek, D.C., and Zigas, V., Pathology of kuru, *Lab Invest*, 8, 799–847, 1959.
135. Elliott, H., Gubbins, S., Ryan, J., et al., Prevalence of scrapie in sheep in Great Britain estimated from abattoir surveys during 2002 and 2003, *Vet. Rec.*, 157, 418–419, 2005.
136. Bessen, R.A. and Marsh, R.F., Biochemical and physical properties of the prion protein from two strains of the transmissible mink encephalopathy agent, *J. Virol.*, 66, 2096–2101, 1992.
137. Doherr, M.G., Bovine spongiform encephalopathy (BSE)—Infectious, contagious, zoonotic or production disease?, *Acta Vet. Scand. Suppl.*, 98, 33–42, 2003.
138. Pearson, G.R., Wyatt, J.M., Gruffydd-Jones, T.J., et al., Feline spongiform encephalopathy: Fibril and PrP studies, *Vet. Rec.*, 131, 307–310, 1992.

Section III

Control of Microbial Food Contamination

11

Kosher and Halal Food Laws and Potential Implications for Food Safety

Joe M. Regenstein, Muhammad M. Chaudry, and Carrie E. Regenstein

CONTENTS

The information in this chapter is as accurate as possible at the time of submission. However, the final decision on any application rests with the religious authorities providing supervision. The ruling of the religious authorities may differ from the information presented here.

11.1   Introduction

The objective of this chapter is to describe the kosher and halal laws as they apply in the food industry, particularly the United States, with a special emphasis on how these laws might affect food safety and related issues. To understand their potential impact on food safety, one must have some understanding of how kosher and halal foods are produced, and how important kosher and halal compliance is to consumers.

11.1.1   Kosher and Halal Laws

The kosher (kashrus) dietary laws determine which foods are "fit" or "proper" for consumption by Jewish consumers who observe these laws. The laws are Biblical in origin, coming mainly from the original five books of the Holy Scriptures, the Torah, which has remained unchanged since then but responds to modern needs. At the same time that Moses received the Ten Commandments on Mount Sinai, Jewish tradition teaches that he also received the oral law, which was eventually written down many years later in a text know as the Talmud. This oral law is as much a part of the Biblical law as the written text. Over the next 3500 years, the meaning of the Biblical kosher laws have been interpreted and extended by the rabbis to protect the Jewish people from violating any of the fundamental laws, and to address new issues and technologies. The system of Jewish law is referred to as *halacha*.

The halal dietary laws determine which foods are "lawful" or permitted for Muslims. These laws are found in the Quran and the books of Hadith, the Traditions, which together constitute the Sunna of Muslim law. Islamic law is referred to as Shari'ah and has been interpreted by Muslim scholars over the years. The basic principles of the Islamic laws remain definite and unaltered. However, their interpretation and application may change according to the time, place, and the circumstances. Besides the two basic sources of Islamic law, the Quran and the Hadith, other sources of jurisprudence are used in determining the permissibility of food, when a contemporary situation is not explicitly covered in the basic sources. The third source of guidance is called Ijihad, or to exert oneself fully to derive an answer to the problem. This could be accomplished by one or both of the following processes:

1. Ijma, meaning a consensus of opinion, and
2. Qiyas, meaning reasoning by analogy.

Current issues of genetically modified organisms (GMO), animal feed, hormones, etc., are discussed in the light of these two concepts and several other lesser sources of Islamic jurisprudence. Unconventional sources of ingredients, synthetic materials, and innovations in animal slaughter and meat processing are some of the issues Muslim scholars are dealing with in helping the consumers make informed choices.

Why do Jews follow the kosher dietary laws? Many explanations have been given. The following explanation by Rabbi I. Grunfeld summarizes the most widely held ideas about the subject (Grunfeld, 1972).

It is important to note that, unlike the kosher laws that are not health laws, the health aspects of eating are an important consideration with the halal laws. These food laws are viewed by the Jewish community as given to the community by G-d without a need for explanation. Only in modern times have some people felt a need to try to justify them as health laws. For example, the claim that trichinosis in pork was a reason for these laws. There are only two problems with this idea—mummified pork obtained from the Egyptian pyramids did not have any signs of the trichinosis cyst and the incubation period for trichinosis is 10–14 days—making it very unlikely that the cause and effect needed for such a rule would have been figured out at that time. For a more complete discussion of why the kosher laws are not health laws, please see Regenstein (1994).

> "And ye shall be men of a holy calling unto Me, and ye shall not eat any meat that is torn in the field" (Exodus XXII:30). Holiness or self-sanctification is a moral term; it is identical with ... moral freedom or moral autonomy. Its aim is the complete self-mastery of man.
>
> To the superficial observer it seems that men who do not obey the law are freer than law-abiding men, because they can follow their own inclinations. In reality, however, such men are subject to the most cruel bondage; they are slaves of their own instincts, impulses and desires. The first step towards emancipation from the tyranny of

animal inclinations in man is, therefore, a voluntary submission to the moral law. The constraint of law is the beginning of human freedom. ... Thus the fundamental idea of Jewish ethics, holiness, is inseparably connected with the idea of Law; and the dietary laws occupy a central position in that system of moral discipline which is the basis of all Jewish laws.

The three strongest natural instincts in man are the impulses of food, sex, and acquisition. Judaism does not aim at the destruction of these impulses, but at their control and indeed their sanctification. It is the law which spiritualizes these instincts and transfigures them into legitimate joys of life.

Why do Muslims follow the halal dietary laws? The main reason for the observance of the Islamic faith including the halal laws is to follow the Divine Orders.

O ye who believe! Eat of the good things wherewith WE have provided you, and render thanks to ALLAH if it is He whom ye worship. (Quran II:172)

God reminds the believers time and again in the Holy Scripture to eat what is *Halal-un-Tayyaban*, meaning "permitted and good or wholesome."

O, Mankind! Eat of that which is Lawful and Wholesome in the earth ... (Quran II:168)

Eat of the good things. We have provided for your sustenance, but commit no excess therein. (Quran XX:81)

Again in the Quran, Sura 6 entitled "Cattle," Muslims are ordained to eat the meat of animals upon which Allah's name has been invoked. This is generally interpreted as requiring that an invocation be made at the time of slaughtering an animal.

Eat of that over which the name of Allah hath been mentioned, if ye are believers in His revelations. (Quran VI:119)

Although Muslims eat what is permitted specifically or by implication or by deliberate omission, albeit without comment, they avoid eating what is specifically disallowed, such as

And eat not of that whereupon Allah's name hath not been mentioned, for lo, It is abomination. Lo! The devils do inspire their minions to dispute with you. But if ye obey them, ye will be in truth idolators. (Quran VI:122)

The majority of the Islamic scholars are of the opinion that this verse deals with proper slaughtering of the allowed animals.

Since Muslim dietary laws relate to divine permissions and prohibitions, if anyone observes these laws, he/she is rewarded in the hereafter and if one violates these laws, he/she may receive punishment accordingly. The rules for those foods that are not specifically prohibited may be interpreted differently by various scholars. The things that are specifically prohibited are few in number, and are summarized in the following verses:

> Forbidden unto you are: carrion and blood and swine flesh, and that which hath been dedicated unto any other than Allah, and the strangled, and the dead through beating, and the dead through falling from a height, and that which hath been killed by the goring of horns, and the devoured of wild beasts saving that which ye make lawful, and that which hath been immolated to idols. And that ye swear by the divining arrows. This is abomination. (Quran V:3)

Although these permissions and prohibitions are enough for a Muslim to observe the laws, it is believed that the dietary laws are based on health reasons that suggest the impurity or the harmfulness of the prohibited foods.

11.1.2   Kosher and Halal Market

Why are we concerned about kosher and halal in the secular world? Because both kosher and halal are important components of the food business and impact how a company does its food processing, with potential positive and negative benefits to food safety. Most people, even in the food industry, are not aware of the breadth of foods that are under religious supervision. This section provides a short background on the economic aspects that make it important for the food industry to have a better understanding of kosher and halal.

The kosher market according to Integrated Marketing, an advertising agency specializing in the kosher food industry, comprises almost 75,000 products in the United States, about $180 billion worth of products are estimated to have a kosher marking on them. The deliberate consumers of kosher food, i.e., those who specifically look for the kosher mark before purchasing, are estimated to be over 10 million Americans. They are purchasing almost $10 billion worth of kosher product. Annually, almost 10,000 companies produce kosher products and the average U.S. supermarket has 13,000 kosher products. Less than one-third (possibly as low as 20%) of the kosher consumers are Jewish (900,000 year-round consumers). Other consumers who at times find kosher products helpful in meeting their dietary needs include Muslims, along with others such as Seventh Day Adventists, vegetarians, vegans, people with various types of allergies—particularly to dairy, grains, and legumes (which are carefully addressed through Passover products)—and general consumers who value the quality of kosher products, even though there is rarely a one-to-one correlation between kosher and these consumers' needs.

Over the past 30 years many halal markets and ethnic stores have sprung up in the United States, mainly in the major metropolitan areas. Most of the 6–8 million Muslims in North America observe halal laws, particularly the avoidance of pork, but the food industry has, for the most part, ignored this consumer group. Although there are excellent opportunities to be realized in the North American halal market, even more compelling opportunities exist on a worldwide basis as the food industry moves to a more global business model. The number of Muslims in the world is over 1.3 billion and trade in halal products is over $150 billion (Egan, 2002). In many countries halal certification has become necessary for products to be imported.

Although many Muslims purchase non-meat kosher food in the United States, these foods, as we see in Section 11.6, do not always meet the needs of the Muslim consumer. The most common areas of concern for the Muslim consumer when considering purchasing kosher products are the use of various questionable gelatins in products produced by more lenient kosher supervisions and the use of alcohol as a carrier for flavors, as well as a food ingredient in all kosher products. The detailed concerns for both of these ideas will be developed later in this paper.

11.2 Kosher

11.2.1 Kosher Dietary Laws

The all-year-round kosher dietary laws predominantly deal with three issues, all focused on the animal kingdom:

1. The allowed animals
2. The prohibition of blood
3. The prohibition of mixing of milk and meat

Additionally, for the week of Passover (in late March or April) restrictions on *chometz*, the prohibited grains (wheat, rye, oats, barley, and spelt) in other than unleavened form—and the rabbinical extensions of this prohibition—lead to a whole new set of regulations, focused in this case on the plant kingdom.

In this chapter we also discuss additional laws dealing with special issues such as grape juice, wine, and alcohol derived from grape products; Jewish supervision of milk; Jewish cooking, cheese making, and baking; equipment kosherization; purchasing new equipment from non-Jews; and old and new flour.

The kosher laws are an internally consistent logic system and have an implied science behind them—which may or may not agree with modern science. This system is the basis upon which rabbis work through problems and come up with a solution.

11.2.2 Allowed Animals

Ruminants with split hoofs that chew their cud, the traditional domestic birds, and fish with fins and removable scales are generally permitted. Pigs, wild birds, sharks, dogfish, catfish, monkfish, and similar species are prohibited as are all crustacean and molluscan shellfish. Almost all insects are prohibited such that carmine and cochineal, which are used as natural red pigments, are not permitted in kosher products by most rabbinical supervisors. However, honey and shellac (lac resin) are permitted, as discussed later in this section.

Four classes of prohibited animals are specifically described in the Torah. These are simply those animals that have one kosher sign but not both. For example, the rock badger, the hare, and the camel chew their cud but do not have a split hoof; the pig has a split hoof but does not chew its cud. Neither category is more or less non-kosher than other non-kosher animals; none are kosher, and they are listed specifically only to clarify the text. In modern times, the prohibition of pork has often been the focus of most people with respect to both the kosher and halal laws, since pork is such a major item of commerce.

With respect to poultry, the traditional domestic birds, i.e., chicken, turkey, squab, duck, and goose are kosher. Birds in the rattrie category (ostrich, emu, and rhea) are not kosher as the ostrich is specifically prohibited in the Bible (Lev. XI:16). Another issue deals with tradition, e.g., newly discovered birds may not be acceptable. Some rabbis do not accept wild turkey (and a few even the domesticated turkey), while some are not accepting the featherless chicken (a natural genetic mutant).

The only animals from the sea that are permitted are those with fins and scales. All fish with scales have fins, so the focus is on the scales. These must be visible to the human eye and must be removable from the fish skin without tearing the skin. A few fish remain controversial, especially swordfish, whose scales do not seem to belong to any of the biologists standard scale types. The Conservative movement also permits sturgeon, which most Orthodox authorities consider non-kosher.

Most insects are not kosher. The exception includes a few types of grasshoppers, which are acceptable in the parts of the world where the tradition of eating them has not been lost. The edible insects are all in the grasshopper family identified as permitted in the Torah due to their unique "jumping" movement. Again, only visible insects are of concern; an insect that spends its entire life cycle inside a single food is not of concern, e.g., many rule that the cod and seal worms fit this category. The recent development of exhaustive cleaning methods to prepare prepackaged salad vegetables eliminates a lot of the insects that are sometimes visible, rendering the product kosher and, therefore, usable in kosher foodservice establishments and in the kosher home without requiring extensive special inspection procedures. Presumably, this whole produce of washing and insect removal should make these products cleaner and safer, especially with some of the concerns for hand washing by workers in the fields. However, most recently some rabbis have been questioning the validity of the process. Kosher consumers have appreciated the use of pesticides to keep products insect free. Modern integrated pest management (IPM) programs that increase the level of insect infestation in fruits and vegetables can cause problems for the kosher consumer. Honey and other products from bees are covered by a unique set of laws that essentially permits honey and beeswax. Most rabbis extend this permission to the use of lac resin or shellac, which is used in candy and fruit coatings to provide a shine.

11.2.3   Prohibition of Blood

Ruminants and fowl must be slaughtered according to Jewish law by a specially trained religious slaughterman (*shochet*) using a special knife designed for the purpose (*chalef*). The knife must be extremely sharp and have a very straight blade that is at least twice the diameter of the neck of the animal to be slaughtered. It is the process itself, and the strict following of the law, that makes a product kosher, and not the presence or absence of a blessing over the food. However, prior to slaughter the shochet does make a blessing. The animal is not stunned prior to slaughter. If the slaughter is done in accordance with Jewish law and with the highest standards of modern animal handling practices, the animal will die without showing any signs of stress. In 1958, the U.S. Congress declared kosher slaughter and similar systems, (e.g., such as halal) to be humane, but included an exemption for preslaughter handling of the animal prior to kosher and halal slaughter. To deal with problems due to inappropriate preslaughter handling, the Food Marketing Institute, the trade association for many North American supermarkets, and the National Council of Chain Restaurants are developing a set of animal welfare-based kosher and halal standards for upright slaughter based on the American Meat Institutes guidelines that have existed for a number of years. Some of the more fervently Orthodox groups do require upside down slaughter, and appropriate systems and procedures for this system are being developed in conjunction with the rabbis.

Slaughtered animals are subsequently inspected for visible internal organ defects by rabbinically trained inspectors. If an animal is found to have a defect, the animal is deemed unacceptable and becomes *treife*. There is no "trimming" of defective portions as generally permitted under secular law. This is viewed by some consumers as a reason to choose kosher, i.e., problem animals are eliminated from the kosher food supply. The general rule is that the defect would not lead to a situation where the animal could be expected to die within a year. Some rabbis invoke these rules in dealing with issues related to veterinary practices, e.g., injections into certain parts of the animal's anatomy such as the neck of a chicken. This can at times limit the options for dealing with animal health of producers for these markets.

As the major site of halachic defects, the lungs must always be inspected. Other organs are spot-checked or examined when a potential problem is observed. Meat that meets this strict standard is referred to as *glatt kosher*, referring to the fact that the animal's lungs (specifically large animals such as cattle) do not have more than two adhesions (*sirkas*). The *bodek*, or the inspector of the internal organs, looks for lung adhesions both before and after the lungs are removed from the lung cavity. All *sirkas* are removed and then the lung is blown up using normal human air pressure. The lung is then put into a water tank and the *bodek* looks for air bubbles. If the lung is still intact, it is kosher. At this time we do not have a full understanding of what animal handling practices lead to higher incidences of lung adhesions, although pneumonia in the calf is certainly one consideration. However, the concept is that kosher leads to the use of healthier animals. For practical reasons, i.e., because they cannot pass this inspection, culled dairy cows are not generally slaughtered and so the threat of mad cow disease (BSE) is reduced.

Meat and poultry must be further prepared by properly removing certain veins, arteries, prohibited fats, blood, and the sciatic nerve. This process is called *nikkur* in Hebrew and *treiboring* in Yiddish. In practical terms, this means that only the front quarter cuts of kosher red meat are used in the United States and most Western countries. These are the cheaper cuts and have at times led to the use of higher USDA meat grades, e.g., prime and choice, which are more highly marbled, a possible health concern.

To further remove the prohibited blood, red meat and poultry must then be soaked and salted (*melicha*) within 72 h of slaughter. If this is not possible, then non-glatt meat is specially washed (*begissing*) and this wash procedure may be repeated for up to two more times, each time within 72 h of the previous washing. The soaking is done for a half an hour in cool water, thereafter, the salting is done for 1 h with all surfaces, including cut surfaces and the inside cavity of a chicken, being covered with ample amounts of salt. The salted meat is then rinsed three times. The salted meat must be able to drain throughout and all the blood being removed must flow away freely.

Once the meat is properly koshered, any remaining "red liquid" is no longer considered blood according to *halacha* and the meat can be used without further concern for these issues.

Work by Jim Marsden's group at Kansas State University (Hajmeer et al., 1999) has shown that this salting process does lead to a lower bacterial count so that the process may in fact be an antimicrobial treatment. The other antimicrobial treatments used for meat safety are receiving mixed reviews from the rabbis. The use of heat (steam or hot water) and some of these chemicals before salting and soaking (which usually does not occur until after the meat has been chilled) are not permitted.

The salt used for koshering must be of a crystal size that is large enough so that the crystals do not dissolve within an hour and must be small enough to permit complete coverage of the meat. The salt industry refers to this size of crystal as kosher salt. Although most salt is religiously kosher, the term "kosher" in this case is referring to the grain size. The specific process of salting and soaking meat to make it ready for use is also referred to as koshering meat.

Because of its high blood content, liver cannot be soaked and salted, but must instead be broiled to at least over half cooked using special equipment reserved for this purpose. The liver is then rinsed, after which the liver can be used in any way the user wishes.

Some concern has been raised about the salt level in kosher meat given the interest in low salt diets. Note that only the surfaces are salted, generally using primal cuts, i.e., 20–40 lb pieces of meat, and that the penetration of the salt is less than a half centimeter in red meat (NY Department of Agriculture and Markets, personal communication). Many pieces of meat, as consumed, have therefore not been directly subjected to the salt treatment. If salt content in a diet is a very important consideration, then one should cut off all surfaces and not use any of the drippings that come out during cooking. However, much of the salt that goes into the meat at the surface is lost during cooking.

Any ingredients or materials that might be derived from animal sources are generally prohibited because of the difficulty of obtaining them from kosher animals. This includes many products that might be used in foods and dietary supplement, such as emulsifiers, stabilizers, and surfactants, particularly those materials that are fat-derived. Very careful rabbinical supervision would be necessary to ensure that no animal-derived ingredients are included in kosher food products. Almost all such materials are available in a kosher form derived from plant oils. A possible exception might be a normative mainstream gelatin, which is now being produced from *glatt kosher* beef hides or fish (see Section 11.7.1.1). Also some rennet, the cheese-coagulating enzyme, is obtained from the dried fourth stomach of a kosher slaughtered milk-fed calf, but the regular supply is not acceptable. Biotechnology derived chymosin is generally kosher (see Section 11.7.1.2).

11.2.4 Prohibition of Mixing of Milk and Meat

> Thou shalt not seeth the kid in its mother's milk. (Exodus XXIII:19, Exodus XXXIV:26, Deuteronomy XIV:21)

This passage appears three times in the Torah, and is therefore considered a very serious admonition. As a result, the law cannot be violated even for non-food uses such as pet food. Neither can one derive benefit from such a mixture. Therefore, one cannot own a cheeseburger business. The meat side of the equation has been rabbinically extended to include poultry and religiously slaughtered game (not fish) as both meat and poultry need to be inspected, deveined, salted, and soaked. The dairy side includes all milk derivatives.

Keeping meat and milk separate in accordance with kosher law requires that the processing and handling of all materials and products fall into one of three categories:

1. A meat product.
2. A dairy product.
3. A neutral product called "pareve," "parve," or "parev." For words that are transliterations of Hebrew—like pareve—multiple English spellings are acceptable.

The pareve category includes all products that are not classified religiously as meat or dairy. All plant products are pareve along with eggs, fish, honey, and lac resin (shellac). These pareve foods can be used with either meat products or dairy products. However, if they are mixed with meat or dairy they take on the identity of the product they are mixed with, i.e., an egg in a cheese soufflé becomes dairy.

A special set of rules apply to fish. Fish can be eaten at the same meal at which meat is eaten, but it cannot be mixed directly with the meat. The dishes used with the fish are generally kept separate and rinsed before they are used with meat, or vice versa. The original law in the Talmud speaks of a specific concern that one particular type of fish caused people to get sick when they mixed that fish with meat. Since we do not know what fish that is and have no modern evidence that such a problem exists, this rabbinical health concern is no longer valid or necessarily valid according to the Conservative Jewish movement. This rule is a very specific exception to the generalization that kosher laws are not health laws, but this is a rabbinical extension and not a Biblical mandate. Another exception with respect to handling fish: One of the very traditional Chassidic Orthodox groups, Lubavitch or Chabad, also has a tradition of not mixing milk with fish, e.g., not permitting a fish gelatin to be used in yogurt.

To assure the complete separation of milk and meat, all equipment, utensils, pipes, steam, etc., must be of the properly designated category. If plant materials, like fruit juices, are run through a dairy plant, they would be considered dairy under kosher law. Some kosher supervision agencies would permit such a product to be listed as "dairy equipment (D.E.)" rather than "dairy." The D.E. tells the consumer that it does not contain any intentionally added dairy ingredients, but that it was made on dairy equipment (see Section 11.5). If a product with no meat ingredients is made in a meat plant, like a vegetarian vegetable soup, it may be marked "meat equipment (M.E.)." A significant wait is normally required to use a product with dairy ingredients after one has eaten meat. This can range from 3 to 6 h depending on the customs (*minhag*) of the area from which the husband came.

With the D.E. listing, the consumer can use the D.E. product immediately before or after a meat meal but not with a meat meal. Following dairy, the wait before eating meat is much less, usually from a "rinse of the mouth" with water to 1 h. Certain dairy foods do require the full wait of 3–6 h, i.e., when a hard cheese is eaten, the wait is the same as that for meat to dairy. A hard cheese is defined as a cheese that has been aged for over 6 months or one that is particularly dry and hard like many of the Italian cheeses. Thus, most companies producing kosher cheese usually age their cheese for less than 6 months although with proper consumer packaging marking this is not a religious requirement.

If one wants to make an ingredient or product truly pareve, the plant equipment must undergo a process of equipment kosherization (see Section 11.4.1). From a marketing stand point, a pareve designation is most desirable since it has the most uses, both for the kosher and for the non-kosher consumers.

11.3   Kosher: Special Foods

11.3.1   Grape Products

To be kosher, all grape juice-based products can only be handled by Sabbath-observing Jews from grape-pressing to final processing. If the juice is pasteurized (heated or *mevushal* in Hebrew), then it can be handled by any worker, as an ordinary kosher ingredient. If a liquid bottling line, e.g., a soda line, uses a product with non-kosher grape juice, the line would have to be cleaned (rinsed) out before proceeding to make kosher products.

11.3.2   Jewish Cheese (*Gevinas Yisroel*)

Similar to the laws concerning kosher wine production, most kosher supervision organizations require that the supervising rabbi add the coagulating agent, i.e., the agent that makes the cheese form curd, into the vat to ensure that the cheese is kosher. Any cheese that does not meet this requirement is unacceptable.

If all the ingredients and equipment used during cheese making are kosher, the whey will be kosher as long as the curd and whey have not been heated above 120°F (49°C) before the whey is drained off. This is true even if a rabbi has not added the coagulant. Thus, there is much more kosher whey available in the United States than kosher cheese. To produce kosher whey, several manufacturers of Swiss cheese, which has one of the most desirable, whitest wheys, have reduced the temperature at which they work the curds in the hot whey. Instead of using the traditional 125°F–127°F (52°C–53°C), they are using a temperature under 120°F (49°C) to work the curds and to obtain a kosher whey. But there are other challenges to be overcome to make kosher whey. Much of the whey is produced in spray driers, which are among the most difficult pieces of equipment to kosherize.

Another problem deals with whey cream. Any cream that is separated from cheese at above 120°F (49°C) is subject to the restrictions that come with cheese and is generally not considered kosher. This cream has recently been used to produce butter, which is therefore not considered kosher. Most rabbis had traditionally accepted butter as kosher without supervision as is still the case with milk. The transition to requiring kosher supervision of butter has been difficult. A more detailed article on this, and closely related kosher dairy issues, has been published in 2002 (Regenstein and Regenstein, 2002a,b,c).

11.3.3 *Cholev Yisroel*

Some kosher-observant Jews are concerned about possible adulteration of milk with the milk of non-kosher animals, such as mare's milk or camel's milk, and therefore require that the milk be watched from the time of milking. This *cholev yisroel* milk is required by some of the strict kosher supervision agencies for all dairy ingredients. Rabbis who accept non-*cholev yisroel* milk in the United States do so for two reasons. First, they believe that the laws in the United States and many other countries are strong enough to assure that adulteration with other milks does not occur. Second, the non-kosher milks are worth more money than kosher milks, so there is no incentive to add non-kosher milk to the milk of kosher species.

11.3.4 *Yashon* (Old) and *Chodesh* (New) Flour

On the second day of Passover, Jews traditionally brought a grain offering to the Temple in Jerusalem. This served to bless all of the flour that was growing or had already been harvested on that day. Such flour has attained the status of *yashon* (old) flour. All wheat for flour that has not started to grow by the second day of Passover is considered *chodesh* (new) and should not be used until the next Passover. For all intensive purposes, the new grain should have been planted more than 14 days before the second day of Passover, the minimum time assumed necessary for the seeds to germinate. All winter wheat from the northern hemisphere is automatically considered *yashon*. It is more difficult to assure the *yashon* status of spring wheat, which generally is harvested in August.

11.3.5 Early Fruit

Another kosher law concerning plants is the requirement that tree fruits not be harvested for benefit until the fourth year. This has been particularly problematic with respect to papaya, a tree fruit that is often not kept alive for 4 years! Discussion and disagreement remains at this time.

11.3.6 Passover

The Passover holiday occurs in spring and requires observant Jews to avoid eating most products made from five prohibited grains: wheat, rye, oats, barley, and spelt (Hebrew: chometz). Those observing kosher laws can only eat the specially supervised unleavened bread from wheat (Hebrew: *matzos*) that are prepared especially for the holiday. Once again, some matzos, i.e., *schmura* (watched) matzos are made to a stricter standard with rabbinical inspection beginning in the field. For other Passover matzo the supervision does not start until the wheat is about to be milled into flour. Matzo made from oats and spelt are now available for consumers with allergies.

Special care is taken to assure that the matzo does not have any time or opportunity to "rise." In some cases this literally means that products are made in cycles of less than 18 min. In continuous large-scale operations, the equipment is constantly vibrating so that there is no opportunity for the dough to rise.

Why 18 min? Note that the word for "life" is the two letter Hebrew word *chai*. The drinking toast among Jews is *L'Chaim*, "to life." Since the Hebrew alphabet is "mapped" to numbers (e.g., Aleph = 1, Bet = 2), the word *chai* equals the number 18! Thus during fermentation, "life" is considered to require 18 min to occur. Anything made in less than 18 min has not fermented and has, therefore, not violated the prohibitions of Passover.

In the middle ages, the rabbis of Europe also made products derived from corn, rice, legumes, mustard seed, buckwheat, and some other plants (Hebrew: *kitnyos*) prohibited for Passover. In addition to the actual flours of these materials, many contemporary rabbis also prohibit derivatives such as corn syrup, cornstarch, and cornstarch derivatives such as citric acid. A small number of rabbis permit the oil from kitnyos materials, or liquid kitnyos products and their derivatives such as corn syrup. The major source of sweeteners and starches used for production of sweet Passover items is either real sugar or potato-derived products such as potato syrup.

Rabbis are concerned with other foodstuffs that are being raised in areas where wheat and other Passover grains are grown. Because of possible cross-contamination some crops such as fennel and fenugreek are also prohibited for Passover.

During the dark ages, the Jewish communities within Christian countries did not have regular contact with Jews living in Muslim countries. The laws governing these two communities began to drift apart. As a result, today's European, or Ashkenazic Jewish community has significantly different laws and customs from the Sephardic Jewish community, which included Spain, North Africa, and the Middle East. Sephardic custom, which is the default in Israel, includes among other rules, no ban on all or some of the kitnyos materials like rice, a *beit yosef* meat standard of absolutely no lung adhesions for all animals, and a willingness to use hind-quarter that has been correctly subject to *nikkur* or deveining, including removal of the sciatic nerve.

Passover is a time of large family gatherings but requires two additional sets of dishes specifically for Passover, one meat and one dairy. Overall, 40% of kosher sales for the traditional kosher companies such as Manischewitz, Rokeach, and Kedem occur for the week of Passover. Stores generally begin to make Passover products available to consumers between 4 and 6 weeks before Passover. Consumers who regularly use products such as dietary supplements, and non-life threatening drugs will be concerned about obtaining a version of their favorite and required product that is acceptable for Passover. For drugs, the prohibition of chometz is of special concern since many Jews do not want any manner of chometz in their home, including drugs, pet feeds, and non-food items such as rubbing alcohol.

The most stringent kosher consumers only eat whole unbroken matzos on the first 7 days of Passover, the 7 days observed by Jews everywhere including Israel. Thus, any prepared food for those 7 days (the Biblically commanded time) may need to be made without the use of any matzo meal or matzo flour, i.e., no *gebruckts* (no broken matzos, no wetting). However, on the eighth day—which is a rabbinical extension of Passover outside of the land of Israel—these people will also eat products made with less than whole matzos.

It is a challenge to make Passover food products that are tasty and have a decent texture with all the limitations of Passover. The kosher community welcomes the assistance of food scientists and the food industry to develop more and better Passover products.

11.4   Kosher: Other Processing Issues

11.4.1   Equipment Kosherization

There are three ways to make equipment kosher or to change its status back to pareve from dairy or meat. Rabbis generally frown on going from meat to dairy or vice versa. Most industrial conversions are from dairy to pareve or from *treife* to one of the categories of kosher. There are a range of process procedures to be considered, depending on the equipment's prior production history.

After a plant, or a processing line, has been used to produce kosher pareve products, it can be switched to either kosher dairy or kosher meat without a special equipment kosherization step. It can also subsequently be used for halal production (from pareve or dairy lines, not always from meat lines), and then, finally, for non-kosher products. In many cases, a *mashgiach*, i.e., the rabbinically approved kosher supervisor, is needed on site for equipment kosherization, so it normally is beneficial to minimize the number of change-overs from one status to another.

The simplest equipment kosherization occurs with equipment that has only been handled cold. This requires a good liquid caustic or liquid soap cleaning, i.e., the type of cleaning done normally in most food plants. Some plants do not normally do a wet clean-up between runs, e.g., a dry powder packing plant or a chocolate line, and these would need to seek specific rabbinical guidance for the change-over. In recent years, allergy concerns have eliminated some such conversions. Materials such as ceramics, rubber, earthenware, and porcelain cannot be koshered because they are considered not "capable" of releasing the flavors trapped within them during the equipment kosherization process. If these materials are found in a processing plant, new materials may be required for production.

Most food processing equipment is operated at cooking temperatures, generally above 120°F (49°C), the temperature that is rabbinically defined as "cooking." However, the exact temperature for cooking depends on the individual rabbi, in that it is the temperature at which he must immediately remove his hand when he puts it into hot water. Recently, through an agreement by the major four mainstream American kosher certifying agencies, most normative kosher supervision agencies in the United States have settled on 120°F (49°C) as the temperature at which foods are cooked and this figure is used throughout this paper (see Section 11.7.2.1).

Equipment that has been used with cooked product must be thoroughly cleaned with liquid caustic or soap before being kosherized. The equipment must then be left idle for 24 h, after which it is "flooded" with boiling water being defined as water between 190°F (88°C) and 212°F (100°C), in the presence of a kosher supervisor. The details depend on the equipment being kosherized. In some cases, particularly foodservice establishments, a "pogem" (bittering agent, often ammonia) is used in boiling water in lieu of the 24 h wait and followed up with an immersion in clean boiling water. All these special activities, therefore, lead to extra cleaning of food plant equipment.

The principles concerning koshering by *hagalah* (boiling water) or *irui* (boiling water poured over a surface) are based on an ancient understanding of the movement of *taam* (flavor) in and out of solid materials. The concepts of *taam* and its movement between products are also used to analyze the many possible combinations of kosher meat, kosher dairy, and non-kosher products interacting accidentally, i.e., for analysis only "after the fact" (*b'de-eved*) and unintentionally. For real accidents, the rabbis are able to be more lenient than they might be for things that are done intentionally (*l'chatchilla*, i.e., planned ahead of time). In modern times, where kosher supervision in the United States is active, i.e., the rabbis are operating with a contractual agreement and ongoing inspections, there is less room to use leniencies. In Europe, where rabbis may only make informal visits to plants and report on their visits to their congregants and the greater Jewish community, the rules with respect to after the fact nullification can sometimes be used more freely—since the rabbi cannot control any changes made in the processing after he has left the plant, i.e., between visits.

In the case of ovens or other equipment that uses fire, or dry heat, kosherization involves heating the metal until it glows. Again, the supervising rabbi is generally present while this process is taking place. In the case of ovens, particularly large commercial ovens, issues related to odor/vapors and steam must also be considered. Sometimes the same oven can be used sequentially for alternating pareve and dairy baking. The details are beyond the scope of this paper and require a sophisticated rabbinical analysis to determine which ovens can be used for more than one status without requiring kosherization.

The procedures that must be followed for equipment kosherization, especially for hot equipment, can be quite extensive and time consuming—so the fewer status conversions, the better. Careful formulating of products and good production planning can minimize the inconvenience. If a conversion is needed, it is often scheduled for early Monday morning, before the production week starts.

11.4.2   Jewish Cooking and Jewish Baking

In some cases it is necessary for the rabbis to "do" the cooking (*Bishul Yisroel*). Often this means turning on the pilot light. As long as the pilot light remains lit, the rabbi does not have to be present; if it goes out, he must return. With electrical equipment and appliances, it is possible to keep electricity on all the time, using the lowest setting when actual heating is not taking place.

Baking generally requires Jewish participation, *Pas Yisroel*, i.e., the Jew must start the ovens. In addition, if the owner of the bakery is Jewish, there may be a requirement for "taking challah," a portion of the dough that is removed and needs to be specially handled. Again, the details need to be worked out with the supervising rabbi.

Note that a company that is over 50% Jewish management or Jewish ownership is subject to stricter rules, e.g., the taking of challah and the need to observe the Sabbath and other Jewish holidays. To work with the less strict rules, some owners sell their business to a gentile for the period of concern, even a single day each week. This is a legally binding contract and, in theory, the gentile owner can renege on his or her informal agreement to legally sell it back. On Passover, the need to do this can be more critical: Any chometz in the possession of a Jew during Passover is forever prohibited in a kosher home, i.e., if a Jewish grocery store receives a shipment of bread during Passover, that bread, even if marked as kosher, though obviously non-Passover, can never be used by an observant kosher-observing Jew.

11.4.3   Toveling (Immersing Equipment Purchased from a Gentile)

When a Jewish company purchases or takes new or used equipment from gentiles, the equipment must be immersed in a ritual bath (*mikvah*) before the equipment is kosherized. Equipment made from metal and glass requires a blessing; complex items that contain glass or metal may need to be toveled but may not need a blessing. A *mashgiach* needs to be present for this activity. A natural body of water can be used instead of the indoor *mikvah*, especially with large equipment.

11.4.4 Tithing and Other Israeli Agricultural Laws

In ancient times, products from Israel were subject to special rules concerning tithing for the priests, their helpers, the poor, etc. These are complex laws that only affect products from Israel. The land of Israel is also subject to the Sabbath (sabbatical) years, i.e., crops from certain years cannot be used. These additional requirements challenge kosher consumers in the United States who are interested in purchasing and using Israeli products. Rabbis in Israel arrange for companies to tithe when the products are destined for sale in Israel, but rarely for exports. The details of this process are beyond the scope of this paper.

11.5   Kosher and Allergies

Many consumers use the kosher markings as a guideline to determine whether food products might meet their special needs including allergies. There are, however, limitations that the particularly sensitive allergic consumer needs to keep in mind.

1. When the equipment is kosherized—or converted from one status to another—the procedure may not yield 100% removal of previous materials run on the equipment. This became an issue some years ago when rabbis discovered that the special procedures being used to convert a dairy chocolate line to a pareve chocolate line led to enough dairy contamination that consumers who were very sensitive to dairy allergens were having problems. These lines are koshered without water: either a hot oil or pareve chocolate is run through the line in a quantity sufficient to remove any dairy residual as calculated by the supervising rabbi.

Both Islam and Judaism do not permit practices to occur that will endanger life. As a result, rabbis decided that none of the current religiously acceptable methods for equipment kosherization of chocolate are effective enough to move between dairy and pareve production. Therefore, mainstream kosher supervision agencies no longer permit this conversion. Another problem with plants running both types of chocolate is the possible cross-contamination by powdered milk dust. This would not affect the kosher status of the product but is obviously not acceptable for allergenic concerns.

2. Kosher law does permit certain ex post facto (after the fact) errors to be negated. Trace amounts of materials accidentally added to a

food can be nullified if the amount of "offending" material is less than 1/60 by volume under very specific conditions, i.e., truly added by accident. However, some items can never be negated, e.g., strong flavor compounds that make a significant impact on the product even at less than 1/60. In deference to their industrial client company's desire to minimize negative publicity, many kosher supervision agencies do not announce when they have used this procedure to make a product acceptable. When there is a concern about allergic reactions, however, many rabbis are now more willing to alert the public as soon as possible for health and safety reasons.

Products that might be made in a dairy plant—e.g., pareve substitutes for dairy products and some other liquids like teas and fruit juices—may be produced in plants that have been kosherized, but may not meet a very critical allergy standard. Care in consuming such products is recommended.

3. Labels that say "dairy and meat equipment": There are no intentionally added dairy or meat ingredients, but the product is produced on a dairy or meat line without any equipment kosherization. The product is considered to be like pareve with some additional use restrictions in a kosher home. Again, the more sensitive the allergy, the more caution is advised.

4. In a few instances where pareve or dairy products contain small amounts of fish, such as anchovies in Worcestershire sauce, this ingredient may be marked as part of the kosher supervision symbol. Many certifications do not specifically mark this if the fish in the initial material is less than 1/60 by volume. Someone who is allergic should always read the ingredient label.

5. At Passover there is some dispute about derivatives of kitnyos materials, the non-grain materials that are also prohibited for Ashkenazic Jews. A few rabbis permit items like corn syrup, soybean oil, peanut oil, and similarly derived materials from these extensions. The "proteinaeous" part of these materials is generally not used. Consumers with allergies to these items can therefore purchase these special Passover products from supervision agencies that do not permit kitnyos derivatives. With respect to equipment kosherization: supervising rabbis tend to be very strict about the clean-up of the prohibited grains (wheat, rye, oats, barley, and spelt) so these Passover products come closest to meeting potential allergy concerns; this may not be the case with respect to the products subject to the extended kitnyos prohibitions.

Consumers should not assume that kosher markings ensure the absence of trace amounts of the ingredient to which they are allergic. It is a useful first screen, but products should be carefully tested before assuming everything is okay, i.e., the allergic person should eat a small portion of the product, and increase the amount consumed slowly, over time, to ensure no adverse reaction. People with allergies should get into the habit of checking lot numbers on products and purchasing stable goods with a single lot number in sufficient quantity to meet anticipated needs within the shelf-life expectations of the goods.

How thoroughly are dairy ingredients kept out of a pareve line? The current standard for kosher may not meet the needs of allergic consumers since the dairy powder dust in the air may be sufficient to cause allergy problems? With the new U.S. allergy regulations, a company might indicate that these are religiously pareve, but may not be sufficiently devoid of dairy allergens for very allergic consumers.

11.6   Halal

11.6.1   Halal Dietary Laws

The halal dietary laws define food products as halal (permitted), *haram* (prohibited), and a few items go into the category of *makrooh* (questionable to detestable). The law deals with the following five issues; all but the last are in the animal kingdom:

1. The prohibited animals
2. The prohibition of blood
3. The method of slaughtering/blessing
4. Prohibition of carrion
5. Prohibition of intoxicants

The Islamic dietary laws are derived from the Quran, a revealed book; the Hadith, the traditions of Prophet Muhammad; and through extrapolation of and deduction from the Quran and the Hadith, by Muslim jurists.

There are 11 generally accepted principles pertaining to halal and haram in Islam for providing guidance to Muslims in their customary practices.

1. The basic principle is that all things created by Allah are permitted, with a few exceptions that are prohibited. Those exceptions include pork, blood, meat of animals that died of causes other than proper slaughtering, food that has been dedicated or immolated to someone other than Allah, alcohol, intoxicants, and inappropriately used drugs.
2. To make lawful and unlawful is the right of Allah alone. No human being, no matter how pious or powerful, may take it into his hands to change it.

3. Prohibiting what is permitted and permitting what is prohibited is similar to ascribing partners to Allah. This is a sin of the highest degree that makes one fall out of the sphere of Islam.

4. The basic reasons for the prohibition of things are due to impurity and harmfulness.

A Muslim is not supposed to question exactly why or how something is unclean or harmful in what Allah has prohibited. There might be obvious reasons and there might be obscure reasons. The following rationales might be considered:

Carrion and dead animals are unfit for human consumption because the decaying process leads to the formation of chemicals harmful to humans.

Blood that is drained from an animal contains harmful bacteria, products of metabolism, and toxins.

Swine serves as a vector for pathogenic worms to enter the human body. Infections by *Trichinella spiralis* and *Traenia solium* are not uncommon.

Intoxicants are considered harmful for the nervous system, affecting the senses and human judgment, leading to social and family problems and in some cases even death.

Immolating food to someone other than Allah may imply that there is somebody as important as Allah, that there could be two Gods. This would be against the first tenet of Islam: There Is but One God.

These reasons and explanations, and many more like these, may be acceptable as sound, but the underlying principle behind the prohibitions remains the Divine order: "Forbidden Unto You Are. ..."

5. What is permitted is sufficient and what is prohibited is then superfluous. Allah prohibited only things that are unnecessary or dispensable while providing better alternatives. People can survive and live better without consuming unhealthful carrion, unhealthful pork, unhealthful blood, and the root of many vices, alcohol.

6. Whatever is conducive to the prohibited is in itself prohibited. If something is prohibited, anything leading to it is also prohibited.

7. Falsely representing unlawful as lawful is prohibited. It is unlawful to make flimsy excuses, to consume something that is prohibited, such as drinking alcohol for supposedly medical reasons.

8. Good intentions do not make the unlawful acceptable. Whenever any permissible action of the believer is accompanied by a good intention, his action becomes an act of worship. In the case of

haram, it remains haram, no matter how good the intention or how honorable the purpose may be. Islam does not endorse employing a haram means to achieve a praiseworthy end. The religion indeed insists not only that the goal be honorable, but also that the means chosen to achieve it be lawful and proper. Islamic laws demand that the right should be secured solely through just means.

9. Doubtful things should be avoided. There is a gray area between clearly lawful and clearly unlawful. This is the area of "what is doubtful." Islam considers it an act of piety for the Muslims to avoid doubtful things, for them to stay clear of the unlawful. Prophet Muhammad said:

> The halal is clear and the haram is clear. Between the two there are doubtful matters concerning which people do not know whether they are halal or haram. One who avoids them in order to safeguard his religion and his honor is safe, while if someone engages in a part of them, he may be doing something haram - - -

10. Unlawful things are prohibited to everyone alike. Islamic laws are universally applicable to all races, creeds, and sexes. There is no favored treatment of privileged class. Actually, in Islam, there are no privileged classes; hence, the question of preferential treatment does not arise. This principle applies not only among Muslims, but between Muslims and non-Muslims as well.

11. Necessity dictates exceptions. The range of prohibited things in Islam is quite limited, but emphasis on observing the prohibitions is very strong. At the same time, Islam is not oblivious to the exigencies of life, to their magnitude, or to human weakness and capacity to face them. A Muslim is permitted, under the compulsion of necessity, to eat a prohibited food to ensure survival—but only in quantities sufficient to remove the necessity and avoid starvation.

11.6.2 Prohibited and Permitted Animals

Meat of pigs, boars, and swine is strictly prohibited, as are the carnivorous animals like lions, tigers, cheetahs, cats, dogs, and wolves. Also prohibited are birds of prey like eagles, falcons, osprey, kites, and vultures.

Meat of domesticated animals like ruminants with split hoof, e.g., cattle, sheep, goat, lamb, is allowed for food, as are camels and buffaloes. Also permitted are the birds that do not use their claws to hold down food, such as chickens, turkeys, ducks, geese, pigeons, doves, partridges, quails, sparrows, emus, and ostriches. Some of the animals and birds are permitted only under special circumstances or with certain conditions. Horse meat may be allowed to be consumed under some distressing conditions, discussion of which is beyond the scope of this book. The animals fed unclean or filthy feed, e.g., formulated with biosolids (sewage) or protein from tankage, must be quarantined and placed on clean feed for a period varying from 3 to 40 days before slaughter to cleanse their systems.

Foods from the sea—namely, fish and seafood—are the most controversial among various denominations of Muslims. Certain groups only accept fish with scales as halal, while others consider as halal everything that lives in the water all the time. Consequently, prawns, lobsters, crabs, and clams are halal, but may be detested (*Makrooh*) by some and hence, not consumed. Animals that live both in water and on land (amphibians) such as frogs, turtles, crocodiles, and seals are also not consumed by the majority of observant Muslims.

There is no clear status of insects established in Islam except that locust is specifically mentioned as halal. Insects are generally considered neutral. However, from deduction of the laws, it seems that both helpful insects like bees, ants, and spiders, and harmful or dirty creatures like lice, flies, and mosquitoes are all prohibited as food. Among the byproducts from insects, use of honey was very highly recommended by Prophet Muhammad, PBUH. Other products like royal jelly, wax, shellac, and carmine are acceptable for use without restrictions by most; however, some may consider shellac and carmine *Makrooh* are offensive to their psyche.

Eggs and milk from permitted animals are also permitted for Muslim consumption. Milk from cows, goats, sheep, and buffaloes is halal. Unlike kosher, there is no restriction on mixing meat and milk.

11.6.3 Prohibition of Blood

According to the Quranic verses, blood that pours forth is prohibited for consumption. It includes blood of permitted and non-permitted animals alike. Liquid blood is generally not offered for sale or consumed by Muslims or non-Muslims, but products made with and from blood are available. There is general agreement among Muslim scholars that anything made from blood is unacceptable.

11.6.4 Proper Slaughtering of Permitted Animals

There are special requirements for slaughtering the animal:

1. An animal must be of a halal species.
2. It must be slaughtered by an adult and sane, i.e., mentally competent Muslim.
3. The name of Allah must be pronounced at the time of slaughter.
4. Slaughter must be done by cutting the throat in a manner that induces rapid and complete bleeding, resulting in the quickest death. The generally accepted method is to cut at least three of

the four passages, i.e., carotids, jugulars, trachea, and esophagus. Some Muslim leaders do accept machine slaughter, particularly of poultry. In recent years, however, the trend has gone back toward requiring hand slaughter of these animals.

The meat of animals thus slaughtered is called *zabiha* or *dhabiha* meat.

> Verily Allah has prescribed proficiency in all things. Thus, if you kill, kill well; and if you perform dhabha, perform it well. Let each one of you sharpen his blade and let him spare suffering to the animal he slays (Khan, 1991).

Islam places great emphasis on gentle and humane treatment of animals, especially before and during slaughter. Some of the conditions include giving the animal proper rest and water, avoiding conditions that create stress, not sharpening the knife in front of the animals, using a very sharp knife to slit the throat, etc. Only after the blood is allowed to drain completely from the animal and the animal has become lifeless can the dismemberment, cutting off horns, ears, legs, etc. commence. Thus, the Muslim community has been quite supportive of efforts to improve religious slaughter within the religious framework. Unlike kosher, soaking and salting of the carcass is not required for halal; halal meat is therefore treated like other commercial meat. Animal-derived food ingredients like emulsifiers, tallow, and enzymes must be made from animals slaughtered by a Muslim to be halal.

Hunting of permitted wild animals (like deer) and birds (like doves, pheasants, and quail) is allowed for the purpose of eating but not merely for deriving pleasure out of killing an animal. Hunting during the pilgrimage to Makkah and within the defined boundaries of the holy city of Makkah is strictly prohibited. Hunting is permitted with any tools, e.g., guns, arrows, spears, or trapping. Trained dogs may also be used for catching or retrieving the hunt as long as they do not take even a single bite out of the hunt. The name of Allah may be pronounced at the time of releasing the tool rather than catching of the hunt. The animal has to be bled by slitting the throat as soon as the hunt is caught. If the blessing is made at the time of pulling the trigger or shooting an arrow and the hunted animal dies before the hunter reaches it, it would still be halal as long as slaughter is performed and some blood comes out. Fish and seafood may be hunted or caught by any reasonable means available as long as it is done humanely and no blessing needs to be said.

The requirements of proper slaughtering and bleeding are applicable to land animals and birds. Fish and other creatures that live in water need not be ritually slaughtered. Similarly, there is no special method of killing the locust.

The meat of the allowed land animals that die of natural causes—e.g., diseases, being gored by other animals, being strangled, falling from a height, through beating, or killed by wild beasts—is unlawful to be eaten, unless one saves such animals by slaughtering before they actually become lifeless. Fish that dies naturally and is floating on water or lying out of water is still halal as long as it does not show any signs of decay or deterioration.

11.6.5   Meat of Animals Killed by the *Ahl-al-Kitab*

There has been much discussion and controversy among Muslim consumers as well as Islamic scholars about the permissibility of consuming meat of animals killed by the Ahl-al-Kitab or people of the book, meaning Jews and Christians. The issue focuses on whether meat prepared in the manner practiced by either faith would be permitted for Muslims.

In the Holy Quran, this issue is presented only once in Sura V, verse 6, in the following words:

> This day all good things made lawful for you. The food of those who have received the Scripture is lawful for you, and your food is lawful for them.

This verse addresses the Muslims and seems to establish a social context where Muslims, Jews, and Christians could interact with each other. It points toward two sides of the issue, first, "the food of the people of the book is lawful for you" and second, "your food is lawful for them."

In most discussions, scholars try to deal with the first part (food of Ahl-al-Kitab) and ignore the second part (food of Muslims) altogether, leaving that decision to the people of the book.

As far as the first part of the ruling is concerned, Muslims are allowed to eat the food of the Jews and Christians as long as it does not violate the first part of this verse, "this day all good and wholesome things have been made lawful for you." *Quran 5:6*.

The majority of Islamic scholars are of the opinion that the food of the Ahl-al-Kitab must meet the criteria established for halal and wholesome food including proper slaughter of animals. They believe that the following verse establishes a strict requirement for Muslims.

> And eat not of that whereupon Allah's name hath not been mentioned, for lo! It is abomination. [Quran VI:121]

However some Islamic scholars are of the opinion that the above verse does not apply to the food of Ahl-al-Kitab and there is no need to mention the name of God at the time of slaughtering (Al-Qaradawi, 1984). It is up to the regulatory agencies in the halal food importing countries, halal certifiers for export or domestic consumption, or the individual Muslim consumers to decide how to interpret these verses. However, for clarity in understanding the modern day practices of Ahl-al-Kitab, we would like to offer the following analysis.

1. Christians do not follow a strict food code.
2. Orthodox Jews, who are the only ones slaughtering animals (ruminants and poultry) in their proscribed manner, prepare all kosher meat currently marketed.
3. Orthodox Jewish slaughterers say a blessing at the beginning of a slaughter session but do not pronounce the name of God at the actual time of slaying of each animal although recent rabbinical rulings suggest that a Jewish slaughterman could say the required Muslim prayer at the time of slaughter.

For the Muslims who want to follow requirements of verse VI:121, meat (red meat and poultry) of the Ahl-al-Kitab may not meet halal standards. In addition, as discussed elsewhere in this chapter, processed products, whether meat, dairy, or pareve kosher products may contain alcohol (e.g., in flavors) and some more lenient kosher supervisions as defined above will permit products that contain animal-based ingredients that may also be unacceptable to the halal observing consumer.

11.6.6 Prohibition of Alcohol and Intoxicants

Consumption of alcoholic drinks and other intoxicants is prohibited according to the Quran (V:90–91), as follows:

> O you who believe! Strong drinks and games of chance, and idols and divining arrows are only an infamy of Satan's handiwork. Leave it aside in order that you may prosper. Only would Satan sow hatred and strife among you, by alcohol, and games of chance, and turn you aside from the remembrance of Allah, and from prayer: Will you not, therefore, abstain from them?

The Arabic term used for alcohol in the Quran is *khamr*, which means "that which has been fermented" and implies not only to alcoholic beverages like wine, beer, whiskey, and brandy, but to all things that intoxicate or affect one's thought process. Although there is no allowance for added alcohol in any beverage like soft drinks, small amounts of alcohol contributed from food ingredients may by considered an impurity and hence ignored. Synthetic or grain alcohol may be used in food processing for extraction, precipitation, dissolving, and other reasons, as long as the amount of alcohol remaining in the final product is very small, generally below 0.1%. Each importing country may have its own guidelines, which must be understood by the exporters and strictly adhered to.

In the west, food may be cooked in alcohol to enhance the flavor or to impart distinctive flavor notes. Wine is the most common form of alcohol used in cooking. While one may think that all of the added alcohol evaporates or burns off during cooking, the fact is that it does not. The alcohol retained in the food products varies depending upon the cooking method. The following table gives some of the retained alcohol content of foods prepared by different cooking methods, as reported by the U.S. Department of Agriculture (Larsen, 1995):

Added to boiling liquid and removed from heat	85%
Cooked over a flame	75%
Added without heat and stored overnight	70%
Baked for 25 min without stirring	45%
Mixed then baked or simmered for 15 min	40%
Mixed then baked or simmered for 30 min	35%
Mixed then baked or simmered for 1 h	25%
Mixed then baked or simmered for 2 h	10%
Mixed then baked or simmered for 2½ h	5%

Even after cooking for 2.5 h, up to 5% alcohol remains in the food. Although there is little chance of intoxication by eating such food, the use of alcoholic drinks in cooking is categorically prohibited.

11.6.7   Halal Cooking, Food Processing, and Sanitation

Alcohol may not be used in cooking. Otherwise, there are no restrictions about cooking in Islam, as long as the kitchen is free from haram foods and ingredients.

In food companies, haram materials should be kept segregated from halal materials. The equipment used for non-halal products has to be thoroughly cleansed using proper techniques of acids, bases, detergents, and hot water. As a general rule, kosher cleaning procedures would be adequate for halal too. If the equipment is used for haram products, it must be properly cleaned, sometimes by using an abrasive material, blessed by a Muslim inspector, and finally rinsed with hot water seven times.

11.7   Both Kosher and Halal

11.7.1   Science

11.7.1.1   Gelatin

Important in many food products, gelatin is probably the most controversial of all modern kosher and halal ingredients. Gelatin can be derived from pork skin, beef bones, or beef skin. In recent years, some gelatins from fish skins have also entered the market.

Most currently available gelatins—even if called kosher—are not acceptable to the mainstream U.S. kosher supervision organizations and to the

Muslim community. Many are, in fact, totally unacceptable to halal consumers because they may be pork-based gelatin.

A recent development has been the manufacture of kosher gelatin from the hides of kosher slaughtered cattle. Similarly, at least two major manufacturers are currently producing certified halal gelatin from cattle bones of animals that have been slaughtered by Muslims.

One finds a wide range of attitudes toward gelatin among the lenient kosher supervision agencies. The most liberal view holds that gelatin, being made from bones and skin, is not being made from a food (flesh). Further, the process used to make the product goes through a stage where the product is so unfit that it is not edible by man or dog, and as such becomes a new entity. Rabbis holding this view may accept pork gelatin. Most water gelatin desserts with a generic "K" follow this ruling.

Other rabbis only permit gelatin from beef bones and hides, and not pork. Still other rabbis only accept "India dry bones" as a source of beef gelatin. These bones, found naturally in India from the animals that fall and die in the fields, because of the Hindu custom of not killing the cows, are aged for over a year and are "dry as wood." Again, none of these products is accepted by the mainstream kosher or halal supervisions, and are therefore not accepted by a significant part of the kosher and halal community.

11.7.1.2 Biotechnology

Rabbis and Islamic scholars currently accept products made by simple genetic engineering, e.g., chymosin (rennin) was accepted by the rabbis about half a year before it was accepted by the FDA. The basis for this decision involves the fact that the gene isolated from a non-kosher source is far below "visible." Subsequently, it is copied many times in vitro and then eventually injected into a host that is then reproduced many times. Thus, the original source of the gene is essentially totally lost by the time the food product appears. The production conditions in the fermenters must still be kosher or halal, i.e., the ingredients and the fermenter, and any subsequent processing must use kosher or halal equipment and ingredients of the appropriate status. A product produced in a dairy medium, e.g., extracted from cow's milk, would be dairy. Mainstream rabbis may approve porcine lipase made through biotechnology when it becomes available, if all the other conditions are kosher. The Muslim community is still considering the issue of products with a porcine gene; although a final ruling has not been established, the leaning seems to be toward rejecting such materials. If the gene for a porcine product were synthesized, i.e., it did not come directly from the pig, Muslim leaders must still rule on its acceptability. The religious leaders of both communities have not yet determined the status of more complex genetic manipulations and genetic manipulation of animals; such a discussion is therefore premature.

11.7.1.3   Pet Food

Jews who observe the kosher laws can feed their domestic animals pet food that contains pork or other prohibited meats. They cannot feed their animals with products that contain a mixture of milk and kosher meat. On Passover, their pet food can contain kitnyos, but not chometz. Although pets, even in a halal observant home, can be fed anything, many individual Muslims prefer to use pet foods without pork and other prohibited materials.

11.7.1.4   Health

As described above, the Muslim halal laws are focused on health. Although many people believe that the kosher laws are also considered to be among the laws that were given for people's benefit; this is not the case.

11.7.2   Regulatory

11.7.2.1   Dealing with Kosher and Halal Supervision Agencies

In practical terms, the food industry works with kosher and halal supervision agencies to obtain permission to use the supervision agency's trademark symbol on their products. In this way the industry can make claims in the marketplace that are legal and more important, credible to those intentionally purchasing these products, i.e., this is a third-party audit system. This potential choice provides a significant potential opportunity.

Kosher or halal supervision is taken on by a company to expand its market opportunities. It is a business investment that, like any other investment, must be examined critically in this era of total quality management, just-in-time production, strategic suppliers, etc.

What criteria should a company use to select a supervision agency? Supervision fees must be taken into account, and the agency's name recognition is a consideration. Other important considerations include (1) responsiveness in handling paperwork, in providing *mashgiachs* or Muslim inspectors at the plants as needed on a timely basis, and in doing routine inspections at a defined frequency during the year (anywhere from twice a year to every day including continuous) depending on the nature of the production; (2) willingness to work with the company on problem solving; (3) ability to clearly explain their kosher or halal standards and their fee structure. And, of course, one should consider (4) if the "personal" chemistry is right and (5) if their religious standards meet the company's needs in the marketplace.

One of the hardest issues for the food industry to deal with in day-to-day kosher activities is the existence of so many different kosher supervision agencies. Halal has fewer agencies but still has many standards. How does this impact the food companies? How do the Jewish kosher or Muslim halal consumers perceive these different groups? Because there has not been a central ruling authority for many years in either religion, different rabbis and Muslim inspectors follow different traditions with respect to their dietary standards. Some authorities tend to follow the more lenient standards, while others follow more stringent standards. The trend in the mainstream kosher community today is toward a more stringent standard, because some of the previous leniencies were considered undesirable but were tolerated when fewer alternatives were available. The mainstream Muslim community also seems to be moving toward tighter standards so that approved products are acceptable to a larger audience.

One can generally divide the kosher supervision agencies into three broad categories. First there are the large organizations that dominate the supervision of larger food companies, i.e., the OU (Union of Orthodox Jewish Congregations, Manhattan), the OK (Organized Kashrus Laboratories, Brooklyn), the Star-K (Baltimore), and the Kof-K (Teaneck, New Jersey), all four of which are nationwide and mainstream.

A quick digression to explain the concept of "normative mainstream kosher supervision": The concept of a normative mainstream U.S. kosher standard is the de facto kosher standard in the United States. There are numerous trademarked kosher symbols, over 850 at last count (Wikler, 2006), used around the world. Some are more lenient than the "normative" standard, while others are stricter. The letter "K" cannot be trademarked; any person or company can put a "K" on a product for any reason.

In addition to the national supervision agencies, there are smaller private organizations and many local community organizations that provide equivalent religious standards of supervision. As such, products accepted by any of the normative mainstream organizations will, with an occasional exception, be accepted by other similar organizations.

The second category of kosher supervision (more stringent than normative mainstream) is generally associated with the Hassidic communities, i.e., groups with standards beyond the normative Orthodox standard. Many of the products used in these communities require continuous rabbinical supervision rather than the occasional supervision used by the mainstream organizations for production-line products.

The third level is mainly individual rabbis who are more lenient than the mainstream standard. Many of these rabbis are Orthodox; some may be Conservative. Their standards are based on their interpretation of the kosher laws. Employing a more lenient rabbi means that the food processor cuts out more of the mainstream and stricter markets; this is a retail marketing decision that each company makes for itself. More lenient supervisions are sometimes the only ones that will certify a product with a special problem that causes other supervisions to reject it.

The Muslim community has only one mainstream agency at this time, the Islamic Food and Nutrition Council (IFANCA, Chicago), which is also recognized by many Muslim countries. Other Muslim groups are entering the field, but their standards are not as well defined. Some groups and individuals have resorted to certifying their own products. If one has any interest in exporting to Muslim countries or countries with a significant Muslim population, it is extremely important to know which countries will accept the supervision of which agencies.

In recent years we have started to see products that have dual halal and kosher certification. The first were the military MRE (meals ready-to-eat) meals (Jackson, 2000).

Ingredient companies should be particularly careful in selecting a supervision agency. They should try to use a mainstream kosher or halal supervision agency because most kosher or halal food manufacturing companies will require such supervision. The ability to sell to as many customers as possible requires a broadly acceptable standard. Unless an ingredient is acceptable to the mainstream, it is almost impossible to gain the benefit of having a kosher ingredient for sale. Ingredient companies need to pay attention to the status of the kosher product, i.e., a pareve product is preferred over a dairy product because it has broader potential use.

Food companies will have to pay increasingly more attention to halal standards. In many cases, a few changes make it possible to permit kosher products to also serve the halal community, e.g., the true absence of animal products and care to assure that any residual alcohol in products is below 0.1%. Again a supervision standard acceptable in all or most Muslim countries is desirable. Note that the 0.1% alcohol in finished product standard is used by IFANCA and seems to be acceptable to the leadership of most halal communities. However, many halal consumers are not familiar with this standard at this time, so further education may be necessary.

A system of certification letters is used to provide information from the certifying rabbi concerning the products he has approved. To prevent fraud, it is helpful if these letters are renewed every year and dated with both a starting date and an ending date. Obviously a kosher supervision agency will only accept letters from agencies they find acceptable. That decision depends on two components: the actual kosher standards of the other agency, and an assessment of how well they operate and enforce their supervision. To make this process work better, more agencies are automating this process and computer systems are improving.

There are, of course, periodic recalls of specific products for various kosher defects that would prevent their use. KASHRUS magazine, or its Web site www.kashrusmagazine.com and www.kashrut.com, all try to provide up-to-date listings of products with problems, both of consumer items and industrial ingredients. Such a system of certification letters is also used in the Muslim community. Sometimes these recalls highlight secular (FDA/USDA) problems with products, i.e., when the kosher status is inconsistent with the ingredients labeling, the problem is sometimes with the ingredients label!

The kosher or halal symbol of the certifying agency or an individual doing the certification may appear on the packaging. In some industrial situations, where kosher and non-kosher (or halal and non-halal) products are similar, some sort of color-coding of product labels and packages may also be used. Most of these symbols are trademarks that are duly registered.

Three additional notes about kosher and halal markings on products:

1. To ensure that labels are marked properly, it is the responsibility of the food company to show its labels to its certifying agency before printing. This responsibility includes both the agency symbol and the documentation establishing its kosher status, e.g., dairy or pareve. It is the responsibility of the kosher supervision agency to review these labels carefully.

2. The labels for private label products with specific agency symbols on their labels should not be moved between plants and cannot be used if supervision changes.

The Toronto Rabbinical Council (COR) requires that each label has a plant number on it. This prevents the movement of labels between plants of the same company. This is the only agency that currently requires this additional safeguard.

In many cases a generic halal symbol, i.e., the word Halal in Arabic in a circle, has been used indiscriminately. Muslim consumers do not have much faith in such a symbol. The Islamic Food and Nutrition Council of America uses a registered trademark logo of the letter "M" inside a closed Crescent. Another agency, the Muslim Consumer Group, uses a triangle 'H' as their logo. Many other halal logos have started to appear on the packages in North America, usually on imported foods.

11.7.2.2   State Regulations

Approximately 20 states, some U.S. counties, and a few cities have laws specifically regulating the claim of kosher. Many of these laws refer to Orthodox Hebrew Practice or some variant of this term, e.g., reference to specific Jewish documents, and the U.S. Supreme Court has ruled (by accepting the decision of the Second Court of Appeals) that this is a violation of the first amendment to the Constitution. In recent years, six states have also passed halal laws.

The newer laws focus specifically on "consumer right to know issues" and "truth in labeling." They avoid having the state define kosher or halal. Rather, the food producer defines its terms and is held to that standard. Religious foods supervisors (or anyone else) providing supervision must then declare the information that a consumer needs to know to make an informed decision.

11.7.2.3   Animal Welfare

The largest fast-food chains in the United States have developed a set of animal welfare standards that determine their product purchasing.

The Food Marketing Institute (FMI, the trade association for many of the supermarkets in North America) and the National Council of Chain Restaurants (NCCR) then appointed an animal welfare committee to come up with a single national animal welfare standard for each species as well as for animal slaughter and poultry slaughter including religious slaughter. These religious slaughter issues are discussed in Regenstein and Grandin (2002) along with recommendations for auditable religious slaughter standards that will be used by the FMI/NCCR auditors. These standards are consistent with the American Meat Institute requirements that religious slaughter preferably be done with the animals in an upright position (for mammals) although a proper upside down pen will be accepted. The standard shackling line is also permitted for poultry religious slaughter.

References and Additional Readings

Al-Qaradawi, Y. 1984. *The Lawful and Prohibited in Islam*, The Holy Quran Publishing House, Beirut, Lebanon.

Blech, Z. 2005. Royal jelly. In *Kosher Food Production*. Blackwell Publishing, Ames, Iowa.

Chaudry, M.M. 1992. Islamic food laws: Philosophical basis and practical implications. *Food Technol*. 46(10):92.

Chaudry, M.M. and J.M. Regenstein. 1994. Implications of biotechnology and genetic engineering for kosher and halal foods. *Trends Food Sci. Technol*. 5:165–168.

Chaudry, M.M. and J.M. Regenstein. 2000. Muslim dietary laws: Food processing and marketing. *Encyclopedia of Food Science and Technology*, John Wiley, New York City, pp. 1682–1684.

Egan, M. 2002. Overview of halal from agri-Canada perspective. Presented at the Fourth International Halal Food Conference, Sheraton Gateway Hotel, Toronto, Canada, April 21–23.

Grunfeld, I. 1972. *The Jewish Dietary Laws*. pp. 11–12. The Soncino Press. London.

Hajmeer, M.N., J.L. Marsden, B.A. Crozier-Dodson, and J.J. Higgins. 1999. Reduction of microbial counts at a commercial beef koshering facility. *J. Food Sci.*, 64(4): 719–723.

Jackson, M.A. 2000. Getting religion—For your product, that is. *Food Tech*. 54(7):60–66.

Khan, G.M. 1991. *Al-Dhabah, Slaying Animals for Food the Islamic Way*, pp. 19–20. Abul Qasim Bookstore, Jeddah, Saudi Arabia.

Larsen, J. 1995. Ask the dietitian. Hopkins Technology, LLC., Hopkins, Minnesota. (http://www.dietitian.com/alcohol.html).

Ratzersdorfer, M., J.M. Regenstein, and L.M. Letson. 1988. Appendix 5: Poultry plant visits. In *A Shopping Guide for the Kosher Consumer*, J.M. Regenstein, C.E. Regenstein, and L.M. Letson (Eds.). For Governor Cuomo, Governor, State of New York.

Regenstein, J.M. 1994. Health aspects of kosher foods. *Activities Report and Minutes of Work Groups and Sub-Work Groups of the R & D Associates*. 46(1):77–83.

Regenstein, J.M. and T. Grandin. 2002. "Kosher and halal animal welfare standards." *Institute of Food Technologists Religious and Ethnic Foods Division Newsletter*. 5(1):3–16.

Regenstein, J.M. and C.E. Regenstein. 1979. An introduction to the kosher (dietary) laws for food scientists and food processors. *Food Technol.* 33(1):89–99.

Regenstein, J.M. and C.E. Regenstein. 1988. The kosher dietary laws and their implementation in the food industry. *Food Technol.,* 42(6):86, 88–94.

Regenstein, J.M. and C.E. Regenstein. 2000. Kosher foods and food processing. *Encyclopedia of Food Science,* pp. 1449–1453.

Regenstein, J.M. and C.E. Regenstein. 2002a. The story behind kosher dairy products such as kosher cheese and whey cream. *Cheese Reporter* 127(4):8, 16, 20.

Regenstein, J.M. and C.E. Regenstein. 2002b. What kosher cheese entails. *Cheese Marketing News* 22(31):4, 10.

Regenstein, J.M. and C.E. Regenstein. 2002c. Kosher byproducts requirements. *Cheese Marketing News* 22(32):4, 12.

Wikler, J. 2006. The 2007 Kosher Supervision Guide. *Kashrus Magazine* (Oct.), 36.

12

Control of Foodborne Pathogens and Spoilage Microorganisms by Naturally Occurring Antimicrobials

Larry R. Beuchat

CONTENTS

12.1 Introduction

Prevention of human illnesses caused by foodborne pathogens is a major goal of public health agencies, food manufacturers, and food service facilities. The importance of food safety in many countries is evidenced by recent federal and local regulations based on the principles of hazard analysis critical control point (HACCP) systems. Although industrially synthesized food antimicrobials are perceived by some consumers to have toxicological problems, their safety is ensured by regulatory authorities. Nevertheless, synthetic antimicrobial compounds may be considered less desirable by a segment of the consuming public than are naturally occurring antimicrobials. This has resulted in widespread interest in the food industry to exploit natural antimicrobials for the purpose of controlling the growth of spoilage microorganisms as well as microorganisms known to produce toxins or cause human infections. There are numerous natural compounds in plants and animals that are known to prevent the growth of these microorganisms. For ease of presentation here, these antimicrobials have been placed in two groups: those of plant origin and those of animal origin. For more extensive coverage of naturally occurring antimicrobials, the reader is referred to reviews by Burt (2004), Dillon and Board (1994), Johnson and Larson (2005), López-Malo et al. (2000), López-Malo Vigil et al. (2005), Sofos et al. (1998), and Stopforth et al. (2005).

12.2 Antimicrobials of Plant Origin

Naturally occurring antimicrobial compounds are present in plant leaves, stems, barks, roots, flowers, and fruits. Information on the antimicrobial activity of plant substances, particularly spices and herbs, has been available for centuries (Beuchat, 1994). In many instances, however, concentrations of compounds in spices and herbs necessary for inhibiting microorganisms exceed those resulting from normal usage in foods (Shelef et al., 1984). Nevertheless, naturally occurring substances in plants do indeed play a role in controlling the growth of foodborne spoilage and pathogenic microorganisms in foods. The following is a brief review of naturally occurring plant substances that have antimicrobial activity. The reader is referred to publications by López-Malo Vigil et al. (2005) and Sofos et al. (1998) for more extensive coverage of this topic.

12.2.1 *Allium* Species

Garlic (*Allium sativum*), onion (*A. cepa*), and leek (*A. porrum*) are probably the most widely consumed foods that have substantial antimicrobial activity. Garlic has been used for medicinal purposes for centuries, but it was not until the 1940s that scientific evidence confirmed that garlic does indeed possess antimicrobial and medicinal properties. Cavallito and Bailey (1944) and Cavallito et al. (1945) were the first to isolate the major antimicrobial component from garlic bulbs. They identified allicin, a diallyl thiosulfinate (2-propenyl-2-propenethiol sulfinate), as an antimicrobial and described it as an extremely pungent colorless oil responsible for the principal odor and taste of garlic and onion. Allicin was reported to be bactericidal, at concentrations of 1:85,000 in laboratory broth, to a wide range of gram-negative and gram-positive organisms.

Tissues of garlic and other *Allium* species do not contain allicin while in an intact state, but do contain the precursor, alliin (*S*-allyl-L-cysteine-*S*-oxide). Alliin undergoes hydrolysis to yield allicin, pyruvate, and ammonia by the action of the phosphopyridoxal enzyme, allinase, when tissue of the bulb is disrupted (Stoll and Seebeck, 1949). Garlic extracts inhibit alkaline phosphatase, invertase, urease, and papain activities (Wills, 1956). Allicin inhibits sulfhydral enzymes but very few nonsulfhydral enzymes. Sulfhydral enzymes can be protected by cysteine or glutathione against inhibition by allicin, but only partial recovery of enzyme activity is obtainable after the allicin and enzyme have been in contact. Inhibition of sulfhydryl enzymes is thought to be associated with the presence of the —SO—S— grouping and not —SO—, —S—S, or —S— groups (Wills, 1956). He demonstrated that most of the sulfhydryl enzymes were inhibited by 0.0005 M allicin. These included succinic dehydrogenase, urease, papain, xanthine oxidase, choline esterase, hexokinase, choline oxidase, glyoxylase, triose phosphate dehydrogenase, and alcohol dehydrogenase. Other sulfhydryl enzymes (carboxylase, adenosine triphosphatase, and β-amylase) were unaffected by 0.0005 M allicin. Among the nonsulfhydryl enzymes inhibited were dehydrogenase, alkaline phosphatase, and tyrosinase.

Work on antimicrobial activity of garlic and other *Allium* species has been done using foodborne pathogenic bacteria, mycotoxigenic molds, and spoilage microorganisms in general. Since sulfhydryl enzymes are common to all of these microorganisms, the spectrum of activity of *Allium* extracts is broad. Early studies revealed that allicin, at dilution of 1:125,000, prevented growth of *Staphylococcus aureus* and *Bacillus* species (Cavallito and Bailey, 1944). Mantis et al. (1978) studied the effect of garlic extract on *S. aureus* in culture media. They reported that 5% garlic extract solution had a lethal effect, whereas concentrations of garlic extract equal to or greater than 2% were inhibitory and concentrations less than 1% were not inhibitory. Garlic extract was generally more inhibitory at 37°C and pH 7.4 than at 28°C and pH 6.0. These researchers concluded that sausage containing greater than 1% garlic was not a favorable environment for the growth of *S. aureus*, especially after the pH is reduced as a result of fermentation. Tynecka and Gos (1973) observed that aqueous dilution (1:256) of garlic juice was inhibitory to *S. aureus*, while lethal effect was exhibited by 1:32 dilution. Garlic extract prevented growth of *Streptococcus* at much lower concentration (1:125,000 dilution) in a laboratory medium (Cavallito and Bailey, 1944).

At concentrations of 3%, 5%, and 10%, aqueous extracts from fresh garlic bulbs inhibit growth of *Bacillus cereus* on nutrient agar plates by 31.3%, 58.2%, and 100%, respectively (Saleem and Al-Delaimy, 1982). Extracts from garlic bulbs stored at −18°C were slightly more inhibitory than extracts from bulbs stored at 15°C–35°C for 6 months. Gamma irradiation of bulbs at a dose of 0.47 kGy, with subsequent freezing before extraction decreased activity up to 50%. Exposing extracts to heat treatments at 80°C–90°C for 5 min completely destroyed the activity.

DeWitt et al. (1979) investigated the effect of garlic and onion oils on toxin production by *Clostridium botulinum* type A in meat slurry. A concentration of 1500 μg/g inhibited toxin production at 20°C. Inhibition was incomplete and toxin production by *C. botulinum* type B and type E was not inhibited. It was concluded that garlic and onion oils should not be applied in the meat industry for the purpose of inhibiting toxin production by clostridia because of their apparent ineffectiveness against nontype A *C. botulinum*.

Growth of *Lactobacillus plantarum* in laboratory broth containing higher than 1% extract was reported by Karaioannoglou et al. (1977) to be inhibited. Growth at 30°C and pH 6.6 was less inhibitory than at 37°C and pH 7.4. It was concluded that garlic extract concentrations greater than 1% are inhibitory to *L. plantarum* while concentrations less than 1%, under favorable conditions of pH and temperature, are less inhibitory and may permit growth if large populations (>10^6 cells/mL) are initially present.

A large number of gram-negative bacteria are also inhibited by extracts from *Allium* species. Sirvastava et al. (1982) compared fresh garlic extract to ampicillin for activity against 21 strains of gram-negative bacteria, including *Citrobacter, Enterobacter, Escherichia, Klebsiella, Proteus, Pseudomonas, Salmonella, Serratia,* and *Shigella*. Extract was more effective than 30 μg/mL ampicillin for inhibiting all test bacteria except *Salmonella arizonae* and *Shigella cloacae*. The inhibitory effect of boiled extract was similar to that of the unheated extract. However, the antibacterial properties of garlic extract diminished during storage. Lee et al. (2004) reported that aqueous extracts of Chinese leeks at concentrations as low as 2 μg/mL inhibit the growth of *Campylobacter* species. Activity was stable at pH 2.0–8.0 but was diminished by heating at >75°C.

The bactericidal activity of freshly reconstituted, dehydrated onion and garlic at concentrations of 1% and 5% (w/v), respectively, against *Salmonella typhimurium* and *Escherichia coli*, was reported by Johnson and Vaughn (1969). Maximal death rates occurred with concentrations of 5% and 10%. At the higher concentrations, decimal reduction times at 37°C were 1.1 and 1.2 h, respectively, for resting *S. typhimurium* cells and 1.8 and 2.1 h, respectively, for growing cells. Of the major volatile aliphatic disulfide compounds in onions, *n*-propyl allyl and di-*n*-propyl, at a concentration of 0.1%, showed a comparable activity against resting cells. Growing cells of *E. coli* were more susceptible than those of *S. typhimurium* to garlic, but apparently more resistant to onion. Tynecka and Gos (1973) reported that *E. coli* was inhibited by a 1:28 dilution and killed by a 1:64 dilution of garlic juice.

Juices and solvent extracts of garlic, onion, and *Allium kurrat* were reported by Abdou et al. (1992) to prevent growth of *E. coli, Pseudomonas pyocyaneus,* and *S. typhimurium*. Inhibition by crude juices appeared to be greater than inhibition by ether, chloroform, or ethanol extracts. It was concluded that both garlic and onion are strong antiseptics and could be used for medicinal applications.

Yeasts and molds are also susceptible to the inhibitory action of *Allium* extracts. Tynecka and Gos (1973) reported that garlic juice was very potent against *Candida albicans* and speculated that fungal skin diseases could be effectively treated with garlic extract. The yeast was inhibited by a 1:512 dilution of juice and killed by juice diluted 1:256. Barone and Tansey (1977) attributed inhibition of 39 of 41 strains of *C. albicans* by aqueous extracts of garlic to destruction of thiols such as L-cysteine and glutathione. They hypothesized that additional lethal or inhibitory effects of allicin are due to its ability to inactivate proteins by oxidation of essential thiols to the disulfide and to competitively inhibit the activity of these sulfhydryl compounds by combining them. Extract heated at 121°C for 10 min retained no anticandidal activity. Activity was unaffected at pH 2.0–6.0 but reduced at pH 9.0 and eliminated at pH 12.0.

Moore and Atkins (1977) reported that a variety of yeast-like fungi representing the genera *Cryptococcus*, *Rhodotorula*, *Torupolsis*, and *Trichosporon* were inhibited in vitro by aqueous extract of garlic at concentrations diluted as much as 1:1024. In addition, they observed that 22 actively pathogenic isolates of *C. albicans* were inhibited. Kim et al. (2004) reported that minimum inhibitory concentrations of garlic oil, onion oil, diallyl trisulfide, diallyl tetrasulfide, and dimethyl trisulfide for yeasts range between 2 and 45 µg/mL. Stability was not influenced by pH.

Conner and Beuchat (1984a) investigated the inhibitory effects of 32 essential oils from plants on 13 food spoilage yeasts. Garlic oil was a potent inhibitor of growth at concentrations as low as 25 µg/mL. Onion oil was also strongly inhibitory. Resuscitation of heat-stressed yeasts representing several food spoilage yeasts (*Candida lipolytica*, *Debaryomyces hansenii*, *Hansenula anomala*, *Kloeckera apiculata*, *Lodderomyces elongisporus*, *Rhodotorula rubra*, *Saccharomyces cerevisiae*, and *Torulopsis glabrata*) was less inhibited by garlic oil than by onion oil (Conner and Beuchat, 1984b; Conner and Beuchat, 1985). Essential oil and oleoresin of garlic adversely affected ethanol production by *S. cerevisiae* (Conner et al., 1984) and garlic oil delayed sporulation of *H. anomala*.

Aflatoxin-producing molds, namely *Aspergillus flavus* and *Aspergillus parasiticus*, are effectively inhibited by various extracts of onion, including ether extracts, lachrymatory factor (thiopropanal-S-oxide) and steam-distilled onion oil (Sharma et al., 1979). Ethyl acetate was ineffective. Exposure of onions to γ-irradiation with a sprout-inhibiting dose (6 krad) did not alter the inhibitory potency of the onion extracts which, however, appeared to be heat labile. In another study, Sharma et al. (1981a) reported that germinated conidia were more susceptible to inhibition by onion extracts than were ungerminated conidia. The lethal effect of extract against conidia of *A. parasiticus* was lost by heating, freeze-drying, dehydration, and aeration. The effect of garlic on mycelial growth and aflatoxin production by *A. flavus* was studied by Mabrouk and El-Shayeb (1981). Minced garlic was more effective than garlic extract in inhibiting aflatoxin formation. Heat treatment at 121EC reduced the

potency of minced garlic. Sharma et al. (1981b) demonstrated that spor-
icidal activity of onion extracts against *A. parasiticus* could be retained by
freezer drying.

Extracts of garlic and onion inhibit the growth of many other molds, some
of which are known to spoil grains, legumes, and processed foods (Coley-
Smith and King, 1969; Appleton and Tansey, 1975; Tansey and Appleton,
1975). Even when growing in soil, garlic and onion can influence the microflora in the rhizosphere. Timonin and Thexton (1950), for example, observed
that the rhizosphere soil in proximity to garlic and onion harbored 11 and
12 times, respectively, more bacteria and 6 and 13 times more actinomycetes
than control soil. The microflora profile in soil adhering to garlic and onion
bulbs and roots as they were taken from the field for processing may
therefore be substantially different than profiles in soil adhering to the
bulbs or roots of other plants.

Fliermans (1973) described the inhibition of *Histoplasma capsulatum* by
extracts of the garlic plant. The mycelial phase of the organism was inhibited by both volatile and water-soluble components of garlic at concentrations of 254 ng/mL. The problem of *H. capsulatum* infectivity is most
significant in soils which have been exposed to bird excreta, a situation
common in soils adjacent to bird roosting sites. Although they did not
extrapolate laboratory results to a field situation, application of the active
component of garlic to infected soils may cause inhibition of the organism.
Inhibition of growth of *H. capsulatum* has also been reported by Tansey and
Appleton (1975).

12.2.2 Spices and Herbs

Many spices and herbs also exhibit antimicrobial activity (Table 12.1).
Compounds present in spices and herbs that are largely responsible for
antimicrobial activity include many simple and complex derivatives of
phenol which are volatile at room temperature. Concentrations of these
compounds necessary for inhibiting growth or various metabolic activities
in microorganisms often exceed those normally used in foods. Nevertheless,
the preservative effects of these seasoning agents should not be discounted.

Among the spices having highest antimicrobial activity are cinnamon,
clove, and allspice. The antimicrobial principles are often present in the
essential oil of these spices. Cinnamic aldehyde (3-phenyl-2-propenal) has
been shown to be the major antimicrobial compound in cinnamon. In
addition to exhibiting antibacterial activity (Deans and Richie, 1987), cinnamic aldehyde also inhibits mold growth and mycotoxin production.
Hitokoto et al. (1987) reported that cinnamon bark had a strong inhibitory
effect on fungi, including *A. parasiticus*. Bullerman (1974) reported that a
1%–2% concentration of ground cinnamon in broth would allow some
growth of *A. parasiticus* but reduced aflatoxin production by 99%. In a
later study, Bullerman et al. (1977) demonstrated that the essential oil of
cinnamon at a concentration of 200 g/mL was inhibitory to growth and

TABLE 12.1

Plants Used as Spices and Herbs Containing Compounds Possessing
Antimicrobial Activity

Achiote	Dill	Oregano
Allspice (pimenta)	Elecampane	Paprika
Almond (bitter)	Fennel	Parsley
Angelica	Fenugreek	Pennyroyal
Anise	Garlic	Pepper
Basil (sweet)	Ginger	Peppermint
Bay (laurel)	Horseradish	Pimento
Bergamot	Leek	Rosemary
Calmus	Lemon	Sage
Cananga	Lemongrass	Sassafras
Caraway	Licorice	Savory
Cardamon	Lime	Spearmint
Celery	Mace	Star anise
Chenopodium	Mandarin	Tarragon (estragon)
Cinnamon	Marjoram	Tea
Citronella	Musky bugle	Thyme
Clove	Mustard	Turmeric
Cocoa	Nutmeg	Vanilla
Coffee	Onion	Verbena
Coriander	Orange	Wintergreen

Source: Adapted from Burt, S., *Int. J. Food Microbiol.*, 94, 223, 2004;
Boonchird, C. and Flegel, T.W., *Can. J. Microbiol.*, 28, 1235, 1982; Conner, D.E.
and Beuchat, L.R., *J. Food Sci.*, 49, 429, 1984a; Maruzzella, J.C. and Liguori, L.,
J. Am. Pharm. Assoc., 47, 250, 1958; Huhtanen, C.N., *J. Food Prot.*, 43, 195, 1980;
López-Malo, A., Alzamora, S.M., and Guerrero, S. in Alzamora, S.M., Tapia,
S.M., and López-Malo, A., (Eds.), *Minimally Processed Fruits and Vegetables.
Fundamentals, Aspects and Applications*, Aspen Publishers, Gaithersburg, MD,
2000, 237–264.

subsequent toxin production by *A. parasiticus*, and that cinnamic aldehyde
(150 μg/mL) was inhibitory. Other saturated aldehydes (citral and citronellol), an unsaturated alcohol (geraniol), and a terpene alcohol (menthol)
exhibit various degrees of antimycotic activity (Moleyar and Narasimham,
1986). Geraniol and citronellol also inhibit growth of *Erwinia* (Scortichini
and Rossi, 1991), a bacterium often responsible for spoilage of raw fruits and
vegetables.

Eugenol [2-methoxy-4-(2-propenyl)phenol], a major constituent in clove
oil and present in considerable amounts in the essential oil of allspice,
possesses antimicrobial activity. Karapinar and Aktug (1987) reported that
eugenol was more effective against *S. typhimurium*, *S. aureus*, and *Vibrio
parahaemolyticus* than was thymol, anethol, or menthol. Clove powder
(1200 μg/mL) and eugenol (200 μg/mL) have been shown to adversely
affect the rate of germination of *Bacillus subtilis* spores (Al-Khayat and
Blank, 1985; Blank et al., 1987). Spores of the same bacterium had increased
heat sensitivity when exposed to clove powder (64%–98% relative humidity,

25°C–35°C) before treatment (Blank et al., 1988). Eugenol and carvacrol solubilized in nonionic surfactant micelles have been reported to inhibit the growth of *E. coli* O157:H7 and *L. monocytogenes* (Gaysinsky et al., 2005).

Clove oil at 250 μg/mL has been shown to inhibit growth and toxin production of *A. parasiticus* (Bullerman et al., 1977); eugenol was inhibitory at a concentration of 125 μg/mL. Hitokoto et al. (1980) observed ground cloves to completely inhibit the growth of toxigenic aspergilli. The essential oils and oleoresins of cinnamon, clove, and allspice are known to inhibit the growth of several food spoilage and fermentation yeasts (Conner and Beuchat, 1984a). Resuscitation of heat-stressed yeast cells was impaired in media containing as low as 25 μg/mL of essential oil of cinnamon (Conner and Beuchat, 1984b, 1985).

Vanillin (4-hydroxy-3-methoxybenzaldehyde), a major constituent in vanilla beans, is structurally similar to eugenol and is also antimycotic. The compound has been shown to inhibit or retard the growth of yeasts (Boonchird and Flegel, 1982) and molds (Maruzzella and Liguori, 1958). Vanillin is also inhibitory to *L. monocytogenes* (Delaquis et al., 2005).

Thymol [5-methyl-2-(1-methylethyl) phenol], present in the essential oils of thyme, oregano, savory, sage, and several other herbs, is among the compounds having a wide spectrum of antimicrobial activity. Beuchat (1976) reported that essential oils of thyme and oregano are inhibitory to *V. parahaemolyticus*. Of 50 plant essential oils examined by Deans and Richie (1987), thyme oil was the most inhibitory against 25 genera of bacteria. The level of inhibitory activity of extracts from thymol-containing herbs against *Shigella* is affected by pH and temperature (Bagamboula et al., 2003). Alcoholic extracts of these spices as well as those of rosemary and turmeric were shown to inhibit germination, growth, and toxin production by *C. botulinum* when used at a concentration of 500 μg/mL (Huhtanen, 1980). The presence of 500 μg/mL ethanolic extract of thyme inhibits the growth of *S. aureus* (Aktug and Karapinar, 1986); growth of *V. parahaemolyticus* was inhibited by 1000, 5000, and 6000 μg/mL of powdered thyme, bay leaves, and mint, respectively. Thyme extract has been reported to inhibit salmonellae, *E. coli* O157:H7, *Yersinia enterocolitica*, *Shigella flexneri*, *L. monocytogenes*, and *S. aureus* (Rota et al., 2004). Sage is inhibitory to *V. parahaemolyticus* (Shelef et al., 1980), *B. cereus*, *S. aureus*, and *S. typhimurium* (Shelef et al., 1984).

Thymol has been shown to inhibit growth of phytopathogenic molds (Boyraz and Özcan, 2006) and food spoilage yeasts (Conner and Beuchat, 1984b; Elgayyar et al., 2001), and toxin production by mycotoxigenic molds (Ray and Bullerman, 1982; Benjilali et al., 1984; Akgul and Kivanc, 1988). Thymol concentrations of ≥500 μg/mL were shown to completely inhibit the growth of *A. parasiticus*, while lower concentrations caused partial or transitory growth and toxin production patterns (Buchanan and Shepherd, 1981). Hitokoto et al. (1980) reported that a 2% concentration of oregano in potato dextrose agar completely inhibited the growth of seven mycotoxigenic molds. Maruzzella and Liguori (1958) reported that the volatile oils (essential oils) from origanum (oregano), savory, and thyme possessed substantial antifungal activities against 18 pathogenic and nonpathogenic fungi when tested in vitro using a standard zone of inhibition test. Carvacrol, a major component of essential oil of oregano and thyme, is lethal to *S. cerevisiae* (Knowles and Roller, 2000). Extracts of rosemary and oregano inhibit the growth of *Aspergillus niger* and *C. albicans* (Santoyo et al., 2005, 2006).

Thyme and oregano can have a stimulatory effect on lactic acid production by *L. plantarum* and *Pediococcus cerevisiae* (Zaika and Kissinger, 1981; Zaika et al., 1983). Manganese was identified as a factor in these and other spices responsible for the enhancement of acid production by meat starter bacteria (Zaika and Kissinger, 1984). Farbood et al. (1976) reported that rosemary spice extractive at 1000 μg/mL substantially inhibited the growth of *S. typhimurium* and *S. aureus*. A concentration of 3000 μg/mL of sage or rosemary in culture media inhibited the growth of 20 foodborne gram-positive bacteria, whereas a concentration of 5000 μg/mL was considered bactericidal (Shelef et al., 1980).

Bhavanti Shankar and Sreenivasa Murthy (1979) investigated the effect of turmeric on the growth of intestinal and pathogenic bacteria. They reported that the oil fraction of turmeric was inhibitory toward numerous bacteria including *B. cereus, S. aureus, E. coli,* and *L. plantarum*. Changes in membrane permeability and interference with enzyme function may be involved in the lethal mode of action of phenolic compounds in spices and herbs. Thongson et al. (2005) showed that commercial essential oil of turmeric inhibits the growth of *L. monocytogenes* but not *S. typhimurium*. Energy depletion in yeasts caused by allyl hydroxycinnamates (Baranowski et al., 1980) and essential oils of allspice, clove, cinnamon, oregano, thyme, and savory (Conner et al., 1984) have been reported. Ethanol production, respiratory activity, and sporulation of yeasts can also be influenced by essential oils of spices and herbs.

Many other plant parts and extracts used as spices and herbs are known to contain volatile compounds that possess antimicrobial activity. Allyl isothiocyanate, a nonphenolic compound naturally occurring in plants belonging to the *Crucifereae* family, for example, has been successfully used to control or eliminate *E. coli* O157:H7 in ground beef (Nadarajah et al., 2005a,b) and alfalfa seeds intended for sprout production (Park et al., 2000). Other foodborne pathogenic bacteria adversely affected by a wide range of compounds present in these seasoning agents include *C. botulinum, B. cereus, L. monocytogenes, S. typhimurium, Shigella, S. aureus, V. parahaemolyticus,* and *Y. enterocolitica*. Growth of the mycotoxigenic molds such as, *A. flavus, A. parasiticus, Aspergillus versicolor, Aspergillus ochraceus, Penicillium urticae,* and *Penicillium roquefortii* (Azzouz and Bullerman, 1982), as well as food-spoilage molds, yeasts, and bacteria is also retarded or inhibited in the presence of many commonly used spices and herbs.

12.2.3 Plant Pigments

The antimicrobial properties of several compounds responsible for color of plant tissues have been demonstrated. Anthocyanin pigments are present in almost all higher plants and are predominant in flowers and fruits. These pigments consist of an aglycone (anthocyanidin) portion esterified with one or more sugars. All anthocyanidins are derivatives of flavylium cation and have various degrees of hydroxylation and methyoxylation. Pelargonidin, cyanidin, delphinidin, plonidin, petunidin, and malvidin are among the most important anthocyadins in terms of contributing to the sensory quality of foods. Although anthocyanin pigments are better known for their food-coloring capabilities, they are also inhibitory to some bacteria. Hartman (1959) reported that pelargonidin 3-monoglucoside and its degradation products inhibit the growth of *E. coli* and *S. aureus*, and Powers et al. (1960) observed that certain anthocyanins were inhibitory to *E. coli, S. aureus*, and *Lactobacillus casei*. Similar observations were made by Zimmerman (1959) with *Lactobacillus acidophilus*. Pratt et al. (1960) showed that monoglucosides of cyanidin, perlargonidin, and delphinidin not only increased that lag phase of bacteria, but also decreased the maximum growth attained. Marwan and Nagel (1986) observed that flavanols and proanthocyanidins in cranberries are highly inhibitory to yeasts.

Researchers have studied the mechanism of antimicrobial activity of anthocyanins. Carpenter et al. (1967) reported that anthocyanins had an inhibitory effect of certain bacterial enzymes. The chelating ability of anthocyanins described by Somaatmadja et al. (1964) may partially explain their inhibitory action on bacterial enzymes. The unavailability of these metals could render these enzymes inactive, thus resulting in growth inhibition since the activity of many enzymes is dependent on metal ions. The role of anthocyanins as chelators was substantiated by Somaatmadja et al. (1964), who reported that the addition of magnesium and calcium ions reversed bacterial inhibition cause by malvidin 3-monoglucoside.

All higher plants contain chlorophylls *a* and *b*. Upon degradation, chorophyllides, phylophytins, pheaphorbides, and pyrrole compounds are formed. Beuchat et al. (1966) reported that chlorophyllide *a* inhibited growth of *E. coli, Pseudomonas fluorescens*, and *B. subtilis*.

Galindo-Cuspinera et al. (2003) observed that annatto extracts inhibit the growth of *B. cereus, C. perfringens*, and *S. aureus*, with minimum inhibitory concentrations of 0.08, 0.31, and 0.16% (vol/vol), respectively. *Listeria monocytogenes*, lactic acid bacteria, and yeasts were more resistant to antimicrobial activities of the extracts.

12.2.4 Other Phenolic Compounds

There are at least six major phenolic components in ethyl acetate extracts of green olives (Fleming et al., 1969), among them a phenolic glycoside (oleuropein) and the aglycone of oleuropein. The hydrolysis products of oleuropein, which contains glucose, β-3,4-dehydroxyphenylethyl alcohol, and an acid, are β-3,4-dihydroxyphenylethyl elenolic acid and the oleuropein aglycons. Oleuropein may not be antimicrobial but the aglycone and elenolic acids inhibit the growth of lactic acid bacteria (Fleming et al., 1973). Inhibition of *Lactobacillus, Leuconostoc mesenteroides,* and fungi, including *Geotrichum candidum, Rhizopus* spp., and *Rhizoctonia solani,* has been reported (Juven and Henis, 1970). Zanichelli et al. (2005) found that inhibition of *S. aureus* by oleuropein is largely due to hydrogen peroxide production as a result of tryptone oxidation. The presence of these compounds is thought to be responsible for occasional abnormal fermentation patterns of green olives. Degradation products of oleuropein are surface active, causing leakage of cytoplasmic constituents such as glutamate, potassium, and inorganic phosphate from bacterial cells (Juven et al., 1972). Aflatoxin production by *A. parasiticus* and *A. flavus* is greatly reduced in the presence of oleuropein (Gourama and Bullerman, 1987) and ethanolic extracts of olive callus tissues (Paster et al., 1988). Reduction in the amount of aflatoxin produced is not correlated with reduction in mycelium formation.

Phenolic compounds such as caffeic, chlorogenic, *p*-coumaric, ferulic, and quinic acids, are present in plant parts used as spices (Beuchat and Golden, 1989). Depending upon the botanical species, the antimicrobial activity of these and other hydroxycinnamic and cinnamic acids has been shown to retard microbial invasion and delay rotting of fruits and vegetables. Gram-positive and gram-negative bacteria, molds, and yeasts commonly encountered as food-spoilage organisms are sensitive to hydroxycinnamic acid derivatives (Davidson and Branen, 1981). Caffeic, ferulic, and *p*-coumaric acids, for example, inhibit *E. coli, S. aureus,* and *B. cereus* (Herald and Davison, 1983). Vanillic acid has been shown to inhibit *L. monocytogenes* (Delaquis et al., 2000) and *E. coli* O157:H7 (Moon et al., 2006). Baranowski et al. (1989) reported that ferulic acid and, to a lesser extent, *p*-coumaric acid inhibited growth of *S. cerevisiae,* suggesting that naturally occurring hydroxycinnamic acids may interfere with the fermentation of fruit juices by this yeast. Paster et al. (1988) observed that caffeic acid and *o*-coumaric acid inhibited aflatoxin production by *A. flavus* and coumaric-inhibited growth.

Other phenolic compounds have been demonstrated to exhibit antimicrobial activity. Tannins and tannic acid are present in bark, rinds, and other structural tissues of plants and known to possess antimicrobial activity. Beuchat and Heaton (1975) attributed the toxic effect of pecan packing tissue on *Salmonella senftenberg* to a high concentration of tannins. Tannic acid is inhibitory to *L. monocytogenes, E. coli, S. enteritidis, S. aureus, A. hydrophila,* and *Streptococcus faecalis* (Chung and Murdock, 1991). Singleton and Esau (1969) predicted that the antimicrobial effect of red and white wines should be proportional to flavonoid tannin content. Recent research has focused on evaluating antimicrobial activities of extracts of aromatic plants not necessarily used as foods. Extracts of sumac (Nasar-Abbas and Halkman, 2004), gardenia and cedar wood (Friedman et al., 2002), and *Lamiaceae* species (Araujo et al., 2003), for example, have been shown to exhibit inhibitory activities against foodborne pathogenic and spoilage microorganisms.

Extracts of blueberries, crabapples, strawberries, red wines, grape juice, apple juice, and tea were studied for their antiviral activity by Konowalchuk and Speirs (1976a,b, 1978a,b). Some of these extracts inactivated poliovirus, coxsackievirus, echovirus, and reovirus and herpes simplex virus. The primary inhibitors were thought to be tannins. Tannic acid was antiviral against echovirus, poliovirus and herpes simplex virus. Cliver and Kostenbader (1979) reported that the antiviral activity of grape juice was reversible.

12.2.5 Organic Acids

A major factor influencing survival and growth of microorganisms is the acidity of the environment. Foodborne bacteria capable of causing illness will not grow at pH less than 3.9–4.0, so any food containing sufficient acid to result in lower pH values are essentially protected against bacterial pathogens. Fruits, which contain citric, malic, tartaric, and other acids, generally fall in this range. Benzoic acid occurs in cranberries, prunes, plums, apples, and strawberries (Chipley, 1993) and is synthesized commercially for use as a preservative in foods (Sofos and Busta, 1992; Sofos, 1994). Its antimicrobial activity is greater against yeasts and molds than against bacteria. However, benzoic acid does inhibit growth of bacterial pathogens, including *V. parahaemolyticus, S. aureus, B. cereus,* and *L. monocytogenes* (Chipley, 1993). Sorbic acid also occurs naturally in fruits, e.g., rowan berries, and is used extensively to control microbial growth in foods (Sofos and Busta, 1981; Sofos, 1989). Acetic, lactic, and propionic acids are produced in various fermented foods, often playing a major role in preventing the growth of pathogenic bacteria.

Hop (*Hummulus lupulus*) vine flowers are used to impart desirable bitter flavor to beer. Resins, i.e., α-acids, represented by humulone and its congeners (cohumulone, adhumulone, prehumulone, and posthumulone), and β-acids, represented by lupulone and its congeners (colupulone, adlupulone, prelupulone, and postlupulone), are the major compounds responsible for this flavor. Most of these compounds are also known to inhibit microbial growth. Gram-positive bacteria and some fungi are most sensitive (Schmalreck et al., 1975; Mizobuchi and Sato, 1985). *Lactobacillus* species that may contaminate pitching yeasts are known to develop resistance to humulone. Richards and Macrae (1964) reported that several strains of lactobacilli acquired an 8- to 20-fold increase in resistance to 100 µg/mL humulone after two to four subcultures. Undissociated molecules are mainly responsible for inhibition of *Lactobacillus brevis* (Simpson and Smith, 1992). Hops may contribute very little to the microbial stability of beer, since resistant populations retain a degree of stability upon subculture in the absence of humulone.

Germination of conidia and the rate of colony development by *Aspergillus niger*, *Aspergillus glaucus*, and a *Penicillium* species are adversely affected by 1.5% hop extract in a laboratory medium (Engelson et al., 1980). The effects are more pronounced as the a_w of the medium is reduced by adding glycerol. These researchers suggested that the combined effect of reduced a_w and hop extract may be used to impart biological stability to intermediate moisture foods.

12.2.6 Coffee, Tea, Kola, and Cocoa

Several commonly consumed beverages are based on plant products containing antimicrobial compounds. Caffeine (1,3,7-trimethylxanthine) is present in coffee and cocoa beans, tea, and kola nuts and is antimycotic as well as antibacterial. Inhibition of growth of several mycotoxigenic *Aspergillus* and *Penicillium* species has been documented (Buchanan et al., 1981; 1983a; Lenovich, 1981). Caffeine adversely affects the production of aflatoxin, ochratoxin A, sterigmatocystin, citrinin, and patulin. The mechanism by which caffeine inhibits polyketide mycotoxin synthesis and other metabolic activities of fungal cells has not been clearly defined. Tortora et al. (1982) reported that caffeine, but not theophylline or papaverine, uncoupled the regulation of glycolysis and glucogenesis in *S. cerevisiae*. Buchanan et al. (1983b) reported that inhibition of growth of *A. parasiticus* by caffeine is due in part to an alteration in purine metabolism, but inhibition of aflatoxin synthesis apparently does not involve an inhibition of cyclic AMP phosphodiesterase or a chelation of key metal ions. Evidence does suggest that caffeine may restrict glucose uptake by *A. parasiticus*, resulting in decreased aflatoxin production (Buchanan and Lewis, 1984). In a preliminary examination of the effect of caffeine on patulin production by *Penicillium urticae*, Buchanan et al. (1983a) suggested that activity does not involve a generalized inhibition of lipid synthesis.

The effects of caffeine on lactobacilli, the predominant group of microflora isolated from a commercial instant coffee processing facility, were studied by Vanos and Bindschedler (1985). *L. plantarum* was the dominant species. Total inhibition of growth was obtained at 15 mg/mL caffeine and at 60% total nondecaffeinated coffee solids. *Staphylococcus aureus*, *Salmonella*, *E. coli*, *Streptococcus faecalis*, and *B. cereus* failed to grow in 2% (w/v) reconstituted decaffeinated and nondecaffeinated coffee. Pearson and Marth (1990c) investigated the effect of caffeine on *L. monocytogenes*. At a concentration of 0.5% in skimmed milk, growth at 30°C occurred although the lag phase was extended to 6–9 h compared to less than 3 h in milk not containing caffeine.

Theophylline (1,3-dimethylxainthine) and theobromine (3,7-dimethylxanthine) are present in tea and cocoa. Theophylline is present in manufactured tea at a concentration range of 0.23–0.44 mg/100 g whereas the theobromine content is about 50 mg/100 g in manufactured tea (Lunder, 1979). Theobromine is the principal alkaloid in cocoa beans (1.5%–3%) and is also present in kola nuts. Pearson and Marth (1990b) observed that the addition of cocoa to milk enhanced the growth of *L. monocytogenes*. In another study (Pearson and Marth, 1990a), the pathogen was observed to have a longer lag phase in milk containing cocoa, but reached a higher population than in milk without cocoa. The neutralization effect of casein on antilisterial activity of cocoa (Pearson and Marth, 1990a) is in agreement with observations reported by Zapatka et al. (1977) on *S. typhimurium*, who reported that the addition of 3%–5% casein to 5% cocoa in distilled water resulted in 44%–57% survival of the organism compared to no survival in the absence of casein. Buchanan and Fletcher (1978) reported that neither theophylline nor theobromine appear to have much effect on aflatoxin production.

Vanos et al. (1987) observed that growth of *S. typhimurium*, *E. coli*, *S. aureus*, and *B. cereus* are adversely affected in a 2% (total solids) instant tea infusion. Inhibition of *L. planatrum* was observed in a 10% tea infusion. It was concluded that a flavanol (catechin) plus caffeine complex was the only natural inhibitor of lactobacilli in instant tea. Friedman et al. (2006) evaluated seven green tea catechins and four black tea theaflavins, generally referred to as flavonoids, for inhibitory activity against *B. cereus*. Eight of the compounds showed antibacterial activity at nanomolar levels. The linden flower, used to prepare tea in the near East, has been reported to inhibit the growth of *S. aureus* and, to a lesser extent, *S. typhimurium* and *V. parahaemolyticus* (Gonul and Karapinar, 1987).

12.2.7 Phytoalexins

Phytoalexins are low molecular weight compounds produced by higher plants in response to microbial infection and naturally occurring elicitors (Dixon et al., 1983). Production of phytoalexins by plant cell cultures was reviewed by Whitehead and Threlfall (1992) and Walker (1994). The mechanism of action of phytoalexins is not fully understood, though evidence suggests that they alter properties of plasma membranes. Phytoalexins are known to occur in leaves, fruits, seeds, roots, and tubers of a wide range of plants. Glyceollin, coumestrol, and glycinol, all phytoalexins produced by soybeans, inhibit microbial membrane-associated processes. The major antibacterial phytoalexins produced in soybeans inoculated with *Erwinia carotovora* and *S. cerevisiae* is glycinol, which has been hypothesized to inhibit the growth of a wide range of other bacteria and fungi. Exposure of *E. coli* membrane vesicles to glycinol results in inhibition of respiration-linked transport (Weinstein and Albersheim, 1983). Numerous other phytoalexins are produced in soybeans and other legumes (Rizk and Wood, 1980). Low molecular weight antimicrobial compounds are also known to be produced by green beans, broad beans, garden peas, cowpeas, and alfalfa. A broad range of fungi and bacteria are sensitive to these stress metabolites. Capsidiol from bell peppers (Stoessel et al., 1972), rishitin, lubimin, and phytuberin from potatoes and auberginone from eggplant (Dixon et al., 1983) are also known to exhibit antimicrobial activity.

The formation of dihydroisocoumarin, chromone, and scopoletin in carrot roots is induced by invasion with various spoilages (Coxin et al., 1973). Two other phytoalexins, β-glucosides of 6-methoxymellein and 6-hydroxymellein, are also produced by carrot cells (Kurosaki et al., 1984). 6-Methoxymellein production is elicited by fungal invasion (Kurosaki and Nishi, 1983; Amin et al., 1986a) and also by partial hydrolysis of carrot cells (Kurusaki and Nishi, 1984). The compound is toxic to bacteria as well as fungi. Inhibition of gram-positive (*S. aureus*, *Streptococcus pyogenes*, and *B. subtilis*) and gram-negative bacteria (*S. typhimurium*, *Shigella sonnei*, *E. coli*, *Klebsiella pneumoniae*, *Serratia marcescens*, and *Proteus vulgaris*) has been reported when cells are exposed to 0.05–0.5 mM 6-methoxymellein (Kurusaki and Nishi, 1983). The mechanism of action of this phytoalexin apparently involves interference with membrane-associated functions. Alteration of membrane permeability (Weinstein and Albersheim, 1983; Amin et al., 1988), mitochondria (Boydston et al., 1983), cyclic nucleotide phosphodiesterase activity, and multilamellar liposomes (Amin et al., 1986b) has been documented.

Beuchat and Brackett (1990) reported that viability of *L. monocytogenes* decreased upon contact with raw carrots but not with cooked carrots, indicating that the lethal compounds are heat labile. In a study using *L. monocytogenes*, *L. innocua*, *L. ivanovii*, *L. seeligeri*, and *L. welshimeri*, Nguyen-the and Lund (1991) confirmed that a lethal component existed in raw, sliced, and macerated carrots. It was subsequently shown that antilisterial activity of carrot slices was suppressed by anaerobioses, thiol compounds, and bovine serum albumin but not by sodium ascorbate, propyl gallate, catalase, superoxide dismutase, or chelating agents (Nguyen-the and Lund, 1992).

Differentiation and aflatoxin formation by *A. parasiticus* are inhibited by extracts of carrot roots (Batt et al., 1980). Geraniol, citrol, and terpineol in the volatile fraction of carrot seed oil prevent growth, while limonene and terpinene do not affect growth but do inhibit aflatoxin production (Batt et al., 1983). It is not known whether these compounds would also influence the growth patterns of microflora naturally present in carrots and other fresh produce.

12.2.8 Propolis

Propolis is a mixture of resinous material collected by honeybees from buds, blossoms, and leaves of plants, pollen, and enzymes secreted by the bees. The antimicrobial activity of propolis has been attributed to flavonoids and esters of phenolic acids (Sforcin et al., 2000), as well as other components (Kujumgiev et al., 1999). Ethanolic extracts of propolis has been reported to inhibit *S. aureus* at concentrations as low as 7.5 μg/mL

(Lu et al., 2005). Cells in late-exponential phase are most susceptible and acidic pH enhances activity.

12.3 Antimicrobials of Animal Origin

Enzymes and other polypeptides with antimicrobial activity occur naturally in animals as well as plants. These polypeptides are often classified as functioning by oxygen-dependent or -independent mechanisms. The inhibition or killing of microorganism by oxygen dependent means involves enzymes or metabolic processes generating toxic metabolites of oxygen such as hydrogen peroxide, superoxide ions, or hydroxyl radicals, and decreasing production of halides (Sofos et al., 1998). Oxygen-independent mechanisms utilize peptides and proteins that react with the cell surface and disrupt structural surface layers or membranes. This group includes lytic enzymes, hydrolases, and cationic peptides and proteins.

12.3.1 Lytic Enzymes

Lysozyme, a mucopeptide glycohydrolase, and other lytic enzymes are found in many foods and in various secretions such as egg albumen, tears, and milk. Lysozymes act by cleaving the glycoside bond between C_1 of N-acetylmuramic acid and C_4 of acetylglucosine in the bacterial cell wall (Tranter, 1994). Some lysozymes hydrolyze chitin or possess esterase activity. Lysozyme in the albumen of chicken egg contributes to up to 3.5% of the protein content. Its lysing activity has been demonstrated against *L. monocytogenes* and *C. botulinum* (Hughey and Johnson, 1987). Ethylenediaminetetraacetic acid (EDTA) is known to act as a synergist with lysozyme to lyse pathogenic and spoilage bacteria, including *Salmonella, E. coli, Yersinia*, and *Pseudomonas* (Repaske, 1958). Mono-, di-, and trivalent salts, however, can reduce the antibacterial efficacy of lysozyme–chelator combinations. Boland et al. (2004) observed that inhibitory activities of EDTA, disodium pyrophosphate, and pentasodium tripolyphosphate in combination with lysozyme were lost in the presence of ≥ 1 mM Ca^{2+} and Mg^{2+} at pH 7.

Enzymes other than lysozyme cleave carbohydrate or peptide linkages. These include glycosidases specific for the glycoside bond between alternating sugars in the polypeptide backbone of microbial cells and an amidase which releases the tetrapeptide from N-acetylmuramic acid, endopeptidases, and lipases. Nielsen (1991) reported that lytic enzymes lysed *Campylobacter, E. coli, Salmonella*, and *V. parahaemolyticus*, indicating their potential use as natural food antimicrobials to reduce the risk of foodborne illness.

Encapsulation of lysozyme in phospholipid liposomes has been shown to enhance efficacy against *L. monocytogenes* (Were et al., 2004), indicating the potential of liposomes to serve as delivery vehicles for antimicrobials in foods. High-pressure homogenization increases the sensitivity of gram-negative and gram-positive bacteria to lysozyme (Vanninni et al., 2004). It was hypothesized that the interaction between pressure and lysozyme is associated with conformational modifications of proteins.

12.3.2 Peroxidases and Oxidases

Peroxidases are widespread in nature and oxidize molecules at the expense of hydrogen peroxide. Lactoperoxidase is the most abundant enzyme in bovine milk and is also produced in salivary glands of mammals. Lactoperoxidase oxidizes thiocyanate or halogens, thereby producing toxic metabolites. In raw milk, the lactoperoxidase system (LPS) inhibits lactic acid bacteria but is bactericidal to gram-negative spoilage psychrotrophs and *Salmonella* (Reiter and Harnulv, 1984; Leyer and Johnson, 1993). The LPS is also active against gram-positive pathogens such as *L. monocytogenes* (Siragusa and Johnson, 1989), *S. aureus* (Kamau et al., 1990b), and *B. cereus* (Zajac et al., 1981).

Duy Le Nguyen et al. (2005) studied the effectiveness of the LPS in controlling the growth of disease-causing microorganisms in mangoes. Application of LPS inhibited the growth of *Xanthomonas campestris*, *Botryodiplodia theobromae*, and *Colletotrichum gloeosporioides*, the major causes of bacterial black rot, stem-end rot, and anthracnose, respectively, in mangoes. High pressure is known to enhance the antibacterial activity of lactoperoxidase (Vannini et al., 2004).

Glucose oxidase catalyzes a reaction between glucose and oxygen to yield gluconic acid or D-glucono-S-lactone and hydrogen peroxide. The enzyme is used commercially to remove glucose from eggs, prevent Maillard browning reactions, and remove oxygen from beverages (Frank, 1992). Inhibition of growth of *Salmonella infantis*, *S. aureus*, *Clostridium perfringens*, and *B. cereus* by glucose oxidase was reported by Tiina and Sandholm (1989).

12.3.3 Transferrins

Survival and growth of foodborne pathogens depend on the availability of iron ions, although the absolute requirement has yet to be determined (Sofos et al., 1998). Sequestration of iron through chelation by iron-binding polypeptides, especially the transferrins and related proteins, is the mechanism of control of iron-dependent microorganisms. Ovotransferrin (conalbumin) comprises about 13% of the protein in egg white, and has been known to inhibit the growth of *S. aureus*, *E. coli*, and *Shigella* since the early 1940s (Schade and Caroline, 1944). Lactoferrin, present in milk, is another transferrin known to inhibit or kill foodborne pathogenic and spoilage microorganisms (Arnold et al., 1980; Tomita et al., 1992; Hoek et al., 1997).

References

Abdou, I.A., A.A. Abdou-Zeid, M.R. El-Sherbeeny, and Z.H. Abou-El-Gheat. 1972. Antimicrobial activity of *Allium Sativum, Allium cepa, Barbanus sativus, Capsicum frutescens, Eruca sativa,* and *Allium kurrat* on bacteria. *Qual. Plant Mater. Veget.* 22:29–35.

Akgul, A. and M. Kivanc. 1998. Inhibitory effects of Turkish spices and oregano components on some foodborne fungi. *Int. J. Food Microbiol.* 6:263–268.

Aktug, S.E. and M. Karapinar. 1986. Sensitivity of some common food poisoning bacteria to thyme, mint and bay leaves. *Int. J. Food Microbiol.* 3:349–354.

Al-Khayat, M.A. and G. Blank. 1985. Phenolic spice-components sporostatic to *Bacillus subtilis. J. Food Sci.* 50:971–974, 980.

Amin, M., F. Kurosaki, and N. Nishi. 1986a. Extracellular pectinolytic enzymes of fungi elicit phytoalexin accumulation in carrot suspension culture. *J. Gen. Microbiol.* 132:771–777.

Amin, M., F. Kurosaki, and N. Nishi. 1986b. Inhibition of cyclic nucleotide phospho-diesterase by carrot phytoalexin. *Phytochemistry* 25:2305–2307.

Amin, M., F. Kurosaki, and N. Nishi. 1988. Carrot phytoalexin alters the membrane permeability of *Candida albicans* and multilamellar liposomes. *J. Gen. Microbiol.* 134:241–246.

Appleton, J.A. and M.R. Tansey. 1975. Inhibition of growth of zoopathogenic fungi by garlic extract. *Mycologia* 67:882–885.

Araujo, C., M.J. Sousa, M.F. Ferreira, and C. Leao. 2003. Activity of essential oils from Mediterranean *Lamiaceae* species against food spoilage yeasts. *J. Food Prot.* 66:625–632.

Arnold, R.R., J.E. Russell, W.J. Champion, and J.J. Gauthier. 1980. Bactericidal activity of human lactoferrin: Influence of physical conditions and metabolic state of the target microorganism. *Infect. Immun.* 32:655–660.

Azzouz, M.A. and L.B. Bullerman. 1982. Comparative effects of selected herbs, spices, plant compounds, and commercial antifungal agents. *J. Food Prot.* 45:1298–1301.

Bagamboula, C.F., M. Uyttendaele, and J. Debevere. 2003. Antimicrobial effect of spices and herbs on *Shigella sonnei* and *Shigella flexneri. J. Food Prot.* 66:668–673.

Baranowski, J.D., P.M. Davidson, C.W. Nagel, and A.L. Branen. 1980. Inhibition of *Saccharomyces cerevisiae* by naturally occurring hydroxycinnamates. *J. Food Sci.* 45:592–594.

Barone, F.E. and M.R. Tansey. 1977. Isolation, purification, identification, synthesis and kinetics of activity of the anticandidal component of *Allium sativum* and a hypothesis for its mode of action. *Mycologia* 69:793–825.

Batt, C., M. Solberg, and M. Ceponis. 1980. Inhibition of aflatoxin production by carrot root extract. *J. Food Sci.* 45:1210–1213.

Batt, C., M. Solberg, and M. Ceponis. 1983. Effect of volatile components of carrot seed oil on growth and aflatoxin production by *Aspergillus parasiticus. J. Food Sci.* 48:762–768.

Benjilali, B., A. Tantaoui-Elaraki, A. Ayadi, and M. Ihlal. 1984. Method to study antimicrobial effects of essential oils: Application of six Moroccan essences. *J. Food Prot.* 47:748–752.

Beuchat, L.R. 1976. Sensitivity of *Vibrio parahaemolyticus* to spices and organic acids. *J. Food Sci.* 41:899–902.

Beuchat, L.R. 1994. Antimicrobial properties of spices and their essential oils. In R.G. Board and V. Dillon (Eds.), *Natural Antimicrobial Systems in Food Preservation*. CAB International, Wallingford, Oxon, UK, pp. 167–179.

Beuchat, L.R. and D.A. Golden. 1989. Antimicrobials occurring naturally in foods. *Food Technol.* 43(1):134–142.

Beuchat, L.R. and R.E. Brackett. 1990. Inhibitory effects of raw carrots on *Listeria monocytogenes*. *Appl. Environ. Microbiol.* 56:1734–1742.

Beuchat, L.R. and E.K. Heaton. 1975. *Salmonella* survival on pecans as influenced by processing and storage conditions. *Appl. Microbiol.* 29:795–801.

Beuchat, L.R., R.V. Lechowich, S.W. Schanderl, D.Y.C. Co, and R.F. McFeeters. 1966. Inhibition of bacterial growth by chlorophyllide a. *Quart. Bull. Mich. Agric. Expt. Sta.* 48:411–416.

Bhavanti Shankar, T.N. and V. Sreenivasa Murthy. 1979. Effect of turmeric (*Curcuma longa*) fractions on the growth of some intestinal and pathogenic bacteria *in vitro*. *J. Expt. Biol.* 17:1363–1366.

Blank G., M. Al-Khayat, and M.A.H. Ismond. 1987. Germination and heat resistance of *Bacillus subtilis* produced on clove and eugenol based media. *Food Microbiol.* 4:35–42.

Blank, G., G. Akomas, M. Henderson, and J. Zawistowski. 1988. Heat sensitization of *Bacillus subtilis* spores by selected spices. *J. Food Safety* 9:83–96.

Boland, J.S., P.M. Davidson, B. Bruce, and J. Weiss. 2004. Cations reduce antimicrobial efficacy of lysozyme-chelator combinations. *J. Food Prot.* 67:285–294.

Boonchird, C. and T.W. Flegel. 1982. *In vitro* antifungal activity of eugenol and vanillin against *Candida albicans* and *Cryptococcus neoformans*. *Can. J. Microbiol.* 28:1235–1241.

Boydston, R., J.D. Paxton, and D.E. Koeppe. 1983. Glyceollin, a site-specific inhibitor of electron transport in isolated soybean mitochondria. *Plant Physiol.* 72:151–155.

Boyraz, N. and M. Özcan. 2006. Inhibition of phytopathogenic fungi by essential oil, hydrosol, ground material and extract of summer savory (*Satureja hortensis* L.) growing wild in Turkey. *Int. J. Food Microbiol.* 107:238–242.

Buchanan, R.L. and A.M. Fletcher. 1978. Methylxanthine inhibition of aflatoxin production. *J. Food Sci.* 43:654–655.

Buchanan, R.L. and A.J. Shepherd. 1981. Inhibition of *Aspergillus parasiticus* by thymol. *J. Food Sci.* 46:976–977.

Buchanan, R.L. and D.F. Lewis. 1984. Caffeine inhibition aflatoxin synthesis: Probable site action. *Appl. Environ. Microbiol.* 47:1216–1220.

Buchanan, R.L., G. Tice, and D. Marino. 1981. Caffeine inhibition of ochratoxin A production. *J. Food Sci.* 47:319–321.

Buchanan, R.L., M.A. Harry, and M.A. Gealt. 1983a. Caffeine inhibition of sterigmatocystin, citrinin and patulin production. *J. Food Sci.* 48:1226–1228.

Buchanan, R.L., D.J. Joover, and S.B. Jones. 1983b. Caffeine inhibition of aflatoxin production: mode of action. *Appl. Environ. Microbiol.* 46:1193–1200.

Bullerman, L.B. 1974. Inhibition of aflatoxin production by cinnamon. *J. Food Sci.* 39:1163–1165.

Bullerman, L.B., F.Y. Lieu, and S.A. Seier. 1977. Inhibition of growth and aflatoxin production by cinnamon and clove oils, cinnamic aldehyde and eugenol. *J. Food Sci.* 42:1107–1109, 1116.

Burt, S. 2004. Essential oils: Their antibacterial properties and potential applications in foods: A review. *Int. J. Food Microbiol.*, 94:223–253.

Carpenter, J.A., Y.P. Wang, and J.J. Powers. 1967. Effect of anthocyanin pigments on certain enzymes. *Proc. Soc. Exp. Biol. Med.* 124:702–706.

Cavellito, C.J. and J.H. Bailey. 1944. Allicin, the antibacterial principle of *Allium sativum*. I. Isolation, physical properties and antibacterial action. *J. Am. Chem. Soc.* 16:1950–1951.

Cavellito, C.J., J.H. Bailey, and J.S. Buck. 1945. The antibacterial principle of *Allium sativum*. III. Its precursor and "essential oil of garlic." *J. Am. Chem. Soc.* 67:1032–1033.

Chipley, J.R. 1993. Sodium benzoate and benzoic acid. In P.M. Davidson and A.L. Branen (Eds.), *Antimicrobials in Foods*. 2nd ed. Marcel Dekker, Inc., New York, pp. 11–48.

Chung, K.T. and C.A. Murdock. 1991. Natural systems for preventing contamination and growth of microorganisms in foods. *Food Microstruct.* 10:361.

Cliver, D.O. and K.D. Kostenbader. 1979. Antiviral effectiveness of grape juice. *J. Food Prot.* 42:100–104.

Coley-Smith, J.R. and J.E. King. 1969. The production of species of *Allium* of alkyl sulphides and their effect on germination of sclerotia of *Sclerotium cepivorum* Berk. *Ann. Appl. Biol.* 64:289–301.

Conner, D.E. and L.R. Beuchat. 1984a. Effects of essential oils from plants on growth of food spoilage yeasts. *J. Food Sci.* 49:429–434.

Conner, D.E. and L.R. Beuchat. 1984b. Sensitivity of heat-stressed yeasts to essential oils of plants. *Appl. Environ. Microbiol.* 47:229–233.

Conner, D.E. and L.R. Beuchat. 1985. Recovery of heat-stressed yeasts in media containing plant oleoresins. *J. Appl. Bacteriol.* 59:49–55.

Conner, D.E., L.R. Beuchat, R.W. Worthington, and H.L. Hitchcock. 1984. Effects of essential oils and oleoresins on plants of ethanol production, respiration and sporulation of yeasts. *Int. J. Food Microbiol.* 1:63–74.

Coxin, D.T., R.F. Curtis, K.R. Price, and G. Levett. 1973. Abnormal metabolites produced by *Daucas carota* roots stored under conditions of stress. *Phytochemistry* 12:1881–1885.

Davidson, P.M. and A.L. Branen. 1981. Antimicrobial activity of non-halogenated phenolic compounds. *J. Food Prot.* 44:623–632.

Davidson, P.M. and A.L. Branen (Eds.). 1993. *Antimicrobials in Foods*. Marcel Dekker, Inc., New York.

Deans, S.G. and G. Ritchie. 1987. Antibacterial properties of plant essential oils. *Int. J. Food Microbiol.* 5:165–180.

Delaquis, P., K. Stanich, and P. Toivonen. 2005. Inhibition of *Listeria* spp. by vanillin and vanillic acid. *J. Food Prot.* 68:1472–1476.

DeWitt, J.C., S. Notermans, N. Gorin, and E.H. Kempelmacher. 1979. Effect of garlic oil or onion oil on toxin production by *Clostridium botulinum* in meat slurry. *J. Food Prot.* 42:222–224.

Dillon, V.M. and R.G. Board. 1994. *Natural Antimicrobial Systems and Food Preservation*. CAB International, Wallingford, Oxon, UK, 328 pp.

Dixon, R.A., P.M. Dey, and C.J. Lamb. 1983. Phytoalexins: Enzymology and molecular biology. *Adv. Enzymol.* 55:1–136.

Duy le Nguyen, D., M.-N. Ducamp, M. Dornier, D. Montet, and G. Loiseau. 2005. Effect of the lactoperoxidase system against three major causal agents of disease in mangoes. *J. Food Prot.* 65:1497–1500.

Elgayyar, M., F.A. Draughon, D.A. Golden, and J.R. Mount. 2001. Antimicrobial activity of essential oils from plants against selected pathogenic and saprophytic microorganisms. *J. Food Prot.* 64:1019–1024.

Engelson, M., M. Solbert, and E. Karmas. 1980. Antimycotic properties of hop extract in reduced water activity media. *J. Food Sci.* 45:1175–1178.

Farbood, M.I., J.H. McNeil, and K. Ostovar. 1976. Effect of rosemary spice extractive on growth of microorganisms in meat. *J. Milk Food Technol.* 39:675–679.

Fleming, H.P., W.M. Walter, Jr., and J.L. Etchells. 1969. Isolation of a bacterial inhibitor from green olives. *Appl. Microbiol.* 18:856–860.

Fleming, J.P., W.M. Walter, Jr., and J.L. Etchells. 1973. Antimicrobial properties of oleuropein and products of its hydrolysis from green olives. *Appl. Microbiol.* 26:777–782.

Fliermans, C.B. 1973. Inhibition of *Histoplasma capsulatum* by garlic. *Mycopath. Mycol. Applicata* 50:227–231.

Frank, H.K. 1992. *Dictionary of Food Microbiology.* Technomic Publishing Co., Lancaster, PA.

Friedman, M., P.R. Henika, and R.E. Mandrell. 2002. Bacterial activities of plant essential oils and some of their isolated constituents against *Campylobacter jejuni, Escherichia coli, Listeria monocytogenes,* and *Salmonella enterica. J. Food Prot.* 65:1545–1560.

Friedman, M., P.R. Henika, C.E. Levin, R.E. Mandrell, and N. Kozukue. 2006. Antimicrobial activities of tea catechins and theaflavins and tea extracts against *Bacillus cereus. J. Food Prot.* 69:354–361.

Galindo-Cuspinera, V., D.C. Westhoff, and S.A. Rankin. 2003. Antimicrobial properties of commercial annatto extracts against selected pathogenic, lactic acid and spoilage microorganisms. *J. Food Prot.* 66:1074–1078.

Gaysinsky, S., P.M. Davidson, D.B. Bruce, and J. Weiss. 2005. Growth inhibition of *Escherichia coli* O157:H7 and *Listeria monocytogenes* by carvacrol and eugenol encapsulated in surfactant micelles. *J. Food Prot.* 68:2549–2566.

Gonul, S.E.A. and M. Karapinar. 1987. Inhibitory effect of linden flower (tilia flower) on the growth of foodborne pathogens. *Food Microbiol.* 4:97–100.

Gourama, H. and L.B. Bullerman. 1987. Effects of oleuropein on growth and aflatoxin production *Aspergillus parasiticus. Lebensm. Wiss. Technol.* 20:226–228.

Hartman, G.D. 1959. The effect of anthocyanin pigment, pelargonidin-3-monoglucoside, and its heat degration products on growth of selected bacteria. M.S. Thesis, University of Georgia, Athens.

Herald, P.J. and P.M. Davidson. 1983. Antibacterial activity of selected hydroxycinnamic acids. *J. Food Sci.* 48:1378–1379.

Hitokoto, H., S. Morozumi, T. Wauke, S. Sakai, and I. Veno. 1978. Inhibitory effects of condiments and herbal drugs on the growth and toxin production of toxigenic fungi. *Mycopathologia* 66:161–167.

Hitokoto, H., S. Morozumi, T. Wauke, S. Sakai, and H. Kurata. 1980. Inhibitory effects of spices on growth and toxin production of toxigenic fungi. *Appl. Environ. Microbiol.* 39:818–822.

Hoek, K.S., J.M. Milne, P.A. Grieve, D.A. Dionysius, and R. Smith. 1997. Antibacterial activity in bovine lactoferrin-derived peptides. *Antimicrob. Agents Chemother.* 41(1):54–59.

Hughey, V.L. and E.A. Johnson. 1987. Antimicrobial activity of lysozyme against bacteria involved in food spoilage and foodborne disease. *Appl. Environ. Microbiol.* 53:2165–2170.

Huhtanen, C.N. 1980. Inhibition of *Clostridium botulinum* by spice extracts and aliphatic alcohols. *J. Food Prot.* 43:195–196.

Johnson, M.G. and R.H. Vaughn. 1969. Death of *Salmonella typhimurium* and *Escherichia coli* in the presence of freshly reconstituted dehydrated garlic and onion. *Appl. Microbiol.* 17:903–905.

Johnson, E.A. and A.E. Larson. 2005. Lysozyme. In P.M. Davidson, J.N. Sofos, and A.L. Branen (Eds.), *Antimicrobials in Food*, 3rd ed., Taylor and Francis Group, Boca Raton, FL, pp. 361–387.

Juven, B. and Y. Henis. 1970. Studies on the antimicrobial activity of olive phenolic compounds. *J. Appl. Bacteriol.* 33:721–732.

Juven, B., Y. Henis, and B. Jacoby. 1972. Studies on the mechanism of the antimicrobial action of oleuropein. *J. Appl. Bacteriol.* 35:559–567.

Kamau, D.N., S. Doores, and K.M. Pruitt. 1990b. Enhanced thermal destruction of *Listeria monocytogenes* and *Staphylococcus aureus* by the lactoperoxidase system. *Appl. Environ. Microbiol.* 56:2711–2716.

Karaioannoglou, P.G., A.J. Mantis, and A.G. Panetsos. 1977. The effect of garlic extract on lactic acid bacteria (*Lactobacillus plantarum*) in culture media. *Lebensm. Wiss. Technol.* 10:148–150.

Karapinar, M. and S.E. Aktug. 1987. Inhibition of foodborne pathogens by thymol, eugenol, menthol and anethole. *Int. J. Food Microbiol.* 4:161–166.

Kim, J.W., Y.S. Kim, and K.H. Kyung. 2004. Inhibitory activity of essential oils of garlic and onion against bacteria and yeasts. *J. Food Prot.* 67:499–504.

Knowles, J. and S. Roller. 2001. Efficacy of chitosan, carvacol, and a hydrogen peroxide-based biocide against foodborne microorganisms in suspension and adhered to stainless steel. *J. Food Prot.* 64:1542–1548.

Konowalchuk, J. and J.I. Speirs. 1967a. Antiviral activity of fruit extract. *J. Food Sci.* 14:1013–1017.

Konowalchuk, J. and J.I. Speirs. 1967b. Virus inactivation of grapes and wines. *Appl. Environ. Microbiol.* 32:757–763.

Konowalchuk, J. and J.I. Speirs. 1978a. Antiviral effect of commercial juices and beverages. *Appl. Environ. Microbiol.* 35:1219–1220.

Konowalchuk, J. and J.I. Speirs. 1978b. Antiviral effect of apple beverages. *Appl. Environ. Microbiol.* 36:798–801.

Kujumgiev, A., I. Tsvetkova, Y. Serkedjieva, V.V. Bankova, R. Chrostov, and S. Popov. 1999. Antimicrobial, antifungal and antiviral activity of propolis of different geographical origin. *J. Ethnopharmacol.* 64:235–240.

Kurosaki, F. and A. Nishi. 1983. Isolation and antimicrobial activity of the phytoalexin 6-methoxymellein from cultured carrot cells. *Phytochemistry* 22:669–672.

Kurosaki, F. and A. Nishi. 1984. Elicitation of phytoalexin production in cultured carrot cells. *Physiol. Plant Pathol.* 24:169–176.

Kurosaki, F., K. Matsui, and A. Nishi. 1984. Production and metabolism of 6-methoxymellein in cultured carrot cells. *Physiol. Plant Pathol.* 25:313–322.

Lee, C.-F., C.-K. Han, and J.-L. Tsau. 2004. *In vitro* inhibitory activity of Chinese leek extract against *Campylobacter* species. *Int. J. Food Microbiol.* 94:169–174.

Lenovich, L.M. 1981. Effect of caffeine on aflatoxin production of cocoa beans. *J. Food Sci.* 46:655–656.

Leyer, G.L. and E.A. Johnson. 1993. Acid adaptation induces cross-protection against environmental stress in *Salmonella typhimurium*. *Appl. Environ. Microbiol.* 59:1842–1847.

López-Malo, A., S.M. Alzamora, and S. Guerrero. 2000. Natural antimicrobials in plants. In S.M. Alzamora, S.M. Tapia, and A. López-Malo (Eds.), *Minimally Processed Fruits and Vegetables. Fundamentals, Aspects and Applications*, Aspen Publishers, Gaithersburg, MD, pp. 237–264.

López-Malo Vigil, A., E. Palou, and S.M. Alzamora. 2005. Naturally occurring compounds-plant sources. In P.M. Davidson, J.N. Sofos, and A.L. Branen (Eds.), *Antimicrobials in Food*, 3rd ed., Taylor and Francis Group, Boca Raton, FL, pp. 429–451.

Lu, L.-C., Y.-W. Chen, and C.-C. Chou. 2005. Antibactyerial activity of propolis against *Staphylococcus aureus*. *Int. J. Food Microbiol*. 102:213–220.

Lunder, T.L. 1979. *Tea: History–Botany–Chemistry–Manufacture–Nutritional Value*. Centre de Documentation Technique, Nestle, Vevey, Switzerland.

Mabrouk, S.S. and N.M.A. El-Shayeb. 1981. The effects of garlic on mycelial growth and aflatoxin formation by *Aspergillus flavus*. *Chem. Mikrobiol. Technol. Lebensm*. 7:37–41.

Mantis, A.J., P.G. Karaiannoglou, G.P. Spanos, and A.G. Panetsos. 1978. The effect of garlic extract on food poisoning bacteria in culture media. I. *Staphylococcus aureus*. *Lebensm. Wiss. Technol*. 11:26–28.

Maruzzella, J.C. and L. Liguori. 1958. The *in vitro* antifungal activity of essential oils. *J. Am. Pharm. Assoc*. 47:250–254.

Marwan, A.G. and C.W. Nagel. 1986. Microbial inhibitors in cranberries. *J. Food Sci*. 51:1009–1013.

Mizobuchi, S. and Y. Sato. 1985. Antifungal activities of hop bitter resins and related compounds. *Agric. Biol. Chem*. 49:399–403.

Moleyar, V. and P. Narasimham. 1986. Antifungal activity of some essential oil components. *Food Microbiol*. 3:331–336.

Moon, K.D., P. Delaquis, P. Toivonen, S. Back, K. Stanich, and L. Harris. 2006. Destruction of *Escherichia coli* O157:H7 by vanillic acid in unpasteurized juice from apple cultivars. *J. Food Prot*. 69:542–547.

Moore, G.S. and R.D. Atkins. 1977. The fungicidal and fungi-static effects of an aqueous garlic extract on medially important yeast-like fungi. *Mycologia* 69:341–348.

Nadarajah, D., J.H. Han, and R.A. Holley. 2005a. Inactivation of *Escherichia coli* O157:H7 in packaged ground beef by allyl isothiocyanate. *Int. J. Food Microbiol*. 99:269–279.

Nadarajah, D., J.H. Han, and R.A. Holley. 2005b. Use of mustard flour to inactivate *Escherichia coli* O157:H7 in ground beef under nitrogen flushed packaging. *Int. J. Food Microbiol*. 99:257–267.

Nasar-Abbas, S.M. and A.K. Halkman. 2004. Antimicrobial effect of water extract of sumac (*Rhus coriara* L.) on the growth of some food borne bacteria including pathogens. *Int. J. Food Microbiol*. 97:63–69.

Nguyen-the, C. and B.M. Lund. 1991. The lethal effect of carrot on *Listeria* species. *J. Appl. Bacteriol*. 70:479–488.

Nguyen-the, C. and B.M. Lund. 1992. An investigation of the antibacterial effect of carrot on *Listeria monocytogenes*. *J. Appl. Bacteriol*. 73:23–30.

Nielsen, H.K. 1991. Novel bacteriolytic enzymes and cyclodextrin glycosyl transferase for the food industry. *Food Technol*. 45(1):102–104.

Park, C.M., P.J. Taormina, and L.R. Beuchat. 2000. Efficacy of allyl isothiocyanate in killing enterohermorrhagic *Escherichia coli* O157:H7 on alfalfa seeds. *Int. J. Food Microbiol*. 56:13–20.

Paster, N., B.J. Juven, and H. Harshemesh. 1988. Antimicrobial activity and inhibition of aflatoxin B_1 formation by olive plant tissue constituents. *J. Appl. Bacteriol.* 64:293–297.

Pearson, L.J. and E.H. Marth. 1990a. Inhibition of *Listeria monocytogenes* by cocoa in a broth medium and neutralization of this effect of casein. *J. Food Prot.* 53:38–46.

Pearson, L.J. and E.H. Marth. 1990b. Behavior of *Listeria monocytogenes* in the presence of cocoa, carrageenan and sugar in a milk medium incubated with and without agitation. *J. Food Prot.* 53:30–32.

Pearson, L.J. and E.H. Marth. 1990c. Behavior of *Listeria monocytogenes* in the presence of methylxanthines—caffeine and theobromine. *J. Food Prot.* 53:47–50.

Powers, J.J., D. Somaatmadja, D.E. Pratt, and M.K. Hamdy. 1960. Anthocyanins. II. Action of anthocyanin pigments and related compounds on the growth of certain microorganisms. *Food Technol.* 14:626–632.

Pratt, D.E., J.J. Powers, and D. Somaatmadja. 1960. Anthocyanins. I. The influence of strawberry and grape anthocyanins on the growth of certain bacteria. *Food Res.* 25:26–32.

Ray L.L. and L.B. Bullerman. 1982. Preventing growth of potentially toxic molds using antifungal agents. *J. Food Prot.* 45:953–963.

Reiter, B. and B.G. Harnulv. 1984. Lactoperoxidase antibacterial system: Natural occurrence, biological functions and practical applications. *J. Food Prot.* 47:724–732.

Repaske, R. 1958. Lysis of Gram-negative organisms and the role of versene. *Biochim. Biophys. Acta* 30:225–232.

Richards, M. and R.M. Macrae. 1964. The significance of the use of hops in regard to the biological stability of beer. II. The development of resistance to hop resins by strains of lactobacilli. *J. Inst. Brew.* 70:484–488.

Rizk, A.-F. and G.E. Wood. 1980. Phytoalexins of leguminous plants. *CRC Crit. Rev. Food Sci. Nutr.* 13:245–295.

Rota, C., J.J. Carraminana, J. Burello, and A. Herrera. 2004. *In vitro* antimicrobial activity of essential oils from aromatic plants against selected foodborne pathogens. *J. Food Prot.* 67:1252–1256.

Saleem, Z.M. and K.S. Al-Delaimy. 1982. Inhibition of *Bacillus cereus* by garlic extracts. *J. Food Prot.* 45:1007–1009.

Santoyo, S., S. Cavero, L. Jaime, E. Ibanez, F.J. Senorans, and G. Reglero. 2005. Chemical composition and antimicrobial activity of *Rosmarinus officinalis* L. essential oil obtained via supercritical fluid extraction. *J. Food Prot.* 68:790–795.

Santoyo, S., S. Cavero, L. Jaime, E. Ibanez, F.G. Senorans, and G. Reglero. 2006. Supercritical carbon dioxide extraction of compounds with antimicrobial activity from *Origanum vulgare* L.: Determination of optimal extraction parameters. *J. Food Prot.* 69:369–375.

Schade, A.L. and L. Caroline. 1944. Raw hen egg white and the role of iron in growth inhibition of *Shigella dysenteriae, Staphylococcus aureus, Escherichia coli*, and *Saccharomyces cerevisiae. Science* 100:14–15.

Schmalreck, A.F., M. Teuber, W. Reininger, and A. Hartl. 1975. Structural features determining the antibiotic potencies of nature and synthetic hop bitter resins, their precursors and derivatives. *Can. J. Microbiol.* 21:205–212.

Scortichini, M. and M.O. Rossi. 1991. *In vitro* susceptibility of *Erwinia amylovora* (Burrill) Winslow et al. to geraniol and citronellol. *J. Appl. Bacteriol.* 71:113–118.

Sforcin, J.M., A. Fernandes, Jr., C.A.M. Lopes, V. Bankova, and S.R.C. Funari. 2000. Seasonal effect of Brazilian propolis antibacterial activity. *J. Ethnopharmacol.* 73:243–249.

Sharma, A., G.M. Tewari, A.J. Shrikhande, S.R. Padwal-Desai, and C. Bandyopadhyay. 1979. Inhibition of aflatoxin-producing fungi by onion extracts. *J. Food Sci.* 44:1545–1547.

Sharma, A., S.R. Padwal-Desai, G.M. Tewari, and C. Bandyopadhyay. 1981a. Factors affecting antifungal activity of onion extractives against aflatoxin-producing fungi. *J. Food Sci.* 46:741–744.

Sharma, A., G.M. Tewari, C. Bandyopadhyay, and S.R. Padwal-Desai. 1981b. Sporicidial activity of onion extracts against aflatoxin-producing fungi. *Lebensm. Wiss. Technol.* 14:21–22.

Shelef, L.A., O.A. Naglik, and D.W. Bogen. 1980. Sensitivity of some common foodborne bacteria to the spices sage, rosemary and allspice. *J. Food Sci.* 45:1042–1044.

Shelef, L.A., E.K. Jyothi, and M.A. Bulgarelli. 1984. Growth of enteropathogenic and spoilage bacteria in sage-containing broth and foods. *J. Food Sci.* 49:737–740, 809.

Simpson, W.J. and A.R.W. Smith. 1992. Factors affecting antibacterial activity of hop compounds and their derivatives. *J. Appl. Bacteriol.* 72:327–334.

Singleton, V.L. and P. Esau. 1969. *Phenolic Substances in Grapes and Wine, and Their Significance.* Academic Press, New York.

Siragusa, G.R. and M.G. Johnson. 1989. Inhibition of *Listeria monocytogenes* growth by the lactoperoxidase-thiocyanate-H_2O_2 antimicrobial system. *Appl. Environ. Microbiol.* 55:2802–2805.

Sirvastava, K.C., A.D. Perera, and H.O. Saridakis. 1982. Bacteriostatic effects of garlic sap on Gram negative pathogenia bacteria—an *in vitro* study. *Lebensm. Wiss. Technol.* 15:74–76.

Sofos, J.N. 1989. *Sorbate Food Preservatives.* CRC Press, Inc., Boca Raton, FL.

Sofos, J.N. 1994. Antimicrobial agents. In A.T. Tu and J.A. Maga (Eds.), *Handbook of Toxicology. Volume 1. Food Additive Technology.* Marcel Dekker, Inc., New York, pp. 501–529.

Sofos, J.N. and F.F. Busta. 1981. Antimicrobial activity of sorbate. *J. Food Prot.* 44:614–622.

Sofos, J.N. and F.F. Busta. 1992. Chemical food preservatives. In A.D. Russell, W.B. Hugo, and G.A.J. Ayliffe (Eds.), *Principles and Practice of Disinfection, Preservation and Sterilization.* 2nd ed. Blackwell Scientific Publications, London, UK, pp. 351–386.

Sofos, J.N., L.R. Beuchat, P.M. Davidson, and E.A. Johnson. 1998. *Naturally Occurring Antimicrobials in Food.* Task Force Report No. 132, Council for Agricultural Science and Technology, Ames, IA. 103 pp.

Somaatmadja, D., J.J. Powers, and M.K. Hamdy. 1964. Anthocyanins. VI. Chelation studies on anthocyanins and other related compounds. *J. Food Sci.* 29:655–660.

Stoessel, A., C.H. Unwin, and E.W.B. Ward. 1972. Post-infectional inhibitors from plants. I. Capsidol, and antifungal compounds from *Capsicum frutescens. Phytopathol. Z.* 74:141–152.

Stoll, A. and E. Seebeck. 1949. Uber aliin, die genuine muttersubstantz des knoblauchols. *Helv. Chim. Acta* 31:189–210.

Stopforth, J.D., P.N. Skandamis, P.M. Davidson, and J.N. Sofos. 2005. Naturally occurring compounds—animal sources. In P.M. Davidson, J.N. Sofos, and A.L. Branen. (Eds.), *Antimicrobials in Food,* 3rd ed., Taylor and Francis Group, Boca Raton, FL, pp. 453–505.

Tansey, M.R and J.A. Appleton. 1975. Inhibition of fungal growth by garlic extract. *Mycologia* 67:409–413.

Thongson, C., P.M. Davidson, W. Mahakarnchanakul, and P. Vibulsresth. 2002. Antimicrobial effect of Thai spices against *Listeria monocytogenes* and *Salmonella typhimurium* DT104. *J. Food Prot.* 68:2054–2058.

Tiina, M. and M. Sandholm. 1989. Antibacterial effect of the glucose oxidase-glucose system on food poisoning organisms. *Int. J. Food Microbiol.* 8:165–174.

Timonin, M.I. and R.H. Thexton. 1950. The rhizosphere effect of onion and garlic on soil microflora. *Soil Sci. Soc. Proc.* 15:186–189.

Tomita, M., W. Bellamy, M. Takase, K. Yamaguchi, H. Wakabayashi, and K. Kawase. 1992. Potential antibacterial peptides generated from pepsin digestion of bovine lactoferrin. *J. Dairy Sci.* 74:4137–4142.

Tortora, P., N. Burlini, G.M. Hanozet, and A. Guerritore. 1982. Effect of caffeine on glucose-induced inactivation of gluconeogenetic enzymes in *Saccharomyces cerevisiae*: A possible role of cyclic AMP. *Eur. J. Biochem.* 126:617–622.

Tranter, H.S. 1994. Lysozyme, ovotransferrin and avidin. In V.M. Dillon and R.G. Board (Eds.), *Natural Antimicrobial Systems and Food Preservation*. CAB International, Wallingford, Oxon, UK, pp. 65–97.

Tynecka, Z. and Z. Gos. 1973. The inhibitory action of garlic (*Allium sativum* L.) on growth and respiration of some microorganisms. *Acta Microbiol. Pol. Ser. B.* 5:51–62.

Vannini, L., R. Lanciotti, D. Baldi, and M.E. Guerzoni. 2004. Interactions between high pressure homogenization and antimicrobial activity of lysozyme and lactoperoxidase. *Int. J. Food Microbiol.* 94:123–135.

Vanos, V. and O. Bindschedler. 1985. The microbiology of instant coffee. *Food Microbiol.* 4:19–33.

Vanos, V., S. Hofstaetter, and L. Cox. 1987. The microbiology of instant tea. *Food Microbiol.* 2:187–197.

Walker, J.R.L. 1994. Antimicrobial compounds in food plants. In V.M. Dillon and R.G. Board (Eds.), *Natural Antimicrobial Systems and Food Preservation*. CAB International, Wallingford, Oxon, UK, pp. 181–204.

Weinstein, L.I. and P. Albersheim. 1983. Host-pathogen interactions. XXIII. The mechanisms of the antibacterial action of glycinol, a pterocarpan phytoalexin synthesized by soybeans. *Plant Physiol.* 72:557–563.

Were, L.M., B. Bruce, P.M. Davidson, and J. Weiss. 2004. Encapsulation of nisin and lysozyme in liposomes enhances efficacy against *Listeria monocytogenes*. *J. Food Prot.* 67:922–927.

Whitehead, I.M. and D.R. Threlfall. 1992. Production of phytoalexins by plant tissue cultures. *J. Biotechnol.* 26:63–81.

Wills, E.D. 1956. Enzyme inhibition of allicin, the active principle of garlic. *Biochem. J.* 63:514–520.

Zaika, L.L. and J.C. Kissinger. 1981. Inhibitory and stimulatory effects of oregano on *Lactobacillus plantarum* and *Pediococcus cerevisiae*. *J. Food Sci.* 46:1205–1210.

Zaika, L.L. and J.C. Kissinger. 1984. Fermentation enhancement by spices: identification of active component. *J. Food Sci.* 49:5–9.

Zaika, L.L., J.C. Kissinger, and A.E. Wasserman. 1983. Inhibition of lactic acid bacteria by herbs. *J. Food Sci.* 48:1455–1459.

Zajak, M., L. Bjorck, and O. Claasson. 1981. Antibacterial effect of the lactoperoxidase system against *Bacillus cereus* (from milk). *Milchwissenschaft* 38:417–418.

Zanichelli, D., T. Baker, M.N. Clifford, and M.R. Adams. 2005. Inhibition of *Staphylococcus aureus* by oleuropein is mediated by hydrogen peroxide. *J. Food Prot.* 68:1492–1496.

Zapatka, F.A., G.W. Varney, and J. Skinskey. 1977. Neutralization of the bactericidal effect of cocoa powder on salmonellae by casein. *J. Appl. Bacteriol.* 42:21–25.

Zimmerman, V.C. 1959. The influence of anthocyanin pigments on certain bacteria *in vitro*. M.S. Thesis, University of Georgia, Athens.

13

Intervention Technologies for Food Safety and Preservation

Vijay K. Juneja, Shiowshuh Sheen, and Gaurav Tewari

CONTENTS

13.1   Introduction

Food preservation has been a long lasting desire of human beings. The significant development in food preservation started the day fire was discovered by prehistoric humans, which was followed by indigenous methods of food preservation such as pickling, oiling, and salting of different food-types, whether raw or processed. Some of the earlier techniques still prevail and are available in several commercial formats. The major developments in and need for food processing and preservation started during wars when extended shelf life of foods became a necessity. As such, several food processing techniques, such as ready-to-eat food in pouches, aseptic processing of milk and liquid foods with particles, ohmic or electric resistance heating of foods, were developed to achieve extended shelf life of foods for soldiers in wars. A technology transfer effort occurred for consumers, when consumers started demanding a food product with fresh-like characteristics along with extended shelf life. Over the years, consumers became more and more educated on added food preservatives and their adverse effects on long-term health. This all resulted in advances in research and development and finally led to commercialization of innovative food preservation techniques. This also gave birth to several nonthermal food preservation techniques, of which ultra-high pressure processing has started to see its commercialization since late 1990s. Irradiation is also getting limited acceptability by consumers for several food products. Thermal food preservation techniques are being revisited and are being modified to provide consumers with a variety of food products with the characteristics of home-cooked meals.

Nevertheless, the ubiquity of potentially life-threatening pathogens in our environment and their contamination in our foods is an enormous problem. The ability of some of these pathogens to survive and proliferate under refrigeration and in reduced oxygen atmospheres, and for some of them, the low number necessary for food poisoning outbreaks, indicate a potential public health hazard. Moreover, microorganisms, previously unknown, or not known to be causes of foodborne disease, have recently been linked with documented outbreaks of illness. The U.S. Public Health Service has estimated that foodborne diseases caused by pathogenic bacteria such as *Salmonella, Campylobacter, Escherichia coli*, and *Vibrio*, as well as *Toxoplasma gondii* and other parasites may cause as many as 9000 deaths and 6.5 million to 81 million cases of diarrheal diseases in the United States annually (Lee, 1994). The annual economic losses in relation to medical costs, loss of productivity, loss of business and possible legal action associated with foodborne diseases may be as large as $5 billion to $6 billion (CAST, 1996). The Centers of Disease Control and Prevention (CDC) have estimated that 2500 cases of listeriosis may occur each year, resulting in 500 deaths, in the United States alone (Mead et al., 1999). Recently (August, 2006), the outbreak of *E. coli* O157:H7 in the prewashed and packaged spinaches has caused 3 deaths and more than 100 illnesses in the United States. These food safety concerns are magnified because of consumer preferences for high quality, minimally processed convenient meals that require minimal preparation time. Accordingly, the need for better control of foodborne pathogens has been paramount in recent years.

Strategies for control of foodborne pathogens include established microbicidal treatments such as ionizing radiation and heating. Microorganisms can also be destroyed by the emerging methods of modified thermal and innovative nonthermal technologies, such as application of high hydrostatic pressure, or a combination of physical processes such as heat–irradiation, heat–high hydrostatic pressure, etc. Each of the novel technologies has specific applications in terms of the types of food that can be processed. This chapter deals with a variety of conventional and novel food processing technologies for controlling foodborne pathogens and enhancing the safety and shelf life of foods.

13.2   Irradiation of Food

Food irradiation improves the safety of meat, poultry, and other foods by destroying indigenous microflora, and thereby extending the shelf life of these products during refrigerated storage. Sources of ionizing radiation come from x-rays with a maximum energy of 5 MeV, electrons with a maximum energy of 10 MeV, and γ-rays emitted by the radioisotopes cobalt-60 or cesium-137. However, those from cesium-137 are not used for food irradiation. The food is exposed to doses of ionizing radiation sufficient to create positive and negative charges leading to death of bacteria and other pathogens in foods. It is the rapidly growing cells of pathogenic and spoilage bacteria or parasites that are killed when food is irradiated. Ionizing radiation affects organisms by damaging the genetic material, i.e., DNA base damage, single-strand and double-strand DNA breaks, and cross linking between bases. As a consequence of this damage, microorganisms are unable to replicate DNA and reproduce, leading to their death. In addition to DNA damage, ionizing radiation may damage bacterial membranes and cause other changes leading to sublethal injury. Another irradiation source used the electron beam, which is similar to the old television set. The electrons are generated and accelerated to nearly the speed of light by electricity. When the products were irradiated, the electron beam accelerator was turned on, the products then passed through the stream of electrons. Electron-beam process is also known as the electronic pasteurization. There are no radioactive materials involved in this process.

13.2.1   Absorbed Doses

There are several terms that must be known with regard to the application of radiation to foods. These terms include the following:

1. Curie
   A curie is a quantity of radioactive substance in which 3.7×10^{10} radioactive disintegrations occur per second.
2. Rad
   A rad, used in the past, is a unit equivalent to the absorption of 100 ergs energy/g of irradiated material.
3. Gray
   The presently used unit of absorbed dose is the Gray (Gy); 1 Gy is the energy absorption on 1 joule/kilogram (1 Gy = 100 rads = 1 J/kg; 1 kGy = 10^5 rads; 1 J = 10^7 ergs).

TABLE 13.1

Ionizing Radiation Dose Requirements for Various Applications
of Food Irradiation

Application	Dose Requirement (kGy)
Inhibition of sprouting potatoes and onions	0.03–0.12
Insect disinfestation of seed products, flours fresh and dried fruits, etc.	0.2–0.8
Parasite disinfection of meats and other foods	0.1–3.0
Radurization of perishable food items (fruits, vegetables, meat, poultry, fish)	0.5–10
Radicidation of frozen meat, poultry, eggs, and other foods and feeds	3.0–10
Reduction or elimination of microbial populations in dry food ingredients (spices, starch, enzyme preparations, etc.)	3.0–2.0
Radappertization of meat, poultry, and fish products	25–60

Source: Adapted from Farkas, J., in *Handouts of IFFIT International Training Course on Food Irradiation,* Intern. Facility for Food Irradiation Technol., Wageningen, the Netherlands, 1980, 1–7.

Depending upon the dose, a variety of desirable effects can be achieved (Table 13.1). Like all processing technologies, excessive doses can produce adverse effects. Sudarmadji and Urbain (1972) estimated threshold doses of irradiation (5°C–10°C) for an organoleptically detectable "off-flavor" in foods of animal origin (Table 13.2). Higher doses can be used without adverse effects by exclusion of oxygen or by irradiation with the product in the frozen state.

Goresline et al. (1964) devised the following terms to describe the applications of irradiation in food processing:

TABLE 13.2

Threshold Doses of Irradiation
at 5°C–10°C for Foods of Animal Origin for
an Organoleptically Detectable "Off-Flavor"

Food	Threshold Dose (kGy)
Beef	2.5
Chicken	2.5
Turkey	1.5
Lamb	6.25
Pork	1.75
Shrimp	2.5

Source: Adapted from Sudarmadji, S., Urbain, W.M., *J. Food Sci.* 37, 671, 1972.

4. Radicidation

   Radicidation is considered equivalent to pasteurization of milk and, accordingly, referred to as "irradiation pasteurization." It is intended to reduce the number of specific, viable, non-spore forming pathogens including parasites, other than viruses, to non-detectable levels as determined by any standard method (radicidation; <10 kGy dose).

5. Radurization

   Radurization may be considered as equivalent to pasteurization. It is intended to considerably reduce the population densities of specific viable spoilage microbes with an aim to extend the shelf life of foods (radurization; <10 kGy dose).

6. Radappertization

   Radappertization is considered as equivalent to sterilization or rendering the food "commercially sterile" as it is known in the canning industry (radappertization; >10 kGy dose). If the food has been enzyme inactivated and has been irradiated while hard frozen in vacuo it will be shelf stable and of excellent quality.

13.2.2   Safety and Consumer Acceptance

Food exposed to ionizing radiation is never in contact with any radioactive material. None of the sources of radiation, such as γ-rays, x-rays, or electrons can render the food radioactive. There is little effect on the food itself since the cells in the food are not multiplying. Extensive research using animal models has provided sufficient evidence that ingestion of irradiated foods is completely safe and that the nutritive value remains essentially unchanged (CAST, 1996).

Some vitamins, e.g., vitamin B_1 and C, however, are sensitive to radiation. Factors affecting the amount of vitamin loss include dose, temperature, presence of oxygen, and the type of food. Packaging of foods in the absence of oxygen and exposing to radiations at low temperatures minimizes any vitamin loss and further loss can be prevented by storage at low temperatures in sealed packages (WHO, 1994). It has been estimated that only 2.3% of vitamin B_1 in the American diet would be lost if all the pork in the United States were to be irradiated (CAST, 1996). Also, irradiation causes a small amount of ascorbic acid in fruits to be converted (oxidized) to dehydroascorbic acid. This compound is as biologically active as its reduced form and is converted back to the reduced form during storage of the fruits or vegetables.

When molecules absorb ionizing energy, they become reactive and form ions or free radicals that react to form stable radiolytic products (Woods and Pikaev, 1994). The CAST (1989) estimated that a dose of 1 kGy will break fewer than 10 chemical bonds for every 10 million such bonds present (cooking produces similar changes in chemical bonds). Researchers have developed methodologies to detect irradiated foods and have identified alkylcyclobutones in some irradiated foods that were not detected in unirradiated foods. However, Crawford and Ruff (1996) reported that no radiolytic product of toxicological significance has been found in irradiated foods. The committee on the wholesomeness of irradiated foods convened by the Food and Agriculture Organization of the United Nations, the World Health Organization, and the International Atomic Energy Agency concluded, based on decades of research, that irradiated foods are safe and wholesome at any radiation dose (WHO, 1997). However, consumer acceptance remains one of the major factors of applying irradiation in foods. The other important factor is the cost. Nayga (2004) concluded that if the consumers were properly educated about what irradiation is and why it is done, approximately 80% will buy irradiated products even paying roughly 10 cents more per pound of ground beef.

13.2.3 Radiation Susceptibility of Microorganisms

Several factors influence the survival of microbial cells when exposed to ionizing radiation. These include the following: (1) Dose of ionizing radiation: the higher the dose, the greater is the destruction of microorganisms. However, the microbicidal efficacy of irradiation is lower under anaerobic conditions than in the presence of oxygen; this effect is attributed to the slower rate of oxidizing reactions, such as the formation of radicals due to the interaction of ionizing energy with water molecules. (2) Food processing treatments such as curing, high hydrostatic pressure, temperature, decreased pH, and added preservatives (sodium benzoate, potassium sorbate, sodium salt of methyl and propyl esters of parahydroxy benzoic acid, etc.) increase the efficiency of the ionizing radiation by decreasing the number of surviving organisms. However, the reduction of water activity or a decrease in the moisture content, a common preservation method, exhibits a protective effect against the lethal effect of ionizing radiation as a result of reduced free-radical formation due to lower moisture content (Thayer et al., 1995). Similarly, freezing causes a substantial increase in the resistance of vegetative cells, due to reduced availability of reactive water molecules; the radical formation is practically inhibited. Microbial radiation resistance in frozen foods is about two- to threefold higher than at ambient temperature. The composition of the food, in addition to its thickness and particle size, also plays an important role in determining the survival of microorganisms and the extent of the dose required to achieve the desired microbiological lethal effect. Bacterial cells are more protected against the lethal effects of irradiation in solid foods than in phosphate buffer. This is because of greater competition of the medium components in food matrix for the free radicals formed from water and activated molecules, thereby protecting the microorganisms. Accordingly, it is not advisable to predict the dose required to kill the microorganisms in one food based on the dose quantified in other foods. (3) Microorganisms vary considerably in their sensitivity to ionizing radiation. In general, the simpler is the organism, the more resistant it is to the effects of ionizing radiation. For example, viruses are more resistant than bacteria, which are more resistant than yeasts, which are more resistant than molds. Within bacteria, gram-negative cells are more sensitive than gram-positive bacteria, and rods are more sensitive than cocci. Spores are very resistant to irradiation because of their low water content.

13.2.4   Reduction or Elimination of Microorganisms

Foodborne pathogens and food spoilage microflora can be destroyed by irradiation. The D_{10} value is the radiation dose required to destroy 90% of bacterial population. Of the gram-negative bacterial pathogens of public health significance such as *Escherichia coli*, *Yersinia enterocolitica*, *Aeromonas hydrophila*, and *Campylobacter* species, *Salmonella* is the most resistant to irradiation, with a *D*-value of 0.6 kGy. Recommended doses for reduction of most resistant serotype of *Salmonella* by about 3 log-cycles (99.9%) to 5 logs (99.999%) are 3–5 kGy for frozen poultry, and 1.5–2.5 kGy for chilled poultry (Kampelmacher, 1984). For *E. coli* O157:H7, elimination of 90% of the viable cells in mechanically deboned chicken meat was achieved using 0.27 kGy at 5°C (Thayer and Boyd, 1993). Clavero et al. (1994) reported D_{10} values of 0.241–0.307 kGy for *E. coli* O157:H7 in ground beef. Thus, irradiation at dose levels of <2 kGy can effectively eliminate at least 6 logs of *E. coli* O157:H7 in ground beef.

Both gram-positive and gram-negative spoilage bacteria are easily destroyed by irradiation pasteurization doses. Irradiation doses to 2.5 kGy reduced the levels of aerobic and anaerobic bacteria by 4 and 5 $\log_{10}$, respectively, in chilled ground beef (Niemand et al., 1983). In an earlier study, Niemand et al. (1983) reported that the shelf life of vacuum-packaged beef was increased by 6 weeks after irradiation at 2 kGy (shelf life: 4 weeks for non-irradiated product versus 10 weeks for irradiated product). Lefebvre et al. (1992) reported that ground beef irradiated at doses of 2.5 kGy exhibited a 3 $\log_{10}$ reduction in psychrotropic aerobic bacteria, with a shelf-life extension of 9 days. Fish fillets treated with 1 kGy ionizing radiation had a refrigerated shelf-life of 15 days longer than non-irradiated fillets (Nickerson et al., 1983; Pryzbylski et al., 1989). Novak et al. (1966) reported that oysters, when irradiated with 2 kGy had a shelf-life of 23 days compared to non-irradiated oysters that began to spoil after 7 days.

13.2.4.1   Parasite Disinfestation

Doses of 0.15–0.30 kGy are required to eliminate the risk of contamination by *Trichinella spiralis*, a pork parasite. Ionizing radiations act by rendering the parasite sexually sterile, and blocking the maturation of ingested larvae in the hosts gut (Sivinski, 1985). The U.S. Food and Drug Administration consequently approved the use of irradiation to control *T. spiralis* in pork at a minimum absorbed dose of 0.3 kGy and not to exceed 1.0 kGy (FDA, 1985). Similarly, doses of 0.3–0.7 kGy are required to kill *Toxoplasma gondii* and render the pork safe for human consumption (Dubey and Thayer, 1994). Gamma irradiation of *Cysticercus bovis*–infected beef, with a dose of 0.4 kGy, prevents development of this parasite in the human host (King and Josephson, 1983).

13.3 Retorting of Liquid Foods with or without Particulates

13.3.1 Introduction

Sterilization of canned foods is essential to ensure safety to the consumer by assuring destruction of microbial growth. Thermal processing is the most important means of achieving commercial sterilization of canned foods; therefore heat transfer in canned food systems has been a matter of interest to researchers. During heating of foods, microbial destruction is also accompanied by nutrient degradation, which is of particular concern to the process designer. This problem can be overcome by high temperature–short time (HTST) process for sterilization of canned foods as this process ensures quality retention because of minimization of nutrient degradation and maintenance of degree of sterilization (Stoforos, 1988). Agitation of canned liquid foods (with or without particulates [solid-food particles]) results in high heat transfer rates. Thus thermal processes with high heat transfer rates from the heating source to the food result in better quality. Traditional methods of sterilization, i.e., retort method and aseptic method are two thermal processing techniques for commercial sterilization of canned foods. Convection is the main mode of heat transfer between heat source and fluid; and also at fluid–particle interface, during these thermal processing techniques.

The traditional method of sterilization of food, i.e., retort method, involves sterilization after filling of food in a can. This results in many problems such as the low rate of heat penetration to the slowest heating point in the container, the long processing time required to deliver the required lethality, destruction of the nutritional and sensory characteristics of the food, low productivity, and high energy costs (Ball and Olson, 1957; Smith et al., 1990; Ramaswamy et al., 1995). Hence, there is significant commercial interest in retort pouch technology.

In the retort method, the main focus has been to determine the effect of various parameters on heat transfer coefficients. The published research related to the determination of heat transfer coefficients in the retort processing technique is reviewed below.

13.3.2 Retort Method: Liquid System

13.3.2.1 Mathematical Treatment

Under the assumption that temperature of fluid surrounding the can is uniform, an energy balance for liquid inside the can yields:

$$hA_c(T_m - T_f) = m_f C_{pf} \frac{dT_f}{dt} \tag{13.1}$$

where h = overall heat transfer coefficient between the external medium and the internal liquid, if T_m is temperature of heating medium (K) or internal heat transfer coefficient between the can wall and inside liquid, if T_m is temperature of the can wall (W m^{-2} K^{-1}),

A_c = total can surface area (m^2)
T_f = uniform temperature of liquid inside the can at time t (K)
m_f = mass of liquid inside the can (kg)
C_{pf} = specific heat of liquid inside the can (J kg^{-1} K^{-1})
t = time (s)

Equation 13.1 can be used to determine h during retort processing of liquid-filled cans.

13.3.3 Effect of Mode of Rotation

In the retort method, cans filled with liquid food are heated by a heating medium (water or steam) for commercial sterilization. Rotation of the can affects the interaction between the liquid molecules and the can wall; thereby the heating rate is enhanced. Conley et al. (1951) reported the impact of rotation of cans on increase of heat transfer rates and the resulting decrease of sterilization times. Many researchers (Tsurkerman et al., 1971; Quast and Siozawa, 1974; Naveh and Kopelman, 1980; Anantheswaran and Rao, 1985) studied the effect of mode of rotation (axial and end-over-end) on heat transfer coefficients. Quast and Siozawa (1974) and Tsurkerman et al. (1971) working with Newtonian fluids (sucrose solutions) and non-Newtonian fluids (carboxyl-methyl-cellulose) reported that heat transfer rates for cans being axially rotated were two to four times the rates for stationary processing.

Naveh and Kopelman (1980) used specially constructed brass cylindrical cans (filled with glucose syrup) for heat transfer experiments. They examined the effect of end-over-end and axial rotation on overall heat transfer coefficient and reported two to three times greater overall heat transfer coefficient for end-over-end rotation than for axial rotation. The end-over-end rotation involves rotation of the central axis of the can around an axis perpendicular to the central axis of the can, i.e., end-over-end agitation is the motion imparted to a can when one end is in contact with the circumference of a revolving drum (Conley et al., 1951).

Quast and Siozawa (1974) reported that there was no significant effect of reversing the direction of rotation on heat transfer rates, whereas Hotani and Mihori (1983) reported that reversing the direction of rotation every 15–45 s (from clockwise to counterclockwise or vice-versa) resulted in higher heat transfer rates and more uniform heating. Hotani and Mihori (1983) conducted their tests when the fluid was at temperatures less than 70°C, which may have caused different heat transfer rates because parameters affecting heating characteristics are generally more dominant at early stages of heating when fluid temperature is high. Quast and Siozawa (1974) made observations at later stages of heating when the fluid temperature reached 96°C.

Anantheswaran and Rao (1985) also studied the effect of end-over-end rotation on heat transfer rates to Newtonian fluids with two copper cans (length to diameter ratio of 0.73 and 1.37) over the range of 0–38.6 rpm and 0–14.9 cm radius of rotation. The test fluids were distilled water, aqueous sucrose solutions, and glycerin. A laboratory agitating sterilizer was used for heat transfer studies. Steam at atmospheric pressure (757 mmHg) was used as the heating medium. They reported that end-over-end rotation of the cans improved the heat transfer rates to the test fluids (from 49% to 79%). The above results are attributed to the fact that for a given liquid the more vigorous the mixing, the more the interaction among the fluid molecules, the higher the fluid velocity, and thus higher heat transfer rates.

13.3.3.1 Effect of Rotational Speed

Clifcorn et al. (1950) performed experiments by rotating a can containing liquid at different speeds to obtain the maximum rate of heat penetration. They found that selection of proper speed may give more turbulence within the can contents and thus high heat transfer rates. They calculated the optimal rotational speed by using the formula $RN^2 = 35{,}196$ (centrifugal force = gravity force), where R is the distance from axis of rotation to the center of can's contents (in.), and N is the speed of rotation (rpm). They used tomato pulp of varying viscosities and reported that optimum rotational speed is a function of fluid viscosity and concluded that for more viscous fluids, the rotational speed must be decreased to achieve optimum conditions in order to allow time for the headspace volume to travel around the lower half of the can and through the center. Conley et al. (1951) reported that as the speed of rotation increases beyond the optimum, the centrifugal forces created decrease the mobility of the contents and thus decrease the heat transfer rates.

Naveh and Kopelman (1980) reported that increasing the rotational speed (0–120 rpm) resulted in a continuous increase of the overall heat transfer coefficient during heating processes, whereas asymptotic values of heat transfer coefficient were obtained with cans agitating at relatively low speeds of 40–70 rpm during the cooling phase. Their experiments were carried out in transparent plexiglass cylinders filled with glucose solutions of varying viscosities (0.12–18 poise). They attributed their observations to the fact that the viscosity of the liquid is higher during cooling phase compared to that during heating (Clifcorn et al., 1950 made observations during cooling phase). These studies (Clifcorn et al., 1950; Conley et al., 1951; Naveh and Kopelman, 1980) were conducted using Newtonian fluids. Anantheswaran and Rao (1985) working with non-Newtonian fluids (aqueous guar gum solutions) found that the overall heat transfer coefficients continuously increased with an increase in rotational speed from 0 to 38.5 rpm. The above observations can be attributed to the fact that the more the agitation, the more the interaction among fluid molecules, and the higher the heat transfer rates.

13.3.3.2   Effect of Distance between Can and Axis of Rotation

Clifcorn et al. (1950) reported that the distance between center of can and axis of rotation affects the rate of heating. Conley et al. (1951) studied the effect of speed of rotation on the cooling rate of a can containing 6:1 orange concentrate when cooled from 96°C to 38°C in 21°C water and reported that the optimum speed of rotation was dependent on the distance between the bottom of can and axis of rotation.

Naveh and Kopelman (1980) reported an increase in overall heat transfer coefficient when rotating cans move from central to off-center axis of rotation. Anantheswaran and Rao (1985) studied the effect of distance between center of can and axis of rotation on the heat transfer rates with 60% sucrose solution during the end-over-end rotation and reported that there is no significant effect of this distance on the heat transfer rates, but their investigation was based on a limited range of distance between the center of can and axis of rotation (0–14.9 cm). In a commercial end-over-end agitating retort, the heating rates were independent of distance between the center of can and axis of rotation (Anonymous, 1983).

13.3.3.3   Effect of Headspace

Headspace volume (total volume of can − volume of the can filled with liquid) is one of the important factors that influence the heat transfer rates during processing of rotating canned liquids. Quast and Siozawa (1974) found that the overall heat transfer coefficient increased significantly with an increase in headspace for viscous fluids, but it decreased slightly for fluids with low viscosity. This can be attributed to the fact that less headspace in more viscous fluids means less agitation, i.e., less interaction among molecules of rotating fluids, and thus results in low heat transfer coefficient. Naveh and Kopelman (1980) reported that the overall heat transfer coefficient approaches a constant value with increasing headspace volume (2%–3% of total internal can volume).

Anantheswaran and Rao (1985) reported that the headspace volume between 3% and 9% did not affect the heat transfer rates. Berry and Kohnhorst (1985) studied the effect of headspace on heat transfer rates by performing tests on commercial cans filled with a homogeneous, milk-based concentrate. A multistage preheat process that increased the product temperature in steps was used in this investigation. After heating to 123.9°C for less than 1 min, the cans were cooled rapidly by continuously spraying water at the top. They reported that agitation of the product was enhanced by the presence of headspace. Decreasing headspace resulted in lower heat transfer rates. They also pointed out the headspace effects were more significant for more viscous products (15 cps).

13.3.3.4 *Effect of Fluid Viscosity*

Fluid viscosity is the most important parameter affecting the heat transfer coefficient. The effect of viscosity on the heat transfer coefficient appears in correlation equation among Nusselt, Reynolds, and Prandtl numbers (Kramers, 1946; Ranz and Marshall, 1952; Whitaker, 1972; Anantheswaran and Rao, 1985).

Quast and Siozawa (1974) reported that heat transfer increased for decreasing viscosities. Many other researchers (Peralta Rodriguez and Merson, 1983; Anantheswaran and Rao, 1985; Rao et al., 1985) also found similar results. This can be explained by the fact that more viscous fluids result in less agitation and thus low heat transfer rates.

13.3.4   Retort Method: Liquid Foods with Particulate

13.3.4.1 *Mathematical Treatment*

An energy balance on the can contents yields

$$U_oA_c(T_{st} - T_f) = m_fC_{pf}\frac{dT_f}{dt} + m_pC_{pp}\frac{dT_p}{dt} \tag{13.2}$$

where
   U_o = overall heat transfer coefficient (W m^{-2} K^{-1})
   T_{st} = temperature of the heating medium (say steam) (K)
   T_p = temperature of particle (K)
   m_p = mass of particles inside the can (kg)
   C_{pp} = specific heat of particles inside the can (J kg^{-1} K^{-1})

Boundary condition at particle surface is

$$m_pC_{pp}\frac{dT_p}{dt} = h_{fp}A_p(T_f - T_p) \tag{13.3}$$

where
   h_{fp} = fluid-to-particle heat transfer coefficient (W m^{-2} K^{-1})
   A_p = surface area of particle (m^2)

Equations 13.2 and 13.3 can be used to determine U_o and h_{fp} during the retort processing of liquid foods with particulates.

13.3.5   Effect of Mode of Rotation

Many researchers (Lenz and Lund, 1978; Hassan, 1984; Deniston et al., 1987; Stoforos, 1988) determined fluid-to-particle heat transfer coefficient (h_{fp}) for canned liquid foods containing particles processed in agitated retort, but they did not compare the effect of different modes of rotation (end-over-end rotation, axial rotation) on h_{fp}.

Lekwauwa and Hayakawa (1986) determined h_{fp} for spheroidal potato particles in water during end-over-end rotation. They matched the center time–temperature profile of a potato particle predicted using a computer model, developed to simulate thermal responses of a packaged liquid–solid food, with the measured data and determined h_{fp} values between 60 and 2613 W m^{-2} K^{-1}.

Chang and Toledo (1990) determined h_{fp} by measuring the time–temperature history at the center of a 2 cm potato cube heated at 75°C in a stationary retort and found a h_{fp} value of 400 W m^{-2} K^{-1}. Weng et al. (1991) also determined h_{fp} from water to spherical polyacetal and nylon particle (2 cm diameter) in static retort and found h_{fp} value of 103 W m^{-2} K^{-1}.

13.3.5.1   Effect of Rotational Speed

The heat transfer coefficient increases with an increase in can rotational speed (Lenz and Lund, 1978; Hassan, 1984; Deniston et al., 1987) because it affects the relative particle-to-fluid velocity, which in turn affects h_{fp}. Lenz and Lund (1978) studied heat transfer and lethality in canned liquid (water or 60% sucrose solution) foods containing particles processed in an agitated retort at a steam temperature of 121°C. The fluid-to-particle heat transfer coefficient (h_{fp}) was determined for spherical lead particles, immobilized in the center of a rotating can. Changing the rotational speed from 3.5 to 8 rpm resulted in an average increase of h_{fp} by 150 W m^{-2} K^{-1}.

Hassan (1984) studied heating of potatoes, Teflon, and aluminum spheres in deionized water and silicone fluids of various kinematic viscosities (1.5×10^{-6}, 50×10^{-6}, and 350×10^{-6} m^2/s at 25°C) in a single can rotating axially. He reported that varying the can rotational speed (9.3–55.5–101 rpm) had a negligible effect on h_{fp} than on the overall heat transfer coefficient. He was unable to explain the reason behind this negligible effect.

Deniston et al. (1987) determined the heat transfer rates to steam heated, axially rotating cans containing potato spheres in water. They attributed the insensitivity of h_{fp} to can rotational speed (9.3–29.1–101 rpm) to three experimental conditions resulting in a small change in relative particle-to-fluid velocity: (1) closeness of density of potato particle (1063 kg/m^3) to that of water, so that particle settling due to gravity was minimal; (2) since the particle was located at the can center, centrifugal force acting on it was small; and (3) stiffness of the thermocouple wire hindered the particle motion.

Stoforos (1988) reported that increasing the rotational speed resulted in higher h_{fp} as long as the increasing rpm affects the relative particle-to-fluid velocity. At high rotational speeds (100 rpm), the can contents in his experiments behaved as a solid body due to centrifugal forces and he found tremendous drop in h_{fp} (from 2071 to 410 W m^{-2} K^{-1}) when Teflon particles heated in silicone fluid at about 50°C were rotated at 100 rpm instead of 54.5 rpm.

13.3.6   Effect of Fluid Viscosity

Lenz and Lund (1978) found lower h_{fp} for particles processed in a 60% aqueous sucrose solution (high viscosity) than for solids processed in water (low viscosity). Hassan (1984) reported that the overall heat transfer coefficient (U_o) and h_{fp} decreased as the fluid viscosity increased. He demonstrated that under equal processing conditions, the U_o and h_{fp} of Teflon particles were lowered when more viscous fluids (silicone oils of kinematic viscosities 1.5×10^{-6}, 50×10^{-6}, and 350×10^{-6} m^2/s) were used instead of water. The same pattern was observed for aluminum particles. Stoforos (1988) visualized a decrease in U_o and h_{fp} with increasing fluid viscosity. This can be attributed to the fact that more viscous fluids result in less agitation, i.e., low particle-to-fluid relative velocity and thus low heat transfer.

13.3.7   Effect of Particle Interaction

The presence of particulate matter during agitated processing alters the flow pattern of pure fluid (Rao and Anantheswaran, 1988). The amount of solid in the can influences the relative particle-to-fluid velocity and thus the heat transfer rates.

Lenz and Lund (1978) added real food (peas, carrot, or radish) particles of equal diameter to the test system containing lead spheres and simulated more closely the velocities and interactions of particles and fluids under real processing conditions and reported no significant effect on the h_{fp}. They immobilized test particles in the rotating cans, which might have caused particle to particle interaction different from a real processing condition. They reported a decrease in U_o for liquid with particles. They attributed this to the decreased relative particle-to-fluid velocity due to the drag exerted on the fluid by the particles.

Deniston et al. (1987) reported a slight increase in h_{fp} with increasing particle volume fraction, which was lowered for higher particle contents. They attributed this to the tight packing in the can (higher particle volume fraction), which restricted the particle's free movement. Stoforos (1988) mentioned that the mixing effect by moving particles contributes to a homogeneous temperature distribution in the can, especially for highly viscous products.

13.3.8 Effect of Particle Properties

The fluid-to-particle heat transfer coefficient (h_{fp}) will remain unaffected by the type of particle as long as the specific properties of particle under study (such as density or surface roughness) do not affect the particle–fluid pattern. When particles are allowed to move freely in the can, their different densities can influence their behavior in the fluid and thus result in different h_{fp} values. Hassan (1984) found higher h_{fp} for potato than for Teflon particles processed in water. Also, Teflon particles exhibited higher h_{fp} than aluminum particles of the same size, when processed in silicone fluids. Stoforos (1988) also reported similar results. He contributed this to high thermal diffusivity of the aluminum particles, which resulted in faster heat conduction in the aluminum particles as compared to Teflon particles.

13.3.9 Effect of Particle Size

Hassan (1984) and Lenz and Lund (1978) studied the effect of different sizes (2.22–3.49 cm) of potato, Teflon, and aluminum spheres on heat transfer coefficients. They reported an increase in both overall U_o and h_{fp} with an increase in particle diameter for particles heated in water. Also, Lekwauwa and Hayakawa (1986) reported higher h_{fp} with an increase in particle size (from 0.89 to 2.30 cm). They also reported that the temperature difference between the fluid and particles increased as the particle size increased. Deniston et al. (1987) reported that potato particle size (2.22, 2.86, or 3.5 cm diameter) did not influence h_{fp}.

The retorting process has not evolved much since its inception by Nicholas Appert in the 1800s, except for better quality retorts, temperature monitoring software and hardware, and different options for agitating cans in the retort during the heating process to get better and uniform heat transfer. However, the concept of retorting is moving toward retorting pouches versus cans for a better quality product, and to overcome issues such as over-heating of food products around walls in the can, and longer time required to accomplish the required lethality values. Whereas in pouches, the greater surface area results in a short time to achieve the required lethality values, which results in better quality products. With commercial innovations in retort pouches, we can see several products in the market at institutional and retail levels utilizing retort pouch technology. Although, nonthermal processing technologies are also gaining interest in the commercial world, retorting still remains the most cost-effective means to achieve shelf-stable low-acid foods.

13.4 Thermal Inactivation—Aseptic Processing

The use of heat treatment to kill bacteria is the most common food preservation process in use today. Heat treatment designed to achieve a specific lethality for foodborne pathogens in the specific target food is fundamentally important to assure the shelf life and microbiological safety of such thermally processed foods. The heat resistance of bacteria is described by two parameters: D- and Z-values. The D-value is defined as the heating time required at a specific temperature to destroy 90% of the viable cells or spores of a specific organism. The Z-value is defined as the change in heating temperature needed to change the D-value by 90% (1 log cycle). The Z-value provides information on the relative resistance of an organism to different destructive temperatures in a given substrate. D- and Z-values are invaluable tools in the design of heat processing requirements for desirable destruction of microorganisms in specific target food products.

13.4.1 Historical Aspects of Aseptic Processing

The concept of aseptic processing originated as a measure of solving the problems associated with the conventional "in-container" sterilization of foods. Aseptic processing was initiated in 1927 at the American Can Company Research Department in Maywood, Illinois under the direction of C.O. Ball (Mitchell, 1988). The result was the development of the HCF (heat-cool-fill) process for which Ball was granted a patent in 1936. The HCF process was targeted at low viscosity liquid and semiliquid foods. In 1938, two HCF units were installed for the commercial production of a chocolate-flavored milk beverage. The product was heated to 148°C in less than 15s, immediately cooled, and filled into sterile cans (Ball and Olson, 1957). The process was not a commercial success because of the associated high cost of the equipment, inflexibility with respect to can size, and the frequent blockages of the can-closing machine. Despite these problems, Ball is considered the pioneer of the aseptic process (Mitchell, 1988).

The Avocet process was another development in the field of aseptic processing credited to George Grindord at the Avocet plant located at San Joaquin of California (Ball and Olson, 1957). A cream product was introduced under the Avocet label in 1942. This process is unique in that the filling and closing area was treated to eliminate bacteria and further protection was accomplished by ultraviolet (UV) lamps (Mitchell, 1988). Sterilization was achieved by direct steam injection to a temperature of 125.4°C–136.4°C. The Avocet process is no longer in operation, but nevertheless it was another milestone in the development of aseptic processing.

Real progress in the commercial development of aseptic processing technology of food began with the invention of the Martin-Dole process in the late 1940s in California by the Dole Engineering Company (Lopez, 1987). The process could be used for the sterilization of any low-acid or high-acid fluid. Technical success was not, however, accompanied by the expected high level of exploitation; because the package, a metal can, had nothing to differentiate it from conventional "in-container" foods. Product heating and cooling was achieved by heat exchangers based on the principles of HTST sterilization, while the containers were sterilized by superheated steam

(Mitchell, 1988). The first commercial Dole system was installed in the early 1950s in California for the production of sauces and split-pea soup. Another historic development was brought about in the early 1960s by Loelinger and Regez of Switzerland, who successfully used hydrogen peroxide (H_2O_2) to sterilize flexible packaging materials used in the manufacture of milk containers (Lopez, 1987). Obtaining better quality products than those in conventional processing was the main objective of the Martin-Dole process, whereas extending the shelf life of fresh milk without refrigeration using low-cost containers was the goal of Loelinger and Regez process. In Europe, the technique developed by Loelinger and Regez is still prevalent in aseptic processing of food. Tetra Pak (a Sweden-based multinational company) is highly specialized and holds monopoly in the application of aseptic packaging techniques to different food products.

13.4.2   Requirements for Aseptic Processing and Packaging

Sterilization of products can be done by the following methods:

Direct heating—It can be achieved either by steam injection or steam infusion.

Indirect heating—It can be achieved using a suitable heat exchanger (plate, tubular, or scraped surface heat exchanger), in which the product is indirectly heated by the heating medium (steam, hot water).

Ohmic heating—It is a novel sterilization process in which heat is generated within a food by the passage of electric current, making it possible for particles to heat at the same or faster rate than fluids (an ideal ohmic process), whereas in a practical scenario, heating rates depend on the electrical (electrical conductivity) and thermal properties of both particle and liquid. This technique utilizes the principle that heat can be generated throughout the material by the passage of electric current, using the inherent electrical resistance of the material. The ohmic heating process is described in detail elsewhere (de Alwis et al., 1990).

Sterilization of packages can be done by hot air, superheated steam, hydrogen peroxide spray, and hot air drying (Table 13.3).

13.4.3   Latest Developments in Aseptic Processing Research

Aseptic processing has been commercially used for liquid foods; the major hurdle to be overcome in the use of this technology is the assurance of microbiological safety of the liquid foods with particulates. Determination of aseptic process schedules is rather complicated, due to difficulties involved in accurate measurement of temperature within the large particles

TABLE 13.3

Different Techniques for Sterilizing Aseptic Packages

Techniques	Types of Packages	Benefits/Limitations
Superheated steam	Metal cans/containers	High temperature can be applied at atmospheric pressure Microorganisms are resistant as compared to saturated steam
Dry hot air	Metal cans/containers	High temperature can be applied at atmospheric pressure Microorganisms are resistant as compared to saturated steam
Hot hydrogen peroxide (H_2O_2)	Plastic/laminated foil containers	Highly efficient
Hot hydrogen peroxide (H_2O_2) + UV light	Preformed plastic containers	More efficient due to UV
Ethylene oxide	Glass/plastic containers	Restricted use (residual problem)
Coextrusion heat process	Plastic containers	Chemically safe
Radiation	Plastic containers (heat sensitive)	Useful for heat sensitive packages Expensive

moving with a continuously flowing fluid in a closed system under pressure. For this reason, mathematical modeling of heat transfer is necessary for process design, which requires the knowledge of h_{fp}. Therefore, research has been done in various food processing research institutions all over the world to ensure "a safe aseptic processing of liquid foods with particulate". Tewari and Jayas (1997) have reviewed the work done in this area, which is summarized in the following paragraphs.

Researchers have made several assumptions to devise a mathematical model for aseptic processing of liquid foods with particulates. de Ruyter and Brunet (1973) developed a mathematical model for a food product containing spherical particles processed in a swept-surface heat-exchanger system. Their model assumes an infinite convective heat transfer coefficient at the particle–fluid interface. Manson and Cullen (1974) developed a thermal process simulation model for aseptic processing of foods containing cylindrical particles (assuming an infinite heat transfer coefficient). Sawada and Merson (1985) developed a model for particulate sterilization using water fluidized beds. Sastry (1986) developed a model for aseptic processing of particulate foods, which considered the effects of particle size, residence time distribution, and estimated values of convective coefficients, while being applicable to particles of regular and irregular shapes. He assumed a Nusselt number of 2.0 (for a steady-state heat conduction process for a sphere) in the simulation, i.e., finite h_{fp}.

The models discussed above require h_{fp} as an input parameter. Unfortunately, the determination of h_{fp} is a difficult exercise because of the difficulty in monitoring the time–temperature data within a particle.

Monitoring time–temperature data in a particulate food system is quite difficult because of difficulty in measuring surface or center temperature of moving particles. To monitor time–temperature data, researchers (Heppell, 1985; Chandarana et al., 1990; Stoforos and Merson, 1991; Ganesan et al., 1992; Balasubramaniam and Sastry, 1994a, b, c, d; Zitoun and Sastry, 1994) have used different techniques, which are listed below. Readers may find more information in the references.

Stationary particle method (Sastry, 1990).

Moving particle method
  Microbiological indicators (Hunter, 1972; Weng et al., 1991).
  Moving thermocouple method (Sastry, 1990).
  Time–temperature integrator (TTI) (Balasubramaniam and Sastry, 1994d).
  Thermal memory cell (Ganesan et al., 1992; Balasubramaniam and Sastry, 1994d).
  Melting point indicator (Mwangi et al., 1993).
  Temperature pill method (Balasubramaniam and Sastry, 1996).
  Liquid crystal method (Cooper et al., 1975; Stoforos, 1988; Balasubramaniam and Sastry, 1994d, 1995).

Relative velocity method (Kramers, 1946; Ranz and Marshall, 1952; Whitaker, 1972; Sastry, 1990).
  Transmitter particle technique (Bhamidipati and Singh, 1994, 1995).

13.5 Microwave Heating

Microwave heating of foods was first envisioned by Dr. Percy Spencer who patented the idea in 1945. By 1991, microwave heating had become so popular that in North American homes alone there were over 60 million microwave ovens (Owusu-Ansah, 1991). Microwave techniques were developed originally for military requirements. The objective was to design and manufacture microwave radar, navigation, and communications during the Second World War. After the war, many peacetime uses of microwaves were developed, including microwave processing systems as well as domestic and commercial microwave ovens.

In food heating operations, microwave heating offers several distinct advantages when compared to conventional heating methods. The advantages include speed of heating, energy saving, precise process control, and faster start-up and shut down times (Decareau, 1985). Other advantages include higher quality product in terms of taste, texture, and nutritional content.

13.5.1 Theory and Characteristics

Microwaves are nonionizing, time varying electromagnetic waves of radiant energy with frequencies ranging from 300 MHz to 300 GHz, i.e., wavelengths ranging from 1 mm to 1 m in free space. Due to possible interferences with television and radio waves, microwave ovens operate at 915 and 2450 MHz, allocated by the International Telecommunications Union. Domestic ovens operate at 2450 MHz. Microwaves travel similar to light waves; they are reflected by large metallic objects, absorbed by some dielectric materials and small strips of metal, and transmitted through other dielectric materials. For example, water and carbon absorb microwaves well; on the other hand, glass, ceramics, and most thermoplastics allow microwaves to pass through with little or no absorption. They can also be refracted when traveling from one dielectric material to the next, analogous to the way light waves bend when passing from air into water.

13.5.2 How Microwaves Produce Heat

There are two main mechanisms by which microwaves produce heat in dielectric materials: ionic polarization and dipole rotation. Ionic polarization occurs when ions in solution move in response to an electric field. Kinetic energy is given up to the ions by the electric field. These ions collide with other ions, converting kinetic energy into heat. When the electric field is rotating at 2.45×10^9 Hz, numerous collisions occur, generating a great deal of heat.

However, the dipole rotation mechanism is more important. It is dependent on the existence of polar molecules. The most common polar material found in foods is water. Water molecules are randomly oriented under normal conditions. In the presence of an electric field, the polar molecules line up with the field. As mentioned above, the electric field of a microwave system alternates at 2.45×10^9 Hz, so that while the molecules try to align themselves with this changing field, heat is generated. When the field is removed, the molecules return to their random orientation.

In capacitive or radio-frequency heating, the material is usually placed between electrodes, whereas in microwave heating a closed cavity or oven is used. When microwaves interact with polar or polarizable molecules in foods, the polar or polarizable (p/p) molecules try to reorient themselves to follow the field. This results in heat generation by the p/p molecules if the time for the establishment and decay of their polarization is comparable to the period of the high oscillation provided by the microwave frequency. The classical view of microwave heating is to consider the heating process as due to the rotation of a dipolar molecule in a viscous medium dominated by friction (Stuchley and Stuchley, 1983). Heating may also result from the movement of electrically charged ions within foods (Giese, 1992). In essence, microwave heating of foods results from interaction of the microwaves with ionic or dipolar content of the food. Water, proteins, and carbohydrates are among the dipolar ingredients in food. In foods, these are volumetrically distributed within the food material. Consequently, microwave heating results in volumetric heating. The effectiveness of this volumetric heating and the depth to which it occurs is determined by the dielectric properties of the material and the frequency of the microwave. The dielectric properties of the material determine the amount of incident microwaves reflected, transmitted, or absorbed by the material.

For low-moisture hygroscopic foods (such as egg-white powder), Adu and Otten (1993) suggested that the increase in product hygroscopicity due to moisture loss, which increases the latent heat of vaporization during heating, will require heating equations that account for changes in product hygroscopicity to accurately predict the microwave heat and mass transfer characteristics of foods during mathematical modelling of microwave heating for dry foods.

13.5.3   Dielectric Properties of Foods

The dielectric property most important in the microwave heating of foods is the ratio of the dielectric properties expressed as ratios of the dielectric properties of free space. This gives the relative dielectric constant and relative dielectric loss factor. The relative dielectric constant governs the amount of incident power absorbed or reflected, while dielectric loss factor measures the amount of absorbed energy dissipated or transmitted within the food.

The relevant electrical property is the complex permittivity (ε^*), which is defined by the following equation:

$$\varepsilon^* = \varepsilon' - j\varepsilon''$$

where
   ε' is the dielectric constant
   ε'' is the dielectric loss factor

The dielectric properties of foods at microwave frequencies are related to their chemical composition. They are also highly dependent on the frequency of the applied electric field, the moisture content, temperature, and bulk density (Metaxas and Meredith, 1983; Decareau, 1985). The dielectric constant at any given frequency increases with moisture content. The loss factor may increase with moisture content depending on temperature, moisture content, and frequency. The loss factor remains approximately constant for moisture contents below the critical moisture content of the material. At constant temperatures, the loss factor increases with increasing moisture content for most solid foods with moisture content greater than their critical moisture content. The loss factor may however increase or decrease with temperature. In materials where the loss factor increases with increase in temperature, uneven heating intensified runaway and thermal runaway may result. The other physical properties of food should be taken into account carefully when predicting the temperature rise during microwave heating. For example, fat and water show a similar temperature increase trend when heated in a 2450 MHz microwave oven, since fat has a lower heat capacity (specific heat) to compensate the lower dielectric loss factor. Unfortunately, most of the dielectric property data for foods remain unavailable, which further impact the design of user-friendly products. Nowadays the majority of household microwave ovens are used for food reheating. In order to overcome the complexities of the food system and the difficulties in predicting its response in microwave heating, Swain et al. (2004) reported the development of food simulants, for microwave oven testing, which provide reliable and reproducible characterization of heating performance of microwave ovens (2450 MHz), specially when heating chilled convenience meals.

The power supply is a significant part of the capital cost of a microwave oven. A magnetron requires anywhere from 4 to 10,000 V to operate. Therefore, the generator must step up the voltage from the electrical outlet (110 V) to the operating requirements. The magnetron creates the microwave signal, which is fed into the cavity (in the case of an industrial process, this might be a conveyor belt).

A microwave oven, compared to a conventional oven is more efficient. For example, if you want to bake in an oven, you must first heat about 15 kg of steel and the air in it, finally the hot air is transferred to the potato. By the time the potato is cooked, you only get about 2% efficiency. In a microwave oven, there is about 50% efficiency in the oven cavity, and almost all of it will be used to cook the potato (Buffler, 1986).

13.5.4 Microwave Food Processing

Microwave food processing activities that have shown great promise include thawing and tempering, reheating, drying, cooking, baking, sterilization and pasteurization, and blanching.

The first industrial scale microwave process was introduced in the early 1960s. This process was for the drying of fried potato chips. The first lightweight counter-top oven was designed in 1965. Some of the first oven sales were to research laboratories of food manufacturers, universities, and government laboratories, where studies were conducted on blanching of vegetables, coffee roasting, freeze-drying, etc.

In general, microwave equipment is more expensive to purchase than conventional technology. However, the use of microwaves industrially is more economical than conventional methods. In addition, capital costs of industrial microwave ovens have been reduced due to recent advances in equipment design. Cooking times of microwaves are one-quarter of the time or less than conventional methods. Presently, microwaves are used to achieve quick internal heating, and conventional heat sources are used to produce the desired surface browning or crispness.

On top of being flexible, microwave processing offers the user a high degree of control; for instance, no-lag startup heating, flatter temperature profiles in the finished product, rapid response to the removal of heat. Microwaves have the ability to heat products while they are still in sealed packages even if the packaging acts as an insulator, and are capable of volume expansion within a closed container as well as generating pressure (Sanio and Michelussi, 1986).

Some commercially proven applications include dehydration of low-moisture solids, precooking of meat products, and tempering of frozen foods. Other microwave operations such as vacuum drying, pasteurization, sterilization, baking, blanching, and rendering are less significant.

13.5.4.1 Thawing and Tempering

Tempering of foods requires raising the temperature of the food item from a solidly frozen condition to about −2°C, where it is still in a firm state so that it can be easily sliced or separated. Conventional tempering of frozen foods is a long and arduous process taking from several hours to a few days to complete depending on the size, type, and initial temperature of the food product. Disadvantages of conventional thawing and tempering include large cold-storage areas, large inventories of frozen products, bacterial growth resulting from the long durations of thawing, large amounts of drip loss, adverse color changes, surface oxidation, and high consumption of fresh water (in cases requiring the use of water as the thawing liquids) (Rosenberg and Bogl, 1987). Microwave tempering eliminates many of these disadvantages. Thus thawing and tempering has become one of the most important applications of microwave technology in the food industry.

Microwave tempering is defined as taking a product from freezer temperature to a condition between −4°C and −2°C in which the product is not frozen but is still firm. Tempering at this temperature avoids overheating and results in minimal quality deterioration, and tremendous energy savings. The lower microwave tempering temperatures and shorter tempering durations eliminate the conditions for microbial growth. In addition, the shorter time for microwave tempering eliminates the need for large temperature-controlled storage areas and large inventories of frozen products. Drip loss reduction of up to 10% adds to the advantages (IFT, 1989). Additional benefit includes being able to process products while they are still in their original container.

Most microwave tempering units operate at 915 MHz due to the higher penetration depth that this frequency provides over 2450 MHz frequency. The high penetration depths are of extreme importance since the target materials are usually fairly large, for example, frozen meat blocks or blocks of butter (Richardson, 1992).

13.5.4.2 Reheating

Reheating is the process of increasing the temperature of previously cooked or heat processed food from ambient temperature to a higher temperature.

The ability of microwave heating to provide faster volumetric heating without the need to heat the container or package material of the foods has made reheating one of the most frequent microwave processing applications. It is this advantage that has resulted in the tremendous success of microwave energy use in domestic and food retail-service centers.

13.5.4.3 Drying

Drying refers to processes that result in the reduction or removal of moisture from a material up to the point where it attains moisture equilibrium with its environment. Microwave drying has been shown to be possible for a number of food products, but the cost of such systems makes it impractical for total drying operations. Consequently, they are mostly applied in combination with hot air or other conventional heating techniques.

Microwave drying is mainly employed during the falling-rate period for finish drying or precise control of final moisture content. This is because during the falling-rate period, the rate limiting step results from the resistance provided by the solid material to the supply of moisture to the surface of the product for evaporation. During the falling-rate period of drying, conventional drying becomes a slow process as heat must first be conducted through already-dried material to the evaporating front inside the material before moisture can migrate to the surface. Microwaves operate directly on the polar water molecules. Consequently, microwave drying is able to speed up the moisture-migration process. Moreover the selective heating of wet portions of the food reduces case hardening and surface browning.

Pasta drying by microwave energy has now become an industry (Giese, 1992). The process is a combination of conventional hot air drying followed by a microwave and hot air stage. Freshly extruded pasta with a moisture content of approximately 30% is hot air dried at 71°C–82°C to around 18%. Combined microwave and hot air drying then lowers the moisture level to about 13%. Microwave vacuum has been used for the production of fruit juice concentrates and microwave freeze drying has been tried for various food products including fruits, coffee and tea, mushrooms, meat, and fish proteins.

Other microwave drying applications include systems for soybean drying and dehusking as a further step toward oil extraction (Decareau, 1986). When soybeans are conventionally dried they have to be kept from 3 to 5 days for the moisture within the seed to equilibrate. Moreover, the seed coat of the dried beans needs to be split for effective dehulling before oil extraction. The volumetric heating resulting from microwaves eliminates the undesirable moisture gradient and thus eliminates the need for the moisture equilibration. Microwaves effectively split the seed coat resulting in effective dehulling.

13.5.4.4 Cooking

Microwave cooking has been found to result in yield increases of 25%–38% of bacon because none of the product is lost by overcooking (IFT, 1989). In addition, the process produces high-quality rendered fat as a by-product. Two alternative systems for bacon cooking are available. The bacon may first be preheated with hot air before cooking with microwave energy. The second alternative uses microwave energy alone for the whole process. The bacon so processed is mainly supplied as precooked bacon to food service operations.

13.5.4.5 Blanching

The heat treatment applied to food material to inactivate cell activity and enzymes is known as blanching. In food processing, this treatment is commonly applied to fruits and vegetables. Blanching serves to prevent development of off-flavors and off-color in frozen fruits and vegetables. For most fruits and vegetables, microwave blanching does not produce significant improvements over conventional steam blanching (IFT, 1989). However, a more successful application may be found for the enzyme inactivation of selected products like tomatoes or whole soybeans (Klingler and Decker, 1989). Metaxas and Meredith (1983) reported that microwave energy effectively inactivates the growth inhibitor enzyme antitrypsin at a temperature of 105°C in 2 min. The minimum time to achieve the same result was 30 min when conventional heating methods were used.

13.5.4.6 Baking

Microwave baking has been successful for several flour-base foods. As mentioned earlier, the main disadvantage of microwave baking is the lack of crust formation and surface browning in baked foods for which crust formation and browning are important. Consequently, in most applications, combined microwave and hot air baking reduced oven time for baking by up to 66% (Richardson, 1992). Decareau (1985) reported that microwave baking resulted in a good retention of the yeasty flavor and attributed this to the lower ambient temperature conditions. The development of microwave susceptor has much enhanced the surface browning and crispiness. The susceptor is widely used in the frozen baked food products that may be reheated in the household microwave oven.

Another application of microwave energy in the baking industry is in enhancing or speeding up the proofing of yeast-raised dough products. Microwave proofing has reduced the total proofing time for yeast-raised doughnuts to an average of 4 min as compared to the conventional 25–35 min (IFT, 1989).

13.5.4.7 Sterilization and Pasteurization

Sterilization refers to the complete destruction of microbial organisms. Commercially, sterility means that all pathogenic, toxic-producing

TABLE 13.4

Microwave Food Processing Applications

Application	Frequency (MHz)	Power (kW)	Products
Tempering—batch or continuous	915	30–70	Meat, fish, poultry
Drying—vacuum or freeze drying	915 or 2450	30–50	Pasta, onions, snack foods, fruit juices
Precooking	915	50–240	Bacon, poultry, sausages, meat patties, sardines
Pasteurization/ sterilization	2450	10–30	Fresh pasta, milk, semi-solid foods, pouch-packages foods
Baking	915	2–10	Bread, doughnut proofing

Source: From IFT, *Food Technol.* 43, 117, 1989.

organisms and spoilage organisms have been destroyed or reduced to safe levels. Microwave sterilization operates in the temperature range of 110°C–130°C. Pasteurization is a gentle heat treatment usually at temperatures between 60°C and 82°C. Microwave sterilization and pasteurization has been applied to several foods including fresh pasta, bread, granola, milk, and prepared meals. The main advantage of microwave sterilization or pasteurization is the effective reduction in the time required for the heat to penetrate to the food center. Table 13.4 gives a summary of microwave food processing applications. Sweet potato purees were aseptically processed using a continuous flow microwave system to obtain a shelf-stable product reported by Coronel et al. (2004). A pilot scale test was conducted in a 60 kW microwave unit where the product was heated to 135°C and held at that temperature for 30 s. The products were shelf-stable with no detectable microbial count during a 90-day storage period at room temperature. The color and puree viscosity were not significantly affected by this process. The authors also claimed that this is the first report of aseptically packaged vegetable puree processed by a continuous flow microwave heating system.

13.5.4.8 Precooking

Precooking combines microwaves with steam or hot air techniques in the commercial cooking of beef patties, bacon, poultry, battered and breaded fish, etc. Some of the advantages of microwave precooking are reducing production time, floor space, shipping and refrigeration costs; increased yield provides less product waste (sanitation problems); and labor needs.

13.5.5 Microwave Food Process Design

In designing microwave food processes and packaging, various factors that affect microwave heating of foods should be taken into consideration if the effect of uneven heating associated with the use of microwaves is to be kept under control. These factors fall into two broad categories. The first one is thermophysical properties of the food. The second is factors associated with the dielectric characteristics of food and the field intensity distributions provided by various microwave energy applicators and heating systems.

13.5.5.1 Physical Factors

The thermophysical factors that require serious consideration in the design of microwave food processes and packaging systems are

Size and shape of food: The physical size and shape of foods affect the temperature distribution within the food. This results from the fact that the intensity of the wave decreases with depth as it penetrates the food. If the physical dimension of the food is greater than twice the penetration depth of the wave, portions of the food nearer the surface can have very high temperatures while the mid portions are still cold. On the other hand, if the dimension of the food is much lower than the penetration depth of the wave, the center temperature can be far higher than the temperature at the surface. This situation normally results in "the focussing effect", which results from the combined intensity of the wave (in three space dimensions) being higher at the inner portions than the outer portions of the product.

   Some shapes reflect more microwaves than others. In addition, some shapes prevent increasing amounts of the waves from leaving the material by reflecting them back into the interior. For most spherical and cylindrical foods, wave focussing occurs for product diameters between 20 and 60 mm. In rectangular foods, focussing causes the overheating of corners. Thus in package design, sharp corners are avoided and tube shaped pans have been suggested (Giese, 1992). Moreover in foods with corners, packages are designed using metals or aluminum foils to reflect microwave energy away from corners and thus selectively heating some portions more.

Surface area: In microwave heating, the product temperature rises above its ambient temperature due to volumetric heating. Higher product surface area therefore results in higher surface heat loss rate and more rapid surface cooling. During microwave heating, the highest temperature is not at the surface of the product (despite the higher intensity of power absorbed there) but somewhere in the interior.

Specific heat: How much a food product will heat given a specific amount of energy depends on its heat capacity. The implication of this for microwave heating is that different food products heated together have different temperature histories. To control this, some microwave food packages are sealed tight to allow heat transfer between hotter and colder foods, thus giving similar temperature history for different foods in the same package.

Dielectric properties: The dielectric behavior of foods affects their heating characteristics. As stated earlier, the dielectric properties of some foods increase with temperature while for others they decrease. When foods with opposite dielectric behaviour are heated together, temperature differences between them intensify with time. Thus foods with similar dielectric characteristics are put together or special packages are designed to facilitate heat transfer between dissimilar foods.

13.5.6 Microbial Safety with Microwave Heating

It is generally accepted that the microbial kill during the microwave heating follows the principles of thermal inactivation. The lethality, therefore, may be calculated using the Z-value of a microbe, especially the pathogens, and the time–temperature history of the microwave heating process. Due to the uneven heating occurring in the microwave cooking and the complexities of the food system (compositions, shapes, and packaging, etc.), locating the coldest point may become a major challenge for food developers (product development) and food processors (process development). FDA (2000) has published an article with useful information regarding the microwave applications and microbial safety concerns. Also, the recent development of magnetron with better designed control devices has increased the microwave power and efficiency for industrial food heating applications.

13.6 Hydrostatic High-Pressure Processing

13.6.1 Introduction

Nonthermal food processing techniques are regarded with special interest by the food industry presently. Among nonthermal techniques (pulse-electric field pasteurization, high intensity pulsed lights, high intensity pulsed-magnetic field, ozone-treatment), high-pressure processing (HPP) is also gaining in popularity with food processors not only because of its food preservation capability but also because of its potential to achieve interesting functional effects (Leadley and Williams, 1997). High-pressure processing has had application for years in other industries that process or use ceramics, carbon graphite, diamond, steel/alloy, and plastics. Hite et al. (1914) were the first researchers who reported the effects of HPP on food microorganisms by subjecting milk to pressures of 650 MPa and obtaining a reduction in the viable numbers of microbes. For the last 15 years, the use of HPP has been explored extensively in the food industry and related research institutions due to the increased demand by consumers for improved nutritional and sensory characteristics of food without loss of "fresh" taste. In recent years, HPP has been extensively used in Japan, and a variety of food products like jams and fruit juices have been processed (Cheftel, 1995). There have been 10–15 types of pressurized foods on the Japanese market, but several have disappeared, and those that remain are so specific that they would have little interest to European or American markets. Nevertheless, interest in HPP derives from its ability to deliver foods with fresh-like tastes without added preservatives. In the recent development, Avomex Inc. (Keller, Texas) has successfully produced commercially and marketed the avocado paste, which has set the new quality standard for HPP-treated products. The Grupo Jumex (Mexico) also introduced the HPP-treated juices. Other commercialized products available in the United States include fruit smoothies, salsa, oysters, ham, chicken strips, etc. The cost of high pressure processed products may be up to 10 cents per pound more than those made by thermal process depending on the production scale. The cost from HPP is expected to decrease as the technology becomes more mature and market expands in the coming years.

13.6.2   Mechanism of HPP

Any phenomenon in equilibrium (chemical reaction, phase transition, change in molecular configuration), accompanied by a decrease in volume, can be enhanced by pressure (Le Chatelier's Principle: Leadley and Williams, 1997). Thus, HPP affects any phenomenon in food systems where a volume change is involved and favors phenomena that result in a volume decrease. The HPP affects non-covalent bonds (hydrogen, ionic, and hydrophobic bonds) substantially as some non-covalent bonds are very sensitive to pressure, which means that low molecular weight food components (responsible for nutritional and sensory characteristics) are not affected, whereas high molecular weight components (whose tertiary structure is important for functionality-determination) are sensitive. Some specific covalent bonds are also modified by pressure. The other principles that govern HPP are the *Isostatic Principle*, which implies that the transmittance of pressure is uniform and instantaneous (independent of size and geometry of food), however, transmittance is not instantaneous when gases are present; and the *Microscopic Ordering Principle*, which implies that at constant temperature, an increase in pressure increases the degree of ordering of the molecules of a substance (Heremans, 1992). Another interesting rule concerns the small energy needed to compress a solid or liquid to 500 MPa as compared to heating to 100°C, because compressibility is small. HPP offers several advantages: reduced process times; minimal heat penetration and heat damage problems; freshness, flavor, texture, and color are well retained; there is no vitamin C loss; multiple changes in ice-phase forms resulting in pressure-shift freezing; and functionality alterations are minimized compared with traditional thermal processing

(Farr, 1990; Mertens, 1992; Williams, 1994; Cheftel, 1995; Knorr, 1995; Leadley and Williams, 1997).

13.6.3 Microbial Inactivation

Application of HPP as a method for microbial inactivation has stimulated considerable interest in the food industry. The effectiveness of HPP on microbial inactivation has to be studied in great detail to ensure the safety of food treated in this manner. Currently, research in this area has concentrated mainly on the effect of HPP on spores and vegetative cells of different pathogenic bacterial species. Detectable effects of HPP on microbial cells include an increase in the permeability of cell membranes and possible inhibition of enzymes vital for survival and reproduction of the bacterial cells (Farr, 1990). To design appropriate processing conditions for HPP of food materials, it is essential to know the precise tolerance levels of different microbial species to HPP and the mechanisms by which that tolerance level can be minimized. Acknowledgment of critical factors that affect the baroresistance of different bacterial species will help in the development of more effective and accurate high-pressure processors. Inappropriate use of a variety of parameters like pressure range, processing temperature, initial temperature of sample, holding time, and packaging type may adversely affect the outcome of HPP. Thus, a thorough understanding of the effect of a variation in critical factors on the intracellular changes undergone by pressure-treated microbial species is essential for documentation of a safe HPP. The physicochemical environment can adversely change the resistance of a bacterial species to pressure. In most cases, the effect of HPP on gram-positive bacteria is less pronounced than on gram-negative species. Factors such as the water activity and pH also influence the extent to which foods need to be treated to eliminate pathogenic microorganisms.

Hoover et al. (1989) reported that most bacteria are baroduric, i.e., they are capable of enduring high pressures but grow well at atmospheric pressures. Hauben et al. (1997) studied HPP resistance development in *Escherichia coli* MG1655 mutants. Three barotolerant mutants (LMM1010, LMM1020, and LMM1030) were isolated and pressure treated. Mutants showed 40%–85% survival at 200 MPa for 15 min (ambient temperature) and 0.5%–1.5% survival at 800 MPa for 15 min (ambient temperature). In contrast, survival of the parent strain (MG1655) decreased from 15% at 220 MPa to 2×10^{-8}% at 700 MPa. It should be noted that pressure sensitivity of the mutants increased from 10°C to 50°C, as opposed to the parent strain that showed minimum sensitivity at 40°C. This research indicated that the development of high levels of barotolerance should be properly understood in order to predict the safety of HPP. Similar studies are needed to document the barotolerance of other potentially pathogenic bacterial species.

Maggi et al. (1994) studied the effects of HPP on the heat resistance of fungi in apricot nectar and distilled water. They reported complete inactivation of *T. flavus* ascospores at 900 MPa for 20 min at 20°C, a 2 log cycle reduction in *N. fischeri*, but no effect was seen on *B. fulva* and *B. nivea* populations. In contrast, preheating apricot nectar (50°C) followed by pressure treatment of 800 MPa for 1–4 min resulted in complete inactivation of all four species. Also, lower pressure resistance was observed in distilled water samples.

13.6.3.1 Factors Affecting Microbial Inactivation

Several theories on the effect of HPP on bacterial species have been proposed over the years to explain the mechanism behind microbial inactivation and to better optimize HPP of foods. The processing conditions (initial sample temperature, circulating water temperature, pressurizing medium, holding time) under which high pressures are applied significantly influence the level of inactivation as well as the overall effect on the nutritional and sensory characteristics of food. Ye et al. (1996) studied the pressure tolerance of *Saccharomyces cerevisiae*, *Escherichia coli*, and *Staphylococcus epidermidis* in various media (agar, broth, apple jam, and juice), by subjecting the inocula to a pressure of 300 MPa at 5°C–25°C for 1–20 min. They reported that media pH played a very important role in the destruction of microbes; *S. epidermidis* was inhibited >90% at 300 MPa in 11.2 min at pH 7.2 and in 4.8 min at pH 4.0. Variations in the pH and water activity of foods can result in different levels of lethality to a particular bacterium for the same high-pressure processing parameters. Studies conducted by Timson and Short (1965) on *B. subtilis* showed that the pressure resistance of the bacterium (when subjected to 483 MPa for 30 min) was decreased as the pH in milk medium was lowered or raised from a pH value of 8. This value is not a constant for all microorganisms and the survival of *B. subtilis* at a specific pH can vary with the pressure and temperature of treatment. The type of culture medium used for growing the microbial species can also have a significant impact on the pressure and heat resistance of any microorganism. In general, the richer the growth medium, the better the baroresistance of the microorganisms. This is thought to be because of the increased availability of essential nutrients and amino acids to the stressed cell. It must be kept in mind that the parameters governing pressure tolerance are not constant for every bacterial species; they vary from one bacterium to another, and may also be different for a single species grown under different conditions or in different growth media. It is very likely that the application of pressure affects a multitude of functions in a cell, thus interacting to retard or even kill the cell (Hoover et al., 1989). Therefore, studies related to the inactivation of bacterial species during HPP should specifically describe and document the processing conditions under which the inactivation took place. Also, specific information should be given about the variation in sample temperature during HPP.

Hayakawa et al. (1994) compared the pressure resistance of spores of six *Bacillus* strains. The spores were cultivated on nutrient agar and suspended in cold, sterile, distilled water with the filtrate being heated for

30 min at 80°C to destroy any vegetative cells. Spores of these six strains were then treated under pressures ranging from 196 to 981 MPa at 5°C–10°C for holding times of 20–120 min. It was found that *B. stearothermophilus* IAM 12043, *B. subtilis* IAM 12118, and *B. licheniformis* IAM13417 had the most resistance to pressure, but *B. coagulans* was actually activated when treated with high pressures. There was no actual correlation between pressure and heat resistance, although they chose rightly a number of spore-forming bacteria varying widely in heat resistance. This could be due to applications of very low pressure in most cases. However, variables including initial and final spore levels and dilution levels were not specified, which may help understanding the results better. It should also be noted that, in most cases, the reference heat treatment is much more inactivating than the pressure treatment to be compared, therefore, direct comparisons between heat resistance and pressure resistance are not possible.

Patterson et al. (1995) studied the sensitivity of vegetative pathogens (*Yersinia enterocolitica* 11174, *Salmonella typhimurium* NCTC 74, *Salmonella enteritidis*, *Staphylococcus aureus* NCTC 10652, *Listeria monocytogenes*, *Escherichia coli* O157:H7) in buffer (pH 7.0), UHT milk, and poultry meat to high pressures up to 700 MPa at 20°C. A 10^5 reduction in numbers was obtained in all cases when pressures in the range of 275–700 MPa for 15 min were applied at 20°C. Different strains of *L. monocytogenes* and *E. coli* O157:H7 showed significant variation in pressure resistance, which were further used to examine the effect of substrates on pressure sensitivity, and indicated that the substrate affected the baroresistance of the microorganisms significantly.

The pH of a food material plays a very important role in determining the extent to which HPP affects the microorganisms under study. Several studies have documented and analyzed changes in heat resistance of organisms grown under different pH conditions, but there have not been very many studies on the pressure resistance of spores at different pH values. Roberts and Hoover (1996) investigated the effects of changes in pH values combined with a variety of other factors on the pressure-resistance of *B. coagulans* ATCC 7050. They reported an increase in the effectiveness of pressurization as the pH of the buffer was lowered. A decrease of an additional 1.5 log was observed as the pH was decreased from 7.0 to 4.0. On the basis of these results, it is highly probable that, other factors remaining constant, a neutral pH value is most conducive to high-pressure resistance in the cells. Earlier, Timson and Short (1965) observed that at high pressure the spores were most resistant at neutral pH; and at low pressure, most sensitive to neutral pH. That is perfectly in line with other findings that a pressure between 50 and 200 MPa enhances germination followed by kill and direct killing at high pressures above 900 MPa. In contrast, Sale et al. (1970) reported that the inactivation of bacterial spores by pressurization was maximum when the buffer was at a pH near neutral and was lowest at extreme values of pH. The difference in pH was thought to affect membrane ATPase and intracellular functions of the spore, thereby destabilizing the microorganisms (MacDonald, 1992). This effect of pH on the pressure resistance of any microorganism is accentuated by other factors like the addition of salts, temperature conditions, and general process parameters. A better understanding of the exact process by which the variations in the pH affects the stability of the spore is still awaited and should give a better overall picture of the effect of high pressures. Therefore, studies to examine the effect of pH variation on the inactivation of different types of spores by HPP need to be done.

The water activity (a_w) of cells also affects the in-pressure resistance. It is reported that the lower the a_w, the higher the pressure resistance of cells. Palou et al. (1996, 1998) studied the combined effect of HPP and a_w on *Zygosaccharomyces bailii* inhibition. They reported complete inhibition of yeast at $a_w > 0.98$, and an increase in the surviving fraction with a decrease in a_w. They concluded that addition of sucrose (to decrease a_w) acts as a baroprotective layer, preventing inhibition of yeast even at high pressures. Such a mechanism can be utilized to prevent inhibition of favorable microbes during HPP. More work is also needed in this area.

13.6.4 Combined Processes

13.6.4.1 Pressure and Temperature

Alpas et al. (1998) studied the interaction of pressure, time, and temperature on the viability of *Listeria innocua* strain CWD47 in peptone solution, by subjecting samples to pressures in the range of 138–345 MPa, temperature in the range of 25°C–50°C, and exposure times of 5–15 min. They showed that the combination of 345 MPa, 50°C, and 9.1 min could reduce the microbial population by 7 logs, with a Z-value (temperature change in degree Celsius causing a 10-fold reduction in D-value; here it stands for pressure in MPa needed to reduce D-value by 10-fold) of 173 MPa. Such studies resulting in description of Z-values for a specific microbial species are aimed toward a standardization of HPP parameters, which will facilitate commercialization of HPP.

Maggi et al. (1995) studied the use of HPP for inactivation of *Clostridium pasteurianum* spores isolated from peeled tomato and inoculated into tomato serum. They reported that high-pressure treatments of 900 MPa for 5 min at 60°C completely destroyed the spores (which was not obtained at temperatures <60°C). Pressures of 700 or 800 MPa for 5 min at 60°C resulted in D-values of 2.4 and 3.4 min, respectively. They also studied spore inactivation using pressure pretreatment followed by heat treatment and found that a pretreatment of 300 or 500 MPa for 1 min at 60°C reduced heat resistance of spores by one-third and half, respectively. Their documented D-values for *C. pasteurianum* may be used for developing a database for pressure-temperature-time requirements for complete destruction of different types of spores. Roberts and Hoover (1996) studied the inactivation of *Clostridium sporogenes* PA3679 and *Bacillus subtilis* 168 using a combination of pressure, temperature, acidity, and nisin. They exposed the samples (buffer at pH 4–7, inoculated with spores) to 405 MPa at different temperatures (25°C–90°C) for 15 or 30 min. After pressure treatment, spores were pour plated onto agar with or without nisin. They reported an increase in spore inactivation with a decrease in pH. Also, sterilization was achieved using higher temperatures and pressures, e.g., pressurization to 405 MPa at 45°C for 30 min resulted in complete inhibition of *Clostridium sporogenes* at pH 4, whereas at 90°C it yielded complete inhibition over a pH range of 4–6. *Bacillus subtilis* was completely inhibited by pressurization to 405 MPa at 70°C for 15 min at pH 4. Addition of nisin resulted in further reduction of microbial numbers. Unfortunately, this study was limited to only one pressure and the *D*-value was not documented. The use of other combinations of pressures and temperatures may have given more promising results.

Maggi et al. (1996) studied the combined effect of pressure and temperature on the inactivation of *Clostridium sporogenes* PA 3679 (ATCC 7953) spores in liquid media at pH 7.0 (beef or carrot broth medium, and phosphate buffer). They reported that 1500 MPa at 20°C for 5 min resulted in no spore-inactivation, whereas 1500 MPa at 60°C fully inactivated the spores, a pressure of just 800 MPa at 80°C–90°C resulted in sterilization of beef or carrot broth. Rovere et al. (1996) studied the effect of high pressure (up to 1500 MPa) and temperature (20°C–88°C) on the destruction of *Clostridium sporogenes* strain PA 3679, ATCC 7955, and reported that total bacterial spore inactivation could be obtained using a combined pressure (1000 MPa) and temperature (50°C–60°C) treatment. Butz et al. (1996) also reported a combined pressure–temperature treatment for the inactivation of *Byssochlamys nivea* DSM 1824 ascopores. Researchers (Clouston and Wills, 1969; Gould and Sale, 1970; Awao and Taki, 1990; Mallidis and Drizou, 1991; Taki et al., 1991; Seyderhelm and Knorr, 1992; Nishi et al., 1994) have also attempted to inactivate bacterial spores (*Bacillus stearothermophilus*, *Bacillus licheniformis*, *Bacillus cereus*, *Bacillus coagulans*, *Clostridium botulinum*) using combined high pressure (>0.7 MPa) and moderate temperatures (>50°C), and found satisfactory results. However, for complete spore inactivation, pressures >100 MPa in combination with temperature 60°C–80°C are required.

Sonoike et al. (1992) examined the death rates of *Lactobacillus casei* Y1T9018 and *Escherichia coli* JCM1649 under various temperatures (0°C–60°C) and pressures (0.1–400 MPa). They reported that death rates of both strains decreased with rising temperatures under a high pressure, and contours of constant death-rates of both strains on the pressure–temperature plane were elliptical and similar with that of free-energy difference for pressure–temperature-reversible denaturation of proteins.

Hashizume et al. (1995) studied the inactivation of yeast using HPP at low temperatures, by subjecting *S. cerevisiae* IFO 0234 to a pressure range of 120–300 MPa at −20°C to 50°C. After performing regression analysis of 43 inactivation rates, they reported that the same degree of inactivation was achieved at higher pressures and higher temperatures as compared with low pressures and low (subzero) temperatures (e.g., the inactivation effect at 190 MPa and −20°C was similar at 320 MPa and room temperature).

They concluded that high-pressure treatment applied at subzero temperatures requires lower pressures than when conducted at high temperatures to achieve the same degree of microbial inactivation. Since only a few studies have been performed using HPP at subzero temperatures, further studies are needed in this area to demonstrate the robustness of HPP at low temperatures, which may lead to interesting results.

13.6.4.2 *Pressure and Other Processes*

Crawford et al. (1996) studied the combined use of pressure and irradiation to destroy *Clostridium sporogenes* spores in chicken breast. They reported a 5 log reduction at ambient temperature (25°C) with a pressure of 689 MPa applied for 60 min; heating samples at 80°C for 20 min before pressurization resulted in the lowest number of survivors. They also reported that a 3.0 kGy irradiation treatment before and after pressurization at 80°C for 1, 10, and 20 min did not show any significant differences in spore numbers between samples that were pressurized and then irradiated or vice versa. However, the irradiation *D*-value of *Clostridium sporogenes* decreased from 4.1 to 2 kGy at high pressures (>600 MPa at 80°C for 20 min); their research showed that high pressure reduced the irradiation dose required to produce chicken with an extended shelf life. They concluded that pretreatment with irradiation (prior to HPP) is a useful technique for inactivating *Clostridium sporogenes* spores, thereby reducing the radiation dose required to eliminate the spores by irradiation alone.

Fornari et al. (1995) studied the inactivation of *Bacillus* spp. using a combination of pressure, time, and temperature. They studied four *Bacillus* spp. (*B. cereus*, SSICA/DA1 [from wheat flour], *B. licheniformis* SSICA/DA2 [from spices], *B. coagulans* SSICA 1881 [from tuna in tomato sauce], and *B. stearothermophilus* SSICA/T460 [from spoiled canned peas]) by subjecting prepared samples to a pressure range of 200–900 MPa for 1–10 min at 20°C, 50°C, 60°C, or 70°C. They also examined the effect of pressure-cycling on spore inactivation (pressure treatment of 200–500 MPa followed by 900 MPa). They found that *B. cereus* spp. were more sensitive to pressure treatment (inactivation of $4 \times 10^{+5}$ endospores/mL was achieved at ambient temperature by treatment at 200 MPa for 1 min followed by 900 MPa for 1 min). However, for other species, a combination of higher pressure and moderate temperature was needed for significant reduction (*B. licheniformis* was inactivated at 800 MPa for 5 min at 60°C; *B. coagulans* was reduced to 10^{-4} endospores/mL at 900 MPa for 5 min at 70°C; *B. stearothermophilus* was inactivated at 70 MPa for 5 min at 70°C).

Aleman et al. (1996) studied the effects of pulsed and static HPP on fruit preservation by inactivating *Saccharomyces cerevisiae* 2407-1a in unsweetened pineapple juice. They applied sinusoidal and step-pressure pulses and compared the inactivation effects with static pressure treatments. They reported that no inactivation was observed after the application of 40–4000 fast sinusoidal pulses (10 cycles/s) at 4–400 s over a pressure range of 235–270 MPa, whereas static pressure treatments of 270 MPa at 40 and 400 s gave 0.7 and 5.1 decimal reductions, respectively. Also, slower 0–270 MPa step pulses at 0.1 (10 pulses), 1 (100 pulses), and 2 (200 pulses) cycles/s with total time of 100 s resulted in 3.3, 3.5, and 3.3 decimal reductions, respectively. They also reported that the ratio of on-pressure time to off-pressure time also affected inactivation (e.g., on-pressure time of 0.6 s and off-pressure time of 0.2 s resulted in a 4 decimal reduction in 100 s). They concluded that slower step pulses resulted in increased effectiveness of HPP as more reduction in microbial numbers was observed in less time in step-pressure processing. However, studies need to be done using step-pressure processing for inactivating other microorganisms and documenting their destruction kinetics. More studies are needed along the same lines for inactivation of other baroresistant microbes (e.g., gram-positive bacteria, spores) using cycled pressure treatment. However, the high resistance of bacterial spores to HPP is still a major outstanding issue and is the subject of a variety of reports (Shimada, 1992; Crawford et al., 1996; Maggi et al., 1996; Roberts and Hoover, 1996).

Shimada (1992) reported that the combined treatment of high pressure and alternating current yields lethal damage in *E. coli* and *B. subtilis* spores. Earlier, Shimada and Shimahara (1985, 1987) found that the exposure of *E. coli* cells to an alternating current (a.c.) of 50 Hz caused the release of intracellular materials located in the nucleus region within the cells, causing a decrease in the resistance to basic dyes. This was believed to have resulted from loss and (or) denaturation of cellular components responsible for the normal function of the cell membrane, which suggested that the lethal damage to microorganisms may be enhanced when the organisms are exposed to a.c. before or after the pressure treatment. Shimada (1992) subjected the *E. coli* cells to 300 MPa for 10 min immediately after a.c. exposure and *B. subtilis* suspension to 400 MPa for 30 min before a.c. exposure. A.C. exposure was carried out at the rate of 0.6 A/cm^2 for *E. coli* cells at 35°C for 2 h, and at the rate of 1 A/cm^2 for spores at 50°C for 5 h. They found that the surviving fractions of *E. coli* cells and *B. subtilis* spores treated with a.c. and pressure were significantly reduced. It was also found that the susceptibility of *E. coli* cells and *B. subtilis* spores to some chemicals increased after the combination treatment, suggesting that the combined use of pressure and a.c. also lowers the tolerance-level of microorganisms to other challenges.

Response to pressure–cycling (Honma and Haga, 1991; Knorr, 1994), ultrasound with pressure (Knorr, 1994), and additives plus pressure (Popper and Knorr, 1990; Papineau et al., 1991; Knorr, 1994) have been studied, and significant interactive effects on microbial inactivation have been found. In addition, sensory and functional characteristics of foods were enhanced. Knorr (1994) reported that neither ultrasonic nor high-pressure treatment alone was capable of inactivating *Rhodoturola rubra*; however, pretreatment of samples with ultrasonic waves (100 W/cm^2, 25°C, 25 min) followed by HPP (400 MPa, 25°C, 15°C) resulted in complete inactivation of *R. rubra*. Popper and Knorr (1990) demonstrated the effectiveness of combinations of enzymes like lysozyme, lactoperoxidase, and glucose oxidase on the inactivation of microbes at atmospheric pressure. It is highly likely that the combination of enzyme pretreatment with HPP may result in significant inactivation of microbes even at low pressures.

The work done in combined pressure–temperature, pressure–a.c. exposure, pressure–cycling, and pressure–ultrasound areas is at a preliminary level and the exact mechanisms of spore inactivation by such combined processes are not well known. There is no doubt that combined high pressure and moderate temperature (60°C–80°C) or high pressure and a.c exposure will have a beneficial impact on the sensory characteristics of heat-sensitive products; yet no such processes can be commercialized until microbial safety can be guaranteed. In most of the studies, researchers did not evaluate the effect of pressure-induced adiabatic heating on sample temperatures, nor did they examine spore inactivation during pressure "come-up" time, both of which may affect inactivation kinetics significantly. Also, the operational efficiency of a high-pressure food processor is very important during combined treatments; therefore, proper equipment maintenance and effective training of personnel are prerequisites for such studies. A detailed evaluation of the database accumulated from studies, which used a combination of pressure and other treatments (temperature, a.c. exposure, cycling) is needed before the commercialization of HPP. Also, corresponding *D*-values for specific microorganisms need to be documented and validated to standardize HPP, before it can be commercialized.

13.7   Conclusions and Outlook to the Future

There is no doubt that novel thermal and nonthermal food processing technologies represent another interesting and promising dimension for food processing because not only they inactivate microorganisms but also they provide opportunities for development of new value-added food products. The need for an alternative to traditional retort processing as the primary means of eliminating pathogenic and spoilage microorganisms is substantial. Nonthermal processing holds promise since food materials treated by this method retain their natural flavor, color, and texture without loss in vitamin or nutrient content. Furthermore, predictable changes in functional characteristics of proteins and complex carbohydrates during novel food processing mean that there are some exciting avenues of work in novel food processing treatment of foods that remain to be explored. Although extensive research has been conducted in the area of novel food processing, a lot still remains to be done in terms of understanding the critical limits of the process and the extent to which this might ensure appropriate treatment of food materials. Research has been done in various research institutions, universities, and food industry R&D laboratories, yet a direct comparison of the data obtained is not possible. There can be no possibility of extensive implementation of this technology unless specific processing parameters are established for each food material treated by novel food processing technologies. The possibility of commercialization of novel food technologies also depends on its economic viability. Therefore, a detailed economic analysis needs to be done by comparing the process costs with the present costs of processing by conventional means and at the same time factoring in the added value of the improved sensory characteristics of novel food technology-treated foods.

Thus far no concerted effort has been made to validate novel food technologies for complete elimination of pathogenic bacteria. It is important that standard operating criteria and processing conditions be established that will ensure the reliability of novel technologies as an alternative to conventional food processing. For example, thermal processing has had standards like D- and Z-values, holding times, and minimum temperatures developed for different foods; likewise, standards need to be set for novel food processing. Very few studies on the novel food processing inactivation of microorganisms discuss inactivation effects in terms of the D-value associated with each particular strain of organism. More research is needed along these lines so that a database of D-values for different microorganisms can be prepared. Without a well-documented database of D-values, there is no means to effectively compare the results of experiments performed with different microorganisms under different processing conditions. There is a need for comparable standards that might indicate the resistance of various microorganisms to pressure and temperature combinations used in novel food processing technologies. Different D-values at constant values of temperature and pressure may be used as an indication of resistance of a particular bacterial species with respect to another species. Thus, an effort should be made to understand and derive both D-values and Z-values so that minimum processing conditions may be developed for contaminants in target foods. Since the general norm followed in the food industry is to subject food products to treatments that ensure a 12D reduction of microorganisms, to ensure that novel food processing is effective in inactivating microorganisms, treatments that result in 12D reduction must be another goal.

The remaining questions are variability of resistance between different strains of the same microbial species; possible protecting effects of food constituents, making it important to study microbial inactivation in given foods; stressed cells and their possible recovery during chilled or ambient storage; effects of high pressure and subzero temperature processing; and effects of pressure–cycling and pressure–a.c. exposure treatments to reduce the microbial viability. An exciting aspect of this technology is its effect on different functional characteristics of foods (starch gelatinization, protein denaturation, and enzyme inactivation). Not only do these areas require further study but also utilizing nonthermal food technologies such as HPP as a method of storage by freezing foods (pressure-shift freezing, rapid thawing, rapid cooling) requires further work. From the methodological standpoint, it would be necessary to monitor temperatures in the food sample, pressure at different positions in the HPP vessel, and to use well-calibrated pressure gauges. Although novel food processing shows promise in its ultimate usefulness for food preservation, limitations with respect to difficulty in data comparison and complexity associated with understanding interactive components of the process currently limit full acceptance of the practice. The only way to fully commercialize novel food processing is to find niche applications of these technologies, which can provide the processors and retailers maximum profit and they may enter into sectors of food industry, which were untapped before.

References

Adu, B. and L. Otten. 1993. Effects of the increasing hygroscopicity on microwave heating of solid foods. Conference of Food Engineers, Paper no. 5B-4.

Aleman, G.D., E.Y. Ting, S.C. Mordre, A.C.O. Hawes, M. Walker, D.F. Farkas, and J.A. Torres. 1996. Pulsed ultra high pressure treatments for pasteurization of pineapple juice. *J. Food Sci.* 61:388–390.

Alpas, H., N. Kalchayanand, F. Bozuglu, and B. Ray. 1998. Interaction of pressure, time and temperature of pressurization on viability loss of *Listeria innocua. World J. Microbiol. Biotech.* 14:251–253.

Anantheswaran, R.C. and M.A. Rao. 1985. Heat transfer to model Newtonian foods in cans during end-over-end rotation. *J. Food Eng.* 4:1–19.

Anonymous. 1983. Process design for rotomots. In: NFPA research laboratories 1983 annual report, National Food Processors Association, Washington, DC, pp. 36–37.

Awao, T. and Y. Taki. 1990. Sterilization of spores of genus *Bacillus* by hydrostatic pressure. *Kagaku kogaku* 54:283–285.

Balasubramaniam, V.M. and S.K. Sastry. 1994a. Liquid-to-particle heat transfer in a non-Newtonian carrier medium during continuous tube flow. *J. Food Eng.* 23:169–187.

Balasubramaniam, V.M. and S.K. Sastry. 1994b. Liquid-to-particle heat transfer in a continuous flow through a horizontal scraped surface heat exchanger. *Trans. I ChemE., Part C, Food and Bioproducts Proc.* 72:189–196.

Balasubramaniam, V.M. and S.K. Sastry. 1994c. Liquid-to-particle heat transfer in continuous tube flow: Comparison between experimental techniques. *Intl. J. Food Science and Tech.* 10:75–82.

Balasubramaniam, V.M. and S.K. Sastry. 1994d. Methods for noninvasive estimation of convection heat transfer coefficients in continuous flow. Paper 946543. *Am. Soc. Agric. Eng.*, St. Joseph, MI. 11p.

Balasubramaniam, V.M. and S.K. Sastry. 1995. Use of liquid crystals as temperature sensors in food processing research. *J. Food Eng.* 26:219–230.

Balasubramaniam, V.M. and S.K. Sastry. 1996. Noninvasive estimation of convective heat transfer between fluid and particle in continuous flow using a remote temperature sensor. *J. Food Proc. Eng.* 19:220–240.

Ball, C.O. and F.C.W. Olson. 1957. *Sterilization in Food Technology*. McGraw Hill, New York.

Berry, M.R., Jr. and A.L. Kohnhorst. 1985. Heating characteristics of homogeneous milk-based formulas in cans processed in an agitating retort. *J. Food Sci.* 50:209–214.

Bhamidipati, S. and R.K. Singh. 1994. Fluid to particle heat transfer coefficient determination in a continuous system. Paper 946542. *Am. Soc. Agric. Eng.*, St. Joseph, MI. 13p.

Bhamidipati, S. and R.K. Singh. 1995. Determination of fluid-particle convective heat transfer coefficient. *Trans. ASAE*. 38(3):857–862.

Buffler, C. 1986. Electromagnetic radiation and microwave power. Proceedings of the workshop on microwave applications in the food and beverage industry. Ontario Hydro, Toronto.

Butz, P., S. Funtenberger, T. Haberditzl, and B. Tauscher. 1996. High pressure inactivation of *Byssochlamys nivea* ascospores and other heat resistant moulds. *Lebensm. Wiss. u Technol.* 29:404–410.

CAST. 1989. Ionizing energy in food processing and pest control: II. Applications, Task Force Report No. 115, Council for Agricultural Science and Technology, Ames, Iowa.

CAST. 1996. Radiation pasteurization of food, Issue paper No. 7. Council for Agricultural Science and Technology, Ames, Iowa.

Chandarana, D.I, A. Gavin, and F.W. Wheaton. 1990. Particle/fluid interface heat transfer under UHT conditions at low particle/fluid relative velocities. *J. Food Proc. Eng.* 13:191–206.

Chang, S.Y. and R.T. Toledo. 1990. Simultaneous determination of thermal diffusivity and heat transfer coefficient during sterilization of carrot dices in a packed bed. *J. Food Sci.* 55(1):199–205.

Cheftel, J.C. 1995. Review: High pressure, microbial inactivation and food preservation. *Food Sci. Technol. Int.* 1:75–90.

Clavero, M.R.S, J.D. Monk, L.R. Beuchat, M.P. Doyle, and R.E. Brakett. 1994. Inactivation of *Escherichia coli* O157:H7, salmonellae and *Campylobacter jejuni* in raw ground beef by gamma irradiation. *Appl. Environ. Microbiol.* 60:2069.

Clifcorn, L.E., G.T. Peterson, J.M. Boyd, and J.H. O'Neil. 1950. A new principle for agitating in processing of canned foods. *Food Technol.* 4(11):450–457.

Clouston, J.G. and P.A. Wills. 1969. Initiation of germination and inactivation of *Bacillus pumilus* spores by hydrostatic pressure. *J. Bacteriol.* 97:684–690.

Conley, W., L. Kaap, and L. Schuhmann. 1951. The application of "end-over-end" agitation to the heating and cooling of canned food products. *Food Technol.* 5(11):457–460.

Cooper, T.E., R.J. Field, and J.F. Meyer. 1975. Liquid crystal thermography and its application to the study of convective heat transfer. Paper presented at AIChE-ASME Heat transfer conference, San Francisco, CA. August 11–13.

Coronel, P., V.D. Truong, J. Simunovic, K.P. Sandeep, and G.D. Cartwright. 2004. Aseptic processing of sweet potato purees using a continuous flow microwave system. *J. Food Sci.* 70(9):E531–E536.

Crawford, L.M. and E.H. Ruff. 1996. A review of the safety of cold pasteurization through irradiation. *Food Control* 7(2):87.

Crawford, Y.J., E.A. Murano, D.G. Olson, and K. Shenoy. 1996. Use of high hydrostatic pressure and irradiation to eliminate *Clostridium sporogenes* spores in chicken breast. *J. Food Prot.* 59:711–715.

de Alwis, A.A.P., Z. Li, and P.J. Fryer. 1990. Modelling sterilisation and quality in the ohmic heating process. In: *Advances in Aseptic Processing Technologies*. Elsevier Applied Science, London, U.K., pp. 103–140.

Decareau, R.V. 1985. *Microwaves in the Food Processing Industry*. Academic Press Inc. Orlando, FL.

Decareau, R.V. 1986. Microwave application in the food industry: A technical overview. Proceedings of the Workshop on Microwave Applications in the Food and Beverage Industry. Ontario Hydro, Toronto.

Deniston, M.F., B.H. Hassan, and R.L. Merson. 1987. Heat transfer coefficients to liquids with food particles in axially rotated cans. *J. Food Science* 52:962–966, 979.

de Ruyter, P.W. and R. Brunet. 1973. Estimation of process conditions for continuous sterilization of foods containing particulate. *Food Technol.* 27(7):44.

Dubey, J.P. and D.W. Thayer. 1994. Killing different strains of *Toxoplasma gondii* tissue cysts by irradiation under defined conditions. *J. Parasitol.* 80:764.

Farr, D. 1990. High pressure technology in the food industry. *Trends Food Sci. Technol.* 1:14–16.

FDA. 1985. Irradiation in the production, processing and handling of food. *Federal Register*, 5014:21 CFR part 179, 29658.

FDA. 2002. "Kinetics of microwave inactivation for alternative food processing technologies—Microwave and radio frequency processing" June 2, 2000. www.cfsan.fda.goc/~comm/ift-micr.html.

Fornari, C., A. Maggi, S. Gola, A. Cassara, and P.L. Manachini. 1995. Inactivation of *Bacillus* endospores by high-pressure treatment. *Ind. Conserve.* 70:259–265.

Ganesan, S.G., K.R. Swartzel, R.W. Hamaker, and R.T. Kuehn. 1992. F_o value determinations of food particles heated under continuous flow: Utilization of novel thermal sensor. Abstract no. 620. Presented at 1992 IFT Annual Meeting, New Orleans, LA.

Giese, J. 1992. Advances in microwave food processing. Food technology special report, pp. 118–123.

Goresline, H.E., M. Ingram, P. Macuch, G. Macquot, D.H. Mossel, C.F. Niven, and F.S. Thatcher. 1964. Tentative classification of food irradiation processes with microbiological objectives. *Nature* 204:237.

Gould, G.W. and A.J.H. Sale. 1970. Initiation of germination of bacterial spores by hydrostatic pressure. *J. Gen. Microbiol.* 60:335–346.

Hashizume, C., K. Kimura, and R. Hayashi. 1995. Kinetic analysis of yeast inactivation by high pressure treatment at low temperatures. *Biosci. Biotech. Biochem.* 59:1455–1458.

Hassan, B.H. 1984. Heat transfer coefficients for particles in liquid in axially rotating cans. Ph.D. Thesis, University of California. Davis. (Cited by Stoforos (1988).)

Hauben, K.J.A., D.H. Bartlett, C.C.F. Soontjens, K. Cornelis, E.Y. Wuytack, and C.W. Michiels. 1997. *Escherichia coli* mutants resistant to inactivation by high hydrostatic pressure. *Appl. Environ. Microbiol.* 63:945–950.

Hayakawa, I., T. Kanno, K. Yoshiyama, and Y. Fujio. 1994. Oscillatory compared with high pressure sterilization on *Bacillus stearothermophilus* spores. *J. Food Sci.* 59:164–167.

Heppell, N.J. 1985. Measurement of the liquid-solid heat transfer coefficients during continuous sterilization of liquid containing solids. Presented at 4th International Congress on Engineering and Foods. Edmonton, Alberta, Canada. July 7–10.

Heremans, K. 1992. From living systems to biomolecules. In: Balny, C., Hayashi, R., Hermans, K., and Masson, P. (Eds.), *High Pressure and Biotechnology*, John Libbey and Co. Ltd., London, pp. 37–44.

Hite, B.N., N.J. Giddings, and C.E. Weakly. 1914. The effect of certain microorganisms encountered in the preservation of fruits and vegetables. *Bull. West Virginia Agr. Exp. Sta.* 146:3–67.

Honma, K. and N. Haga. 1991. Effects of high pressure treatment on sterilization and physical effect of high pressure treatment on sterilization and physical properties of egg white. In: Hayashi, R. (Ed.), *High Pressure Science for Food*, San-Ei Pub. Co., Kyoto, Japan, pp. 317–324.

Hoover, D.G., C. Metrick, A.M. Papineau, D.F. Farkas, and D. Knorr. 1989. Biological effects of high hydrostatic pressure on food microorganisms. *Food Technol.* 43(1):99–107.

Hotani, S. and Mihori, T. 1983. Some thermal engineering aspects of the rotation method in sterilization. In: *Heat Sterilization of Food*. Koseisha-Koseikaku Co. Ltd., Tokyo, Japan, pp. 121–129.

Hunter, G.M. 1972. Continuous sterilization of liquid media containing suspended particles. *Food Technol. Aust.* April: 158–165.

IFT. 1989. Microwave food processing. A scientific status summary by the IFT Expert Panel on Food Safety and Nutrition. *Food Technol.* 43(1):117–126.

Kampelmacher, E.H. 1984. Irradiation of food: A new technology for preserving and ensuring the hygiene of foods. *Fleischwirtschaft* 64:322.

King, B.L. and E.S. Josephson. 1983. Actions of radiations on protazoa and helminths. In: Josephson, E.S. and Peterson, M.S. (Eds.), *Preservation of Foods by Ionizing Irradiation*, Vol 2, CRC Press, Boca Raton, pp. 245–267.

Klinger, R.W. and D. Decker. 1989. Microwave heating of soybeans on laboratory and pilot scale. In: Spiess, W.E.L. and Schubert, H. (Eds.), *Engineering and Food*, Vol. 2. Elsevier Applied Science, London, U.K., pp. 259–268.

Knorr, D. 1994. Hydrostatic pressure treatment of food: microbiology. In: Gould, G.W. (Ed.), *New Methods of Food Preservation*, Blackie Academic and Professional, London, pp. 159–175.

Knorr, D. 1995. Advantages and limitations of non-thermal food preservation methods. In: VTT Symposium 148: New Shelf-Life Technologies and Safety Assessments, Technical Research Center of Finland, Finland, pp. 7–12.

Kramers, H. 1946. Heat transfer from spheres to flowing media. *Physica* 12(2): 61–80.

Leadley, C.E. and A. Williams. 1997. High pressure processing of food and drink-an overview of recent developments and future potential. In: *New Technologies, Bull. No. 14*, Mar., CCFRA, Chipping Campden, Glos, UK.

Lee, P.R. 1994. Irradiation to prevent foodborne illness. From the Assistant Secretary for Health, US Public Health service. *J. Am. Med. Assoc.* 4:261.

Lefebvre, N., Thibault, C., and Charbonneau, R. 1992. Improvement of shelf-life and wholesomeness of ground beef by irradiation. 1. Microbial aspects, *Meat Sci.* 32:203.

Lekwauwa, A.N. and K.I. Hayakawa. 1986. Computerized model for the prediction of thermal responses of packaged solid-liquid food mixtures undergoing thermal processes. *J. Food Sci.* 51:1042–1049.

Lenz, M.K. and D.B. Lund. 1978. The lethality-Fourier number method. Heating rate variations and lethality confidence intervals for forced-convection heated foods in containers. *J. Food Pro. Eng.* 2:227–271.

Lopez, A. 1987. *A Complete Course in Canning and Related Processes*. The Canning Trade Inc. Baltimore, MD.

Macdonald, A.G. 1992. Effect of high hydrostatic pressure on natural and artificial membranes. In: Balny, C., Hayashi, R., Hermans, K., and Masson, P. (Eds.), *High Pressure and Biotechnology*, John Libbey and Co. Ltd., London, pp. 67–75.

Maggi, A., S. Gola, E. Spotti, P. Rovere, and P. Mutti. 1994. High-pressure treatments of ascospores of heat-resistant moulds and patulin in apricot nectar and water. *Ind. Conserve*. 69:26–29.

Maggi, A., A. Cassara, P. Rovere, and S. Gola. 1995. Use of high pressure for inactivation of butyric clostridia in tomato serum. *Ind. Conserve*. 70:289–293.

Maggi, A., S. Gola, E. Spotti, P. Rovere, L. Miglioli, G. Dall'aglio, and N.G. Lonneborg. 1996. Effects of combined high pressure-temperature treatments on *Clostridium sporogenes* spores in liquid media. *Ind. Conserve*. 71:8–14.

Mallidis, C.G. and D. Drizou. 1991. Effect of simultaneous application of heat and pressure on the survival of bacterial spores. *J. Appl. Bacteriol*. 71:285–288.

Manson, J.E. and J.F. Cullen. 1974. Thermal process simulation for aseptic processing of foods containing discrete particulate matter. *J. Food Sci*. 39:1084.

Mead, P.S., L. Slutsker, V. Dietz, L.F. McCaig, J.S. Bresee, C. Shapiro, P.M. Griffin, and R.V. Tauxe. 1999. Food-related illness and death in the United States. *Emerg. Infect. Dis*. 5. Available at: http://www.cdc.gov/ncidod/eid/vol5no5/mead.htm

Mertens, B. 1992. Recent developments in high pressure processing. In: *New Technologies for the Food and Drink Industries, Symposium Proceedings, Part 1, CCFRA*, Chipping Campden, Glos, U.K.

Metaxas, A.C. and R.J. Meredith. 1983. *Industrial Microwave Heating*. Peter Peregrinus Ltd., London.

Mitchell, E.L. 1988. A review of aseptic processing. In: *Advances in Food Research*, Academic Press, Inc. CA, pp. 2–37.

Mwangi, J.M., S.S.H. Rizvi, and A.K. Datta. 1993. Heat transfer to particles in shear flow: Application in aseptic processing. *J. Food Eng*. 19:55–74.

Naveh, D. and I.J. Kopelman. 1980. Effect of some processing parameters on the heat transfer coefficients in a rotating autoclave. *J. Food Process. and Preserv*. 4:66–77.

Nayga, R.M., Jr. 2004. Consumer acceptance of irradiated prepared and processed food. In Irradiation to Ensure the Safety and Quality of Prepared Meals. Proceedings of the 2nd Research Coordination Meeting FAO/IAEA Coordinated Research Project held in Pretoria South Africa, 26–30 April 2004. Reproduced by the IAEA Vienna, Austria, 2004.

Nickerson, J.T.R., J.J. Licciardello, and L.J. Rosivalli. 1983. Radurization and radicidation: Fish and shellfish, In: Josephson, E.S. and Peterson, M.S. (Eds.), *Preservation of Food by Ionizing Irradiation*, Vol 3, CRC Press, Boca Raton, FL, pp. 13–82.

Niemand, J.G., H.J. Van Der Linde, and W.H. Holapfel. 1983. Shelf life extension of minced beef through combined treatments involving radurization. *J. Food Prot*. 46:791.

Nishi, K., R. Kato, and R. Tomita. 1994. Activation of *Bacillus spp.* spores by hydrostatic pressure. *Nippon Shokuhin Kogyo Gakkaishi* 41:542–549.

Novak, A.F., J.A. Liuzzo, R.M. Grodner, and R.T. Lovell. 1966. Radiation pasteurization of Gulf coast oysters. *Food Technol*. 20:201.

Owusu-Ansah, Y.J. 1991. Advances in microwave drying of foods and food ingredients. *J. Inst. Can. Sci. Technol. Aliment.* 24(3/4):102–107.

Palou, E., A. Lopez-Malo, G.V. Barbosa-Canovas, B.G. Swanson, and J. Welti. 1996. Combined effect of high hydrostatic pressure and water activity on *Zygosaccharomyces bailii* inhibition. In: *Institute of Food Technologists Annual Meeting, Book of Abstracts*, p. 57.

Palou, E., A. Lopez-Malo, G.V. Barbosa-Canovas, J. Welti-Chanes, P.M. Davidson, and B.G. Swanson. 1998. High hydrostatic pressure come-up time and yeast viability. *J. Food Prot.* 61:1657–1660.

Papineau, A.M., D.G. Hoover, D. Knorr, and D.F. Farkas. 1991. Antimicrobial effect of water-soluble chitosans with high hydrostatic pressure. *Food Biotechnol.* 5:45–47.

Patterson, M.F., M. Quinn, R. Simpson, and A. Gilmour. 1995. Sensitivity of vegetative pathogens to high hydrostatic pressure treatment in phosphate-buffer saline and foods. *J. Food Prot.* 58:524–529.

Peralta Rodriguez, R.D. and R.L. Merson. 1983. Experimental verification of a heat transfer model for simulated liquid foods undergoing flame sterilization. *J. Food Sci.* 48:726–733.

Popper, L. and D. Knorr. 1990. Applications of high-pressure homogenization for food preservation. *Food Technol.* 44:84–89.

Przybylski, L., M. Finerty, and R. Grodner. 1989. Extension of shelf-life of fresh channel catfish fillets under modified atmosphere packaging and low dose irradiation. *J. Food Sci.* 54:269.

Quast, D.C. and Y.Y. Siozawa. 1974. Heat transfer rates during heating of axially rotated cans. Proceedings of the 4th International Congress on Food Science and Technology. 4:458–468.

Ramaswamy, H.S., K.A. Abdelrahim, B.K. Simpson, and J.P. Smith. 1995. Residence time distribution (RTD) in aseptic processing of particulate foods: A review. *Food Res. Intl.* 28(3):291–310.

Ranz, W.E. and W.R. Jr. Marshall. 1952. Evaporation from drop. *Chem. Eng. Progress.* 48:141.

Rao, M.A., H.J. Cooley, R.C. Anantheswaran, and R.W. Ennis. 1985. Convective heat transfer to canned liquid foods in a steritort. *J. Food Sci.* 50:150–154.

Rao, M.A. and R.C. Anantheswaran. 1988. Connective heat transfer to fluid foods in cans. In: *Advances in Food Research*. v32. Academic Press Inc., San Diego, CA, pp. 39–84.

Richardson, P. 1992. Microwave technology—The opportunity for food processors. *Food Sci. Technol. Today* 5(3):146–149.

Roberts, C.M. and D.G. Hoover. 1996. Sensitivity of spores of *Clostridium sporogenes* PA3679 and *B. subtilis* 168 to combination of high hydrostatic pressure, heat, acidity, and nisin. In: *Institute of Food Technologists Annual Meeting, Book of Abstracts*, pp. 174–175.

Rosenbergy, U. and W. Bogl. 1987. Microwave pasteurization, sterilization, blanching, drying, and baking in the food industry. *Food Technol.* 41(6):85–99.

Rovere, P., D. Tosoratti, and A. Maggi. 1996. Sterilizing trials to 15000 bar to obtain microbiological and enzymatic stability. *Ind. Alimentari.* 35:1062–1065.

Sale, A.J.H., Gould, G.W., and W.A. Hamilton. 1970. Inactivation of bacterial spores by hydrostatic pressure. *J. Gen. Microbiol.* 60:323–334.

Sanio, M. and I. Michelussi. 1986. Microwave applications in the food and beverage industry. Preliminary Report for EnerMark, the Electricity People. Ontario Hydro, Toronto.

Sastry, S.K. 1986. Mathematical evaluation of process schedules for aseptic processing of low-acid foods containing discrete particulate. *J. Food Sci.* 5:1323–1328.

Sastry, S.K. 1990. Liquid-to-particle heat transfer coefficient in aseptic processing. In: Singh, R.K. and Nelson, P.E. (Eds.), *Advances in Aseptic Processing Technologies*. Elsevier Applied Science. Great Britain, pp. 63–72.

Sawada, H. and R.L. Merson. 1985. Estimation of process conditions for bulk sterilization of particulate foods in water-fluidized beds. Presented at Fourth International Congress on Engineering and Food, Edmonton, Alberta, Canada, July 7–10.

Seyderhelm, I. and D. Knorr. 1992. Reduction of *Bacillus stearothermophilus* spores by combined high pressure and temperature treatments. ZFL (*J. Food Ind.*) 43:17–20.

Shimada, K. 1992. Effect of combination treatment with high pressure and alternating current on the lethal damage of *Escherichia coli* cells and *Bacillus subtilis* spores. In: Balny, C., Hayashi, R., Hermans, K., and Masson, P. (Eds.), *High Pressure and Biotechnology*, John Libbey and Co. Ltd., London, pp. 49–51.

Shimada, K. and K. Shimahara. 1985. Leakage of cellular contents and morphological changes in resting *Escherichia coli* B cells exposed to an alternating current. *Agr. Biol. Chem.* 49:3605–3607.

Shimada, K. and K. Shimahara. 1987. Effect of alternating current exposure on the resistivity of resting *Escherichia coli* B cells to crystal violet and other basic dyes. *J. Appl. Bacteriol.* 62:261–268.

Sivinski, J.S. 1985. Control of trichinosis by low-dose irradiation of pork. *Food Irradat. Newsl.* 2:8.

Smith, J.P., H.S. Ramaswamy, and B.K. Simpson. 1990. Developments in food packaging technology, part 1: Processing/cooking considerations. *Trends Food Sci. Technol.* 1(5):106–109.

Sonoike, K., T. Setoyama, Y. Kuma, and S. Kobayashi. 1992. Effect of pressure and temperature on the death rates of *Lactobacillus casei* and *Escherichia coli*. In: Balny, C., Hayashi, R., Hermans, K., and Masson, P. (Eds.), *High Pressure and Biotechnology*, John Libbey and Co. Ltd., London, pp. 297–301.

Stoforos, N.G. 1988. Heat transfer in axially rotating canned liquid/particulate food system. Ph.D. Thesis, University of California, Davis, CA.

Stoforos, N.G. and R.L. Merson. 1991. Measurement of heat transfer coefficients in rotating liquid/particulate systems. *Biotechnol. Prog.* 7:267–271.

Stuchley, S.S. and M.A. Stuchley. 1983. Microwave drying: Potential and limitations. *Adv. Drying* 2:53–71.

Sudarmadji, S. and W.M. Urbain. 1972. Flavor sensitivity of selected raw animal protein foods to gamma radiation. *J. Food Sci.* 37:671.

Swain, L.V.L., S.L. Russel, R.N. Clarke, and M.J. Swain. 2004. The development of food simulants for microwave oven testing. *Intl. J. Food Sci. Tech.* 39:623–630.

Taki, Y., T. Awaao, S. Toba, and N. Mitsuura. 1991. Sterilization of *Bacillus spps.* spores by hydrostatic pressure. In: Hayashi, R. (Ed.), *High Pressure Science for Food*, San-Ei Pub. Co., Kyoto, Japan, pp. 217–224.

Tewari, G. and D.S. Jayas. 1997. Heat transfer during thermal processing of liquid foods (with or without particulates): A review. *Intl. Ag. Eng. J.* 6(1):1–27.

Thayer, D.W. and G. Boyd. 1993. Elimination of *Escherichia coli* O157:H7 in meats by gamma irradiation. *J. Food. Sci.* 57:848.

Thayer, D.W., G. Boyd, J.B. Fox, and L. Jr. Lakritz. 1995. Effects of NaCl, sucrose, and water content on the survival of *Salmonella typhimurium* on irradiated pork and chicken. *J. Food Prot.* 58:490.

Timson, W.J. and A.J. Short. 1965. Resistance of microorganisms to hydrostatic pressure. *Biotechnol. Bioeng.* 7:139–159.

Tsurkerman, V.C., V.I. Rogachev, Q.G. Fromzel, N.M. Pogrebenco, V.I. Tsenkevich, G.M. Evstigneer, and C.F. Kolodyazhnyi. 1971. Preservation of tomato paste in large containers under rotation. Konsewnaya i Ovashchesushi "naya promyshlennost" 11: 11–13 (abstract). (Cited by Quast and Siozawa (1974).)

Weng, Z., M. Hendrickx, G. Maesmans, and P. Tobback. 1991. Immobilized peroxidase: A potential bioindicator for evaluation of thermal processes. *J. Food Sci.* 56(2):567–570.

Whitaker, S. 1972. Forced convection heat transfer correlations for flow in pipes, past flat plates, single cylinders, single spheres, and for flow in packed beds and tube bundles. *AIChE J.* 18(2):361–370.

WHO. 1994. Safety and nutritional adequacy of irradiated food, World Health Organization, Geneva.

WHO. 1997. Food irradiation, Press release WHO/68, September 19, World Health Organization, Geneva.

Williams, A. 1994. New technologies in food preservation and processing, part II. *Nutr. Food Sci.* 1:20–23.

Woods, R.J. and A.K. Pikaev. 1994. Interaction of radiation with matter. In: *Applied Radiation Chemistry: Radiation Processing*, John Wiley & Sons, New York.

Ye, H.Y., H. Wang, J.F. Wang, Q. Xu, and Y.H. Li. 1996. Pressure tolerance of microbes and techniques for high pressure disinfection of acid food (jams etc.) at room temperature. *Food Sci. China* 17:30–34.

Zitoun, K.B. and S.K. Sastry. 1994. Determination of convective heat transfer coefficient between fluid and cubic particles in continuous tube flow using noninvasive experimental techniques. *J. Food Process. Eng.* 17:209–228.

14

Genetic and Biochemical Control of Aflatoxigenic Fungi

Deepak Bhatnagar, Kanniah Rajasekaran, Robert Brown,
Jeffrey W. Cary, Jiujiang Yu, and Thomas E. Cleveland

CONTENTS

14.1 Introduction

Mycotoxins are typically low molecular weight organic compounds produced by fungi and are not considered to be essential to maintaining the life of the fungal cell (reviewed in Bhatnagar et al., 2002). They are called "secondary metabolites" because they are not involved in obtaining energy or synthesizing structural components of the cell. The well-studied mycotoxins are the aflatoxins because they are highly toxic and carcinogenic compounds that frequently contaminate foods and feeds. These compounds

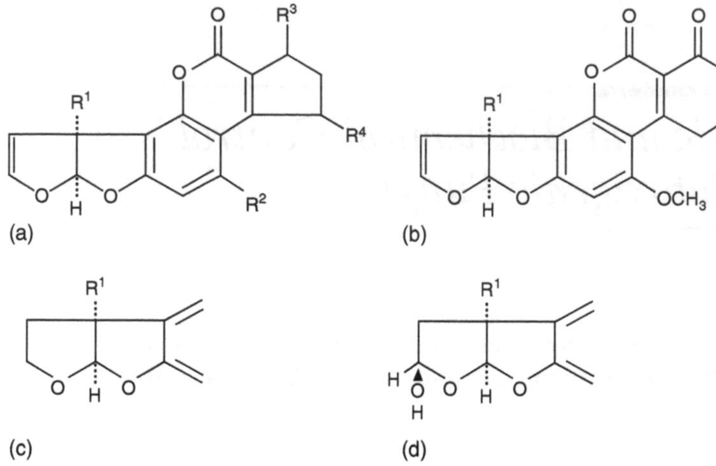

(a)

(b)

(c)

(d)

Aflatoxins	Structure	R^1	R^2	R^3	R^4
B_1	A	H	OCH_3	=O	H
M_1	A	OH	OCH_3	=O	H
P_1	A	H	OH	=O	H
Q_1	A	H	OCH_3	=O	OH
R_0	A	H	OCH_3	OH	H
R_0H_1	A	H	OCH_3	OH	OH
B_2	AC	H	OCH_3	=O	H
B_{2a}	AD	H	OCH_3	=O	H
M_2	AC	OH	OCH_3	=O	H
G_1	B	H	–	–	–
G_2	BC	H	–	–	–
G_{2a}	BD	H	–	–	–
GM	BC	OH	–	–	–

FIGURE 14.1
Chemical structure of aflatoxins. (a) The B-type aflatoxins are characterized by a cyclopentane E-ring. These compounds have a blue fluorescence under long-wavelength UV light. (b) The G-type aflatoxins have a xanthone ring in place of the cyclopentane and fluoresce green under UV light. (c) Aflatoxins of the B_2 and G_2 type have a saturated bis-furanyl ring. Only the bis-furan is shown. (d) Aflatoxins of the B_{1a} and G_{1a} type have a hydrated bis-furanyl structure.

(Figure 14.1) are produced by several species of fungi in the genus *Aspergillus*. *Aspergillus flavus*, the most common species causing crop contamination, is an opportunistic pathogen, which routinely produces aflatoxins B_1 and B_2. *Aspergillus parasiticus* produces two additional toxins, namely G_1, and G_2. Aflatoxin B_1 is both the most common and the most toxic and, as a result, is the aflatoxin most stringently regulated because it is the major toxicosis threat. Presence of aflatoxins in human foods may cause chronic health effects including immune-system suppression, impaired childhood development, and cancer. Acute poisoning can result in death (Wild and Turner,

2002; Gong et al., 2004). In developing countries, where detection and decontamination policies and practices are impractical, aflatoxin contamination is predominantly a food safety issue. Recently Kenya reported a minimum of 125 people killed by consuming aflatoxin-contaminated maize (http://www.cdc.gov/mmwr/preview/mmwr.html/mm533a4.htm). In developed countries, however, aflatoxin remains an economic problem because the contamination is most frequently recognized due to loss in crop value (estimated to be as high as $300 million in direct cost in the United States alone) resulting from strict government regulations on maximum permissible levels in crops and crop-related products (Cotty, 2001; Richard and Payne, 2003; Wu, 2004). In crops intended for human consumption, maximum permitted aflatoxin levels range from 2 ppb aflatoxin B_1 (4 ppb total aflatoxins) in the European Union to 20 ppb total aflatoxins in the United States. Small proportions of crop aflatoxin content are transferred from feed to milk (aflatoxin M_1) causing even food crops to have stringent regulations for use at dairies (van Egmond, 2004; Wu, 2004). Aflatoxin contamination occurrence frustrates not only the agricultural community but also all those that handle, market, or utilize crops from highly vulnerable regions. The crop may have no visible symptoms, and yet contain enough aflatoxins to either severely reduce value or completely eliminate available markets. The same fungal isolates may cause contamination of several crops grown in a given area, such as cottonseed, corn, peanuts, and tree nuts.

No completely effective control strategies are available to prevent aflatoxin accumulation in the field when conditions are favorable for the fungal growth and crop infection. A complete understanding of the host plant–*Aspergillus flavus* interaction and aflatoxin contamination process should help in the development of effective control strategies aimed at interrupting the mechanisms responsible for preharvest aflatoxin contamination for production of a safer, economically viable food and feed supply. Numerous investigations, as reviewed in this chapter, have attempted to gain a better understanding of the relationship between the host plant and the invading fungus, *A. flavus*, because this relationship affects the aflatoxin contamination process. It is now hypothesized that several host plant and fungal genes are probably involved in determining the degree of aflatoxin contamination of the crop. The understanding of the genetic makeup of the fungus that affects its ability to infect crops and produce toxins as well as survive in the field, along with elucidation of the biochemical processes within the affected crops have provided sufficient information for designing effective measures to control fungal invasion of crops by the toxigenic fungus and its ability to make aflatoxins.

14.2 Genetics of *Aspergillus flavus*

It has been well understood in research programs pertaining to aflatoxin contamination that, in order to solve this problem, a comprehensive understanding is needed of the fungus and its environment and the inter-action of the fungus with the host crop; the latter being unique for each crop, even though the fungus is a common factor.

The information derived from the use of tools such as genomics provides us with the best and the quickest opportunity to achieve a clear understand-ing of the survival of toxigenic fungi in the field, the fungal invasion of crops, and the toxin contamination process under various environmental conditions. The fundamental strategy in a genomics approach is to expand the scope of biological investigation from studying single genes to studying all genes at once in a systematic fashion.

Significant progress has been made by many researchers around the world in understanding the genetic makeup of some of the most significant toxin-producing fungi including *Aspergillus flavus*. Progress has also been made in the study of fungal–host crop interactions for these and other fungi. The information available will be used in deriving the requisite information required for developing effective strategies to interrupt the machinery in the fungus required to produce these toxins, as well as to assist in the development of host-resistance against fungal invasion and toxin contami-nation of crops.

14.2.1   Aflatoxin Biosynthesis

Aflatoxins are polyketide-derived bisfurans produced by *A. flavus*, *A. para-siticus*, *A. nomius*, *A. pseudotamarii*, and *A. bombycis*. Some *Aspergillus* spp. related to *A. nidulans*, for example *A. ochraceoroseus*, also produce aflatoxins. AFB_1 is the most toxic in this group and other aflatoxins are less toxic $(B_1 > G_1 > B_2 > G_2)$. Other significant members of the AF family, such as M_1 and M_2, are metabolites of AFB_1 and AFB_2, respectively, and originally isolated from bovine milk (reviewed in Eaton and Groopman, 1994; Bhatnagar et al., 2002).

AFB_1 and AFG_1 biosynthesis requires the expression of at least 27 genes and involves 23 enzymatic steps (Bhatnagar et al., 2003). After formation of the decaketide from a hexanoyl-CoA starter unit, a series of 14 oxidative steps, two methyltransferase steps, and one esterase step are required to convert the anthraquinone norsolorinic acid to AFB_1. The 70 kb biosynthetic gene cluster encodes the oxidative enzymes required, including five cyto-chrome P450 monooxygenases, a desaturase, and several types of oxido-reductases, some unique to the aflatoxin biosynthesis pathway. The pathway-specific regulatory gene (*aflR*) encodes a Gal 4-type DNA-binding protein (reviewed in Bhatnagar et al., 2003). Regulation of AflR activity is complex and involves a coactivator, a possible repressor, and C-terminal serine phosphorylation via a protein kinase A (PKA) signaling pathway. Other transcription factors whose activity is mediated by nitrate metabolism and glucose metabolism also have been shown to be necessary for AflR activity or expression. Defects in aflR and the polyketide synthase gene in the koji molds *A. sojae* and *A. oryzae* respectively, prevent formation of AF in these commercially important fungi (Matsushima et al., 2001).

14.2.2 Regulatory Elements in Aflatoxin Biosynthesis

Aflatoxin biosynthesis in fungi is responsive to environmental cues such as carbon and nitrogen source, stress, plant constituents (i.e., volatiles and tannins), and physical factors such as pH and temperature. These environmental stimuli are transduced via complex signaling cascades that control the expression of both global-acting and AF pathway-specific transcription factors.

Two known AF pathway-specific regulator genes, *aflR* (described earlier) and *aflJ*, have been localized to the AF biosynthetic gene cluster in *Aspergillus flavus* and *A. parasiticus*. These genes are also present in the sterigmatocystin (ST) cluster of *A. nidulans*. AflR protein is a Gal4-type, Zn-finger binuclear cluster, positive-acting transcription factor that is required for expression of all known AF biosynthetic genes (Chang et al., 1993; Payne et al., 1993). AflR activates transcription of AF pathway genes following binding to the conserved 11 bp palindromic sequence, 5'-TCGN5CGR-3', present in the promoter regions of most AF genes (Ehrlich et al., 1999). Fungal isolates in which the *aflR* gene has been inactivated no longer produce AF nor express AF pathway genes while fungi engineered to over-express *aflR* produce increased levels of AF transcripts leading to increased levels of AF production.

AflJ is a second gene in the AF pathway cluster that appears to play a role in regulation of AF biosynthesis. *AflJ* resides adjacent to *aflR* in the AF gene cluster and the two genes are divergently transcribed (Meyers et al., 1998). AflJ protein does not demonstrate significant identity to other proteins of known function in the databases. Interestingly, it was shown that *aflJ* mutants do not produce AF (or only very minute amounts) but they still express AF pathway genes, though at reduced levels. So it appears that AflJ is not functioning like AflR as a transcriptional activator of AF pathway genes. Chang et al. (1999) used a yeast two-hybrid system to show that AflJ can bind to the C-terminal region of AflR. Based on AflJ's ability to bind AflR, it has been proposed that AflJ is either acting as a transcriptional enhancer or coactivator of AflR.

In addition to transcription factors present in the AF gene cluster there are also a number of globally acting transcription factors that are involved in regulation of AF biosynthesis. This is supported by the identification of numerous binding sites (both proven and putative) for these factors in the promoter regions of AF cluster genes including the *aflR–aflJ* intergenic region. Binding sites for both PacC (pH-responsive global regulator) and the nitrogen regulator, AreA, have been identified in the *aflR–aflJ* intergenic region (Chang et al., 2000; Ehrlich et al., 2003). PacC binding sites are consistent with the function of this protein in repressing transcription of acid-expressed genes under alkaline conditions (Tilburn et al., 1995). AF biosynthesis in *A. flavus* occurs in acidic media, but is inhibited in alkaline media. In a different study, Chang et al. (2000) found that, AreA, bound to GATA sites in the *aflR–aflJ* intergenic region, suggesting that nitrogen regulation of AF production could be linked to AreA control of *aflR* and *aflJ* expression. Putative binding sites for global regulatory proteins such as BrlA (developmental regulator) and CreA (regulator of carbon catabolism) have also been identified in the *aflR–aflJ* intergenic region of a number of different AF-producing *Aspergillus* spp. including *A. nidulans* (Ehrlich et al., 2003). It is hypothesized that variability in the number and location of these various transcription factor binding sites within AF gene promoters of these different aspergilli may reflect the need for each of these species to adapt to different environmental stimuli inherent to their particular ecological niche.

A close relationship between AF production and fungal development was first observed by Bennett (1978) when they noted "strain degeneration" in *A. parasiticus* upon repeated subculturing of macerated mycelia. This technique produced morphological variants that gave "fan" and "fluff" phenotypes due to increased mycelial growth. These variants also demonstrated decreased conidiation and AF production compared to the parental strain. Kale et al. (1994, 2003) continued studies on "strain degeneracy" and found that these variants, termed sec- strains for secondary metabolite negative, were stable and did not revert to wild-type levels of AF production or conidiation. Sec- mutants did not express AF biosynthetic genes, and the *aflR* gene expression was from 5- to 10-fold less than that observed in the parental strain. Expanding on the studies of Bennett and Kale, Hicks et al. (1997) identified the genetic mechanism in *A. nidulans* that linked ST (and AF production in *A. parasiticus/flavus*) to fungal development. The mechanism involved a G-protein/cAMP/PKA signaling pathway (Figure 14.2).

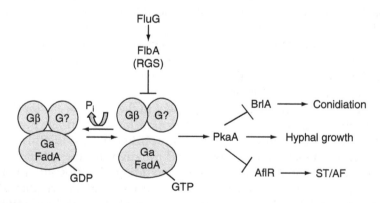

FIGURE 14.2
Schematic of G-protein/cAMP/protein kinase A (PKA) signaling pathway involved in fungal development and AF/ST production in *Aspergillus nidulans* and *A. flavus*. (Adapted from Yu and Keller, *Ann. Rev. Phytopathol.*, 43, 437, 2005.)

FadA is the alpha subunit of the *A. nidulans* heterotrimeric G protein. When FadA is bound to GTP, i.e., in its active form, ST/AF production (and sporulation) is repressed. However, in the presence of FlbA, a protein similar to RGS (regulators of G protein signaling)-type proteins, the intrinsic GTPase activity of FadA is stimulated, thereby, leading to GTP hydrolysis, inactivation of FadA-dependent signaling, and stimulation of ST/AF production and conidiation. The activity of RGS-type proteins is mediated by extracellular signals that begin the signaling process by binding to a cell-surface receptor. For the ST signaling cascade in *A. nidulans*, one possible product is synthesized by a GSI-type glutamine synthetase, FluG. G protein signaling mediates the levels of cAMP, which probably acts as the second messenger, affecting the activity of the protein kinase, PkaA, which in turn, directly modulates the activity of AflR both transcriptionally and posttranscriptionally. AflR protein is inactivated by PkaA-mediated phosphorylation and the transcription of *aflR* is repressed by PkaA activity (Shimizu et al., 2003). Interestingly, certain mutations in genes involved in the FadA signaling pathway also alter cleistothecial development in *A. nidulans* (Shimizu and Keller, 2001) suggesting the existence of an association not only with conidiation and secondary metabolism but also with processes leading to the development of the sexual stage.

Only a few genes are known to be involved in sexual development, one example is the velvet gene, *veA*. The *veA* gene product does not demonstrate homology with any other protein of known function; however, it is known that *veA* mediates a developmental light response in *A. nidulans* (Calvo et al., 2002). In strains of *A. nidulans* containing a wild-type allele of the *veA*, light reduces and delays cleistothecial formation and the fungus develops asexually forming conidia, whereas in the dark, fungal development is directed toward the formation of cleistothecia. In *A. nidulans*, deletion of *veA* blocks cleistothecial production, demonstrating that *veA* is necessary for sexual development (Calvo et al., 2002). Deletion of *veA* also blocks ST production in this fungus by repression of *aflR* (Kato et al., 2003).

veA homologs have been identified in both *A. parasiticus* and *A. flavus* (Duran et al., 2007). Studies showed that *A. flavus veA* deletion strains are unable to produce sclerotia or AF. It was also shown that the blockage in the production of AF in the *veA* deletion strain is related to the absence of expression of both *aflR* and the adjacent gene *aflJ*. Additionally, the *veA* deletion strain showed reduced growth and conidial production, and this also occurred when grown on the natural substrate such as peanut seed. There is also evidence that inactivation of the *veA* gene in *A. flavus* results in significant reduction in the levels of the mycotoxins, cyclopiazonic acid (CPA), and aflatrem (Duran et al., 2007).

Like *veA*, the *laeA* gene first identified in *A. nidulans*, also encodes a global regulator of secondary metabolite production in *Aspergillus* spp. (Bok and Keller, 2004). Loss of LaeA silenced ST and penicillin (PN) production in *A. nidulans* and gliotoxin production in *A. fumigatus*, while overexpression of *laeA* increased PN and lovastatin production in *A. nidulans* and *A. terreus*, respectively. Like VeA, LaeA appears to play a role in fungal development. LaeA is believed to function as a protein methyltransferase that is involved in chromatin modification (reviewed in Keller et al., 2005). A model for LaeA function suggests that secondary metabolite gene clusters such as the ST gene cluster are maintained in silenced heterochromatin (HC) that is surrounded by transcriptionally active euchromatin (EC). It is believed that LaeA functions to initiate a chromatin remodeling process that converts HC to EC by interfering with methylases or deacetylases that are associated with HC. Therefore, LaeA regulation of secondary metabolism in aspergilli may represent a form of epigenetic control of gene transcription and it may provide some insight into the evolution and maintenance of clustering of secondary metabolic genes.

Because of its role in both secondary metabolite production and morphological development, VeA is a good candidate for EST and full genome microarray studies (described later) to elucidate mechanisms controlling mycotoxin and sclerotial production in *A. flavus*. These types of studies are currently underway as a collaborative effort of the USDA-ARS, Southern Regional Research Center, academic institutions and The Institute for Genomic Research.

14.2.3 Genomics of *A. flavus*

Functional genomics is needed to speed up our understanding of the field biology of the fungus in relationship to its interaction with the host plant. But this insight into the behavior of these biological systems first requires the sequence information (structural genomics) of the mycotoxigenic fungi of interest. The entire genomic sequence of *A. flavus* has been completed, and microarrays have been prepared based on this sequence information. Environmental influences on the fungus, ecological/evolutionary significance of fungal propagation, fungal virulence, and toxin formation as manifested by changes in gene expression profiles and global signal transduction within the fungus are now being rapidly analyzed using this genomics information.

The whole genome sequencing of related fungi such as *A. fumigatus*, *A. oryzae*, *A. nidulans*, *A. niger*, *F. oxysporum*, and *F. solani* is also assisting in identifying factors that afford the toxin producing fungi, a unique property of invading crops and producing toxins (comparative or evolutionary genomics).

Many of the early investigations were limited to the study of only one gene or gene product from either the fungus or the plant at a time and could thus be characterized as more targeted genomics studies. The need for the use of genomics and proteomics technologies to study global expression of genes has become more obvious as researchers have discovered that a complex array of multiple fungal and host-plant genes probably govern aflatoxin contamination of crops. In fact, despite the extensive literature on plant and fungal factors that may regulate the aflatoxin contamination process, it is likely that several genes governing the host plant–*A. flavus* interaction and aflatoxin biosynthesis have not yet been identified. These earlier studies provided valuable insights into which categories of fungal and host-plant traits are most important in governing the plant–fungus interaction, thus facilitating the search for additional genes and proteins in expressed sequence tag (EST) or protein databases, respectively.

Aspergillus flavus genomics and proteomics of seed- and kernel-based resistance are investigative tools for simultaneous discovery and analysis of the biochemical function and genetic regulation of the critical genes governing the plant–fungal interaction and aflatoxin biosynthesis. *A. flavus* ESTs and microarray technology have allowed rapid identification of the majority, if not all, of the genes expressed in the fungal genome and helped to understand better the coordinated regulation of gene expression. The *A. flavus* EST and corn kernel proteomics programs at the U.S. Department of Agriculture (USDA)/Agricultural Research Service (ARS)/Southern Regional Research Center (SRRC) are aimed at understanding the genetic control and regulation of aflatoxin biosynthesis by potential regulators upstream of aflR, the mechanism of aflatoxin production in response to internal and external factors, the relationship between primary and secondary metabolism, the basis of fungal pathogenicity, and the mechanism of seed-based resistance to fungal invasion and aflatoxin contamination in corn.

14.2.3.1 Expressed Sequence Tag Technology

As a part of the USDA/ARS/SRRC fungal genomics program, a total of 26,110 normalized *A. flavus* cDNA clones were sequenced by The Institute for Genomic Research and 7218 unique ESTs were identified after annotation (Yu et al., 2004); 30% of these had related sequences in the GenBank database. The fully annotated EST data set was released to the public by Gene Index constructed at TIGR (http://www.tigr.org/tigr-scripts/tgi/T index.cgi? species = a flavus). Among those ESTs, the ones that are potentially involved directly or indirectly in aflatoxin production have been identified based on their functional classifications (Yu et al., 2004). These genes were classified into five categories: (1) genes directly involved in aflatoxin biosynthesis such as structural and regulatory genes in the known aflatoxin pathway gene cluster, (2) genes putatively involved in global regulation and signal transduction such as *laeA*, (3) genes possibly involved in virulence and pathogenicity such as genes encoding hydrolytic enzymes, (4) genes involved in stress response and antioxidation, and (5) genes putatively involved in fungal development and sporulation. Several of the genes of interest are listed in Table 14.1, which has been modified from Yu et al. (2007).

14.2.3.2 DNA Microarrays

DNA microarrays have been constructed at TIGR for functional studies of *A. flavus* biology. Based on the information derived from the EST sequence,

TABLE 14.1
Genes Identified That Could Be Involved in Fungal Development and Secondary Metabolism

EST ID	Hit Accession No.	Putative Function	Organism	% ID	% Similarity	E-Value
Genes Involved in Fungal Development/Sporulation						
NAGBG48TV	GB|BAA35140.1	Chitinase	*Emericella nidulans*	68.55	84.68	1.30E-44
NAGBA10TV	GB|AAD34461.1	Ascus development protein 3	*Neurospora crassa*	36.1	54.29	4.20E-06
NAGBD49TV	SP|P40552	Cell wall protein TIR3 precursor	*Saccharomyces cerevisiae*	27.97	45.45	2.70E-10
NAGBU14TV	SP|P10169	Conidiation-specific protein 8	*Neurospora crassa*	41.11	51.11	5.90E-08
TC10246	SP|P10169	Conidiation-specific protein 8	*Neurospora crassa*	41.11	51.11	5.80E-08
TC11956	SP|P10713	Conidiation-specific protein 10	*Neurospora crassa*	71.60	80.25	2.40E-25
TC12083	SP|P10713	Conidiation-specific protein 10	*Neurospora crassa*	67.86	73.21	7.00E-12
NAFEA74TV	GI|585141	Developmental regulator *flbA*	*Emericella nidulans*	93.00	96.00	1.00E-126
NAGBI96TV	SP|O60032	Conidiophore development protein *hymA*	*Emericella nidulans*	89.66	95.40	4.50E-39
TC8878	SP|O60032	Conidiophore development protein *hymA*	*Emericella nidulans*	90.83	95.83	3.30E-53
Genes Involved in Transport and Drug Resistance						
NAGCB21TV	GB|CAC28822.2	Multidrug resistance-associated protein	*Neurospora crassa*	52.56	67.31	6.70E-30
NAGDC32TV	SP|P32767	Pleiotropic drug resistance regulatory protein 6	*Saccharomyces cerevisiae*	36.43	57.36	1.20E-08
NAFCV74TV	GB|CAD21494.1	Conserved hypothetical protein	*Neurospora crassa*	48.61	70.83	4.80E-11

NAGCB47TV	GB|CAD71016.1	Probable mportin-alpha export receptor	*Neurospora crassa*	51.20	72.80	1.20E-27
TC11203	GB|CAD70375.1	Probable fluconazole resistance protein	*Neurospora crassa*	55.62	69.10	9.00E-51
TC11795	PIR|T30882	Multidrug resistance protein 1	*Aspergillus flavus*	100.00	100.00	0
TC9584	GB|AAA50353.1	Metal resistance protein	*Saccharomyces cerevisiae*	49.70	72.26	4.30E-94
TC9769	SP|P32386	ATP-dependent bile acid permease	*Saccharomyces cerevisiae*	56.28	74.49	9.80E-75
Genes Potentially Involved in Secondary Metabolism						
NAGCA40TV	GB|BAB49569.1	NADH-dependent dehydrogenase	*Mesorhizobium loti*	29.63	50.62	0.038
NAGCB08TV	GB|AAF26281.1	Monooxygenase	*Aspergillus parasiticus*	100.00	100.00	2.30E-26
NAGCB61TV	SP|O47950	NADH-ubiquinone oxidoreductase 19.3 kDa subunit	*Neurospora crassa*	92.42	96.21	1.60E-66
NAGCO63TV	GB|AAF26274.1	NADH oxidase	*Aspergillus parasiticus*	87.32	92.25	1.30E-60
NAGCQ74TV	PIR|T38538	Probable oxidoreductase	*Schizosaccharomyces pombe*	43.07	64.23	4.40E-24
TC10309	GB|BAC20334.1	Monooxygenase	*Aspergillus oryzae*	98.69	99.22	1.20E-213
TC10899	GB|AAF26280.1	Cytochrome P450 monooxygenase	*Aspergillus parasiticus*	98.35	100.00	4.60E-63
TC8634	PIR|S55328	Serine-type carboxypeptidase precursor	*Aspergillus phoenicis*	80.00	85.79	1.40E-79
TC8800	SP|P36060	NADH-cytochrome b5 reductase precursor	*Saccharomyces cerevisiae*	42.72	61.17	3.70E-49
TC10233	SP|P41747	Alcohol dehydrogenase	*Aspergillus flavus*	99.71	99.71	2.10E-184
NAGBA01TV	GB|AAD13655.1	T-2 toxin biosynthesis protein	*Fusarium sporotrichioides*	45.11	63.59	6.50E-32

Source: Modified from Yu, J., Ronning, C.M., Wilkinson, J.R., Campbell, B.C., Payne, G.A., Bhatnagar, D., Cleveland, T.E., and Nierman, W.C., *Food Add. Contam.*, 2007 (in press).

the high-density and high-quality microarray of 6684 short amplicons representing 5002 unique gene elements was constructed which includes the 31 known aflatoxin cluster genes. Gene expression profiling experiments by microarrays have been used by our group and others to successfully identify differentially expressed genes associated with aflatoxin production in *A. flavus* and *A. parasiticus* grown under different nutritional and environmental conditions (O'Brian et al., 2003; Price et al., 2005; Wilkinson et al., 2007). We are also using near-isogenic development and secondary metabolic mutants of *A. flavus* and *A. parasiticus* in the proposed microarray studies that will not require shifts in growth media (Yu et al., 2007). This will allow us to more accurately select specific subsets of differentially expressed genes that are involved in aflatoxin production and fungal development.

14.2.3.3 Whole Genome Sequencing

A national project at the North Carolina State University (PI, Gary Payne), in collaboration with SRRC, to sequence the entire *A. flavus* genome (at TIGR) was initiated in 2003. The sequencing has been completed with a 5 × depth of coverage (79 scaffolds representing 1407 contigs, scaffold size ranging from 4.5 Mb to 1.0 kb). The 36.3 Mb *A. flavus* genome sequence data indicates that the genome contains 11,736 genes (Payne et al., 2006). The annotated sequence data are available to the collaborative laboratories and have recently been also made available to the public at the TIGR Web site (http://www.tigr.org) and the NC State Web site (http://www.aspergillusflavus.org). Based on this sequence, two whole genome *A. flavus* microarrays have been printed. USDA/ARS/SRRC has printed new TIGR arrays containing amplicons of all predicted genes in the *A. flavus* genome, and whole genome Affymetrix arrays have been prepared from USDA/NRI funding awarded to Drs Payne, Keller, Woloshuk, and Yu. These current resources are being used to study the environmental influences on the fungus, ecological/evolutionary significance of *A. flavus* propagation (biodiversity), fungal virulence/pathogenicity factors, and aflatoxin formation as manifested by changes in gene expression profiles and global signal transduction within the fungus.

14.3   Strategies to Control Preharvest Aflatoxin Contamination

14.3.1   Biological Control

Some *A. flavus* isolates that are well adapted to plant-associated niches do not produce aflatoxins yet have the capacity to competitively exclude aflatoxin producers. These atoxigenic strains can serve as biological control agents for management of aflatoxins in crops. Management strategies directed at utilizing atoxigenic strains as biological control agents to limit aflatoxin contamination have been pursued for almost two decades (Cole and Cotty, 1990; Dorner, 2004). These strategies seek to competitively exclude aflatoxin producers from crops with strains of *A. flavus* that do not produce aflatoxins and have the potential to interfere with the contamination process. The displacement results in both reduced incidences of aflatoxin producers throughout the environment and reduced aflatoxin contamination of crops. Aflatoxin prevention technologies based on atoxigenic strains of *A. flavus* and *A. parasiticus* are being developed for several crops (Cotty, 1994; Cotty and Antilla, 2003; Dorner, 2004). Such technologies deliver atoxigenic strains on nutritive solid substrate and handling characteristics for on farm use in target areas (Bock and Cotty, 1999a). Those technologies that have been developed commercially all rely on nutritive substrates to provide the atoxigenic strain initial advantage upon application. In 1996, the first commercial fields were treated with atoxigenic strains under an experimental use permit pesticide registration. Since then, over 50,000 ha of cotton have been treated (Cotty and Antilla, 2003).

The timing of atoxigenic strain applications is key to successful displacement of aflatoxin producers. For atoxigenic strains of *A. flavus* to be useful during crop production, they must be applied at a time and manner that allows successful competition with aflatoxin producers (Cotty 2001; van Egmond, 2004). In theory, application of an atoxigenic strain, when overall *A. flavus* levels are low, provides preferential exposure to the crop and an advantage in competing for crop resources (Orum et al., 1997; van Egmond, 2004). Atoxigenic strains are routinely applied once per crop at 10–20 lb per acre, depending on the crop treated (Cotty and Antilla, 2003; Dorner, 2004).

However, the extent to which atoxigenic strain technology is utilized is dependent on the economics of contamination. Not all areas with some contamination have sufficient contamination to warrant treatments and in areas with frequent contamination, as effective treatments are made, economic justification for continued treatments declines. Thus, in some regions, cost-benefit analyses result in discontinuation of treatments before full and cumulative benefits are reached.

14.3.2 Enhancement of Host-Plant Resistance

Success in conventional breeding for resistance to mycotoxin-producing or phytopathogenic fungi is dependent on the availability of resistance gene(s) in the germplasm. Even when it is available, breeding for disease-resistant crops is very time-consuming, especially in perennial crops such as tree nut crops, and does not lend itself ready to combat the evolution of new virulent fungal races. While it is possible to identify a few genotypes of corn or peanuts that are naturally resistant to *Aspergillus* we do not know whether these antifungal factors are specific to *A. flavus*. In addition, the resistance is often a polygenic trait as in the case of corn (White et al., 1999). In crops such as cotton, there are no known naturally resistant varieties to *Aspergillus*. Availability of transgenic varieties with antifungal traits will be extremely valuable in cotton breeding. Disease-resistant transgenic crops would not only control mycotoxin-producing organisms such as *A. flavus*, *A. parasiticus*, and *Fusarium* spp. but also several other microbial (fungal, bacterial, and viral) diseases which cause significant economic losses in crop production. Above all, transgenic crops resistant to aflatoxin-producing fungi offer not only the promise of negating the adverse effects caused by the toxin on immuno-compromised humans and animals but also provide environmentally safe alternatives from the current practices of using chemicals and pesticides. With the current information available with respect to proteomics of host and genomics and field ecology of the fungus, novel strategies for aflatoxin contamination will emerge based on a clear understanding of the toxin biosynthesis and contamination processes, especially at the molecular level. The following summary provides recent advances in control of preharvest aflatoxin contamination made through conventional breeding and genetic engineering in selected crops vulnerable for contamination.

14.3.2.1 Plant Breeding Strategies

14.3.2.1.1 Peanut

Several sources of resistant peanut germplasm have been identified from a core collection representing the entire peanut germplasm collection (Holbrook et al., 1995). Over 95% of this core collection has been preliminarily screened in a single environment; and 16 genotypes tested over 3 years in two environments still display low levels of aflatoxin. A possible link between low linoleic acid content in peanut and low preharvest aflatoxin production has been indicated (Holbrook et al., 1995). Significant correlations have also been observed between leaf temperature and aflatoxin levels, and visual stress ratings and aflatoxin levels. The preliminary screening of peanut genotypes using either or both of these traits could greatly reduce expenses involved in developing resistant cultivars. Promising germplasm, however, has less than acceptable agronomic characteristics, and is thus being hybridized with those with commercially acceptable features. Resistant lines are also being crossed to pool resistances to aflatoxin production. Thus, some success has been achieved in identifying resistant peanut germplasm, and field studies are being conducted by various researchers to verify this trait.

14.3.2.1.2 Tree Nuts

Among tree nuts, strategies for controlling preharvest aflatoxin formation by breeding for host-resistance have been mostly studied in almonds (Gradziel et al., 1995). The approach employed in this effort is to integrate multiple genetic mechanisms for control of *Aspergillus* spp. as well as navel orange worm, which appears important for initial fungal infection. Resistance to fungal colonization has been shown to be present in the undamaged seed coat of several advanced breeding selections and is further being pursued through breeding/genetic engineering of resistance to *A. flavus* in kernel tissue and also by developing genotypes that produce low amounts of aflatoxin following fungal infections (Gradziel and Dandekar, 1999). Studies have also been conducted with figs and pistachios to identify the mode of infection of the crops by *A. flavus*. McGranahan et al. (1999) reported that evaluation of 26 walnut cultivars, representing a range of germplasm at USDA, WRRC, has resulted in identification of one variety, Tulare, for its consistent low aflatoxin content, possibly due to its intact seed coat. The value of the intact seed coat in preventing aflatoxin contamination was also considered as one of the factors in the low aflatoxin producing variety, Tulare. This variety has been utilized in several crosses with high aflatoxin producing varieties such as Hartley. Upon further analyses, it has been well established by Mahoney and Molyneux (2004) that precursors of hydrolyzable tannins (HT), gallic acid, within the pellicle tissues are responsible for tolerance to *A. flavus* infection in Tulare. Identification of natural sources of resistance to aflatoxin synthesis has helped researchers to evaluate genetics of the trait and to identify genetic components. Once these parameters are clearly understood, strategies could be developed to identify germplasm with agronomically desirable characteristics and resistance to fungal infection (Doster et al., 1995).

14.3.2.1.3   Cotton

Cultivated cottons belong to the following four species—the diploid *Gossypium arboreum* and *G. herbaceum*, often referred to as "old world cottons" and the tetraploid *Gossypium hirsutum* and *G. barbadense*. Systematic study of all cotton genotypes to identify lines resistant to *Aspergillus* has not been done so far and there is no known resistant line among cultivated cotton. Thus, genetic engineering offers a novel means of introducing heterologous resistance traits into cultivated species of cotton (Wilkins et al., 2000; Rajasekaran, 2004).

14.3.2.1.4   Enhancement of Maize Resistance

Several resistant inbreds among the 31 tested in Illinois field trials (Campbell and White, 1995), have been incorporated into a breeding program whose major objective is to improve elite Midwestern maize lines such as B73 and Mo17. In this program, the inheritance of resistance of inbreds in crosses with B73 and Mo17 was determined (Maupin et al., 2003; Walker and White, 2001; White et al., 1995a, 1998; Hamblin and White, 2000). In the case of several highly resistant inbreds, Tex6, LB31, CI2, Oh513, and MI82, genetic dominance was indicated. Overall, results indicated that selection for resistance to *Aspergillus* ear rot and aflatoxin production should be effective. The frequency distribution of ear rot ratings and aflatoxin production in F3 families and in backcrosses to the susceptible self families of

Mo17 × Tex6 and B73 × LB31 pointed to the possibility of success in the development of resistant inbreds for use in breeding commercial hybrids (White et al., 1995b).

Chromosome regions associated with resistance to *A. flavus* and inhibition of aflatoxin production in maize have been identified through restriction fragment length polymorphism (RFLP) analysis in three resistant lines (R001, LB31, and Tex6) in the Illinois breeding program, after mapping populations were developed using B73 and Mo17 elite inbreds as the susceptible parents (White et al., 1995a, 1998). In some cases, chromosomal regions were associated with resistance to *Aspergillus* ear rot and not aflatoxin inhibition, and vice versa, whereas other chromosomal regions were found to be associated with both traits. This suggests that these two traits may be at least partially under separate genetic control. Also, it was observed that variation can exist in the chromosomal regions associated with *Aspergillus* ear rot and aflatoxin inhibition in different mapping populations, suggesting the presence of different genes for resistance in the different identified resistance germplasm. RFLP technology may provide the basis for employing the strategy of pyramiding different types of resistances into commercially important genetic backgrounds, while avoiding the introduction of undesirable traits.

Another quantitative trait loci (QTL) mapping program was undertaken using a mapping population created from a resistant inbred Mp313E and a susceptible one, Va35 (Davis et al., 1999). Here, regions were revealed on the chromosomes associated with resistance to aflatoxin contamination. Similar work to map resistance traits in maize is proceeding in another program, which could ultimately facilitate the pyramiding of insect and fungal resistance genes into commercial germplasm (Guo et al., 2000).

A collaborative research effort between the International Institute of Tropical Agriculture (IITA) in Ibadan, Nigeria, and the USDA-ARS in New Orleans is aimed at developing maize inbreds resistant to aflatoxin contamination and also the identification of resistance markers in these lines (Brown et al., 2003). Initially, a number of inbreds, adapted to the savanna and midaltitude ecological zones of West and Central Africa were selected for moderate to high levels of resistance to ear rot under conditions of severe natural infection in their respective areas of adaptation (Brown et al., 2001). The major ear rot-causing fungi in these environments include *Aspergillus*, *Botryodiplodia*, *Diplodia*, *Fusarium*, and *Macrophomina*. To determine their potential to resist aflatoxin production by *A. flavus*, these lines were sent to ARS-New Orleans to be screened using the laboratory-based kernel screening assay (KSA) (Brown et al., 1995). A relatively large number of these lines were shown to be lower in aflatoxin accumulation than a resistant U.S. check. Therefore, these potentially aflatoxin-resistant lines from IITA and a number of U.S. resistant lines were used as parents for crosses in the collaborative breeding effort. IITA developed a large number of inbred lines from backcross populations with 75% U.S.–25% IITA germplasm and F1 crosses with 50% U.S.–50% IITA germplasm. Over the years, a number of lines in these two backgrounds have been developed, and screened by the KSA. These lines, now in S6 and S7 generations are also being evaluated for agronomic characteristics (Brown et al., 2005). After running confirmation tests of the promising lines using KSA and field testing, the best lines with good agronomic features and resistance to aflatoxin accumulation will be slated for release as potential sources of genes for resistance to aflatoxin production in breeding programs.

The new inbred lines emanating from this project, which combined genes from the two sets of germplasm are potentially new sources of resistance mechanisms that can be used to accelerate the breeding efforts of the national programs in West and Central Africa to combat the problem of mycotoxin contamination (Menkir et al., 2007). Some of these lines could be used directly to develop synthetic varieties that could be deployed to farmers' fields readily to combat the problem of aflatoxin contamination. A potential also exists to generate basic genetic information using some of the near-isogenic lines with contrasting levels of aflatoxin in order to develop a breeding strategy for pyramiding different alleles that confer resistance to mycotoxins. Proteomics is being used on these lines to identify markers through the identification of resistance-associated proteins (RAPs) and their corresponding genes. This would allow breeders to use this germplasm to transfer resistance to other desirable backgrounds through marker-assisted breeding.

14.3.2.1.5   *Identification of Resistance-Associated Proteins through Proteomics*

Developing resistance to fungal infection in wounded as well as intact maize kernels would accelerate solving the aflatoxin problem (Payne, 1992). Studies demonstrating subpericarp (wounded-kernel) resistance in maize kernels have led to research to identify subpericarp resistance mechanisms. In a number of studies, proteins associated with resistance (RAPs) have been identified (Brown et al., 2004). However, to take advantage of the increased reproducibility, map resolution, reliability, and accuracy that 2D PAGE offers over 1D gel electrophoresis (Gorg et al., 1985, 1988), a proteomics approach has been employed to facilitate further identification of RAPs. Proteomics, the analysis of the protein complement of a genome (Pennington et al., 1997; Wilkins et al., 1996), makes use of state-of-the-art analytical software and computers, and the recent acquisition of genomic data for a number of organisms. It involves the systematic separation, identification, and quantification of many proteins simultaneously. 2D electrophoresis is also unique in its ability to detect post and cotranslational modifications, which cannot be predicted from the genome sequence.

Through proteome analysis and a subtractive approach based on comparing aflatoxin-resistant with susceptible genotypes, it may be possible to identify important protein markers associated with resistance, as well as genes encoding these proteins. This could facilitate marker-assisted breeding and genetic engineering efforts. Endosperm and embryo proteins from several resistant and susceptible genotypes have been compared using large format 2D gel electrophoresis, and over a dozen such protein spots, either unique or fivefold upregulated in resistant lines (Mp420 and Mp313E), have been identified, isolated from preparative 2D gels and analyzed using ESI-MS/MS after in-gel digestion with trypsin (Chen et al., 2000, 2002). These proteins are all constitutively expressed. A recent investigation into corn kernel resistance (Chen et al., 2001) determined that both constitutive and induced proteins are required for resistance to aflatoxin production. In fact, one major difference demonstrated between resistant and susceptible maize genotypes is the relatively high level of constitutively expressed antifungal proteins in the former compared to the latter. A function of these high levels of constitutive proteins may be to delay fungal invasion, and subsequent aflatoxin formation, until infection-induced antifungal proteins can be synthesized. Proteins identified in this study can be grouped into three categories based on their peptide sequence homology: (1) storage proteins, such as globulins and late embryogenesis abundant proteins; (2) stress-responsive proteins, such as aldose reductase, a glyoxalase I protein, and a 16.9 kDa heat shock protein; and (3) antifungal proteins. This latter category includes a pathogenesis-related protein, PR-10, that through further characterization was strongly implicated in resistance (Chen et al., 2006a).

During the screening of progeny developed through the IITA–USDA/ARS collaborative project, near-isogenic maize lines from the same backcross differing significantly in aflatoxin accumulation were identified, and proteome analysis of these lines was conducted (Brown et al., 2003). Results demonstrate that proteins expressed fit into the above-three categories. Investigating corn lines from the same cross with contrasting reaction to *A. flavus* should enhance the identification of RAPs clearly without the confounding effect of differences in the genetic backgrounds of the lines.

Heretofore, most RAPs identified have had antifungal activities. However, increased temperatures and drought, which often occur together, are major factors associated with aflatoxin contamination of maize kernels (Payne, 1998). It has also been found that drought stress imposed during grain filling reduces dry matter accumulation in kernels (Payne, 1998). This often leads to cracks in the seed and provides an easy entry site to fungi and insects. Possession of unique or of higher levels of hydrophilic storage or stress-related proteins, such as the aforementioned, may put resistant lines in an advantageous position over susceptible genotypes in the ability to synthesize proteins and defend against pathogens under stress conditions. Therefore, the necessary requirements for developing commercially useful, aflatoxin-resistant maize lines may include, aside from antifungal proteins, a high level of expression of stress-related proteins. Further studies including physiological and biochemical characterization, genetic mapping, plant transformation using RAP genes, and marker-assisted breeding should clarify the roles of stress-related RAPs in kernel resistance. RNAi gene silencing experiments involving RAPs presently being conducted, may also contribute valuable information. (Brown et al., 2003).

The direct involvement of a purported stress-related protein in resistance to aflatoxin accumulation was recently investigated with glyoxalase I (Chen et al., 2004). The substrate for glyoxalase I, methylglyoxal, is a potent cytotoxic compound produced spontaneously in all organisms under physiological conditions from glycolysis and photosynthesis intermediates, glyceraldehydes-3-phosphate, and dihydroxyacetone phosphate. Methylglyoxal is an aflatoxin inducer even at low concentrations; experimental evidence indicates that induction is through upregulation of aflatoxin biosynthetic pathway transcripts including the AFLR regulatory gene. Therefore, glyoxalase I may directly affect resistance by removing its aflatoxin-inducing substrate, methylglyoxal.

14.3.2.2 Genetic Engineering for Resistance to Aspergillus flavus

Transgenic varieties providing resistance to *Aspergillus* spp. are not yet available. As a matter of fact, there is no transgenic variety available with disease resistance traits to phytopathogenic fungi indicating the dire need for the same or the complexity in achieving the goal of host-plant resistance (Rajasekaran et al., 2002; Punja et al., 2004; Rajasekaran et al., 2005a). However, several laboratories are experimenting with potential antifungal gene constructs that offer resistance in vitro, in situ, or in planta to *A. flavus* often stacked with insect-resistant genes. It is often speculated that bollworm or insect injury to cotton bolls serve as an entry point for *A. flavus* spores although concrete evidence is not yet available (Zipf and Rajasekaran, 2003); yet insect control may be useful in preventing the spore entry into the fatty acid-rich cottonseed. For example, studies have shown that aflatoxin contamination is not directly correlated with pink bollworm damage and contamination may occur in the absence of damage (Henneberry et al., 1978; Russell, 1980; Bock and Cotty, 1999b). However, aflatoxin contamination in peanuts (Lynch and Wilson, 1991) or in tree nuts (Gradziel et al., 1995) is positively correlated with insect damage. The following section provides a brief account of different antifungal gene constructs that have been tested using crop or model test plants for resistance to the mycotoxigenic fungi.

14.3.2.2.1 Native Antifungal Genes

A number of potentially useful antifungal enzymes/proteins are produced either constitutively or in response to fungal attack in plants. These include chitinases and β-1,3-glucanases (Broglie et al., 1991; Meins et al., 1992; Cornelissen and Melchers, 1993; Thomma et al., 2002), osmotins (Singh et al., 1989), protease inhibitors (Ryan, 1990), thionins (Bohlmann, 1994), and polygalacturonase inhibitor proteins (PGIPs) (Toubart et al., 1992). Several laboratories have attempted to identify and characterize native antifungal genes from corn. Identifying resistance in corn makes it possible to correlate resistance with many endogenous low molecular weight compounds and biomacromolecules in kernel tissues already implicated as antifungal at various stages of kernel development in grain crops. However, compounds with activity against other fungal species are often ineffective against *A. flavus*, and thus it is important to select the best candidate inhibitory compounds and identify and characterize their respective genes before plant genetic engineering procedures are initiated. A list of candidate antifungal compounds may include RIPs, lectins, relatively small MW polypeptides, cell-surface glycoproteins, hydrolases, and certain basic proteins (Cleveland et al., 1997). For example, trypsin inhibitor (TI) (Chen et al., 1998) has been shown to be correlated with kernel resistance to *A. flavus* infection of corn and when expressed in transgenic tobacco, resulted in enhanced resistance to the tobacco pathogen, *Colletotrichum destructivum* (Rajasekaran et al., 2002). In addition, leaf extracts from transgenic tobacco inhibited the growth of other phytopathogens, such as *Verticillium dahliae*. Evidence from several IITA corn genotypes (progeny of U.S. and African parental lines), resistant to preharvest aflatoxin contamination, indicates that TI plays a key role in imparting this resistance. When cotton was transformed with the TI gene under the control of 35S CaMV promoter, the expression level was sufficient to control *Verticillium* but not *A. flavus* (Rajasekaran et al., 2002). Perhaps higher seed-specific expression of this gene in cottonseed would be helpful. Recently, we identified the usefulness of corn PR-10, a pathogenesis-related protein with antifungal and RNase activities (Chen et al., 2006) and glyoxalase I, a stress-related protein with demonstrated potential to directly inhibit aflatoxin accumulation (Chen et al., 2004). For example, a synthetic version of a corn ribosome-inhibiting protein (RIP) gene (called *mod*1) has been shown to control *A. flavus* in corn and peanuts (Boston et al., 1994, 1996; Weissinger et al., 2003). Lozovaya et al. (1998) reported that the resistance of a corn hybrid to *A. flavus* infection was correlated with an elevated level of α-1–3-glucanase in transgenic cells.

A full-length polyphenol oxidase cDNA from walnut embryos of resistant lines has been identified and is being tested for its antifungal or antiinsect activity. Following the recent demonstration by Mahoney and Molyneux (2004) that a precursor(s) of HT, gallic acid, present within the pellicle tissues is responsible for inhibiting aflatoxin biosynthesis, Dandekar et al. (2000) have initiated a program to identify and isolate genes responsible for HT/gallic acid biosynthesis with the objective of genetic engineering of susceptible walnut lines (and other crops) which lack or underexpress gallic acid in the seed coat.

14.3.2.2.2   Heterologous Antifungal Genes

Small MW peptides have been isolated from organisms other than plants that also show promise as antifungal agents (Rao, 1995; Broekart et al., 1997; Hancock and Chapple, 1999; Reddy et al., 2004); for example, the cecropins (Bowman and Hultmark, 1987) and magainins (Zasloff, 1987) of insect and amphibian origins respectively, and their synthetic analogs (Cary et al., 2000; Rajasekaran et al., 2001; DeGray et al., 2001; Li et al., 2001; Chakrabarti et al., 2003).

Genes coding for haloperoxidases (Wolffram et al., 1988) and their utility for plant disease resistance has been documented in transgenic tobacco plants (Rajasekaran et al., 2000). In bioassays using *A. flavus* as the test organism, addition of a myeloperoxidase greatly enhanced (90-fold) the lethality of H_2O_2 by catalyzing its conversion to sodium hypochlorite (Jacks et al., 1991). A bacterial chloroperoxidase also greatly reduced the viability of *A. flavus* conidia in vitro (Jacks et al., 1999; Rajasekaran et al., 2000). One of the bacterial chloroperoxidases, CPO-P was found to confer antifungal traits against *Aspergillus* spp. and other phytopathogens in transgenic tobacco, cotton, and peanut (Rajasekaran et al., 2000; Jacks et al., 2004; Niu et al., 2004). H_2O_2 is produced by plants under pest attack and it often serves as the substrate for these unique peroxidases in the specific host-plant tissues (Jacks and Hinojosa, 1993; Rajasekaran et al., 2000). In fact, several investigators were attempting to increase host-plant resistance by increasing the level of H_2O_2 production. For example, Wu et al. (1995) introduced a glucose oxidase (GO) gene from *A. niger* to generate large amounts of hydrogen peroxide in transgenic potato plants to augment natural defense mechanisms. The transgenic potato plants showed an increased level of resistance to soft rot caused by *Erwinia carotovora* and to potato late blight caused by *Phytophthora infestans*. In contrast to these observations, a similar attempt with transgenic cottons expressing the *Talaromyces flavus* GO gene resulted in a limited antifungal activity against the root pathogen, *V. dahliae* (Murray et al., 1999). However, these authors also discovered that the expression of GO in cottons resulted in phyto toxicity and reduced yield. Corn embryonic cultures have also been successfully cotransformed with the wheat oxalate oxidase (OXO) gene (Simmonds et al., 1998). OXO is a source of extracellular production of H_2O_2 in plants.

Certain small lytic peptides have demonstrated convincing inhibitory activity against *A. flavus* and show promise for transformation of plants to reduce infection of seed. In our laboratory, we (Rajasekaran et al., 2001; Cary et al., 2000) reported that a synthetic lytic peptide (D4E1) gene, when transformed into tobacco, greatly enhances resistance *in planta* to *Colletotrichum destructivum*. Treatment of germinating *A. flavus* spores with tobacco leaf extracts from plants, transformed with the D4E1 gene, significantly reduced spore viability (colony forming units) relative to results obtained using extracts from nontransformed (control) plants. Similarly, in recent tests with cottonseed expressing the D4E1 gene, we demonstrated resistance to penetration of seed coats by a GFP reporter gene-containing *A. flavus* strain (Rajasekaran et al., 2005b). In addition to inhibiting the germination of *A. flavus* spores, D4E1 caused severe abnormal lytic effects on mycelial wall, cytoplasm, and nuclei (Figure 14.3). The expression of D4E1 gene in the progeny of transgenic cotton was sufficient enough to inhibit the growth in vitro of *Fusarium verticillioides* and *Verticillium dahliae* or *in planta* of *Thielaviopsis basicola* (Rajasekaran et al., 2005b) and provide a good germination stand in a field infected with *Fusarium oxysporum* f. sp. *vasinfectum* (Rajasekaran et al., 2006). Transformation of peanut with another antifungal peptide, D5C, has been reported (Weissinger et al., 1999). Although the pure D5C showed strong activity in vitro against *A. flavus*, it was shown that the transgenic peanut callus showed poor recovery of plants because of possible phytotoxicity of the peptide.

Recently Emani et al. (2003) transformed cotton plants with a cDNA clone encoding a 42 kDa endochitinase from the mycoparasitic fungus, *Trichoderma virens*. Homozygous T2 plants of the high endochitinase-expressing cotton lines showed significant resistance against a soilborne pathogen, *Rhizoctonia solani*, and a foliar pathogen, *Alternaria alternata*.

Peanut is also currently being transformed with antifungal genes; e.g., with a gene encoding for MOD-1, a synthetic version of corn RIP (Weissinger et al., 2003), while walnut has been successfully transformed with barley lectin and nettle lectin antifungal genes (Mendum et al., 1995). Transgenic peanuts expressing the MOD-1 gene have demonstrated antifungal traits when peanut cotyledons were infected with *A. flavus*. Ozias Akins et al. (1999) are also evaluating the potentials of soybean *lox1* gene in suppressing the aflatoxin biosynthetic pathway. Soybean *lox1* gene encodes an enzyme that catalyzes the formation of a specific lipoxygenase metabolite of linoleic acid, 13(*S*)-β-hydroperoxyoctadecadienoic acid (HPODE) that has been shown to suppress the aflatoxin biosynthetic pathway in vitro (Burow et al., 1997; Keller et al., 1999).

In addition to nuclear transformation, we are also exploring the possibility of expressing the antifungal genes in plastids with the objective of higher expression and preventing transgene escape through pollen. For example, the antimicrobial peptide MSI-99, an analog of magainin 2, was expressed via the chloroplast genome (DeGray et al., 2001) of tobacco. Leaf extracts from T2 generation plants showed 96% inhibition of growth against *P. syringae* pv. *tabaci*. In addition, leaf extracts from T1 generation plants inhibited the growth of pregerminated spores of three fungal species, *A. flavus*, *Fusarium verticillioides*, and *Verticillium dahliae*, by more than 95%, compared with nontransformed control plant extracts. *In planta* assays with the bacterial pathogen *P. syringae* pv. *tabaci* resulted in areas of necrosis around the point of inoculation in control leaves, whereas transformed leaves showed no signs of necrosis, demonstrating high-dose release of the peptide at the site of infection by chloroplast lysis. *In planta* assays with the fungal pathogen, *Colletotrichum destructivum*, showed necrotic anthracnose lesions in nontransformed control leaves, whereas transformed leaves showed no lesions. In addition to lytic peptide genes, a variety of other candidate antifungal genes from bacterial, plant, and mammalian sources have a good probability of being active against *A. flavus* upon transformation into plants.

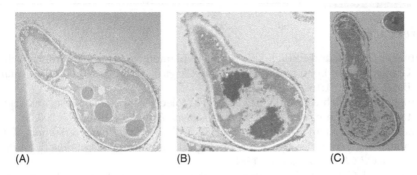

(A) (B) (C)

FIGURE 14.3
Transmission electron micrographs of pregerminated *Aspergillus flavus* spores exposed to the antifungal peptide D4E1. (A) Control in PDB; (B and C) spores exposed to 10 μM D4E1 for 1 h. Note cytoplasmic degradation due to exposure to D4E1 leading to eventual lysis (K. Rajasekaran, unpublished).

14.4 Conclusion

Even though biological control of toxigenic fungi and plant breeding strategies to enhance host-resistance of various crops have proven to be effective strategies for reducing aflatoxin contamination of crops, there is still a lot more work that needs to be done to achieve complete (or near-complete) elimination of toxin from the food supply. Continuing the investigation of the biochemical function and genetic regulation of the genes in a fungal system on a genomic scale will aid in gaining a better understanding of the complex host plant–fungus interaction, which influences aflatoxin contamination and in devising strategies to interrupt the contamination process. Extensive progress has been made in identifying resistance markers through proteomic comparisons of differentially resistant corn varieties, thus identifying protein markers that could be used in breeding or gene insertion technologies to enhance resistance in crops to aflatoxin contamination. In addition, *Aspergillus flavus* EST technology will allow rapid identification of the majority, if not all, of the genes expressed in the fungal genome and promote a better understanding of their functions, regulation, and coordination of gene expression in response to internal and external factors, relationships between primary and secondary metabolism, plant–fungal interactions, and fungal pathogenicity, as well as evolutionary biology. Microarrays made from the EST or whole genome sequences are being used to detect a whole set of genes expressed under specific environmental conditions, for example. This technology allows us to study a complete set of fungal genes, simultaneously, that are responsible for, or related to, toxin production. Microarray technology is expected to provide valuable information on factors that are responsible for turning on and off aflatoxin production during the fungal–plant interaction. These advances will soon allow us to obtain a safer and economically viable food and feed supply worldwide, free of aflatoxin contamination.

References

Bhatnagar D, Yu J, and Ehrlich KC. Toxins of filamentous fungi. In: Breitenbach M, Crameri R, and Lehrer SB (Eds.), *Fungal Allergy and Pathogenicity. Chem. Immunol.* Basel, Karger 81:167–206, 2002.

Bhatnagar D, Ehrlich KC, and Cleveland TE. Molecular genetic analysis and regulation of aflatoxin biosynthesis. *Appl. Microbiol. Biotechnol.* 61:83–93, 2003.

Bennett JW, Silverstein RB, and Kruger SJ. Isolation and characterization of two nonaflatoxigenic classes of morphological variants of *Aspergillus parasiticus. J. Am. Oil Chem. Soc.* 58:952, 1981.

Bock CH and Cotty PJ. The relationship of gin date to aflatoxin contamination of cottonseed in Arizona. *Plant. Dis.* 83:279–285, 1999a.

Bock CH and Cotty PJ. Wheat seed colonized with atoxigenic *Aspergillus flavus*: Characterization and production of a biopesticide for aflatoxin control. *Biocontrol Sci. Technol.* 9:529–543, 1999b.

Bohlmann H. The role of thionins in plant protection. *CRC Crit. Rev. Plant Sci.* 13:1–16, 1994.

Bok JW and Keller NP. LaeA, a regulator of secondary metabolism in *Aspergillus* spp. *Eukaryot. Cell* 3:527–535, 2004.

Bok JW, Hoffmeister D, Maggio-Hall LA, Murillo R, Glasner JD, and Keller NP. Genomic mining for *Aspergillus* natural products. *Chem. Biol.* 13:31–37, 2006.

Boston RS, Bass HW, and O'Brian GR. DNA encoding ribosome inactivating protein. U.S. Patent 5,332,808, 1994.

Boston RS, Bass HW, and O'Brian GR. DNA encoding ribosome inactivating protein. U.S. Patent 5,552,140, 1996.

Bowman HG and Hultmark D. Cell-free immunity in insects. *Annu. Rev. Microbiol.* 31:103–126, 1987.

Broekaert WF, Cammue BPA, Debolle MFC, Thevissen K, Desamblanx GW, and Osborn RW. Antimicrobial peptides from plants. *Crit. Rev. Plant Sci.* 16:297–323, 1997.

Broglie K, Chet I, Holliday M, Cressman R, Biddle P, Knowlton S, Mauvais CJ, and Broglie R. Transgenic plants with enhanced resistance to the fungal pathogen *Rhizoctonia solani. Science* 254:1194–1197, 1991.

Brown RL, Chen Z-Y, Menkir A, Cleveland TE, Cardwell K, Kling J, and White DG. Resistance to aflatoxin accumulation in kernels of maize inbreds selected for ear rot resistance in West and Central Africa. *J. Food Prot.* 64:396–400, 2001.

Brown RL, Chen Z-Y, Menkir A, and Cleveland TE. Using biotechnology to enhance host resistance to aflatoxin contamination of corn—A mini-review. *Afr. J. Biotechnol.* 2:557–562, 2003.

Brown RL, Chen Z-Y, and Cleveland TE. Molecular biology for control of mycotoxigenic fungi. In: Arora D, Bridge P, and Bhatnagar D (Eds.), *Fungal Biotechnology in Agricultural, Food, and Environmental Applications*, Marcel Dekker, Inc., NY, pp. 69–77, 2004.

Brown RL, Chen Z-Y, Menkir A, Bandyopadhyay R, and Cleveland TE. Development of aflatoxin-resistant maize inbreds and identification of potential resistance markers through USA–Africa collaborative research. Proceedings of the USDA–ARS Aflatoxin and Fumonisin Elimination and Fungal Genomics Workshop, Raleigh, NC, p. 78, 2005.

Brown RL, Cleveland TE, Payne GA, Woloshuk CP, Campbell KW, and White DG. Determination of resistance to aflatoxin production in maize kernels and detection of fungal colonization using an *Aspergillus flavus* transformant expressing *Escherichia coli* ß-glucuronidase. *Phytopathology* 85:983–989, 1995.

Burow GB, Nesbitt TC, Dunlap J, and Keller NP. Seed lipoxygenase products modulate *Aspergillus* mycotoxin biosynthesis. *MPMI* 10:380–387, 1997.

Calvo AM, Wilson RA, Bok J-W, and Keller NP. Relationship between secondary metabolism and fungal development. *Microbiol. Mol. Biol. Rev.* 66:447–459, 2002.

Calvo AM, Bok J-W, Brooks W, and Keller NP. VeA is required for toxin and sclerotial production in *Aspergillus parasiticus*. *Appl. Environ. Microbiol.* 70:4733–4739, 2004.

Campbell KW and White DG. Evaluation of corn genotypes for resistance to *Aspergillus* ear rot, kernel infection, and aflatoxin production. *Plant Dis.* 79:1039–1045, 1995.

Cary JW, Rajasekaran K, Jaynes JM, and Cleveland TE. Transgenic expression of a gene encoding a synthetic antimicrobial peptide results in inhibition of fungal growth *in vitro* and in plants. *Plant Sci.* 153:171–180, 2000.

Chakrabarti A, Ganapathi TR, Mukherjee PK, and Bapat VA. MSI-99, a magainin analogue, imparts enhanced disease resistance in transgenic tobacco and banana. *Planta* 216:587–596, 2003.

Chang P-K, Cary JW, Bhatnagar D, Cleveland TE, Bennett JW, Linz JE, Woloshuk CP, and Payne GA. Cloning of the *Aspergillus parasiticus apa-2* gene associated with the regulation of aflatoxin biosynthesis. *Appl. Environ. Microbiol.* 59:3273–3279, 1993.

Chang P-K, Yu J, Bhatnagar D, and Cleveland TE. The carboxy-terminal portion of the aflatoxin pathway regulatory protein AFLR of *Aspergillus parasiticus* activates GAL1::lacZ gene expression in *Saccharomyces cerevisiae*. *Appl. Environ. Microbiol.* 65:2508–2512, 1999.

Chang P-K, Yu J, Bhatnagar D, and Cleveland TE. Characterization of the *Aspergillus parasiticus* major nitrogen regulatory gene, *areA*. *Biochim. Biophys. Acta* 1491:263–266, 2000.

Chen Z-Y, Brown RL, Russin JS, Lax AR, and Cleveland TE. Resistance to *Aspergillus flavus* in corn kernels is associated with a 14-kDa protein. *Phytopathology* 88:276–281, 1998.

Chen Z-Y, Brown RL, Damann KE, and Cleveland TE. Proteomics analysis of kernel embryo and endosperm proteins of corn genotypes resistant or susceptible to *Aspergillus flavus* infection. Proceedings of the USDA-ARS Aflatoxin Elimination Workshop, Yosemite, CA, p. 88, 2000.

Chen Z-Y, Brown RL, Cleveland TE, Damann KE, and Russin JS. Comparison of constitutive and inducible maize kernel proteins of genotypes resistant or susceptible to aflatoxin production. *J. Food Prot.* 64:1785–1792, 2001.

Chen Z-Y, Brown RL, Damann KE, and Cleveland TE. Identification of unique or elevated levels of kernel proteins in aflatoxin-resistant maize genotypes through proteome analysis. *Phytopathology* 92:1084–1094, 2002.

Chen Z-Y, Brown RL, Damann KE, and Cleveland TE. Identification of a maize kernel stress-related protein and its effect on aflatoxin accumulation. *Phytopathology* 94:938–945, 2004.

Chen Z-Y, Brown RL, Rajasekaran K, Damann KE, and Cleveland TE. Evidence for involvement of a pathogenesis-related protein in maize resistance to *Aspergillus flavus* infection and aflatoxin production. *Phytopathology* 96:87–95, 2006a.

Chen Z-Y, Brown RL, Rajasekaran K, Damann KE, and Cleveland TE. Identification of a maize kernel pathogenesis-related protein and evidence for its involvement in resistance to *Aspergillus flavus* infection and aflatoxin production. *Phytopathology* 96:87–95, 2006b.

Cleveland TE, Cary JW, Brown RL, Bhatnagar D, Delucca AJ, Yu J, Chang PK, and Rajasekaran K. Use of biotechnology to eliminate aflatoxin in preharvest crops. Bulletin of the Institute for Comprehensive Agricultural Sciences, Kinki University, Nara, *Japan*. 5:75–90, 1997.

Cole RJ and Cotty PJ. Biocontrol of aflatoxin production by using biocompetitive agents. In: Robens J, Huff W, and Richard J (Eds.), *A Perspective on Aflatoxin in Field Crops and Animal Food Products in the United States: A Symposium*; ARS-83 Department of Agriculture, Agricultural Research Service, Peoria, IL, 62–66, 1990.

Cornelissen BJC and Melchers LS. Strategies for the control of fungal diseases with transgenic plants. *Plant Physiol.* 101:709–712, 1993.

Cotty PJ. Influence of field application of an atoxigenic strain of *Aspergillus flavus* on the population of *A. flavus* infecting cotton bolls and on the aflatoxin content of cottonseed. *Phytopathology* 84:1270–1277, 1994.

Cotty PJ. Cottonseed losses and mycotoxins. In: Kirkpatrick TL and Rothrock CS (Eds.), *Compendium of Cotton Diseases. Part 1. Infectious Diseases*. The American Phytopathological Society, St. Paul, MN, 9–13, 2001.

Cotty PJ and Bayman P. Competitive exclusion of a toxigenic strain of *Aspergillus flavus* by an atoxigenic strain. *Phytopathology* 83:1283–1287, 1993.

Cotty P and Antilla L. Managing aflatoxins in Arizona, United States Department of Agriculture, Agricultural Research Service, New Orleans, LA, 16 pp., 2003.

Dandekar AM, McGranahan G, Vail P, Molyneaux R, Mahoney N, Leslie C, Uratsu S, and Tebbets S. Genetic engineering and breeding of walnuts for control of aflatoxin. Proceedings of the USDA-ARS Aflatoxin Elimination Workshop, Yosemite, CA, pp. 108–109, 2000.

Davis GL, Windham GL, and Williams WP. QTL for aflatoxin reduction in maize. Maize Genetics Conference Abstracts, Lake Geneva, WI. 41(T8): 139, 1999a.

Davis GL, Windham GL, and Williams WP. QTL for aflatoxin reduction in maize. Maize Genetics Conference Abstracts 41(T8): 139, 1999b.

DeGray G, Rajasekaran K, Smith F, Sanford J, and Daniell H. Expression of an antimicrobial peptide via the chloroplast genome to control phytopathogenic bacteria and fungi. *Plant Physiol.* 127:852–862, 2001.

Dorner JW. Biological control of aflatoxin contamination of crops. *J. Toxicol-Toxin Rev.* 23:425–450, 2004.

Doster MA, Michailides TJ, and Morgan DP. Aflatoxin control in pistachio, walnut, and figs: Identification and separation of contamination nuts and figs, ecological relationships, and agronomic practices. Proceedings of the USDA-ARS Aflatoxin Elimination Workshop, Atlanta, GA, pp. 63–64, 1995.

Doster M, Michailides T, Cotty PJ, Holtz B, Bentley W, Morgan D, and Boeckler L. Aflatoxin control in pistachios: Removal of contaminated nuts, ecological relationships, and biocontrol. *Mycopathologia* 155:44, 2002.

Duran RM, Cary JW, and Calvo AM, Production of cyclopiazonic acid, aflatrem, and aflatoxin by *Aspergillus flavur* is regulated by veA, a gene necessary for sclerotial formation. *Appl. Microbiol. Biotechnol.* 73(5):1158–1168, 2007.

Eaton DL and Groopman JD (Eds.), *The toxicology of aflatoxins: Human health, veterinary, and agricultural significance*. Academic Press, San Diego, CA, 1994.

Ehrlich KC, Cary JW, and Montalbano BG. Characterization of the promoter for the gene encoding the aflatoxin biosynthetic pathway regulatory protein AFLR. *Biochim. Biophys. Acta* 1444:412–417, 1999.

Ehrlich KC, Montalbano BG, and Cotty PJ. Sequence comparison of *aflR* from different *Aspergillus* species provides evidence for variability in regulation of aflatoxin production. *Fungal Genet. Biol.* 38:63–74, 2003.

Emani C, Garcia JM, Lopata-Finch E, Pozo MJ, Uribe P, Kim DJ, Sunilkumar G, Cook DR, Kenerley CM, and Rathore KS. Enhanced fungal resistance in transgenic cotton expressing an endochitinase gene from *Trichoderma virens*. *Plant Biotechnol. J.* 1:321–336, 2003.

Gong YY, Hounsa A, Egal S, Turner PC, Sutcliffe AE, Hall AJ, Cardwell K, and Wild CP Postweaning exposure to aflatoxin results in impaired child growth: A longitudinal study in Benin, West Africa. *Environ. Health Persp.* 112:1334–1338, 2004.

Gorg A, Postel W, Gunther S, and Weser J. Improved horizontal two-dimensional electrophoresis with hybrid isoelectric focusing in immobilized pH gradients in the first dimension and laying-on transfer to the second dimension. *Electrophoresis* 6:599–604, 1985.

Gorg A, Postel W, and Gunther S. The current state of two- dimensional electrophoresis with immobilized pH gradients. *Electrophoresis* 9:531–546, 1988.

Gradziel TM and Dandekar A. Endocarp ventral vascular tissue development appears to be the Achilles heel for almond susceptibility to insect damage and aflatoxin contamination. Proceedings of the USDA-ARS Aflatoxin Elimination Workshop, Atlanta, GA, p. 5, 1999.

Gradziel T, Dandekar A, Ashamed M, Hirsh, Driver NJ, and Tang A. Integrating fungal pathogen and insect vector resistance for comprehensive preharvest aflatoxin control in almond. Proceedings of the USDA-ARS aflatoxin Elimination Workshop, Atlanta, GA, p. 5, 1995.

Guo BZ, Widstrom NW, Cleveland TE, and Lynch RE. Control of preharvest aflatoxin contamination in corn: Fungus-plant-insect interactions and control strategies. *Recent Res. Dev. Agric. Food Chem.* 4:165–176, 2000.

Hamblin AM and White DG. Inheritance of resistance to *Aspergillus* ear rot and aflatoxin production of corn from Tex6. *Phytopathology* 90:292–296, 2000.

Hancock REW and Chapple DS. Peptide antibiotics, *Antimicrob. Agents Chemother.* 43:1317–1323, 1999.

Henneberry TJ, Bariola IA, and Russell TE. Pink bollworm: Chemical control in Arizona and relationship to infestations, seed damage, and aflatoxin contamination. *J. Econ. Entomol.* 71:440–448, 1978.

Hicks JK, Yu JH, Keller NP, and Adams TH. *Aspergillus* sporulation and mycotoxin production both require inactivation of the FadA G alpha protein-dependent signaling pathway. *EMBO J.* 16:4916–4923, 1997.

Holbrook CC, Wilson DM, and Matheron ME. An update on breeding peanut for resistance to preharvest aflatoxin contamination. Proceedings of the USDA-ARS Aflatoxin Elimination Workshop, Atlanta, GA, p. 3, 1995.

Jacks TJ and Hinojosa O. Superoxide radicals in intact tissues and in dimethyl sulfoxide-based extracts. *Phytochemistry* 33:563–568, 1993.

Jacks TJ, Cotty PJ, and Hinojosa O. Potential of animal myeloperoxidase to protect plants from pathogens. *Biochem. Biophys. Res. Commn.* 178:1202–1204, 1991.

Jacks TJ, Cary JW, Rajasekaran K, Cleveland TE, and van Pée K-H. Transformation of plants with a chloroperoxidase gene to enhance disease resistance. U.S. Patent 6,703,540, 2004.

Jacks TJ, Delucca AJ, and Morris NM. Effects of chloroperoxidase and hydrogen peroxide on the viabilities of *Aspergillus flavus* conidiospores. *Mol. Cell. Biochem.* 195:169–172, 1999.

Kale SP, Cary JW, Bhatnagar D, and Bennett JW. Isolation and characterization of morphological variants of *Aspergillus parasiticus* deficient in secondary metabolite production. *Mycological Res.* 98:645–652, 1994.

Kale SP, Cary JW, Baker C, Walker D, Bhatnagar D, and Bennett JW. Genetic analysis of morphological variants of *Aspergillus parasiticus* deficient in secondary metabolite production. *Mycological Res.* 107:831–840, 2003.

Kato N, Brooks W, and Calvo AM. The expression of sterigmatocystin and penicillin genes in *Aspergillus nidulans* is controlled by *veA*, a gene required for sexual development. *Eukaryot. Cell* 2:1178–1186, 2003.

Keller NP, Calvo A, and Gardner H. Linoleic acid and linoleic acid derivatives regulate *Aspergillus* development and mycotoxin production. Proceedings of the USDA-ARS 1999 Aflatoxin Elimination Workshop, p. 43, 1999.

Keller NP, Turner G, and Bennett JW. Fungal secondary metabolism—from biochemistry to genomics. *Nat. Rev.* 3:937–947, 2005.

Li QS, Lawrence CB, Xing HY, Babbitt RA, Bass WT, Maiti IB, and Everett NP. Enhanced disease resistance conferred by expression of an antimicrobial magainin analog in transgenic tobacco. *Planta* 212:635–639, 2001.

Lozovaya VV, Waranyuwat A, and Widholm JM. α-1–3-glucanse and resistance to *Aspergillus flavus* infection in maize. *Crop Sci.* 38:1255–1260, 1998.

Lynch RE and Wilson DM. Enhanced infection of peanut, *Arachis hypogaea* L. seeds with *Aspergillus flavus* group fungi due to external scarification of peanut pods by the lesser cornstalk borer, *Elasmopalpus lignosellus*, Zeller. *Peanut Sci.* 18:110, 1991.

Mahoney N and Molyneux RJ. Phytochemical Inhibition of aflatoxigenicity in *Aspergillus flavus* by constituents of walnut, *Juglans regia*. *J. Agric. Food Chem.* 52(7):1882–1889, 2004.

Matsushima K, Chang P-K, Yu J, Abe K, Bhatnagar D, and Cleveland, TE. Pretermination in AFLR of *Aspergillus sojae* inhibits aflatoxin biosynthesis. *Appl. Microbiol. Biotechnol.* 55:585–589. 2001.

Maupin LM, Clements MJ, and White DG. Evaluation of the MI82 corn line as a source of resistance to aflatoxin in grain and use of BGYF as a selection tool. *Plant Dis.* 87:1059–1066, 2003.

McGranahan G, Dandekar A, Vail P, Leslie C, Uratsu S, Tebbets S, and Escobar M. Genetic engineering and breeding of walnuts for control of aflatoxin. Proceedings of the USDA-ARS 1999 Aflatoxin Elimination Workshop, p. 63, 1999.

Meins F, Neuhaus J-M, Sperisen C, and Ryals J. The primary structure of plant pathogenesis-related glucanohydrolases and their genes. In: Boller T, Meins F, (Eds.), Genes Involved in *Plant Defense* pp. 245–282, 1992.

Mendum M, McGranahan G, Dandekar A, and Uratsu S. Progress in engineering walnuts for resistance to *Aspergillus flavus*. Proceedings of the USDA-ARS Aflatoxin Elimination Workshop Atlanta, GA, p. 21, 1995.

Menkir A, Brown RL, Bandyopadhyay R, Chen Z-Y, and Cleveland TE. A U.S.A.–Africa collaborative strategy for identifying, characterizing, and developing maize germplasm with resistance to aflatoxin contamination. *Mycopathologia*-Special Issue "Global Perspectives of Fungal Secondary Metabolite Research", Bhatnagar D and Cary JW (Eds.), 162:225–232, 2006.

Meyers DM, O'Brian G, Du WL, Bhatnagar D, and Payne GA. Characterization of *aflJ*, a gene required for conversion of pathway intermediates to aflatoxin. *Appl. Environ. Microbiol.* 64:3713–3717, 1998.

Murray F, Llewellyn D, McFadden H, Last D, Dennis ES, and Peacock WJ. Expression of the *Talaromyces flavus* glucose oxidase gene in cotton and tobacco reduces fungal infection, but is also phytotoxic. *Mol. Breed.* 5:219–232, 1999.

Niu C, Deng X-Y, Hazra S, Chu Y, and Ozias-Akins P. Introduction of antifungal genes into peanut. Proceedings of the USDA-ARS 17th Aflatoxin Elimination Workshop, p. 33, 2004.

O'Brian GR, Fakhoury AM, and Payne GA. Identification of genes differentially expressed during aflatoxin biosynthesis in *Aspergillus flavus* and *Aspergillus parasiticus*. *Fungal Genet. Biol.* 39:118–127, 2003.

Orum TV, Bigelow DM, Nelson MR, Howell DR, and Cotty PJ. Spatial and temporal patterns of *Aspergillus flavus* strain composition and propagule density in Yuma County, Arizona, soils. *Plant Dis.* 81:911–916, 1997.

Ozias-Akins P, Gill R, Yang H, and Lynch R. Genetic engineering of peanut: Progress with Bt, peroxidase, peptidyl MIM D4E1, and lipoxygenase. Proceedings of the USDA-ARS 1999 Aflatoxin Elimination Workshop, pp. 69–70, 1999.

Payne GA. Aflatoxin in maize. *Crit. Rev. Plant Sci.* 10:423–440, 1992.

Payne GA. Process of contamination by aflatoxin-producing fungi and their impact on crops. In: Sinha KK and Bhatnagar D (Eds.), *Mycotoxins in Agriculture and Food Safety*, Marcel Dekker, New York, pp. 279–306, 1998.

Payne GA and Brown MP. Genetics and physiology of aflatoxin biosynthesis. *Annu. Rev. Phytopathol.* 36:329–362, 1998.

Payne GA, Nystorm GJ, Bhatnagar D, Cleveland TE, and Woloshuk CP. Cloning of the *afl-2* gene involved in aflatoxin biosynthesis from *Aspergillus flavus*. *Appl. Environ. Microbiol.* 59:156–162, 1993.

Payne GA, Nierman WC, Wortman JR, Pritchard BL, Brown D, Dean RA, Bhatnagar D, Cleveland TE, Machida M, and Yu J. Whole genome comparison of *Aspergillus flavus* and *A. oryzae*. *Med. Mycol.* 44 (Suppl. 9–11):1–3, 2006.

Pennington SR, Wilkins MR, Hochstrasser DF, and Dunn MJ. Proteome analysis: From protein characterization to biological function. *Trends Cell Biol.* 7:168–173, 1997.

Price MS, Conners SB, Tachdjian S, Kelly RM, and Payne GA. Aflatoxin conductive and non-conducive growth conditions reveal new gene associations with aflatoxin production. *Fungal Genet. Biol.* 42:506–518, 2005.

Punja ZK. Genetic engineering of plants to enhance resistance to fungal pathogens. In: Punja ZK (Ed.), *Fungal Disease Resistance in Plants: Biochemistry, Molecular Biology, and Genetic Engineering*, Food Products Press, NY, pp. 207–258, 2004.

Rajasekaran, K. *Agrobacterium*-mediated genetic transformation of cotton. In: Curtis, IS (Ed.), *Transgenic Crops of the World—Essential Protocols*. Springer-Verlag, Berlin, pp. 243–254, 2004.

Rajasekaran K, Cary JW, Jacks TJ, Stromberg K, and Cleveland TE. Inhibition of fungal growth *in planta* and *in vitro* by transgenic tobacco expressing a bacterial nonheme chloroperoxidase gene, *Plant Cell Rep.* 19:333–338, 2000.

Rajasekaran K, Stromberg K, Cary JW, and Cleveland TE. Broad-spectrum antimicrobial activity *in vitro* of the synthetic peptide D4E1. *J. Agric. Food Chem.* 49(6):2799–2803, 2001.

Rajasekaran K, Cary JW, Jacks TJ, and Cleveland TE. Genetic engineering for resistance to phytopathogens. In: Rajasekaran K, Jacks TJ, Finley JW (Eds.), *Crop Biotechnol.* American Chemical Society Symposium Series No. 829. Washington, DC: American Chemical Society. pp. 97–117, 2002.

Rajasekaran K, Bhatnagar D, Brown RL, Chen Z-Y, Cary, JW, and Cleveland TE. Enhancing food safety: Prevention of preharvest aflatoxin contamination.

In: Ramasamy C, Ramanathan S, and Dhakshinamoorthy M (Eds.), Perspectives of Agricultural Research and Development, Tamil Nadu Agricultural University Centennial Issue, Coimbatore, India, pp. 434–467, 2005a.

Rajasekaran K, Cary JW, Jaynes JM, and Cleveland TE. Disease resistance conferred by the expression of a gene encoding a synthetic peptide in transgenic cotton, *Gossypium hirsutum* L. plants. *Plant Biotechnol. J.* 3:545–554, 2005b.

Rajasekaran K, Ulloa M, Hutmacher R, Cary JW, and Cleveland, TE. Disease resistance in transgenic cottons. Proceedings of 2006 Beltwide Cotton Conferences. National Cotton Council, Memphis, TN, 2006.

Rao AG. Antimicrobial peptides, *Mol. Plant-Microbe Interact.* 8:6–13, 1995.

Reddy KV, Yedery RD, and Aranha C. Antimicrobial peptides: Premises and promises. *Int. J. Antimicrob. Agents* 24:536–547, 2004.

Richard J and Payne GA. Mycotoxins: Risk in plant, animal, and human Systems. CAST Report 139. p. 199, 2003.

Russell TE. Aflatoxins in cottonseed. Publication Q422, University of Arizona, Cooperative Extension Service, Tucson, AZ, 1980.

Ryan CA. Protease inhibitors in plants: Genes for improving defenses against insects and pathogens. *Annu. Rev. Phytopathol.* 28:425–449, 1990.

Shimizu K and Keller NP. Genetic involvement of cAMP-dependent protein kinase in a G protein signaling pathway regulating morphological and chemical transitions in *Aspergillus nidulans. Genetics* 157:591–600, 2001.

Shimizu K, Hicks J, Huang T-P, and Keller NP. Pka, Ras and RGS protein interactions regulate activity of *AflR*, a Zn(II).2Cys6 transcription factor in *Aspergillus nidulans. Genetics* 165:1095–1104, 2003.

Simmonds J, Cass L, and Lachance J. Genetic transformation of Ontario maize inbreds. Proceedings of the Joint Meeting of the Fiftieth Annual Southern Corn Improvement Conference and the Fifty-Third Annual Northeastern Corn Improvement Conference. Blacksburg, VA, p. 10, 1998.

Singh NK, Nelson DE, Kuhn D, Hasegawa PM, and Bressan RA. Molecular cloning of osmotin and regulation of its expression by ABA and adaption to low water potential. *Plant. Physiol.* 90:1096–1101, 1989.

Thomma BPHJ, Cammue BPA, and Thevissen K. Plant defensins. *Planta.* 216:193–202, 2002.

Tilburn J, Sarkar S, Widdick DA, Espeso EA, Orejas M, Mungroo J, Penalva MA, and Arst HN, Jr. The *Aspergillus* PacC zinc finger transcription factor mediates regulation of both acid- and alkaline-expressed genes by ambient pH. *EMBO J.* 14:779–790, 1995.

Toubart P, Desiderio A, Salvi G, Cervone F, Daroda L, DeLorenzo G, Bergmann C, Darvill AG, and Albersheim P. Cloning and characterization of the gene encoding the endopolygalacturonase-inhibiting protein (PGIP) of *Phaseolus vulgaris* L. *Plant J.* 2:367–373, 1992.

van Egmond HP. Natural toxins: Risks, regulations and the analytical situation in Europe. *Anal. Bioanal. Chem.* 378:1152–1160, 2004.

Walker RD and White DG. Inheritance of resistance to *Aspergillus* ear rot and aflatoxin production of corn from CI2. *Plant Dis.* 85:322–327, 2001.

Weissinger A, Liu Y-S, Scanlon S, Murray J, Cleveland TE, Jaynes J, Mirkov E, and Moonan F. Transformation of peanut with the defensive peptidyl MIM D5C. Proceedings of the USDA-ARS Aflatoxin Elimination Workshop, pp. 66–68, 1999.

Weissinger A, Wu M, and Cleveland TE. Expression in transgenic peanut of maize RIP 1, a protein with activity against *Aspergillus* spp. Proceedings of the USDA-ARS Aflatoxin Elimination Workshop, p. 100, 2003.

White DG, Rocheford TR, Kaufman B, and Hamblin AM. Chromosome regions associated with resistance to *Aspergillus flavus* and inhibition of aflatoxin production in maize. Proceedings of the USDA-ARS Aflatoxin Elimination Workshop, p. 8, 1995a.

White D, Rocheford TR, Kaufman B, and Hamblin AM. Further genetic studies and progress on resistance to aflatoxin production in corn. Proceedings of the USDA-ARS Aflatoxin Elimination Workshop, p. 7, 1995b.

White DG, Rocheford TR, Naidoo G, Paul C, Hamblin AM, and Forbes AM. Inheritance of molecular markers associated with, and breeding for resistance to *Aspergillus* ear rot and aflatoxin production in corn using Tex6. Proceedings of the USDA-ARS Aflatoxin Elimination Workshop, pp. 4–6, 1998.

White DG, Rocheford TR, Naidoo G, Paul C, Rozzi RD, Severns DE, and Forbes AM. Inheritance of molecular markers associated with and breeding for resistance to *Aspergillus* ear rot and aflatoxin production in corn. Proceedings of the USDA-ARS Aflatoxin Elimination Workshop, pp. 7–8, 1999.

Wild CP and Turner PC. The toxicology of aflatoxins as a basis for public health decisions. *Mutagenesis* 17:471–481, 2002.

Wilkins MR, Pasquali C, Appel RD, Ou K, Golaz O, Sanchez JC, Yan JX, Gooley AA, Hughes G, Humphrey-Smith I, Williams KL, and Hochstrasser DF. From proteins to proteomes: Large-scale protein identification by two-dimensional electrophoresis and amino acid analysis. *Biotechnology* 14:61–65, 1996.

Wilkins TA, Rajasekaran K, and Anderson DM. Cotton Biotechnology. *Crit. Rev. Plant Sci.* 19(6):511–550, 2000.

Wilkinson JR, Yu J, Bland JM, Nierman WC, Bhatnagar D, and Cleveland TE. Amino acid supplementation reveals differential regulation of aflatoxin biosynthesis in *Aspergillus flavus* NRRL 3357 and *Aspergillus parasiticus* SRRC 143. *Appl. Microbiol. Biotechnol.* 2007 (in press).

Wolffram C, van Pee K-H, and Lingens F. Cloning and high-level expression of a chloroperoxidase gene from *Pseudomonas pyrrocinia*. *FEBS Lett.* 238:325–328, 1988.

Wu F. Mycotoxin risk assessment for the purpose of setting international regulatory standards. *Environ. Sci. Technol.* 38:4049–4055, 2004.

Wu G, Short BJ, Lawrence EB, Levine EB, Fitzsimmons KC, and Shah DM. Disease resistance conferred by expression of a gene encoding H_2O_2-generating glucose oxidase in transgenic potato plants. *Plant Cell* 7:1357–1368, 1995.

Yu J, Whitelaw CA, Nierman WC, Bhatnagar D, and Cleveland TE. *Aspergillus flavus* expressed sequence tags for identification of genes with putative roles in aflatoxin contamination of crops. *FEMS Microbiol. Lett.* 237:333–340, 2004.

Yu J, Ronning CM, Wilkinson JR, Campbell BC, Payne GA, Bhatnagar D, Cleveland TE, and Nierman WC. Gene profiling for studying the mechanism of aflatoxin biosynthesis in *Aspergillus flavus* and *A. parasiticus*. *Food Add. Contam.* 2007 (in press).

Yu J-H and Keller, N. Regulation of secondary metabolism in filamentous fungi. *Ann. Rev. Phytopathol.* 43:437–458, 2005.

Zasloff M. Magainins, a class of antimicrobial peptides from *Xenopus* skin: Isolation, characterization of two active forms, and partial cDNA sequence of a precursor, *Proc. Natl. Acad. Sci. U.S.A.* 84:5449–5453, 1987.

Zipf AE, and Rajasekaran K. Ecological impact of Bt cotton. *J. New Seeds* 5(2/3):115–135, 2003.

Section IV

Microbial Food Contamination and International Trade

15

Mad Cow Disease and International Trade

Robert A. LaBudde and Edward V. LaBudde

CONTENTS

15.1 Introduction

Transmissible spongiform encephalopathies (TSEs) have become a house-hold word over the last 15 years, and have destroyed major parts of the beef market throughout the world. Starting with "scrapie" or OSE (ovine spongiform encephalopathy) in sheep, discovered some 200 years ago in the United Kingdom, successively CJD in humans (Creutzfeldt–Jakob disease), TME in minks (transmissible mink encephalopathy), BSE in cattle (bovine spongiform encephalopathy or mad cow disease) and CWD in deer and elk (chronic wasting disease) have been discovered.

The literature surrounding these new diseases is now extensive, with good current reviews available online.[1–3] Consequently, a full citation of the literature will not be presented, only a few selected references which is topically relevant to the discussion.

15.1.1 Scrapie

In the eighteenth century, Scottish shepherds noticed an unusual nervous system disease they labeled scrapie, as the sheep frequently rubbed themselves against fences, trees, or other objects as their nerves generated phantom itching feelings. The disease was invariably fatal, and has been found to be horizontally transmissible via placenta and other mechanisms. For the last 50 years, scrapie-infected flocks have consequently been eradicated whenever they have been found, but with little effect or control. Scrapie is endemic to most sheep-farming countries (including the United States), except for isolated island countries such as New Zealand and Australia, being spread by the transport of live animals.

15.1.2 BSE

In 1986, a United Kingdom veterinarian reported a cow with suspicious central nervous system (CNS) symptoms to the Weybridge veterinary laboratory for investigation.[4] The animal was found to be infected with a new TSE, dubbed BSE for "bovine spongiform encephalopathy". Luckily, the United Kingdom had funded a substantial research program into scrapie after World War II, so that the disease was easily recognized as a spongiform encephalopathy by investigators.

Subsequent epidemiological modeling[5,6] has indicated that the index case probably occurred in the late 1970s, but amplification was required to raise the level of incidence to the point that veterinarians would encounter a symptomatic case, as they did in 1986. The cause of the index case has never been discovered, with hypotheses ranging from a hidden variant of scrapie in sheep to imported African or Indian meat-and-bone meal (MBM) to random mutations ("Gibbs hypothesis" originated by the late Clarence Gibbs of the United States National Institutes of Health). It has been conjectured that a modest change in the rendering methods in the United Kingdom in 1981 may have played a role in increasing amplification.

Infectivity amplification and feedback were easy to come by in the United Kingdom, as the industry was feeding 10% or more MBM back to young cattle, keeping dairy cattle to elderly ages and recycling CNS tissue in the process. BSE was found transmissible orally, with as little as 1 g of CNS tissue in an oral one-time dose giving rise to a near certainty of disease.[5] Newer estimates place the oral ID50 as low as 0.1 g down to 1 mg.[7] One animal's brain and spinal cord are therefore theoretically capable of infecting hundreds or thousands of others when fed back through MBM to other cattle.

In July 1988, a ruminant-ruminant feed ban was enacted to eliminate amplification via feedback in rendering. This crucial step was the key to controlling BSE, but its result was not felt for some 5 years, approximately the mean incubation and distributional lag time for the disease. In 1992–1993, at the peak of the epizootic in the United Kingdom, there were more than 30,000 BSE cases per year discovered by clinical referral and laboratory confirmation in a total cattle population of about 10 million.[4] As an example of the pervasiveness of the disease, the Isle of Guernsey incidence rate was an amazing 33% of adult animals per year in 1993.[4,8]

Unfortunately, the United Kingdom exported throughout the world the contaminated MBM they did not allow to be fed to their own cattle. BSE cases started appearing in other countries in the EU, starting with France and Ireland and progressing to almost all other countries in Europe.

The EU imposed a feed ban in 1997, but most countries there are still in the midst of expanding epizootics. The political effect of country after country discovering cases of BSE after years of denial has demolished confidence in government and industry and forced the institution of 100% surveillance by biochemical testing of all adult animals slaughtered. In 2002, more than 10 million such animals were tested with some 2,000 positives found.[9] Subsequently, worldwide case rates have been dropping geometrically by 50% per year, with FAO reporting only 474 cases in 2005.

As of May 2006, BSE affected countries are: Austria, Belgium, Canada, Czech Republic, Denmark, Finland, France, Germany, Greece, Ireland, Israel, Italy, Japan, Liechtenstein, Luxembourg, Netherlands, Poland, Portugal, Slovakia, Slovenia, Spain, Sweden, Switzerland, United Kingdom, and the United States.

15.1.3 Variant Creutzfeldt–Jakob Disease

Complicating the situation was the discovery that BSE was apparently implicated in a new form of human Creutzfeldt–Jakob disease (CJD), dubbed vCJD for variant-CJD, which affects primarily young adults and has claimed more than 190 (160 in the United Kingdom) lives to date.[10] The reason for the connection is still not clear, but is presumed to be related to consumption of beef CNS tissue or medical injections of bovine-based vaccines or other pharmaceuticals. Estimates of the human oral ID50 from BSE-contaminated tissues range up to 2 or 3 g, with the so-called cow-to-human species barrier increasing resistance by 25–1000 times.[7]

TSEs turn the brain to "Swiss cheese" by creating "holes" of abnormal morphology (amyloidal plaque). As the disease progresses, more and more brain and CNS tissue are affected. Initial symptoms involve tremors and twitching. Later symptoms include blindness and loss of memory. Death follows.

The most familiar spongiform encephalopathy is Alzheimer's disease (Creutzfeldt and Jakob worked at Alzheimer's institute for brain diseases). It is conjectured that up to 5%–10% of Alzheimer's disease cases may be in reality misdiagnosed CJD cases.

TSEs are believed to be caused, or at least propagated, by misconformed proteins called prions, which somehow "trick" properly conformed proteins to switch to the abnormal conformation. The conversion results in the amyloidal plaque that gives rise to the "spongy" morphology of the brain tissue. How this mechanism works, and whether it is the sole answer to infectivity, is still not well-understood and is the subject of Nobel prizes and significant current research. The amount of prions in the body increases with age as normal prion protein is slowly converted to the pathological form.

TSEs therefore affect primarily older animals, as it takes significant time to amplify prions to a titer capable of generating clinical symptoms. CJD, the TSE of humans, also primarily affects the elderly.

A nasty property of the prion agent is that the misconformed protein is not as susceptible to enzymatic proteolysis (as in digestion) and is not as easily denatured by heat (as in rendering) or by chemicals (as in sanitation), although some deactivation does occur. Consequently prions can survive common disinfection techniques. Many cases of CJD in humans have been caused by reuse of supposedly clean and sterile neurosurgical instruments.

The causal connection between BSE and vCJD is hypothecated primarily upon the clinical and histopathological symptoms of presentation, incubation period, and molecular fragment electrophoresis patterns.[11] However, the number of strains of spongiform encephalopathies so far discovered is small, and may remain so. It is possible that a match in strains between species is not as highly improbable as originally thought, and multiple strains (i.e., molecular conformations of the prion agent) with different virulence factors may be present in every species population.

Such multiple strains with similarities to human CJD or vCJD strains have been found recently in both sheep and cattle,[12–15] and the latest two confirmed cases of BSE in the United States had an atypical histopathological presentation and appear similar, but not identical, to atypical strains discovered in France, Sweden, and Poland.

The export by the United Kingdom to 14 countries in the EU, Asia, and South America of human blood products possibly tainted by vCJD donors during the 1990s has extended the vCJD problem to countries other than those directly impacted by BSE.

15.1.4 North America

Following the United Kingdom and EU experiences with BSE, the United States and Canada imposed a ruminant-ruminant feed ban in 1997 in order to break the feedback loop in the event of introduction of BSE to North America. This ban was later extended to mammalian-ruminant feedback, although "mammals" for this purpose apparently does not include swine and horse.[16] Until 2003, the only BSE cases found in North America were traced to importation from the United Kingdom, and the animals had been controlled by quarantine.

However, at the end of January 2003, a 6-year-old cow sent for slaughter at a province-licensed packer in Alberta was found to exhibit unusual and possibly CNS-based symptoms. The cow was a "downer" (i.e., could not stand) and was wasted. The animal was condemned and the brain was forwarded to the provincial veterinary laboratory for TSE testing, with a presumptive diagnosis of pneumonia.

Because of the raging CWD (chronic wasting disease in deer and elk, see below) epizootic (5000+ samples per year in Alberta), the laboratory back-shelved the suspect animal's brain in favor of meeting CWD test schedules. It was not until May 16 that the sample was tested and found positive for BSE. The diagnosis was confirmed again at CFIA and finally at the United Kingdom Weybridge laboratory on May 20. So after a delay of nearly 4 months, Canada had discovered its first native case of BSE.

Immediately reactions occurred, affecting exports of Canadian beef and cattle. The United States closed its borders to the substantial trade (some 1.7 million live cattle per year) and other countries in the Far East stopped all imports. Within days the Canadian beef industry had lost major markets.

In the month following the announcement of the BSE case, some 2700 cohort animals had been eradicated and tested. All were found negative.

No cause has been found for the first Canadian BSE case, but the presumption is that the age of the animal is consistent with ingestion of contaminated MBM before the feed ban of 1997 (or rather its effective implementation in 1998), or possibly from feed ingredients imported from the United Kingdom or EU. (Three of the so far Canadian-traceable confirmed BSE cases have since been traced back to a common source of feed.)

Animal raisers and packers in Canada were angry with the United States and other countries for keeping their borders closed to Canadian animals and beef. Obviously such moves benefited the domestic beef industries at the expense of Canada. Canadians felt that the uniformly negative results on the 2700 eradication-cohort animals proved that the observed case was an isolated event, and no scientific grounds existed for keeping the borders closed.

Alberta lobbyists even went to the extent of enlisting U.S. Vice-President Cheney's aid in forcing the USDA to remove the import bans. The political consequences and nontariff trade-barriers resulting from the Canadian BSE case extended to the hotly debated "country-of-origin-labeling" law and United States–Japan trade. (The politics of BSE is discussed further in Section 15.5.)

As of May 2006, a total of 100,000 at-risk cattle have been tested for BSE in Canada, with five cases of BSE so far discovered. Luckily, all of the cases found have involved animals at least 6-years old, which still allows some confidence in the original 1997, and later reinforced, ruminant feed ban.

A comparable calamity to that experienced by Canada occurred in the United States on December 23, 2003, when USDA Secretary Veneman announced the discovery of the first U.S. BSE case from a farm in Washington State. The cow slaughtered was confirmed as the first U.S. BSE-positive animal. Luckily the specified risk material (SRM) of the cow was removed at slaughter because it was selected for evaluation by the USDA veterinarian. All meat from the carcass was subsequently recalled, and all cohort animals and offspring were culled for eradication and testing.

By early January the cow was identified definitively by DNA testing and ID tag tracking as a 6½-year-old animal shipped from a farm in Alberta, Canada.

Within days of the BSE-positive cow's discovery, U.S. meat exports to Asia disappeared and cattle futures plummeted by 30%. Domestic consumption was however unchanged, showing consumers believed the problem confined to the Northwest states close to the Canadian border.

USDA's Animal and Plant Health Inspection Service (APHIS) and Food Safety Inspection Service (FSIS) also announced a new surveillance plan with time-limited testing of primarily suspect (clinical symptoms) and risk (suspicious circumstances) animals over the next 2 years. Unfortunately, FSIS's changes meant that downer (non-ambulatory) cattle would no longer be readily available for selection for BSE testing. With the new rules, these animals would likely be killed and buried on-farm or sent directly to rendering facilities. SRM is currently only defined in the United States for animals 30 months and older: Skulls, brains, spinal cords, eyes, etc. from cattle younger than 30 months and not disabled can still be used for human food in the United States.

Subsequent discovery of two other cases of BSE in Canada in January 2005 further solidified official opinion that the problem of BSE was restricted to Canada, and not to the United States.

From January 2004 to July 2005, more than 400,000 high-risk animals (viz., non-ambulatory, central nervous system disorder suspect, wasted or injured, dead) were tested for BSE using principally the very sensitive Bio-Rad rapid test kit (ELISA-based) in duplicate. During that time, only three presumptive positive cases (euphemistically renamed "inconclusive" by USDA) were found. Subsequent retesting by immunohistochemistry (IHC, a traditional low-sensitivity staining test dubbed by USDA as the "Gold Standard") found all three results as "unconfirmed." Attempts by consumer activists to either get the presumptive positive samples tested by independent laboratories (e.g., Weybridge in the United Kingdom) or by the more commonly used and more sensitive Western blot method proved fruitless.

The American beef supply thus appeared safe from the BSE that plagued its northern neighbor, and the disease (inexplicably) did not appear to cross the border with the tens of millions of Canadian live cattle that had been processed here over the last decade. Unfortunately, this rosy scenario promulgated by USDA and the beef industry was not in accord with scientific expectations.

Firstly, it was extremely unlikely that the Canadian situation would be separable from that of the United States, given the historical strong intermixing of the two national herds. Secondly, even if this were so, more Canadian-derived cases of BSE in the United States would be expected, just as had been found in Canada itself (which was thus far responsible for four cases of BSE in a national herd one-tenth the size of the American one). Thirdly, the USDA changes in slaughtering regulations guaranteed that high-risk animals were of little value to renderers, who now demanded payment for processing instead of paying for the animals. Consequently, ranchers now had little incentive to pass the animals on to rendering. In the words of the Alberta Premier Ralph Klein on the subject of high-risk animal disposal, ranchers should "shoot, shovel, and shut up" when confronted with a high-risk animal. This would guarantee that a considerable proportion of the highest risk animals might, in fact, never be sampled and tested.

Finally, USDA was staunchly opposed to any independent testing for BSE (in stark contrast to all other pathogen testing performed in the food industry for other diseases). Invoking a 1913 law called the Virus Serum Toxin Act, USDA claimed sole authority over how and when cattle may be tested, and announced testing for BSE by any unapproved laboratory would be illegal.

Mishandling of a high-risk carcass in Texas in 2004 led to an investigation of USDA's surveillance program by its inspector general, Phyllis Fung. Her OIG investigation uncovered a number of irregularities, including the fact that the presumptive positive of November 2004 had actually tested positive by another, experimental test, but USDA had not disclosed this to the public or taken further confirmation steps other than the usual IHC, which came back negative.

General Fung directed that USDA retest the three presumptive positive samples by the real gold standard, the Western Blot test. The November 2004 sample came back positive (quickly dubbed by USDA as a "weak positive" in the new "BSE-Speak"). The sample was then sent off to Weybridge in the United Kingdom, where it was indeed confirmed as a BSE-positive.

Other problems with USDA's testing protocols also surfaced, including mishandling and mismarking of samples and the very interesting fact that Weybridge apparently had no difficulty in obtaining an IHC-positive result, as well as Western Blot, on the submitted sample.

The animal involved in the November 2004 BSE-confirmed sample was a southern Texas bred, born, and raised Brahmin cow. The animal was some 12-years old when sent to slaughtering, and she was known never to have visited Canada or even congregated with Canadian cattle. It was also extremely fortuitous that she was actually tested for BSE. The cow had at times some difficulties in standing, but did so during most of her trip to the abattoir. Fortunately for consumers, she died before reaching the slaughterhouse and was then transferred to a renderer, where she was flagged for sampling. This BSE-confirmed positive case could not be attributed to Canada.

On March 15, 2006, a second native-born case of BSE was confirmed for a 10-year-old cow in Alabama. As a testament to the political gridlock still present on this issue in the United States, no trace back of the cow's origin or herd was possible. Its age was estimated from dentition.

Astonishingly, until 2006, FDA policy still allowed high-risk animals to be rendered into swine feed.

As of May 2006, there have been three (two native-born, one Canadian) confirmed cases of BSE in the United States, and two unconfirmed or inconclusive cases. Given the method of rapid testing used by USDA (i.e., two successive Bio-Rad tests), the inconclusive cases should also be taken seriously as indications of incidence in the approximately 450,000 animals in the at-risk category in the United States.

15.1.5 Transmissible Mink Encephalopathy

More than 20 years ago, Wisconsin mink farms were decimated by transmissible mink encephalopathy (TME) in repeated epizootics for which the root cause was never discovered. The chief investigator, Richard Marsh, conjectured that scrapie-infected sheep initiated the outbreaks,[17] but this does not appear to fit the high attack rates observed. A perhaps more logical explanation would have been mink-to-mink feeding, but this activity was uniformly denied by the mink ranchers involved.

No more outbreaks have occurred since, and the mink industry is, in any event, now near extinct in the United States.

15.1.6 Chronic Wasting Disease

In 1967, at a capture-and-release research station in Fort Collins, Colorado, wildlife researchers found that young deer were dying from an unknown "wasting" disease. By 1978, the new disease had been dubbed CWD for "chronic wasting disease" and had been found to be a TSE of cervids. As time has passed, CWD has been found to be an endemic disease of mule deer, white-tailed deer, and elk in Colorado and Wyoming. Incidence is as high as 15% of deer in some areas.

Unfortunately, a burgeoning industry in elk antlers for export to the Far East and game farms for hunting created a substantial and unregulated trade in breeding stock for elks and deer that moved animals freely between the states and between the United States and Canada. As a consequence, CWD has spread to new geographical areas over the last few years, now being firmly entrenched in places such as Alberta, Saskatchewan, Colorado, Wyoming, Nebraska, Oklahoma, Minnesota, and Wisconsin. States as far east as Pennsylvania and Virginia are now surveilling deer herds for CWD.

CWD has a horizontal mode of transmission, conjectured to be similar to that of scrapie. It apparently can cross double-fenced enclosures and transmit by casual contact between animals. The Fort Collins research facility has removed the topsoil from penned areas, but new animals still mysteriously contract CWD when introduced into the area. The feces and saliva from infected deer are conjectured to contain the associated prion agent.[18]

As CWD has decimated the export trade for elk antlers, impoverished ranchers have released animals into the wild, further compounding the spread of the disease.

The number of cases of CWD occurring annually is not apparently available to the public at the current time, but must number in the tens of thousands or more in a national cervid herd of perhaps 30 million in the United States alone. The CWD epizootic currently taking place in North America rivals or exceeds the size of the historical BSE epizootics in the United Kingdom and EU.

Except for hunters and ranchers, few people seem concerned about this raging epizootic of CWD. Governmental budgets for coping with the disease do not exceed $30 million in total for both the United States and Canada combined. Only within the last couple of years have regulations been promulgated affecting the interstate transfer of possibly diseased animals.

As of May 2006, states where CWD has been found in deer or elk include Colorado, Illinois, Minnesota, Montana, Nebraska, New Mexico, New York, Oklahoma, South Dakota, Utah, Wisconsin, West Virginia, and Wyoming. CWD has also been found in Alberta and Saskatchewan, Canada. Typical incidence in random sampling of infected areas is 0.1%–15% positive.

15.2 Simple Semiempirical Model of the United Kingdom Epizootic

15.2.1 United Kingdom Epizootic and Passive Surveillance

The EU countries report results of extensive surveillance testing carried out for BSE in four different categories: (1) animals reported as BSE clinical suspects having central nervous system symptoms; (2) suspicious death and other risk animals—"risk" being defined as fallen stock, emergency slaughtered animals, and sick at inspection; (3) for public protection, all animals at normal slaughter over 24 months of age (or 30 months in the United Kingdom); and (4) cohort animals killed as a result of BSE eradication programs.[9] Although part of the EU, until 2000 the United Kingdom selected animals for testing based solely upon clinical symptoms (suspect) or circumstance (risk).

As recommended by the Office International des Epizooties (OIE),[19] BSE-free (negligible risk) and low-risk (controlled risk) countries may satisfactorily perform testing only on suspect and risk animals.

The originating UK BSE epizootic was extremely large-scale, and has spanned nearly two decades to date. About 180,000 BSE cases have been confirmed in the United Kingdom alone. Figure 15.1 shows the annual case rate for BSE in the United Kingdom based upon only suspect and risk categories of animals. All cases were confirmed by laboratory testing.

The general pattern of the case rate data for the United Kingdom shows a deceptively Gaussian or Lorentzian shape. An exponential rise occurs from the first cases found in 1986 to a relatively sharp peak in 1992–1993. After that an exponential decline in cases occurs. The curve is neither symmetrical nor Gaussian. The United Kingdom imposed a feed ban in July 1988, which led to the eventual peaking and decline of the case rate curve. The delay between the imposition of the ban and the peak measures the mean effect of the disease incubation period and the delays associated with implementation of the ban and the distribution of feed throughout the country.

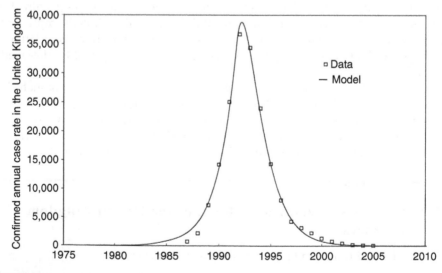

FIGURE 15.1
Annual confirmed case rate for UK BSE epizootic and fitted control system model results.

The mechanism of the BSE epizootic in the United Kingdom has been well-studied by detailed models.[5,6] However, these highly detailed and complex models obscure the basic simplicity of the epizootic phenomenon, and create the illusion that deep understanding of the details of each and every low-level issue must occur before the epizootic case rate can be understood. On the contrary, the epizootic case rate curve can be easily modeled with a very limited understanding of the growth and transmission process of the disease in the host population.

In what follows, the simplest possible mathematical model for the epizootic case rate will be developed, based only on phenomenological properties of the outbreak and top-level control engineering principles associated with a feedback system. The predicted case rate form of the modeling is nearly numerical identical to that of the complex and detailed Andersen model,[5] at least so far as the annual data curve is concerned. (The Andersen model also predicts within-year seasonality and other detail features.)

This method of modeling and analyzing case rate curves in time may be applicable and useful in evaluating and understanding future epidemics and epizootics.

15.2.2 Control Engineering Model

A popular method of applying a control engineering approach to system modeling is to start with a transfer function block diagram.[20] The block diagram expresses the elements of the model as blocks with the frequency response of the element and the interrelations appearing as lines. This approach is very useful at visualizing feedback systems and has been popular with engineers for many years.

In constructing a model for the BSE epidemic we seek the simplest (lowest order) model that will be capable of capturing the physical processes of the spread of the disease. A simple model would contain the following:

1. An integrator to accumulate the total population of sick cattle
2. A switch to model the breaking of the feedback loop by the feed ban
3. A pole to model the capacity of the feed distribution system
4. A gain term to model the number of animals the feed can contaminate
5. A time delay to model the incubation and process transport delays
6. A pole to model the variation in the appearance of sick cattle

If any of these system elements are missing, the United Kingdom epizootic cannot be successfully modeled. A block diagram of this model is shown in Figure 15.2.

The *transfer function* is the ratio of output to input defined as $\frac{\text{Output}}{\text{Input}} = \text{T.F.}$

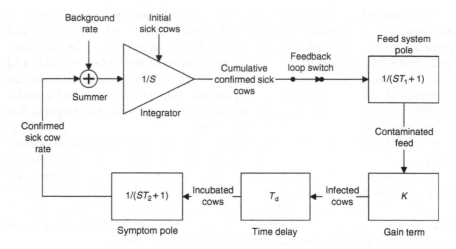

FIGURE 15.2
Block diagram for control system model of the BSE epizootic.

The Laplace variable S is defined as $S = j\omega$, where j is $\sqrt{-1}$ and ω is the time frequency. (This substitution for S converts the Laplace transform of the transfer function into the Fourier transform version.)
A description of each element of the model follows below:

1. *Integrator*: The transfer function is $\frac{\text{Output}}{\text{Input}} = \frac{1}{S}$. The integrator serves as an accumulator of the rate of new sick animals in order to arrive at the total population of sick animals. The integrator has an initial condition that represents the total number of sick cattle at a given point in time. We assume that a single animal entered the system at the start of the epizootic for our initial estimate. We assume an arbitrary provisional initial start date of 15 years prior to the date of the first confirmed case (i.e., 1971) in order to be sure of predating the actual initiating inoculum.

2. *Switch*: The transfer function is $\frac{\text{Output}}{\text{Input}} = 1$ before ban and 0 after ban. The switch serves as a device to open the feedback loop imposed by the feed ban of 1988. We assume the switch is opened in July of 1988.

3. *Feed system pole*: The transfer function is $\frac{\text{Output}}{\text{Input}} = \frac{1}{ST_1 + 1}$. The pole represents the capacitive response of the feed system. The time constant T_1 is interpreted as the time required to fill or deplete the feed system to a level of $1 - 1/e = 63.2\%$ of its capacity. A reasonable starting assumption for this parameter is about 1 year.

4. *Gain*: The transfer function is $\frac{\text{Output}}{\text{Input}} = K$. This gain term represents the number of animals that each sick animal can infect through the feed system (i.e., amplification factor). An upper limit of the gain

can be estimated by assuming a single oral dose of 0.1 g will have a reasonable probability of causing infection. The total weight of infectious material in the cow is about 1000 g and assuming that about 10% of all MBM is fed to other cattle, an upper limit of the gain might be about 1000. A more reasonable value might be two orders of magnitude less, say 10–15, if accounting is made for the expected reduction in infectivity from the rendering process and the low percentage of the feed arriving at the right place and time (viz., weaner calves) for effect.

5. *Time delay*: The transfer function is $\frac{\text{Output}}{\text{Input}} = e^{-ST_d}$. The time delay represents the mean value of all process transport delays in the overall feedback loop, including incubation, processing, and distribution. A starting assumption for this value can be estimated by knowing that animals have a mean incubation period of about 5 years. The mean incubation period includes the sick animal symptom pole. Given an assumption that the pole is about 2 years, the associated time delay would then be about 3 years for incubation. Assuming an additional delay of 6 months for the processing and distribution results in an initial starting estimate of 3.5 years.

6. *Sick animal symptoms pole*: The transfer function is $\frac{\text{Output}}{\text{Input}} = \frac{1}{ST_2+1}$. The pole represents the time required for 63.2% of infected animals to exhibit symptoms after the incubation period. A reasonable estimate of this may be about 2 years.

15.2.3 Results

Numerical results from the model can be achieved in a variety of ways. We used a time domain numerical simulation of the inverse Laplace transform (i.e., the governing ordinary differential equations plus initial conditions) of the model similar to other computer tools.[21] The model was built into a Microsoft Excel workbook so that the add-in Solver (nonlinear optimizer) feature could be used to automatically generate a (nonlinear) least squares fit to actual confirmed annual case rate data. Except for the opening of the feedback loop due to the feed ban, all parameters were held constant during the time simulation.

The latest passive surveillance United Kingdom-confirmed case rate data was obtained from Ref. [22] for the period July 1988–2005.

The initial values of the parameters were determined by a preliminary ad hoc simulation, which led to a reasonable fit to the data. The Solver optimizer function was then used to minimize the mean squared deviations from the data for a variety of values of "Year of start" from 1970 to 1977. It should be noted that the model as posed contains a numerical degeneracy associated with the trade-off of the "Year of start" and "Initial infected cattle" (inoculum). A near equivalency exists for early years with low inoculum and later years

TABLE 15.1

Model Simulation Results

Parameter	Label	Initial Guess	1973.22	1973.36	1973.50
Number of infected cattle/cow	K	15.0	10.1	10.1	10.1
Feed system pole	T1	1.00	1.05	1.68	1.70
Symptom pole	T2	2.00	1.67	1.04	1.04
Initial infected cattle	IC	1.00	6.52	7.13	8.66
Year of start	to	1971	1973.22	1973.36	1973.50
Incubation time delay	Td	3.50	3.20	3.20	3.20
Year of feed ban	YB	1988.5	1988.5	1988.5	1988.5
Rms error of fit		2395	855	854	862

with higher inoculum. This is logical, considering this corresponds to shifting the arbitrary initial conditions along the epizootic case rate curve.

A comparison of parameters associated with the optimum "Year of start" of 1973.36 (i.e., April 1973) and its immediate neighboring solution points are shown in Table 15.1. Figure 15.3 shows the shallow optimum versus "Year of start", and the associated Initial Infected Cattle curve.

The best fit is a "Year of start" around 1973, with an initial inoculum equivalent to 6–9 infected cattle. A dose of this size in ca. 1973 would be sufficient, with the feedback gain of 10.1 animals per recycled animal, to account for the United Kingdom epizootic case rate observed. The optimized parameters indicate that the Total Time Delay is best fit with 3.20 years for all of the optimized models.

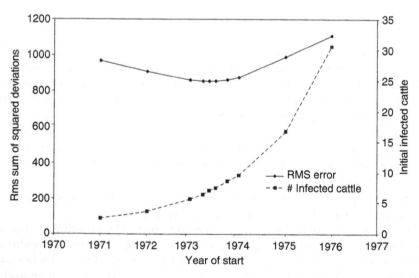

FIGURE 15.3

Root-mean-square deviation of fit versus assumed year of start of the BSE epizootic. Also shown is the associated initial condition for number of infected cattle. Note the shallow optimum between 1973 and 1974.

The model results were achieved without changing any model parameters during the epizootic, thus making it unnecessary to assume, for example, a change in the rendering process in 1981.

The contaminated feed is reduced to less than five equivalent animals by the end of 1999. The model correctly predicts that only about 40 confirmed cases would appear in 2005. The simulation results suggest that the epidemic will end about the year 2011 with less than one confirmed case.

Note that the model derived is the simplest possible which fits the empirical data. This model is top-level only, and cannot predict, for example, within-year seasonality. However, fitting the model requires only annual case rate data and certain salient side information, such as the implementation date of a feed ban. It is instructive that this most simplistic of models fits the annual case rate data to about the same level of error as the most refined and complex model used. This implies that no other assumptions are needed, including the change in rendering practice, to accurately model the UK BSE epizootic case rate data.

The most important lessons that can be learned from this simple model of the UK BSE epizootic are three: (1) A faster than linear rise in the case rate can only happen with feedback and a net amplification greater than one; (2) The epizootic was resolved as soon as the feed ban was instituted in July 1988; and (3) Never live with feedback in a food safety system unless you are absolutely sure you have controlled the gain. In the United Kingdom event, the feed ban reduced the loop gain drastically to below one, eventually quenching the outbreak. The subsequent rise in case rate and exponential decline were artifacts of the inertia of the system, due to capacitive effects of stored feed (particularly for non-ruminants) and already infected animals. Even a poorly implemented (e.g., 90% compliance) feed ban would have "switched off" the epizootic. A 100% feed ban compliance is needed only to drive the final tail of the case rate to zero at the fastest possible rate.

15.2.4 Active Surveillance and Post-Epizootic Artifacts

The model given in the previous section underpredicts the actual total case rate in the United Kingdom for years after 1998. It also overpredicts the case rate for 1988 and earlier.

The overprediction for 1988 and earlier can be attributed to undersurveillance at the beginning of the outbreak. A similar effect is found with the detailed Anderson model.[5]

The underprediction for 1998 and later is due to several factors:

1. In 1999 and after, the United Kingdom instituted an active surveillance program based on random sampling of normally slaughtered cattle. This contributed to additional confirmed cases by a mechanism different from previous surveillance techniques.

2. A maternal mode of vertical transmission has been hypothecated and measured,[4] which would provide additional cases that would

become noticeable as the annual case rate from feed starts to disappear.

3. The feed ban in 1988 was ruminant only. Feed including MBM was still used for other farm animals and persisted in the system. A full mammalian feed ban with full feed security was not instituted until 1996.

4. The United Kingdom sheep population may be a continuing reservoir for BSE (although this appears unlikely).

5. Surveillance was inefficient in the initial years of the outbreak.

Clusters of so-called BARB (born after ruminant ban) BSE cases are still being investigated in the United Kingdom, as they continue to occur up to the present time. Such clusters have so far been attributed mainly to hidden reservoirs of tainted feed.[23]

Finally, in order to emphasize the intrinsic simplicity behind the UK BSE epizootic curve, consider the most simplistic of all hypothetical mechanisms. This corresponds to simple exponential increase with an amplification time constant during the initial phase of the epizootic, rising to a peak value where the delayed switch due to the 1998 feed ban turns off the amplification and discontinuously switches the cases to a simple exponential decline due to the discharge of the BSE-effective cases stored in the existing feed and animal population. This simplistic model does not account for all of the mechanistic features nor the smoothed maximum observed, and does not deal properly with the tails of the epizootic curve. However, it does offer an immediate intuitive and quantitative understanding of the principal effects present.

Figure 15.4 shows a plot of the logarithm of the observed annual number of BSE cases versus year, together with fitted simple exponential straight lines for the ramp up and ramp down portions of the data. Also shown are the results from the mechanistic model described above. Note the usefulness of the exponential lines in understanding and quantifying the shape of the epizootic curve. Also note that the exponential lines are based on the presumed truth of the data, so are unable to suggest substantial underreporting in the early years, as does the simple mechanistic model. The slopes of the simple exponential lines correspond to time constants of 1.17 and 1.79 years, very similar to the 1.04 and 1.68 years found with the control system model. (Thus the graph may be useful in providing initial approximations for key time-constant parameters.).

It is recommended that any analysis of outbreak incidence data starts with plots of the form of Figures 15.1 and 15.4. A linear curve in Figure 15.1 would indicate simple integration (accumulation) as the mechanism, implying simple cumulative feedback. A faster than linear curve in Figure 15.1, but linear in Figure 15.4, would indicate simple exponential gain from feedback. Substantial curvature in both Figures 15.1 and 15.4 would indicate higher-order poles in the underlying mechanism behind the outbreak.

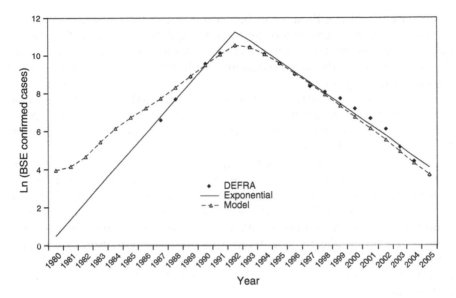

FIGURE 15.4

Plot of the logarithm of UK BSE confirmed annual cases versus year Also shown are the logarithm of the predicted results of the control system model and straight-line (simple exponential model) fits to the logarithm of the data.

This graphical analysis technique does not require understanding of the mechanism of the disease transmission, knowledge of much statistics or numerical analysis, or availability of nonlinear regression tools.

15.3 Passive Surveillance and the EU Testing Experience

15.3.1 The EU Passive and Active Surveillance Results

As mentioned previously, currently the EU countries report results of mandated surveillance testing for BSE based on four different categories: (1) animals reported as BSE clinical suspects; (2) risk, defined as fallen stock, emergency slaughtered animals, and sick at inspection; (3) healthy, or all animals at normal slaughter over 24 months of age (or 30 months in the United Kingdom); and (4) eradication, cohort animals associated with confirmed case animals.

On the other hand, it is common that other countries that are classified as BSE-free (OIE negligible risk) or low risk (OIE controlled risk) for BSE commonly only undertake surveillance only of suspect and risk animals, or so-called passive surveillance. OIE/FAO guidelines require only such passive surveillance.[19] Mass testing of healthy animals (active surveillance) is expensive and not thought to be necessary for public health when BSE case incidence is absent or rare. So far, among the countries outside the EU, only Japan has adopted full active surveillance. The United States and Canada remain on passive surveillance with only a small prototype active surveillance program.

This restriction to passive surveillance has created considerable controversy with public advocacy groups, argue that for extensive surveillance of healthy slaughter animals as necessary to protect the public health (contrary to OIE recommendations).

Given the EU testing experience, which incorporated both passive and active surveillance in a large number of different countries, an opportunity arises to assess the correlation and predictability of passive-only surveillance with respect to missed cases that might have been found in active surveillance of asymptomatic healthy slaughter. The countries in the EU might be considered a theoretical population of inference, which would allow statistical statements to be made about BSE incidence and detection in a hypothetical new EU-like country in similar circumstances.

15.3.2   An Efficacy Model for Passive Surveillance

In order to answer these questions and make the required inferences, an underlying structural model may be posed for the incidence rates observed. Let

$S(k)$ = number of suspect animal BSE positives found in country k,

$R(k)$ = number of risk animal BSE positives found in country k,

$H(k)$ = number of healthy animal BSE positives found in country k, and

$E(k)$ = number of eradication animal BSE positives found in country k

all observed during a period specified. Also let

$A(k)$ = estimated size of adult (>24 months) animal population in country k,

$O(k)$ = cumulative number of healthy animals tested in country k, and

$M(k)$ = cumulative number of eradication animals tested in country k

during the period specified.

Assuming the surveillance methodology in each country is efficient, or at least constant in efficiency, $S(k)$ and $R(k)$ are expected to be proportional to the respective exposure populations $A(k)$. This presumes a constant incidence rate with a Poisson distribution. However, experience suggests that the segregation of referrals as BSE suspect or as risk cases is somewhat a matter of veterinary opinion, and can be expected to vary substantially between countries. Consequently the assumption of constant incidence rate is imposed on the total of $S(k)$ and $R(k)$, not individually:

$$T(k) = S(k) + R(k) \tag{15.1}$$
$$= t(k)\, A(k) \tag{15.2}$$

where $t(k)$ is the incidence rate for BSE in country k.

Similarly, it can be assumed that:

$$H(k) = h(k)\, O(k) \tag{15.3}$$
$$E(k) = e(k)\, M(k) \tag{15.4}$$

where $h(k)$ and $e(k)$ are the respective incidence rates in health and eradication animals in country k. To allow inference about $H(k)$ and $E(k)$ from results $T(k)$, it is necessary to postulate a connection between the incidence rates involved. The simplest such model is

$$H(k) = g\, t(k)\, O(k) \tag{15.5}$$
$$E(k) = z\, t(k)\, M(k) \tag{15.6}$$

where the assumption is made that the $h(k)$ and $e(k)$ are simply proportional to $t(k)$.

The reported results from the 15 EU countries between 2001 and 2002[9] were combined into one dataset (Table 15.2). Only data from the first 2 years of surveillance were used in order to maintain a population of inference, which involved countries that have not had BSE incidence culled by testing of large numbers of healthy animals. Data from seven countries that have reported 0 or 1 positive case in the BSE suspect category were combined to form a composite "country" group, resulting in a total of nine "countries" in the dataset.

The adult population numbers $A(k)$ were scaled by 2.0 to account for the 2-year period of observation in the testing. The resulting 27 data were fitted to the model described (11 unknown parameters: $t(k)$, g, z) using Poisson regression with a log link and deviance scaling using SAS PROC GEN-MOD.[24] Deviance scaling (based on the Pearson formula) was used, due to observed over-dispersion.

15.3.3 Results and Discussion

The combined EU surveillance data are shown in Table 15.2. The results of the Poisson regression are presented in Table 15.3. The deviance decreased from 6423 (26 d.f., intercept only) to 327 (16 d.f., 11 parameters fit), or a difference of 6096 for 10 d.f., which is significant beyond the 0.0001% level.

The value of g found was 1.75, with a 95% C.I. of [1.11, 2.74], based on exponentiation of the fitted parameter in the log-linear model. This can be interpreted as a risk ratio: The incidence rate (probability) of BSE found

TABLE 15.2

Combined Surveillance Data for the EU from January 1, 2001 to December 31, 2002

Country	Total Cattle (M's)[a]	Adult Cattle (M's)[b]	Healthy[f] Tested	Eradication[g] Tested	Suspect[d] Positive	Risk[e] Positive	S + R Positive	Eradication[g] Positive	Healthy[f] Positive
Belgium	3.0	1.5	768,369	6,799	14	24	38	1	45
Germany	14.5	6.5	5,323,692	16,478	18	128	146	7	78
Spain	5.3	3.4	780,327	9,018	26	113	139	7	71
France	20.3	11.1	5,278,407	26,998	132	224	356	4	157
Ireland	7.3	3.5	1,246,932	30,855	231	272	503	8	68
Netherlands	4.0	1.8	945,718	5,558	4	19	23	0	21
Portugal	5.3	0.8	95,105	3,175	85	53	138	4	57
United Kingdom[c]	9.4	5.2	193,470	1,346	1,248	974	2,222	0	15
Combined small	14.8	6.8	2,131,440	13,489	1	43	44	1	54
Totals	83.8	40.5	16,763,460	113,716	1,759	1,850	3,609	32	566

Source: [a] From OIE International Animal Health Code 2002, 10th edition. Appendix 3.8.4: Surveillance and monitoring systems for bovine spongiform encephalopathy. Available online at: http://www.oie.int/eng/publicat/en_code.htm

[b] From Eurostat, BSE testing in the EU, 2006. Available online at: http://ec.europa.eu/food/food/biosafety/bse/mthly_reps_en.htm

[c] Great Britain only.

[d] Animals reported as BSE clinical suspects.

[e] Dead-on-farm animals, emergency slaughtered animals, animals sent for normal slaughter but found sick at ante mortem inspection.

[f] Healthy animals subject to normal slaughter.

[g] Birth and rearing cohorts, feed cohorts, offspring of BSE cases, animals from herds with BSE.

TABLE 15.3

Estimated Parameters and Wald 95% Confidence Intervals

Category	Parameter	Point Estimate	Wald 95% C.I. Low	High	Exponentiated Values Estimate	Low	High
Belgium	$t(1)$	−10.87	−11.89	−9.84	1.91E–05	6.85E–06	5.32E–05
Germany	$t(2)$	−11.48	−12.12	−10.84	1.03E–05	5.45E–06	1.96E–05
Spain	$t(3)$	−10.54	−11.18	−9.91	2.63E–05	1.39E–05	4.97E–05
France	$t(4)$	−11.02	−11.45	−10.59	1.63E–05	1.06E–05	2.51E–05
Ireland	$t(5)$	−9.70	−10.10	−9.30	6.12E–05	4.09E–05	9.17E–05
Netherlands	$t(6)$	−11.68	−13.09	−10.27	8.46E–06	2.07E–06	3.46E–05
Portugal	$t(7)$	−9.11	−9.77	−8.45	1.11E–04	5.73E–05	2.15E–04
United Kingdom	$t(8)$	−8.47	−8.67	8.27	2.10E–04	1.72E–04	2.56E–04
Combined	$t(9)$	−12.08	−13.02	−11.14	5.68E–06	2.22E–06	1.45E–05
Healthy	g	0.557	0.105	1.009	1.75	1.11	2.74
Eradication	z	2.177	0.515	3.840	8.82	1.67	46.53

per average tested healthy animal is 1.75 times the incidence rate (probability) of BSE found per average suspect or risk adult animal per year. This indicates that surveillance of suspect and risk animals is approximately as efficient as sampling 57% of the entire national adult herd, and vindicates the use of these categories as the most effective surveillance program in terms of cost/benefit ratio.

The value of z found was 8.82, with a 95% C.I. of [1.67, 46.53], again based on exponentiation of the fitted parameter in the log-linear model. This indicates the incidence rate (probability) of BSE found per average tested eradication animal is 8.82 times the incidence rate (probability) of BSE found per average suspect or risk adult animal per year. Of more interest is the ratio of z/g, viz., 8.82/1.75 or 5.06. The incidence rate of BSE found in the eradication cohort animals is 5.06 times that found in healthy animals presented at slaughter. Therefore eradication animals do have a modestly higher risk than healthy animals. Whether or not this increase is sufficiently greater to justify the eradication program cost should be investigated further by risk assessment and cost/benefit analysis.

15.3.4 Inferences for BSE-Free and BSE Low-Risk Countries

Consider first the situation of a new, somehow EU-like country that is considered BSE-free due to absence of confirmed native-born cases from surveillance. This might be exemplified by the situation in the United States before 2003.

The United States had a total cattle population of 105 million as of July 1, 2002, with an approximate adult animal population of 45 million.[25] Some 32,117 suspect and risk animals were tested during the period October 1, 2000 to January 31, 2002; all were found negative.[26]

In the units of the EU surveillance data, this suggests that t(USA) is less than 1 case in 45 million per 28/12 years, or less than 9.52×10^{-9} cases per adult animal per year. This would imply the rate in healthy animals presented at slaughter is 1.75 t(USA) or 1.67×10^{-8} cases per healthy animal per year, and with 97.5% confidence no higher than 2.74 t(USA) or 2.61×10^{-8}. Assuming a healthy animal population presented for slaughter of 58 million per year, this would place a 97.5% upper confidence limit of 1.5 animals BSE positive per year, if all were tested.

In fact, assuming an incidence rate of 1.67×10^{-8} cases per healthy animal per year and a Poisson distribution, testing all 58 million healthy animals would give only a 62% confidence of finding at least one BSE positive. Similarly, testing 1 million healthy animals would give only a 1.7% chance of finding a BSE positive. Clearly surveillance of suspect and risk animals is much more effective at discovery than testing healthy animals at slaughter, which is a very expensive proposition in BSE-free countries. (These conclusions depend upon the assumption that all or most risk and suspect animals are examined for the disease.) This was borne out by the actual discovery of the first US BSE case in 2003 (and similarly for Canada).

Note that in our model, the number of veterinary referrals in the suspect and risk categories is not indicative of the level of incidence of BSE in the national herd, even if all were found negative. So whether the United States tested 32,117 or 500,000 animals does not make a practical difference in the degree of confidence of BSE absence. What matters, however, is the size of the national herd adult population, the exposure period tested, and the completeness and objectivity of the surveillance.

Now let us consider the situation of a BSE low-risk country, exemplified by the situation of the United States after 2003.

Some 450,000 suspect and risk animals were tested during the period January 1, 2004, to May 31, 2006, with three confirmed positives and two inconclusive. Combining the confirmed and inconclusive results (a prudent precaution because of the atypical presentation), the discovered incidence is 5 cases in 450,000 tests of the suspect and risk categories over a 17-month period, or an incidence t(USA) of 7.8×10^{-8} cases per adult animal per year, assuming as before an adult cattle population of 45 million. Assuming a Poisson distribution on cases found, the 95% confidence interval for t(USA) is $[3.5 \times 10^{-8}, 18 \times 10^{-8}]$.

This incidence, together with the fitted EU model, implies a rate in healthy animals presented at slaughter in the United States of $h = gt$ of 1.75 t(USA) or 1.37×10^{-8} cases per healthy animal per year, with a rough 95% confidence interval of $[7.9 \times 10^{-8}, 29 \times 10^{-8}]$. Assuming again a healthy animal population presented for slaughter of 58 million per year, this would estimate 7.9 animals BSE positive per year (95% confidence [4.6, 16.8]) in the healthy animals at slaughter that would silently enter the food supply if not tested. These numbers should probably be doubled to account for the loss to passive surveillance of dead animals buried on farm during the testing period analyzed. These asymptomatic BSE cases passing silently into the food supply is the price paid in public health in the United States for 2005 for using passive-only surveillance. Whether or not this cost is considered acceptable is the subject of national risk assessment studies, which is discussed briefly in the next section.

15.4 The vCJD Epidemic

The threat to human public health from BSE is through its presumed causal connection to a human TSE, the so-called new variant CJD or vCJD discussed in Section 15.1.3. The rarity of vCJD (less than 0.5 cases per million population per year even in the United Kingdom or about 1 case per 40,000 population per lifetime), its incidence in otherwise healthy, young adults, and the degradation associated with its clinical manifestation have triggered the fear and paranoia of the consuming public.

Understanding of vCJD is still in its infancy. Substantial issues still remain unresolved as to its causal connection to BSE, the size of the current epidemic, and implications for the future.

15.4.1 Causal Connection of vCJD to BSE

As mentioned in Section 15.1.3, the principal basis for assuming BSE is the cause of human vCJD: (1) similarity of clinical symptoms, incubation period, and histopathological presentation and (2) near identity of molecular fragment electrophoresis patterns. However, as also mentioned in Section 15.1.3, it is possible that only a very few number of stable abnormal prion protein conformations exist, each with its own characteristic clinical symptoms, histopathological presentation, and electrophoresis pattern. Thus BSE and vCJD may be connected only because of basic protein chemistry, not by causality.

Finally, the causality may be inverse, i.e., vCJD may have been a preexisting disease in humans, transferred to cattle via human remains included in MBM. This gives rise to three possible scenarios, each of which must be independently examined:

1. vCJD was a preexisting human disease, not caused by BSE (although BSE may have been caused by vCJD).
2. vCJD was caused by BSE, but now the epidemic is declining.
3. vCJD was caused by BSE, and there will be new outbreaks in the future.

15.4.2 Case A: vCJD Is Not Caused by BSE

When the UK BSE epizootic was discovered, the United Kingdom established the National Creutzfeldt–Jakob Disease Surveillance Unit

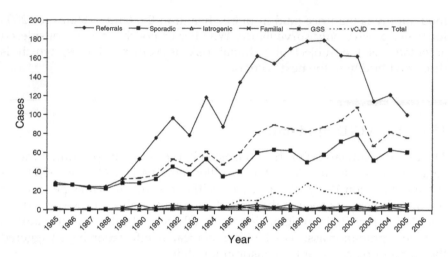

FIGURE 15.5
UK CJD surveillance cases versus year. Separate curves are plotted for clinical referrals, total cases, and breakdown of cases into sporadic, iatrogenic, familial, GSS, and vCJD categories.

(website http://www.cjd.ed.ac.uk/) in order to discover any possible implications for human health. CJD was made reportable and intense surveillance and investigation of cases were instituted. Not infrequently, such increased surveillance generates "surveillance artifacts," such as an apparent increased case rate and discovery of hitherto undetected minor strains. Therefore it is not unlikely that something like vCJD would have been discovered, even if it were not causally related to BSE.

Figure 15.5 shows a plot of the UK CJD surveillance cases[27] versus year. Note that total number of referrals has increased linearly after CJD was made reportable in 1990 to a maximum in 2000–2001, followed by a sharp decline thereafter. This linear ramp-up of referrals represents inflation of reports either due to the "learning curve" of diagnosis and increased public awareness of the disease, or incorporation of cases from an incipient epidemic of a new form of CJD. The subsequent decline in cases represents either the depletion of future cases by earlier heightened surveillance, or the tailing of an epidemic as the delayed impact of remedial hygienic measures, such as the SRM ban and the decline of BSE.

Also note in Figure 15.5 that total cases and sporadic cases also exhibit a linear ramp-up to a maximum in 2002, followed by a current plateau or decline. Following the discovery of vCJD, its confirmed or probable cases linearly increased to a maximum in 2000 and then went into slow decline.

Figure 15.5 therefore supports either the occurrence of short outbreaks of both sporadic and vCJD forms of the disease, both of which are now over, or surveillance artifacts due to change of policy on reporting (see Refs. [27,28]). These artifacts consist of the discovery of the hidden vCJD form and

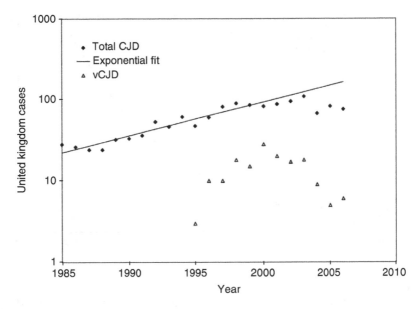

FIGURE 15.6
UK CJD total and vCJD cases logarithmically by year. The fitted straight line for total cases corresponds to exponential growth.

the apparent increase in case rates. The increased surveillance may have "pre-discovered" what future cases would have found, so the apparent decline in case rate may be due to the exhaustion of the undiscovered pool of incubating cases.

Figure 15.6 shows the total vCJD case rate data plotted on a logarithmic scale versus year. Note that the total CJD case increase is consistent with an exponential increase, but not the vCJD data. This is shown more clearly in Figure 15.7, which plots vCJD cases by themselves, where it is clear that the initial growth in vCJD cases is linear, not exponential.

Given that the UK BSE epizootic exhibits strong initial exponential growth, we would expect a vCJD outbreak driven by it to show the same structure, if it were causally related to BSE. This does not seem to have occurred.

Figure 15.8 shows a graph of the US CJD surveillance data. Although there has been no reason to suspect a recent outbreak of vCJD in the United States (there has been only one United Kingdom-imported case reported), the surveillance data for sporadic cases shows an increase to a maximum in 2004 with subsequent slight decline, somewhat similar to that in the United Kingdom data. This supports the idea of a surveillance artifact.

Not shown, and not analyzed here, was a small, concurrent apparent outbreak in the United Kingdom of feline spongiform encephalopathy (FSE), believed also causally related to BSE.

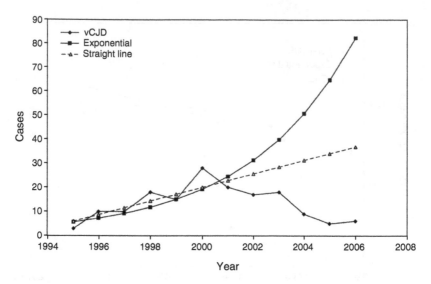

FIGURE 15.7
vCJD cases versus year. Also plotted are linear and exponential fits of the data up to 2002.

In conclusion, the case rate data in the United Kingdom (where 90% of all vCJD cases have occurred) support two possible interpretations: (1) The linear increase and subsequent decline in referrals and cases of all types of CJD are artifacts due to enhanced surveillance; or (2) mini-epidemics of both

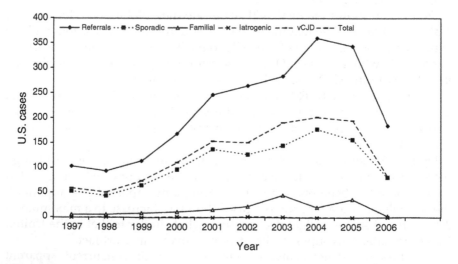

FIGURE 15.8
CJD surveillance in the United States. Note the apparent outbreak in sporadic cases, peaking around 2004.

sporadic CJD and vCJD have occurred and are now resolving. If the latter is true, the epidemic contained within the sporadic category may reflect a hidden outbreak of cases of different (atypical) clinical and histopathological presentation.

So far all cases found of vCJD are methionine-methionine at codon 129 of the prion protein gene, except for one case known to be transmitted by blood, which was methionine-valine. About 40% of the population has the M-M and 40% the M-V genotypes.

The evidence for no causal relation of vCJD to BSE appears to be comprised of (1) a paucity of discovered prion strains; (2) the conflicting information contained in the observed case rates; (3) the dose-dependence of oral infectivity from BSE contamination, coupled with the lack of discovery of an M-V or V-V genotype outbreak; (4) the paradox of vegetarian vCJD (with respect to the oral route); and (5) a simplicity of assumption.

The evidence for BSE causing the vCJD mini-epidemic is (1) BSE is known by experiment to transmit orally to other species; (2) a similar clinical and histopathological presentation; (3) similar electrophoresis patterns; and (4) a coincidence of timing. Given that some of the vCJD cases found were unlikely to have consumed much beef, the route of infection by BSE-contaminated pharmaceuticals may be more plausible than the oral route.

Of course, wise public health policy in the interim is to presume vCJD causally related to BSE, and to maintain all prudent safeguards to prevent new cases. Such is currently the policy in all BSE-affected countries to date.

15.4.3 Case B: vCJD Caused by BSE, but the Epidemic Is Declining

This scenario presumes that the UK vCJD epidemic is resolving due to the feed and SRM bans. The enhancement of the sporadic cases observed may have already included any expected M-V and V-V outbreaks (see Ref. [29,31]).

There have been so far 161 cases of vCJD and approximately 180,000 cases of BSE in the United Kingdom. This implies 1 vCJD case might be expected per 1100 BSE confirmed positives as a rough rule of thumb.

Assuming the upper confidence limit of 16.8 cases of BSE per year in the United States from Section 15.3.4, this would mean the current level of expected associated public health risk of vCJD is about 0.015 cases per year in the United States. Therefore, the vCJD risk in North America would not yet be of significant public health concern. Similar statements could be made for other BSE low-risk countries.

The real risk of BSE in such low-risk countries is not to human food safety, but rather to the cattle and beef industry economic health. Even a single case of BSE found has an immediate impact on beef consumption and exports, due to consumer fear and paranoia, complicated by government and industry duplicity. In the United Kingdom, there probably have been more BSE-related suicides in farmers than deaths from vCJD. This issue of risk assessment is discussed further in Section 15.5.

15.4.4   Case C: vCJD Was Caused by BSE, and There Will Be New Outbreaks in the Future

Under this scenario, the M-M genotype epidemic of vCJD in the United Kingdom has occurred, but it had a smaller incubation time than the same disease for the M-V and V-V genotypes, which then is yet to occur. Or the epidemic so far has been related to a special, small group of genetic susceptibles, which has now been depleted. The large-scale epidemic of vCJD in the general population is yet to come. Or there is a large-scale epidemic of vCJD occurring in the general population, but it is misdiagnosed as Alzheimer's disease.

All of this is extremely speculative and, as yet, is uncorroborated by hard evidence.

15.4.5   An Inconvenient Truth

All of these scenarios are possibilities, and any one of them may eventually prove to be true. Prudent health policy is to "hope for the best, but plan for the worst". It is probably true that a large number of CJD cases are misdiagnosed as Alzheimer's disease, and this will eventually be discovered when routine prion testing of such cases is performed. However, this is not directly germane to BSE and its possible causal connection to vCJD. Certainly vCJD is unlikely to be misdiagnosed as Alzheimer's disease, given the youthful nature of the cases involved.

The most likely scenario is that the vCJD epidemic will remain small, and is perhaps now fully resolved, except for iatrogenic cases (see Refs. [29,30] for more discussion). The simple fact is that the BSE epizootic has been resolved by the feed ban, and therefore BSE contamination in the food supply peaked in 1993 and is very low now. The SRM removal greatly limits the impact of BSE on both the cattle and human food supplies. Incubation period and dose are connected in TSEs, so future cases of vCJD would be expected to be much fewer than those experienced thus far.

Activists promoting hypothetical future calamities fuel the fear and paranoia of the consuming public and make the administration of the public health issues related to BSE and vCJD political instead of scientific, similar to the situation in the early stages of the AIDS epidemic. This is discussed further in the following section.

15.5   BSE and International Trade

In the normal course of events, safety of foodstuffs is handled in a dignified and methodical way by public health authorities, government departments, and industry. Food safety objectives are determined by expert commissions and risk assessment studies, and surveillance and inspection activities are performed by the relevant governmental agencies. Consumers are complacent about food safety, trusting the system to protect them.

BSE has, however, changed all that, and provided a textbook example of how not to carry out public health policy that will probably be studied in the decades or even century to come.

15.5.1 International Guidelines

Food is a product of agriculture, and agriculture has been traditionally the most protected industry in international trade. Government subsidies and nontariff trade barriers related to food have been at the core of numerous trade disputes over the last century.

In 1962, the Joint Food Administration Organization (FAP) of the World Health Organization (WHO) was created with the Codex Alimentarius Commission (CAC) of the World Trade Organization (WTO) as its administrator. The resulting Codex Alimentarius (Codex) adopted by CAC is a collection of food standards enforced in international trade. These standards are a negotiated balance between science-based protection of public health and fair practices in trade between countries.

In 1995, the WTO Sanitary and Phytosanitary Measures Agreement (SPS) was enacted, and applies to all measures that may affect food in international trade. It directs WTO members to harmonize sanitary guidelines and controls. These measures must be based upon risk assessments in accord with international guidelines, such as the Draft Principles and Guidelines for the Conduct of Microbiological Risk Assessment adopted by CAC in 1999.

Article 2 of the SPS states[32]: "Members shall ensure that any sanitary and phytosanitary measure is applied only to the extent necessary to protect human, animal or plant life or health, is based on scientific principles and is not maintained without scientific evidence." In the same manner, the WTO Technical Barriers to Trade (TBT) Agreement says the procedures used to decide whether a product conforms with national standards have to be fair and equitable, and discourages any methods that would give domestically produced goods an unfair advantage.

15.5.2 "Science Goes Out the Door, When Politics Comes Innuendo"

The WTO and Codex agreements are the way food and animal safety is supposed to happen in international trade. Unfortunately, BSE has exemplified the opposite. The Codex is conspicuous by its absence.

As a string of countries has fallen from the BSE free category, in each case almost without exception we have seen (1) the government and national industry denying BSE existed in their national herd; (2) statements that all beef was totally safe; (3) ministers of agriculture taking photo-opportunities eating burgers or feeding one to their child; and (4) protests as to the cost and necessity for implementing feed and SRM bans. A good example of this occurred in the United States, along the lines of "famous last words": The American Meat Institute questioned in February 2003 FDA's change in rendering practice to remove "specified risk materials" from the mammalian feed chain, claiming "science" did not justify the change in rule, as BSE had not yet been found in the United States.[33] Of course, the first U.S. case of BSE was then found later in December of the same year, proving the prudence of FDA's move.

These 100% denials by industry and government, followed by the inevitable discovery of the first national BSE case in each instance, have triggered a justifiable cynicism and skepticism in the consuming public.

At the same time, the rarity and horrific symptoms of vCJD have instilled an irrational fear as well. A substantial collapse in beef prices has invariably resulted.

This fear of consumers has triggered governmental action both externally, where other countries immediately stopped affected importation, and internally, which, happily for the beleaguered cattle and beef industry, usually has included blockage of imports from other BSE-infected or even low-risk countries, as they "don't have the control measures in place that we now do" (cf. France vis-à-vis the United Kingdom.)

In North America, the first Canadian BSE case triggered a closure of the border with the United States, which is still not completely open (viz., no live cattle over 30 months of age), despite the low incidence in Canada, the previous mixing of the two national herds, and the implementation of feed and SRM bans in both countries. Lawsuits have been filed on behalf of the U.S. cattle industry to prevent the USDA from opening the border to live animals. Luckily for Canada, the U.S. meatpacking industry just as strongly wants the border reopened and is slowly winning the protectionist trade battle.

After the discovery of the first BSE cases in Canada and the United States, essentially all trade with the Far East countries (the largest export markets) evaporated. As of May 2006, trade in beef to these countries has not yet regained its previous level. Interestingly, Japan, long-noted for its imposition of nontariff trade barriers, has taken the position that it must protect its population from the dangers of North American beef, despite the occurrence of more than two dozen cases of BSE in its own national herd.

15.5.3 Consumers: A Modest Proposal

The skepticism, fear, and paranoia of consumers have been exploited by anti-meat and advocacy activists to attempt to create a dread of a calamitous vCJD epidemic that looms in the future.

As has been noted previously,[34] people are generally superstitious. If they win the lottery, they are lucky, and other people want to be around them because the luck might "rub off." On the other hand, if an equally rare adverse event befalls them, such as a rare and horrific disease, they are unlucky, and other people avoid them for similar reasons. Unlucky people are presumed to somehow deserve their adversity, as a consequence of some former bad behavior. On the other hand, lucky people are considered special, and somehow favored by fortune. This crowd psychology was clearly exemplified by the AIDS epidemic experience in the last few decades.

Because people do not consider themselves "bad" or deserving of a rare adversity, they naturally look to blame outsiders for their problem. In the case of vCJD, it's (with some justification) the beef industry and the government. Each new case of vCJD discovered will trigger an expensive lawsuit and a calamitous fall in beef consumption by consumers.

In low- and controlled-risk countries the principal threat from BSE is not to consumers, but to the cattle and beef industries. Fear of vCJD cases, and the discovery of the first such native cases, have a severe effect on consumption and the sector economy.

Therefore we suggest that every country now BSE free or every low-risk country institute the following combined industry and government policy:

1. Announce BSE is conceivably present and may occur "here" but only at low levels, or that it has occurred "here," but is under control;

2. vCJD is extremely unlikely, and no more than 1 or 2 native cases are ever expected to occur; and

3. In proof of confidence of this, industry has established a vCJD indemnity fund, which will pay $2 million to the estate of any person living within the country who dies from vCJD. A condition of receiving money from the fund is an agreement to forgo any other legal remedies.

Such an indemnity program would cost 1% or less of the otherwise anticipated damage to the industry from discovery of vCJD cases. vCJD is an insurable risk. If no cases of vCJD are subsequently discovered, there would be no indemnity cost.

15.6 Conclusions

TSEs are now a fact of life in the food animal industries for the indefinite future. Control is achieved by strict feed bans and disposal of SRM to keep it from the animal or human food supplies.

vCJD is, at least to some extent, probably connected causally to BSE via some oral or pharmaceutical route. However, the number of cases worldwide is low and is likely to remain so. The economic and political effects caused by the discovery of this disease are greatly out of proportion to its public health significance.

Except for sporadic continuing cases and discovery of isolated cases in new countries, BSE is now probably a disease of the past. The United Kingdom experience will not be repeated.

Of more significance is CWD, which continues to expand rapidly in North America with no useful control measures known other than herd extermination. The eventual size of this epizootic, and its consequences if the disease is ever found to transmit orally to humans or cattle, is still unknown and dire to contemplate.

15.7 Acknowledgments

The authors would like to offer their sincerest thanks to J. Ralph Blanchfield, Hotz de Baar, and Martin Hugh-Jones for their constant support and encouragement, brilliant insights, and criticism and suggestions.

References

1. Institute of Food Science and Technology, Bovine spongiform encephalopathy (BSE) and variant Creutzfeldt–Jakob disease (vCJD) in humans, 2004. Available online at: http://www.ifst.org/
2. Weston, W. and Bryant, C.M., Transmissible spongiform encephalopathies, *J. Food Sci.* 70(5):R75–R87, 2005. Available online at: http://www.ift.org/cms/
3. Brown, P. et al., Bovine spongiform encephalopathy and variant Creutzfeldt–Jakob disease: Background, evolution and current concerns, *Emerg. Infect. Dis.* 7(1):6–16, 2001.
4. Anonymous, *Bovine Spongiform Encephalopathy in Great Britain*, Ministry of Agriculture, Farms and Fisheries, Surrey, UK. Appendix 1, June 1997.
5. Andersen, R.M. et al., Transmission dynamics and epidemiology of BSE in British cattle, *Nature* 382:779–788, 1996.
6. Donnelly, C.A. and Ferguson, N.M., *Statistical Aspects of BSE and vCJD: Models for Epidemics*, Chapman and Hall, New York, ISBN: 0-8493-0386-9, 1999.
7. Gale, P., BSE risk assessments in the UK: A risk tradeoff? *J. Appl. Micro.* 100:417–427, 2006.
8. Anonymous, Annual incidence rate of BSE in the UK, OIE, 2006. Available online at: http://www.oie.int/eng/info/en_esbru.htm
9. Eurostat, BSE testing in the EU, 2006. Available online at: http://ec.europa.eu/food/food/biosafety/bse/mthly_reps_en.htm
10. National Creutzfeldt-Jakob Disease Surveillance Unit, Monthly Creutzfeldt-Jakob disease statistics, UK Department of Health, 2006. Available online at: http://www.cjd.ed.ac.uk/index.htm
11. Bruce, P. et al., Transmission to mice indicates that 'new variant' CJD is caused by the BSE agent, *Nature* 389:489–501, 1997.
12. Carp, R.I. et al., Scrapie strains retain their distinctive characteristics following passages of homogenates from different brain regions and spleen, *J. Gen. Virol.* 78:283–290, 1997.

13. De Bosschere, H. et al., Atypical case of bovine spongiform encephalopathy in an east-Flemish cow in Belgium, *Inter. J. Appl. Res. Vet. Med.* 2(1):52–54, 2002.
14. Yamakawa, Y. et al., Atypical proteinase K-resistant prion protein (PrPres) observed in an apparently healthy 23-month-old Holstein steer, *J. Infect. Dis.* 56:221–222, 2003.
15. Biacabe, A.G. et al., Distinct molecular phenotypes in bovine prion diseases, *EMBO Rep.* 5(1):110–115, 2004.
16. Anonymous, Animal protein prohibited in ruminant feed, 21 CFR 589, 2000.
17. Marsh, R.F. and Hanson, R.P., On the origin of transmissible mink encephalopathy, in *Slow Transmission Disease of the Nervous System*, Vol. 1, Academic Press, New York, ISBN 0-12-566301-3, 1979.
18. Miller, M.W. and Williams, E.S., Chronic wasting disease of cervids, *Curr. Top. Microbiol. Immunol.* 284:193–214, 2004.
19. *OIE International Animal Health Code 2002*, 10th ed. Appendix 3.8.4: Surveillance and monitoring systems for bovine spongiform encephalopathy OIE, ISBN: 978-9290445562, 2002. Available online at: http://www.oie.int/eng/publicat/en _code.htm
20. Dorf, R.C. and Bishop, R.H., *Modern Control Systems*, 10th ed., Addison Wesley, New York, ISBN 0131457330, 2004.
21. Karayanakis, N.M., *Computer-Assisted Simulation of Dynamic Systems with Block Diagram Languages*, CRC Press, ISBN 0849389712, 1993.
22. Anonymous, BSE Statistics, UK DEFRA, 2006. Available online at: http://www. defra.gov.uk/animalh/bse/statistics/incidence.html
23. Spongiform Encephalopathy Advisory Committee, Minutes of the open session of the 90th meeting held on 24 November 2005. Available online at: http:// www.seac.gov.uk/minutes/final90.pdf
24. SAS for Windows v. 8.01. 2000. SAS Institute Inc., Cary, NC. See online at: http://www.sas.com/
25. Anonymous, Cattle report released July 19, 2002, NASS. Available online at: http://usda.mannlib.cornell.edu/MannUsda/viewDocumentInfo.do?document ID=1017.
26. Detwiler, L., USDA-APHIS, Personal communication, 2003.
27. Anonymous, CJD Statistics, UK National CJD Surveillance Unit, 2006. Available online at: http://www.cjd.ed.ac.uk/figures.htm
28. Ferguson, N.M. et al., Predicting the size of the epidemic of the new variant of Creutzfeldt-Jakob disease, *Brit. Food J.* 101:86–98, 1999.
29. Ghani, A.C. et al., Factors determining the pattern of the variant Creutzfeldt-Jakob disease (vCJD) epidemic in the UK, *Proc. Biol. Sci.* 270:689–698, 2003.
30. Venters, G.A., New variant Creutzfeldt-Jakob disease: The epidemic that never was, *Brit. Med. J.* 323:858–861, 2001.
31. Ghani, A.C., Commentary: Predicting the unpredictable: the future incidence of variant Creutzfeldt-Jakob disease, *Int. J. Epidemiol.* 32:792–793, 2003.
32. WTO. Sanitary and Phytosanitary Measures Agreement. Available online at: http://www.wto.org/English/tratop_e/sps_e/sps_e.htm
33. Anonymous, Science does not support changes to FDA animal feed rules, American Meat Institute, 2003. Available online at: http://www.meatami.com/Template. cfm?Section = BSE&NavMenuID=188&template=TaggedContentFile.cfm& NewsID=629
34. LaBudde, R.A., Why consumers take risks with food safety. *Food Safety Magazine* 9(2):14–17, 2003.

16

Use of Risk Assessment as a Tool for Evaluating Microbial Food Contaminants

Michael D. McElvaine

CONTENTS

16.1 Introduction

Various methods of risk assessment and analysis have been used by engineers, economists, and other scientists since at least the 1930s. In the 1950s and 1960s, risk assessment methods were applied to chemical contaminants that may be in the environment or our food and water.[1] Later, the U.S. Food and Drug Administration (FDA) developed safety assessments, a variation of risk assessment, to evaluate food additives and chemical contaminants.

Statements and opinions in this chapter do not necessarily represent the opinions of the USDA or the Office of Risk Assessment and Cost-Benefit Analysis.

Application of formal risk assessment to biological (multiplying) organisms was not attempted until the 1980s and 1990s. At the time of the first edition of this book, biological risk assessment, including microbial contaminants of food, was literally in its infancy. The science of biological risk assessment has advanced greatly in the intervening years; risk assessments have become more complex and sophisticated. Government regulators have also become more familiar with the methods and have learned how to apply the methods to better inform food safety regulations. Risk assessments of microbial food contaminants and other sanitary and phytosanitary pathogens are routinely required to support any regulation that may restrict trade. USDA was the first government agency specifically required by statute to perform risk analysis and economic analysis for major regulations affecting human health, safety, or the environment.[2]

When applying risk assessment methodology to microbes, there are two related but very different issues. First, we want to know whether a product is contaminated or not, or the probability that each unit may be contaminated. Second, we want to know how many microbes are present. While chemical contaminants are inert for the most part, microbes may increase, decrease, or stay at the same numbers. This is the area of focus for the field of microbial risk assessment. From a human health aspect, we want to use risk assessment methods to evaluate the exposure dose, the dose–response on a population, and the range of health impacts from these exposures. The current focus on food safety and international trade has increased the interest in developing better information about microbial food contaminants in order to improve food safety regulations and to facilitate international trade.

16.2   What Is Risk Assessment?

Risk assessment in itself is not hard science. It is the art of taking scientific information and transforming it into information that is useful as the basis for a decision maker to act upon.[3] There are now several universities in the United States that have degree or certificate programs in environmental or microbial risk assessment. Mostly everyone who practices the art of microbial risk assessment has transferred skills from related fields such as toxicologic risk assessment or food safety and added additional analytic skills and hands-on experience to become skilled in microbial risk assessment. Risk assessment in general and microbial risk assessment in particular have been accepted as the standard of practice for supporting regulations by the United States and by most international regulatory agencies and organizations.

Although most readers now have some idea when the term "risk assessment" is used, it is useful to explain the context in which "microbial risk assessment" will be discussed in this chapter. Risk assessment has been used to evaluate many different types of risks and situations: chemical contaminants, economic impacts, catastrophic events, etc. The fundamental concepts of risk assessment remain the same no matter where they are applied.

In the simplest sense, risk assessment is a methodology for evaluating a given scenario (situation) to determine:[4]

1. What can go wrong?
2. How likely is it?
3. What is the magnitude of the impact?

The general use of risk assessment is not new. In essence, it is the kind of evaluation that our prehistoric ancestors used to determine whether it was worthwhile to face the risk of starvation versus the risk of foraging in the open and possibly being eaten by predators. We all make less dramatic decisions every day, which are in essence risk analysis. Many people drive to work everyday. Do they consciously think about the risk of this activity, or do they take it for granted that the value of earning a salary is greater than the risk of an automobile accident or other corporal risk?

In the context of biological (i.e., microbial) risk assessment, the methodology is an organized framework for presenting information about the risks of a situation, assessing the probability of negative events, and assessing the magnitude of these negative events. The next step, the economic part of the equation, is to compare the magnitude of bad outcomes with the costs of interventions necessary to reduce this magnitude of bad outcomes (we usually translate these magnitudes into dollar values to provide transparency to the decision makers). This is where probability and magnitude provide insight for decision makers.

16.3 Brief Retrospective of Risk Assessment

Risk assessment is an innate part of being human (as far as our ability to reason), and is a basic factor in our lives that guides our actions. It was only in the twentieth century that the art of risk assessment began to be presented in a formalized manner to evaluate scientific and economic questions. In the earlier years of the USDA, various forms of risk assessment methods were used to guide regulatory and programmatic decisions. These methods were primarily descriptive; the descriptive methods became more organized and have been called qualitative risk assessment by some. Only in the last two decades has the USDA begun to accept the organized methods of risk analysis to guide regulatory decisions. The modern use of formal quantitative risk assessment can be traced back to the advent of nuclear power plants in the United States,[5] when quantitative methods using Monte Carlo analysis were used to evaluate new issues arising from their development. Monte Carlo analysis was a significant step in the advancement of quantitative risk assessment methods. This methodology was soon adapted by physicists, economists, and others to evaluate situations where probability and magnitude of impact were factors in decisions. If you have financial advisors who guide you in your investments for retirement, they are probably (pun intended) using these methods to guide their advice.

16.4   Chemical Risk Assessment

In the 1950s and 1960s, there was an awakening as to the toxic effects of chemicals in our environment, which stimulated the development of the chemical risk assessment paradigm. This paradigm was the central focus of the 1983 National Research Council report, *Risk Assessment in the Federal Government: Managing the Process.*[6] This book is commonly referred to as the "red book," and it is in this work where the four components of risk assessment were first laid out:

1. Hazard identification
2. Exposure assessment
3. Dose–response assessment
4. Risk characterization

The FDA also has a long history of development of risk assessment methods for both contaminants of foods and, later, food additives. For both of these issues, the FDA was evaluating what was considered "safe" in the context of food consumption. The concept of "safety" is a value-laden term that can mean very different things in different contexts and to different people, even among those who speak English. When we attempt to translate this concept into other languages, things get even more confused. This increases the challenge for negotiating international agreements related to issues that affect human or environmental safety.

16.5   Risk Assessment for Replicating Organisms

For chemical assessments, we are dealing with inert compounds, which (usually) do not change in concentration. The critical issues here are assessing the exposure dose and the response to that dose. When dealing with microbes, they often are not static, as the number of microbes can change over time. The USDA Agricultural Research Service (ARS) and the Animal and Plant Health Inspection Service (APHIS) both tackled this problem early in the 1990s. ARS constructed a microbial risk assessment modeling program to estimate the levels of microorganisms subjected to various conditions and mitigations.[7] At about the same time, APHIS evaluated the issue of replicating organisms that cause animal diseases. APHIS is charged with protecting the United States from the incursion of foreign animal- and plant-diseases. The agency is thus concerned with whether the pest or microbe is present and whether it could become established in the United States. Because APHIS had traditionally operated under the (unofficial) motto of "If in doubt, keep it out," they have an excellent record of preventing foreign disease outbreaks. This "zero risk" policy has proven useful but is no longer tenable in a modern world guided by the North American Free Trade Agreement (NAFTA) and the General Agreement on Tariffs and Trade (GATT).

APHIS began exploring the use of risk assessment in the early 1990s, using both quantitative and qualitative methods as were appropriate for the specific issues.[8] In recent years, APHIS has used risk assessment as the basis for regionalization to address the risk of foreign animal diseases. APHIS recognition of a country or region used to be viewed as the gold standard for the world to guide trade with other countries or regions before the advent of NAFTA and GATT. Given this large responsibility, APHIS continues to modify and update standards and methodology to be used in evaluating the risks of importing foreign animal diseases from various countries and regions.

16.6 Foodborne Pathogens

It should be obvious at this point that we should apply the methods of risk analysis to microbial pathogens in foods. In the last decade or so, there have been great leaps forward in the sophistication and understanding of methods and analyses for microbial risk assessment. The sanitary and phytosanitary agreements of the GATT[9] point to risk assessment to guide the international trade of animal and plant products. The exact guidance for risk assessments is not contained in the GATT documents, but they do refer to various international organizations as the standard setters. These international organizations continue to refine and update standards for risk assessment. WTO named the Codex Alimentarius Commission (CAC) as the standard-setting organization for microbial risk assessment. The CAC has developed guidelines for risk assessment of foods, which are under review by the Codex Committee on Food Hygiene. Information about the development of these standards is available from the CAC Web site: http://www.codexalimentarius.net

16.7 Microbial Risk Assessment Issues

When we focus on the issue of risk assessment of microbes in food we are faced with a collection of issues. The first question is whether the microbe is present. When a regulatory body sets a policy prohibiting the presence of certain bacteria in food by classifying the bacteria as an adulterant, it has truncated the range of mitigation options. With a regulatory standard of "no" bacteria of a certain species, we have limited our management options to address the broader issue of public health impact. An obvious example of this is the current FDA and USDA Food Safety and Inspection Service (FSIS) policy for zero tolerance of *Listeria monocytogenes* in food.[10] The FDA Center for Food Safety and Applied Nutrition (CFSAN) in cooperation with FSIS has done several risk analyses to evaluate the public health impact of *L. monocytogenes* contamination of foods under different management options.

In the context of international trade, a myriad of issues can be discussed. What is an acceptable level of risk? What is an acceptable level of safety? How do we proceed under GATT? These are all important concerns that need to be addressed within the broader context of risk. The WTO will deal with trade disputes around these issues in the future. Questions that scientific risk assessors need to ask in regard to regulatory issues, particularly international ones, include the following:

1. Is the product contaminated?
2. At what level is the product contaminated?
3. What is the public health impact of this level of contamination?
4. How do we assess equivalency for trade issues?

16.7.1 Is the Product Contaminated?

When we assess a contamination that is infrequent or unacceptable, we want to know if the contaminating pathogen is present. Our goal is to have every unit of product free of pathogens. We estimate the occurrence of contamination (yes/no) and manage the process by not allowing contaminated product to proceed in the product flow. This is the kind of program that the USDA has for *Escherichia coli* O157:H7 in hamburger. This pathogen has been identified as an adulterant by regulation, and no product that is thus contaminated can be offered for sale.[11] It should be noted that currently *E. coli* O157:H7 is only classified as an adulterant in the final ground product; however, the USDA has proposed new guidelines that would classify *E. coli* O157:H7 as an adulterant if found further up in the product stream.

16.7.2 At What Level Is the Product Contaminated?

It is almost impossible to assure that all meat and poultry is free of all pathogens such as *Salmonella*, *Campylobacter*, and others; therefore, the risk assessor wants to determine what levels of pathogen may be present and what mitigations may be needed to reduce these pathogens to a reasonable level. The risk assessor also needs to know what the dose of exposure will be in order to evaluate the potential health impacts.

16.7.3 What Is the Public Health Impact from This Level of Contamination?

For risk assessors and risk managers, this is usually the prime concern, as disease and death are the ultimate negative impacts of contaminated foods. There are multiple factors that have an impact on this area of microbial risk assessment, such as

1. *What is the range of doses?* Predictive microbial risk assessment as well as data on quantity of foods consumed by different population groups provide information to estimate the quantity of pathogens in the exposure dose.
2. *What is the dose–response for the average population?* Many studies have been done over the last 50 years to evaluate the infectious dose of various pathogenic enteric organisms. Unfortunately (for dose–response modelers), these studies were done several decades ago and are difficult to repeat in modern times due to current human studies restrictions. Microbial risk assessors must rely on the old studies, animal models, or information supplied from epidemiologic investigation of foodborne disease outbreaks. There is so much discussion about dose–response issues[12] related to human pathogens that it is almost a subfield of microbial risk assessment.
3. *What is the dose–response for the most sensitive populations?* The most sensitive populations may include very young, very old, or immunocompromised people; people undergoing chemotherapy; transplant patients; and people with other chronic debilitating diseases. These populations have been identified as the target subpopulations to evaluate the safety of microbial pathogens as well as chemicals in our food.

16.7.4 How Do We Assess Equivalency for Trade Issues?

This issue has gained importance as GATT-participating countries become more familiar with the requirements of the Sanitary and Phytosanitary Agreement. Microbial risk assessment will be the tool to address whether a food product processed one way in a particular country can be treated as equivalent to a product processed differently in another country. A pertinent example of this issue is European soft cheeses that are made from unpasteurized milk. The United States requires that the milk used in production of soft (unaged) cheese be pasteurized. Is the European standard of using unpasteurized milk to produce cheese equivalent to the U.S. standards, or is this a technical barrier to trade? Microbial risk assessors will be faced with doing risk assessments that can help national and international decision makers deal with this and other issues in the future.

16.8   Conclusions

Risk assessment is currently recognized as the standard tool for setting policy both at the national and international level. Formal quantitative risk assessment of microbial and other biological contaminants has become more sophisticated in order to provide decision makers the information they need to manage food safety issues in the modern world. Risk assessment does not guarantee that there will be no international trade disputes based on sanitary or phytosanitary issues. However, it does provide a common tool for all parties to use in evaluating scientific information about the risks.

References

1. Morgan, M.G., Risk analysis and management, *Sci. Am.*, July:32–41, 1993.
2. Federal Crop Insurance Reform and Department of Agriculture Reorganization Act of 1994, Public Law 103–354, Title III, Section 304, October 13, 1994.
3. Ruckleshaus, W.D., Risk, science, and democracy, in *Readings in Risk*, Glickman, T.S. and Gough, M. (Eds.), Resources for the Future, Washington, D.C., 1990, pp. 105–119.
4. Kaplan, S. and Garrick, B.J., On the quantitative definition of risk, *Risk Anal.*, 1(1):4–22, 1981.
5. Rasmussen, N.C., The application of probabilistic risk assessment techniques to energy technologies, *Ann. Rev. Energy*, 6:123–138, 1981.
6. National Research Council, *Risk Assessment in the Federal Government: Managing the Process*, National Academy Press, Washington, D.C., 1983.
7. U.S. Department of Agriculture, Agricultural Research Service, Predictive Microbial Risk Assessment Program, Web site: http://ars.usda.gov/Services/docs.htm?docid=6784, August 1, 2007.
8. Chang, L.L., Miller, L., Ahl, A., and McElvaine, M. (Eds.), *What APHIS is Doing in Risk Assessment*, Animal and Plant Health Inspection Service, U.S. Department of Agriculture, Riverdale, MD, 1994.
9. World Trade Organization Agreement on the Application of Sanitary and Phytosanitary Measures, Foreign Agriculture Service, U.S. Department of Agriculture Web site: http://www.fas.usda.gov/itp/policy/gatt/sps_txt.html August 1, 2007.
10. USDA, FSIS, Web site: http://www.fsis.usda.gov/Fact_Sheets/Listeria_monocytogenes/index.asp, August 1, 2007.
11. USDA, FSIS, Web site: http://www.fsis.usda.gov/Fact_Sheets/E_coli/index.asp, August 1, 2007.
12. Wilson, J.D., Of what use are dose-response relationships for human pathogens? *ORACBA News*, 4(1):1–5, 1999.

17

Zoonotic Diseases Risk Assessment and Mitigation

Moez Sanaa and Hussni O. Mohammed

CONTENTS

17.1 Introduction

Several authors and organizations have introduced different definitions for the term zoonosis; however, we believe that the definition adopted by the World Health Organization (WHO) is the one that makes the most sense and which many authors have adopted. The definition of zoonotic diseases adopted by the WHO is "those diseases and infections which are naturally transmitted between vertebrate animals and man" (WHO 1997). This proposed definition captures the essence of the meaning of zoonosis and emphasizes that the transmission of these diseases is under natural circumstances.

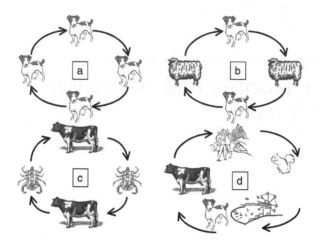

FIGURE 17.1

Classification of zoonotic diseases that is based on the maintenance cycle of the etiologic agent, a, direct zoonosis; b, cyclozoonosis; c, metazoonosis; and d, saprozoonosis.

The word zoonosis is derived from the Greek roots *zoo*, or animal, and *nosos*, or illness, thus, literally, diseases from animals (i.e., not exclusively infectious diseases). Zoonosis may be classified in various ways, including the direction of infection (human to other animals, or vice versa), types of agent (parasitic, viral, bacterial), or according to the role of vectors or external environment in their transmission cycles (e.g., direct, cyclo-, meta-, and saprozoonosis).

Figure 17.1 illustrates the classification of zoonotic diseases based on the maintenance cycle of the etiologic agent. Four classes have been proposed and these include direct zoonosis, cyclozoonosis, metazoonosis, and saprozoonosis. The term direct zoonosis is used to describe diseases where the etiologic agent is perpetuated in nature by a single vertebrate host, examples of such diseases include brucellosis and rabies (Figure 17.1a). Cyclozoonosis is a term used to describe diseases that require more than one vertebrate host for their transmission, e.g., taeniases (Figure 17.1b). There are some etiologic agents that require both vertebrate and invertebrate hosts, e.g., trypanosomiasis (Figure 17.1c), and they are described as metazoonosis. The last category of these four types of diseases is saprozoonotic diseases (Figure 17.4d). These are diseases where the etiologic agent survives and multiplies on inanimate reservoirs as well as vertebrates, e.g., cryptosporidiosis and listeriosis.

Another classification scheme for these zoonotic diseases is based on the direction of the transmission of the etiologic agents between susceptible hosts. If the etiologic agent is able to survive in a broader range of animals, and human, and capable of moving between and within these hosts, then it is described as anthropozoonotic. In these dynamics of infection, humans are generally considered dead-end hosts. Examples of such zoonotic agents could be seen in diseases like rabies and certain infections like cryptosporidiosis (Schwabe 1974). A second type of zoonosis which involves a broader range of hosts, including lower vertebrates, and could be transmitted in either direction is amphixenosis. Example of such zoonotic diseases are staphylococci infections (Schwabe 1974).

These are two common methods of classification of zoonotic disease and there are several other approaches for the classifications (Schwabe 1974). We encourage the reader to review them and adopt the classification that would be appropriate to their interest and their audience. However, we believe that this broad classification is useful in developing the foundation for illustrating the use of the risk assessment and mitigation approaches for the purpose of this chapter and include diseases that could be transmitted between animal and human, through different vectors/reservoirs that require live hosts, i.e., avian influenza and rabies, or could be transmitted through inanimate objects, including food.

The challenge for the scientist would be to provide information on these zoonotic diseases to the decision makers in a format so that risk mitigation measures could be undertaken to manage the associated hazards. Because of the complex and multifactorial nature of these zoonotic diseases, multidisciplinary approaches have to be adopted to identify the factors that lead to their introduction and perpetuation in populations of interest and make recommendations regarding cost-effective prevention and control measures. Two known scientific approaches lend themselves to address this need: epidemiology and risk assessment.

17.2   Epidemiologic Approaches

Epidemiology, the discipline that studies the determinants of health in a population, has three complementary objectives (Schwabe 1974). These objectives are as follows: determining the occurrence of disease in a population, identifying and predicting the factors that lead to its introduction and perpetuation, and shedding light on the strategies that might help controlling and preventing future occurrence. By virtue of its definition and tools, epidemiology doctrine is well suited to help contributing to the body of knowledge on zoonotic diseases.

There are several epidemiologic approaches that can contribute significantly to our understanding of the occurrence of these zoonotic diseases and the factors that might have contributed to their perpetuation and spread in a population. Cross-sectional studies can help in verifying the perception about the occurrence of the zoonotic disease. They are conducted by taking a representative sample from a population of interest and determining the presence of the etiologic agent of interest in the sample (Figure 17.2).

For example, verification of the presence of *Cryptosporidium parvum* among cattle populations in New York City Watershed (Baljer and Wieler 1999;

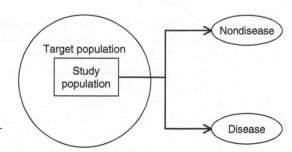

FIGURE 17.2
Conceptual framework for cross-sectional study design.

Wade et al. 2000b) determined the prevalence of the organism among one of the potential sources, i.e., cattle, in the area. Although cross-sectional studies are usually carried out at one point of time or in a short period, they can be used to identify factors that are associated with the presence of the organism (Mohammed et al. 1999a). This association can be used to shed light on the factors that might contribute to the presence of the organism in the population. The advantage of the cross-sectional study is that the study population represents a sample of the target population, and hence the rate of the occurrence of the hazard is a true estimate. Also, the distribution of the risk factors associated with the occurrence of the etiologic agent represents their distribution in the target population. Therefore, it is critical to ensure that the study population is a representative sample of the target population.

Case–control studies are another epidemiologic study design that can contribute significantly to our understanding of the factors that might play a role in the occurrence of these zoonotic diseases in target populations (Schlessleman et al. 1982). In a case–control study design, a sample of individual with the adverse effect of the disease will be compared to another subgroup without the disease with respect to the presence of a risk factor of interest or other related factors (Figure 17.3) .

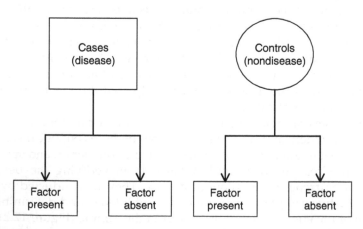

FIGURE 17.3
Schematic design for case–control studies.

Examples of case–control studies can be seen in outbreak investigations, where the interest is on identifying the factors that put individuals at risk of developing a disease and the factors associated with this risk. Gupta and Hass (2004) used data from the Milwaukee outbreak of cryptosporidiosis (1993) to estimate the incubation period for the hazard, *C. parvum*, and the force of infection. Also, case–control studies could help in identifying the factors that are associated with the transmission of the etiologic agent and the susceptible hosts (Kahlor et al. 2002; Naumova et al. 2003; Preiser et al. 2003).

Another epidemiologic approach that has great contributory role in the hazard identification step of the risk assessment is the retrospective cohort study design. Unlike the case–control design, which is also conducted in a retrospective manner, the retrospective cohort design would allow for testing a causal relation between a putative factor and the likelihood of an adverse effect associated with the etiologic agent of interest. Figure 17.4 describes the conceptual approach in the retrospective cohort study design.

In this design a cohort exposed to a factor that might affect the likelihood of the etiologic agent or adverse effect of interest will be selected and the cohort will be followed for a period to see whether the cohort experiences a hypothesized adverse effect in comparison to a group which was not exposed to the factor. The likelihood of the adverse effect in the two groups (exposed and nonexposed) will then be compared using the relative risk (ratio of the risk in the exposed group in comparison to that of the unexposed). Example of the use of retrospective cohort study approach in zoonotic disease identification can be found in the studies that were designed to identify the risk of transmission of *C. parvum* between hospital roommates

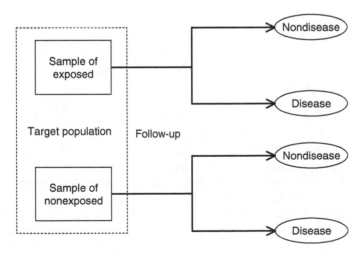

FIGURE 17.4
Schematic presentation of the retrospective cohort studies.

and the causes of mortality among an elk population (Bruce et al. 2000; Pople et al. 2001).

The same retrospective cohort approach could be used in a prospective manner to address specific causal hypothesis between an etiologic agent of a zoonotic disease and hypothesized factor. In the prospective design, the cohorts are selected concurrently and the follow-up is done in a prospective manner, i.e., the investigators age with the cohorts. Estimate of the adverse effect and impact of the factor under investigation is assessed in a similar way as in the retrospective studies.

In conclusion, epidemiologic approaches have the potential to contribute significantly to our knowledge regarding the factors that lead to the introduction and perpetuation of etiologic agents of zoonotic diseases and help us identify strategies to mitigate the associated risk. This knowledge is crucial for building science-based recommendations that are cost effective and have reproducible results. Depending on the resources available and the time line for assessing the risk associated with specific etiologic agent, the investigators could choose among strategies to identify factors or estimate the likelihood of the agent. Sometimes, we do not have all the available resources to carry out a comprehensive approach to understand or delineate the pathway by which these zoonotic agents might cause harmful effect to hosts of interests. Therefore, we might need to complement the observational epidemiologic studies with simulation approaches. This complementary approach could be found in another multidisciplinary approach, the risk assessment.

17.3   Risk Assessment Approaches

Risk assessment is one of the three components of risk analysis—risk assessment, risk communication, and risk management. It is the first step in risk analysis and describes a systematic approach aimed at assessing the likelihood of an adverse effect associated with the zoonotic disease. The adverse effect is a value judgment. Several regional and international organizations and agencies wrestled with the optimal approach to develop systematic guidelines and regulations that encourage participation of the stakeholders and ensure effective implementation of standardized approach for risk assessment. The risk assessment component is intended to identify the risk and quantifies the associated adverse consequence effects in a particular target population. The risk communication component is a continuous step of interaction and exchange of information between the stakeholders and the technical staffs who are involved in the risk management. The risk management component of the risk analysis reflects the process by which the identified risk is mitigated. Although these three components appear independent, they are not mutually exclusive. There is a large interdependency among them. Without initial perception about risk among the stakeholders, excellent communication between the technical/expert staff that would perform the risk assessment and the stakeholders, or intend and goal to mitigate this risk, there is no need to carry out the risk analysis. Successful risk management plans require full participation of all stakeholders and communication with the risk assessors.

Although there is consensus among the international organizations regarding the principles of risk analysis approach, there is still debate regarding the detailed steps of carrying out each component. Since its inception in 1970, the Environmental Protection Agency (EPA) attempted to standardize the approaches for carcinogens risk assessment by publishing a brief and concise guideline. In an attempt to standardize the risk assessment approach, the National Academy of Science (NAS) through the committee of institutional means for assessment of risk to public health of the National Research Council (NRC) developed a standard model (NAS 1983). The purpose was to develop a uniform risk assessment model to be used by all federal regulatory agencies in the United States. The general philosophy of the NRC risk assessment model was based on the characterization of the adverse health effect to humans as a result of exposure to environmental hazard. The NRC model has four steps: hazard identification, release assessment and dose–response, exposure assessment, and risk characterization (Figure 17.5). The report of the committee was published in what has come to be known as the "red book" (EPA 1984).

This model has served the risk assessment for environmental pollutants very well, and was adopted by several national and international organizations as a systematic approach to assess the potential risk. Examples of internationalization of this model can be seen in the guideline recommended by the Codex Alimentarius, the subcommittee of the Food and Agricultural Organization (FAO) for food standards. A minor modification

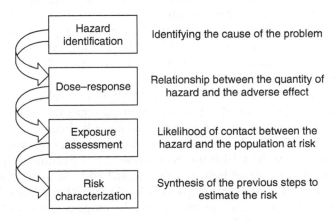

FIGURE 17.5
Steps in the National Research Council model for risk assessment.

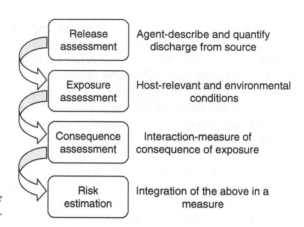

Release assessment	Agent-describe and quantify discharge from source
Exposure assessment	Host-relevant and environmental conditions
Consequence assessment	Interaction-measure of consequence of exposure
Risk estimation	Integration of the above in a measure

FIGURE 17.6
Conceptual   framework   for
Covello–Merkhofer model (1993).

was recommended by the Codex Alimentarius committee that requires full characterization of the etiologic agent of zoonosis.

However, adequacy of the model for different scenarios of adverse effects has been discussed critically over the years regarding its adequacy for different hazards and situations. As a result of these discussions, Covello and Merkhofer (1993) proposed a modification of the NRC model. A conceptual framework of the model is shown in Figure 17.6. The modification emphasizes separation between the hazard and the evidence that the identified hazard has a potential to put the public at risk. In a way, the hazard identification step is an independent step which has to be established first before the risk assessment is carried out. If the hazard is identified then a risk assessment should be carried out. This model is appealing because it puts more emphasis on the process of assessing the risk rather than arguing whether the hazard exists or not. If a consensus among the stakeholders is reached about a particular hazard then a risk assessment can be carried out to assess the potential impact in a particular population. Covello and Merkhofer's (1993) model consists of four steps following the hazard identification and includes release assessment, exposure assessment, consequence assessment, and risk estimation. Although these steps appear to be separate, they constitute an important building block in an integrated process, the risk assessment.

The difference between the original EPA (1983) model and the Covello and Merkhofer (1993) model is that the latter assumes that the hazard has already been identified. If the hazard has already been identified then further discussions should focus on how the hazard is released from its source, the pathways by which the population at risk becomes exposed, the consequence of the contact between the hazard and the susceptible hosts, and integration of the previous steps to estimate the risk associated with the specified hazard. This model represents an advantage over the initial model that was published in 1983.

The first step in Covello and Merkhofer's model focuses on the agent and addresses the potential release of the hazard or agent of interest from the source. The authors' intention was that this step would describe the quantity of hazard discharged from source and the likelihood of putting hosts of interest at risk. In this step the factors affecting release should be identified and their role in the release of the risk should be quantified. For example, if the hazard was identified as a pathogen, the incubation period and the factors that influence the incubation period should be described. Potential sources of the hazard should also be described, i.e., the reservoir hosts that harbor the pathogens and the incubation period of the pathogens in these hosts should be outlined. The conditions that influence the survival and viability of the pathogen (i.e., temperature, humidity, and acidity) in the environment should also be described in this step.

The second step in the Covello and Merkhofer (1993) model focuses on the potential exposure of the host to the identified hazard after release from the source. In this step, the relevant host and environmental factors that increase the likelihood of contact between the released hazard and the pathogen should also be delineated. Such factors include intensity and duration of exposure and how they relate to the transmission and perpetuation of the hazard, the potential routes of exposure, and the population at risk. Other factors that influence interaction between the susceptible host and released agent in the environment should also be described.

Covello and Merkhofer's (1993) model indicated that the exposure assessment step should be followed by the consequence assessment. In this step, measure of consequences of exposure such as health impact on the population at risk (incidence of disease) and ecological impacts (environmental degradation) are described and quantified.

The final step in the Covello and Merkhofer (1993) model is the risk estimation. This step consists of synthesis and integration of the release assessment, exposure, and consequence assessment to produce a single measure of risk associated with the hazard under consideration. In the process, the likelihood of adverse outcome under different scenarios is considered and the uncertainty associated with these scenarios is delineated.

Covello and Merkhofer's model received great attention among risk assessors and international organizations. For example, the Office of International Epizootic (OIE) has adopted the model because of its suitability for disputes in international trades between countries and regions (OIE 1995).

Although the initial model published by the EPA (EPA 1983) and the revised model of Covello and Merkhofer (1994) were used for a long period, there was a feeling that these models should be reviewed for their adequacy for pathogens and biosolids. As part of this review, EPA commissioned the NRC of the National Academy of Sciences to independently review the technical basis of the chemical and pathogen regulations applicable to sewage sludge that is applied to land. In July 2002, the NRC published a report entitled "Biosolids Applied to Land: Advancing Standards and Practices" in response to the EPA's request.

Over the years, the EPA has published several guidelines to standardize the approach in response to specific needs. These guidelines have been under continued review and revision and covered a broad spectrum of issues that included carcinogens; chemical, toxicological, and ecological issues; and pathogens (US EPA 1984, 1991, 1994, 2000) (NRC 1983, 1994). In the process of developing these guidelines, EPA had solicited input from the scientific community and the stakeholders in hope of improving the quality guidelines. The EPA had made it clear that these guidelines are intended to provide guidance only and have no binding effect on the agency or any other regulated entity. Such a provision is intended to provide room for improvement and incorporation of new scientific information and approaches.

Because of the continued concern about the quality of the environment, EPA has developed new guidelines for ecological risk assessment. The conceptual framework for the ecological risk assessment is shown in Figure 17.7. The model aimed to address the potential impact to the environment as a result of discharge of hazardous substance in the environment. The utility of this model has been expanded to be used in conjunction with the Superfund Act. These are funds made available for cleaning the sites that have been used to dump industrial waste in the environment. The model solicits major input from the stakeholder in hazard identification. The hazard identification step is the process of determining whether exposure to an agent (biological or infectious agent in our study) might cause an adverse health effect (disease) to animals and humans. It is a qualitative step through which evidences in the literature are collated and presented in a logical and rational manner to justify the concern regarding the perceived risk of a particular hazard. This step entails examination of the evidence in

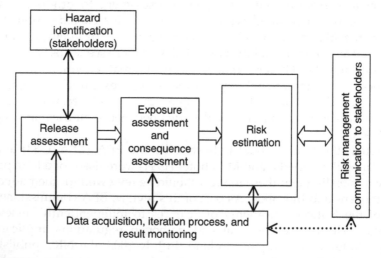

FIGURE 17.7
Steps in the risk assessment for animal and public health.

the literature for causation of disease. In the context of biological hazard in manure, the focus could be on pathogens that originated in agricultural animals, as the sources, and these have a potential to adversely affect human health, i.e., *Escherichia coli* and *Cryptosporidium* spp.

The release assessment step focuses on description and quantification of the potential through which the hazard is released or introduced to the population at risk (human, animal, plant, etc.). This step involves description of the type of hazard, potential sources, likelihood of release from the hosts, amount shed or excreted from the sources, the time, frequency, and length of release. In the process, there is accounting for the factors that might influence the release or introduction of the hazard to the target population. This step focuses mainly on the agent and its characteristics in terms of the host range, incubation period, and its survival on the external environment as it is released from the manure.

Following the release assessment, the model suggested that the exposure and consequence assessments should be investigated simultaneously. Exposure assessment focuses on the host of concern (animal or human) and the likelihood of coming into contact with the hazard (agent). Issues and factors related to the population at risk, routes of exposure, frequency, and intensity and duration of exposure (transmission), and the interaction between host–agent in environment are addressed in this step. The factors are discussed in the context of the likelihood of harmful effect to the susceptible host. In this step, it is important to determine the amount and number of organisms which are likely to constitute exposure taking into consideration the pathway of exposure. For example, the number of pathogens that are released by the source (shed by a calf on farm) in the immediate environment is not likely to be the same that the host at risk is likely to be exposed to in a city (through drinking water).

Consequence assessment is intended to describe and measure the impact of exposure on the population at risk. It entails describing the impact of exposure under a given scenario (incidence) and the potential variation in the response among the hosts of interest.

In the final step, the risk estimation, analysis, and integration of the collated data in the release, exposure, and consequence are performed. The purpose is to produce a quantification of the risk under different scenarios and its impact at the population level. It is the process of estimating adverse effects when taking into consideration different scenarios for the potential release of the pathogen, the dose–response relationship, and the likelihood of the hazard under different exposure circumstances. All associated uncertainties in the collected data and the variability in the computed estimates are captured in the estimations of the risk.

This evaluation process in developing models for the risk assessment emphasizes the fact that there is no "one size fits all" in the approach. And different goals might require different approaches but within the general framework of the risk assessment. One could imagine the challenge for developing a risk assessment for a complex zoonotic disease!

17.4 Possible Approaches for Zoonotic Risk Assessment

Different food safety agencies and authorities are requested to express an opinion on the basis of zoonoses control policies. Specially, technical scientific committees are asked to address assessment of risks related to zoonotic diseases causing major concern to public health. The scientific committees are invited to present a qualitative and, where possible, a quantitative risk assessment. The risk assessment should provide for analysis of different pathogens in relation to specific animal species and the type of their production. On the basis of this analysis, the committees are requested to identify a range of practical options which could be considered to control the presence of zoonotic agents at primary animal production level and throughout the rest of the production system in order to decrease the incidence of foodborne diseases in humans. In principle, controls should cover the whole food chain, from farm to table.

The protection of human health against diseases and infections transmissible directly or indirectly between animals and humans (zoonoses) is of vital importance. Therefore, the objective to investigate a particular zoonosis and zoonotic agents in animal populations should be clearly stated. The objective should take into account the incidence of these zoonoses in animal and human populations, feed and food, their gravity for humans, their potential economic consequences, and the existence of appropriate measures to reduce their prevalence. The risk management options could be strict hygiene barriers (ban importation and commercialization of concerned animal species and their products), cross-contamination avoidance, prevention of fecal contamination of water supplies, monitoring, etc.

Different methodologies to conduct risk assessments have been applied to assess the risk of various types of microbial hazards. In food microbiological risk assessment, the framework developed by Codex Alimentarius is now broadly used (Codex Alimentarius guideline on risk assessment in food). In parallel, the World Animal Health Organization (OIE) developed international standards for animal health and zoonoses. The guidelines are first and foremost designed to prevent the introduction of pathogens to new and susceptible animals and humans into an importing country during trade. The applications are concerned only with risk assessment of importing exotic diseases. In addition, the Terrestrial Animal Health Code does not generally distinguish between measures planned to preserve animal health and those intended to protect human health. There is now a demand to apply the risk assessment paradigm to zoonoses and diseases that are transmissible to humans directly or indirectly, whether or not animals are affected by such diseases.

Currently, no specific international guidelines exist on how to conduct risk assessment for endemic animal diseases or infections. While the methodologies used in any risk assessment are generally similar, the existent EPA, OIE, and Codex Alimentarius guidelines can be modified and adapted for risk assessments of endemic zoonotic diseases without major departure from the basic concepts. Because of the perpetuation of endemic diseases in a population and that several environmental, agent, and host factors play a role in their maintenance, a modification and integration of components from the existing guidelines would help addressing endemic diseases. EPA guidelines contribute on adding ecosystem health component, OIE captures the animal health component, and the Codex Alimentarius captures the food processing and the consumer components. The challenge would be to integrate the terminologies and methods used which vary a lot, among the different organizations and disciplines.

When dealing with zoonotic risk, the approach could differ from one assessment to another depending on the type of zoonoses: microbial hazard type and mode of transmission. According to the zoonoses classification presented in Figure 17.1 and the presence or absence of the disease (endemic vs. exotic) in the region one could use the OIE, Codex Alimentarius, EPA model, or an adaptation of one of the listed models. When the disease is exotic, the goal of risk assessment will be to evaluate the present preventive health system and specially its capacity to prevent the introduction of the disease. The risk assessment will help to define and propose different sorts of management measures:

- Restrict animal importation and contact with wildlife
- Adapt quarantine food inspection system
- Require measures before importing animal or animal products
- Inform travelers

The OIE guidelines are applicable in this case and would address the goal of risk assessment.

On the other hand, when the disease is endemic the goal of risk assessment will be to evaluate options and measures to be implemented to reduce or control the endemic level. The options and measures are intended to break the maintenance cycle (see Figure 17.1); reduce transmission between animals, or between animals and humans. The risk assessment will help to optimize animal health programs, control the contamination of animal products, control food or water contamination, and when relevant, control the spread of the disease within wildlife animals and other possible reservoirs including environmental ones.

As one could see there are several permutations or approaches for conducting zoonotic risk assessment. However, because of the focus of the book on microbial food contamination, we will focus our presentation on risk assessment foodborne zoonoses.

17.5 Risk Assessment of Foodborne Zoonosis

Zoonotic pathogens are the most common cause of foodborne diseases. Most of the serious emerging infections are of food animal origin: *Salmonella* enteritidis and *Campylobacter* from poultry; *Salmonella* Newport, *E. coli* O157:H7, and bovine spongiform encephalopathy (BSE) from cattle; the severe acute respiratory syndrome (SARS) virus originating from palm civet cats; and highly pathogenic avian influenza from ducks, geese, and chickens. The role of companion animals in exacerbating the risk of these diseases should not be ignored. Emerging factors that predispose to these zoonotic diseases are mainly linked to animal production practices. In the following sections we would like to explore the potential pathways for some of the zoonotic diseases.

17.5.1 Pathway

Ideally, risk assessment of foodborne zoonoses should cover the whole food chain, from farm to table (Figure 17.8). Farm animals, affected by the zoonotic diseases, shed the pathogens and carry the pathogens in their gastrointestinal tracts, from where they spread to other animals, their primary products, and farm environment. For example, cows with mastitis can shed huge quantities of bacteria in milk and maintain the infection within the farm via the milking machine. Raw milk may also be contaminated from environmental sources during milking, storage, and transport.

For meat production, cross-contamination can occur during transportation and at preslaughter pens and during processing.

Another source of zoonotic foodborne pathogens is contaminated water, such as inadequately treated or inappropriately applied wastewater, used in

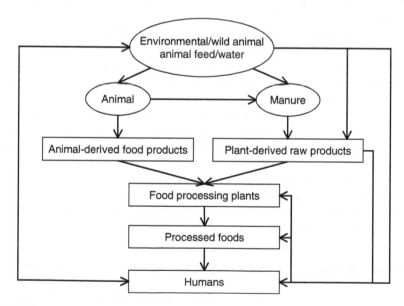

FIGURE 17.8
Zoonotic foodborne risk assessment pathway.

irrigation. Of major concern are waterborne pathogens such as bacteria (*Shigella, E. coli,* and *Campylobacter*), viruses (Norwalk virus), and parasites (such as *Giardia* and *Cryptosporidium*).

After the food leaves the farm, cross-contamination can occur during transportation and processing, i.e., heat treatment or filtration cannot eliminate certain pathogens. It is not unreasonable to control or eliminate the hazard at the source. So far, few safety food strategies center the effort at preharvest stage. Risk management of food safety risks paid more attention on implementing harmonized systems such as Hazard Analysis and Critical Control Point (HACCP), mainly focused on processing. For some microbial hazards, it is crucial to identify preharvest options for preventing hazards from entering the supply chain.

Another likelihood of contamination might take place further down the line for processed foods. After processing, transportation, storage at inadequate conditions, and food handling, certain microbial hazards can increase the level of contamination. In addition, consumer behavior could increase, limit, or eliminate the risk associated with a particular hazard. For example, some consumers like to cook food well done before eating it. This cooking process will no doubt reduce the risk associated with a particular hazard.

When contaminated food is ingested by a consumer, the consequences can have various degrees of severity:

- Microbial hazard fails to infect the consumer and no adverse effect is observed
- Consumer is infected without clinical signs
- Infection presents clinical signs with or without sequelae
- Disease is severe and the issue could be fatal

The degree of severity depends on the interaction between host factors—pathogen factors and environmental factors.

Analyzing every step of the full process from the primary source exposing animals to the human host adverse consequences may be justified.

Today, tools of farming, processing foods, food distribution, and marketing are not simple. Breakdown at a single step could have directly or indirectly catastrophic consequences (contaminated vaccines or feedstuff). We must be constantly aware of likelihood of malfunctions and errors. Traditionally, activities and plants are designed and operated by applying references to codes and standards. Now the trend is a more functional system approach where the focus is on what to achieve, rather than the solution required. Hence, the adequacy of a risk assessment modeling approach could not be assessed by solving a specific problem, but by whether it helps in achieving the goal. It is more pertinent to address the goodness of appropriateness of a specific model to be used in a specific risk analysis and decision contexts. Obviously, a model can be more or less good in describing the system but its capacity to reflect the key feature is more important.

17.5.2 Exposure Assessment

Modular process risk model approach is recognized as an important tool to identifying pathogen pathways and quantifying the presence of the pathogen at the farm, processing, storage and distribution, and consumer handling sectors of the food chain. The objective of the process model is to describe the transmission of the pathogen along the food pathway and develop a quantitative exposure model that meets the risk management goals, which may include animal health risk, occupational risk, trade risk, and foodborne risk (Figure 17.9). In a way, a compartmental approach might be more informative about the system and its relation to the risk of zoonotic diseases. The approach would provide more insight into the system and allow for a better appreciation or understanding of the complexity of the production. Technical experts assigned to each module provide information on the likely pathogen pathways, and the likely impact of current practices on the prevalence and concentration of the pathogen. For each module, the objective is to describe mathematically the relation between the input and output for the number of pathogens per unit of concern (e.g., herd, flocks,

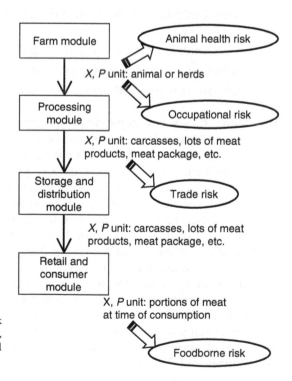

FIGURE 17.9
Example of modular process risk model framework. X: concentration, P: prevalence of the considered hazard.

animal, bulk tank milk, meat, unit of food product, etc.), (X: concentration), and the proportion of contaminated units (P: prevalence).

The on-farm module objective is to evaluate the likelihood of entry and establishment of disease/infection within one farm or spread and transmission to other farms. The output of the farm module could be generated using either empirical approaches or mathematical modeling. Empirical approaches assess, for example, the prevalence of infected animals by observation (cross-sectional and longitudinal studies, monitoring, and surveillance data). Classical statistical analysis techniques or Bayesian techniques could be used to assess uncertainty related to the observable quantities and to describe the variability of the observable quantities between farms, geographical area, and time.

On the other hand, the mathematical modeling approaches assess prevalence of infected animals as a function of a number of observable quantities (animal densities, rate of transmission, animal movements, etc.). Modeling is used to get insight into the pathogen pathways, to identify the risk contributors, and to see the effect of changes.

In the processing module, control of cross-contamination of fresh meat with fecal pathogens remains a priority issue in the slaughterhouse environment. Empirical approaches, although they mimic nature closely, are difficult to implement, time-consuming, and expensive. If time and expense have become major constraints, a viable alternative could be to carry out small experiments at different small processing steps in order to assess statistically the transfer parameter from one carcass to other carcasses by direct or indirect contacts. The transfer parameters, the prevalence of infected slaughtered animals, concentration of the pathogen in fecal material, the growth and survival conditions, and parameters on the microbial hazard are linked mathematically to the processing model outputs (number of infected portion of meat and concentration per gram of meat). The same approaches could also be used to understand a complex step in the system, i.e., storage distribution, retail, and consumer models.

In the mathematical approach, the starting point for all the models or submodels is that we lack perfect knowledge about the observable quantities and we use probabilities to express this lack of knowledge. In addition we should integrate in the model inputs variability and their dynamics (e.g., concentration of the pathogen in meat, cooking time, and temperature are variables). We also use probabilities to describe variability. Simulation models are used to capture probabilistic behavior and allow us to estimate key statistics such as means or tail probabilities of distributions that cannot be derived analytically. Traditionally, simulation models are categorized into two broad categories. Systems simulation models capture the dynamics and behavior of interacting elements of a system, such as a manufacturing facility. These models are driven by changes that occur in the system over time. Monte-Carlo simulation models, on the other hand, are time independent. They involve repeated sampling from probability distributions of model inputs to characterize the distributions of model outputs.

Monte-Carlo simulation models generate distributions of potential out-comes of key model variables along with their likelihood of occurrence.

The simulation models that we need in zoonotic risk assessment applica-tions must combine the two traditional simulation model categories.

17.5.3 Dose–Response Assessment

The biological foundation for dose–response models derives from major steps in the disease process: exposure, infection, illness, and consequences (recovery, sequel, or death). The issue of exposure is the result from the interactions between the pathogen, the host, and the food matrix. Tradition-ally, the concept of minimum infectious dose (MID) is used to measure the infectivity of an organism. MID is an expression of the lowest number of organisms required to initiate an infection in any individual under given circumstances. The term recognizes that each organism has the potential to cause an infection but builds upon the variation that exists in the actual dose required, the virulence of the agent, and the individuals' response. For some pathogenic bacteria, the minimum infectious dose is well established. This traditional interpretation of dose–response information assumes the exist-ence of a threshold level of pathogens that must be ingested in order for the microorganism to produce infection or disease. Attempts to define the numerical value of such thresholds in test populations have typically been unsuccessful.

An alternative hypothesis, due to the potential for microorganisms to grow within the host, is that a single viable infectious pathogenic organism is able to induce infection (single-hit concept). Mathematically, there is always a nonzero probability of infection or illness when a host is exposed to an infectious pathogenic organism. The minimal infectious dose is of value 1 and the probability at this dose is in general very small. Practically, testing experimentally the existence or absence of a threshold, at both the individual and population levels, is impossible. Experiments are usually designed to assess response at relatively high doses (microbial detection limit and limited number of experimental units) and small frequency of infection or illness cannot be precisely assessed. If one assumes the existence of threshold, it cannot be considered as constant and will vary depending on the result from the interaction between the pathogen, the host, and the food matrix.

The threshold model implies a definitive threshold below which no infection would occur. So the nonthreshold model is a more cautious and more appropriate approach than the threshold model in some circumstan-ces. Therefore, we believe that prudent public health protection requires the application of nonthreshold approaches to the assessment of microbial dose–response.

Dose–response model gives the probability of illness according to the amount of ingested pathogenic microorganisms. Among d-ingested microorganisms, some might survive human host barriers and later initiate infection and cause illness. Illness probability was defined as the probability of achieving this sequence of events. If each ingested microorganism has the same probability to provoke illness r, then the number of microorganisms surviving different barriers follows a binomial distribution. If each micro-organism is capable of inducing illness, then the probability of illness given d-ingested microorganisms is the complement of the probability of absence of illness:

$$P_{ill}(d,r) = 1 - (1 - r)^d$$

This model is named single-hit model.

The underlying assumption of the single-hit model is then the absence of interaction between microorganisms where r is an assumed constant, independent of the size of the ingested dose, the state of the microorganisms, the host, and previous exposure to the pathogen.

The exponential and beta-Poisson models are examples of the class of mechanistic models that are derived by assuming that one organism, if it survives to colonize, is sufficient to initiate the infection and disease process. As is the case in all models where the parameters are estimated at the population level, in the exponential model the exposed dose is known at population level and doses at the individual level are assumed random with Poisson probability distribution. The major assumption in this model is that the hazard is randomly distributed in the serving and the probability of ingesting a known number of pathogens in a dose of an average concentration of d is Poisson distributed. Therefore, it is important to remember that the exponential model does not estimate the risk at individual level but at population level and the model assumes that the interaction between the hazard and the host is constant for every individual in the population:

$$P_{ill}(\lambda,r) = \sum_{d=0}^{\infty} \left(1 - [1-r]^d\right) \exp(-\lambda)\frac{\lambda^d}{d!} = 1 - \exp(-r\lambda)$$

The exponential model is an extension of single-hit model that captures the variability in the amount of microbial hazard that is ingested among individuals. It has been used in several incidents to describe the relationship between the amount ingested to a hazard and the reaction of hosts to this amount. The model does not take account of the variability among hosts' responses.

In the beta-Poisson model, we consider, in addition to the variability between doses, the variability between individual r's. Not all hosts respond in a similar way to exposure to a similar dose. As illustrated above, some hosts have a relatively more severe reaction to exposure to a known dose than the others. Assuming that r follows a beta distribution of parameters α and β, the beta-Poisson model is derived on solving the following integral:

$$P_{ill}(\lambda,\alpha,\beta) = \int_{0}^{\infty} (1 - \exp[-r\lambda]) \frac{\Gamma(\alpha+\beta)}{\Gamma(\alpha)\Gamma(\beta)} r^{\alpha-1}(1-r)^{\beta-1}dr$$

This integral has a solution in some circumstances, and leads to a simpler mathematical equation:

$$P_{ill}(\lambda, \alpha, \beta) \approx 1 - \left(1 + \frac{\lambda}{\beta}\right)^{-\alpha} \text{ for } \alpha \ll \beta \text{ and } \beta \gg 1.$$

Therefore, the beta-Poisson distribution would allow us to capture, in addition to the variation in the ingested amount of hazard, the variation in the response to this dose among the hosts.

17.5.4 Risk Characterization

Risk characterization integrates the results of dose–response and exposure assessment into a risk statement that includes one or more quantitative estimates of risk. An essential prerequisite to risk characterization is the clear definition of output. Examples of possible outcomes are expected risk infection to a typical person, expected number of illness or deaths in a community, upper confidence limit to expected number of illness, upper confidence limit for illness to a highly exposed person, or maximum number of illnesses in a community at any one time. The choice between all the possible outcomes has to be decided in relation to the needs of decision maker.

The "annual marginal risk" (AMR) is one of the central possible outcomes. This can be defined as the "expected annual risk of illness for one random individual after one year intake of the considered food product." The term marginal is used as opposed to the term conditional. It refers to the margins of a contingency table and provides information on the average state of the population. So, AMR is here the average of the annual individual risk (AR_i). The latter (AR_i) is conditional to the characteristics of the given individual, e.g., his or her health status and his or her consuming and exposure profile.

The marginal annual risk is also an estimate of the average fraction of individuals affected by the concerned disease after one year of exposure.

The annual risk of illness, AR, of an individual "i" subjected to n exposures could be expressed:

$$AR_i = 1 - (1 - r)^{\sum_{j=1}^{n} d_j}$$

where d_j is the ingested dose during the exposure j ($j = 1, 2, \ldots, n$).

This also implies that the annual risk, given a sum of doses d_j, will be the same whatever the repartition of these doses during the year. A practical approach is suggested in which typical serving with constant serving size of q grams is assessed. Furthermore, only contaminated servings are considered. The amount of contaminated serving is given by $c \times p$, where c is the average number of typical servings consumed per individual per year and p the prevalence of contamination of the typical servings. With the dose ingested at each exposure equal to the product of the mass of a typical serving q and the concentration of microorganisms in those contaminated typical servings at the time of consumption λ_j (colony forming units per gram or CFU/g), the annual risk for a given individual i is given by:

$$AR_i = 1 - (1 - r)^{q \times \sum_{j=1}^{c \times p} \lambda_j}$$

17.5.5 Simple Model for the Annual Marginal Risk

If the conditions of the central limit theorem are fulfilled (large $c \times p$ and λ_j symmetrically distributed), the term $\sum_{j=1}^{c \times p} \lambda_j$ could be simplified in $c \times p \times \bar{\lambda}$, where $\bar{\lambda}$ is the expected value for λ_j in CFU/g. We so obtain what we call the simple model.

If the illness probability r is constant between individual hosts, AMR per consuming individual is

$$AMR = 1 - (1 - r)^D$$

where $D = q \times c \times p \times \bar{\lambda}$.

If there is variability in illness probability between hosts, with the function $f(r)$ being the probability distribution for r, the AMR is given by

$$AMR = \int_0^1 \left[1 - (1 - r)^D \right] f(r)\, dr$$

Assuming that r follows a beta distribution of parameters, α and β, the solution to this integral is

$$AMR = 1 - \frac{\Gamma(\alpha + \beta)\Gamma(\beta + D)}{\Gamma(\beta)\Gamma(\alpha + \beta + D)}$$

where Γ is the gamma function, $\Gamma(s) = \int_0^{+\infty} t^{s-1} e^{-t} dt$. As α and β approach infinity then AMR approaches

$$AMR = 1 - (1 - \bar{r})^D$$

where $\bar{r}$ is the mean illness probability, $\bar{r} = \dfrac{\alpha}{\alpha + \beta}$.

17.5.6 Complex Model for the Annual Marginal Risk

Sometimes, the conditions of the central limit theorem are not fulfilled. This is the case when the product is seldom consumed (c is low), the occurrence of the contamination of the product is rare (p is low), or the distribution of the concentration per typical serving λ_j is not symmetric.

The variability in the concentration values should then be taken into account in the calculation of the AMR:

$$\text{AMR} = 1 - \int\limits_0^1 \int\limits_0^\infty (1-r)^{q \times \sum_{j=1}^{cxp} \lambda_j} \times f(r) \times g(\lambda_j)\, d\lambda_j dr$$

where $g(\lambda_j)$ is the probability distribution function of λ_j. This is what we call the "complex model."

The distribution of λ_j must be a strictly positive and continuous distribution. The lognormal and gamma distributions fulfill those conditions. In both cases, dissymmetry occurs when the dispersion is high. Spatial or temporal high dispersions of microorganisms among typical servings may be due to either clumping phenomena (contamination in or on solid matrix products, production of colonies), variation in the sanitary performance of a process, or within- and between-subject variability in consumer handling and storage. Both the latter causes lead to various recontamination, cross-contamination, and subsequent microbial survival and growth before ingestion.

Two options are possible: use directly the output of exposure assessment simulation model or fit the outcomes using a strictly positive probability distribution.

In contrast to the simple model, the complex models do not have straightforward analytical solutions. To resolve the integration, one could use numerical method using the Monte-Carlo simulation method. Iterations would be performed leading to the distribution of the AR_i , the arithmetic mean of which is an estimate of the AMR.

17.5.7   Model Use

In principle, the modeling approach is used not only to assess the risk distribution but also to provide valuable information on the uncertainty associated with the inputs and control options to be suggested to the risk managers. Sensitivity analysis has to be conducted to identify key contributors to variability and uncertainty in model outputs. In the majority of conducted probabilistic risk assessments, the variability of the output is mainly attributable to variability and uncertainty in a small number of inputs. In identifying those inputs, we are able to suggest targeting research efforts for the characterization of uncertainty in small number of important inputs. In addition to sensitivity analysis, the simulation model could be used to analyze some if-scenarios, and do formal decision analyses, such as multiattributes analyses, cost-benefit analysis, and utility-based analysis. Risk assessment models provide decision support but not hard decisions. The decision maker, risk manager, does his or her analysis in a wider decision-making context.

17.6 Conclusion

Assessing the impact of zoonotic diseases on public health is a daunting task. Nevertheless, the responsibility is unavoidable. The challenge to the scientific community is to develop objective, systematic, science-based, valid, and reproducible methods to address this task. Historical approaches to control and eradicate these zoonotic diseases have relied on prevention and intervention strategies. Nowadays, because of the advances in methodology to address multidisciplinary approaches and acceptability of the concept among scientists who used unidisciplinary approaches, tools like risk assessment could offer an objective approach. The risk assessment approach allows a multidisciplinary team to identify scientists and stakeholders needed to carry an interdisciplinary approach to address the perceived zoonotic problem.

In this spirit, we have proposed a framework for the risk assessment that could be used to address the zoonotic disease problem. The proposed approach builds on existing risk assessment approaches to what we perceive as components of zoonotic diseases, i.e., food safety and animal disease health. Although the primary goal of the food safety risk assessment model is to mitigate the risk of transmission of zoonotic hazard through food and water, it focuses mainly on the transmission stage and does not address the whole cycle of zoonotic diseases. Similarly, the animal health risk assessment model addresses the transmission and perpetuation of the zoonotic pathogens among animal populations which is a component of the zoonotic cycle. In a way, our proposed approach is an attempt toward integrating both the animal health and the food safety models in a complementary approach to address the zoonotic problem. The proposed model encourages scientists and stakeholders to think of the big picture of zoonotic cycle through interdisciplinary approaches to help avert some of the anticipated consequences of these diseases.

Although the proposed zoonotic disease risk model might not have all the answers for the complete cycle of these etiologic agents, it has the potential to highlight the gap in knowledge that is needed to be filled working toward an integrated approach. It is an open invitation for scientists and stakeholders to start thinking about the big picture and develop integrated and iterative approaches rather than sequential approaches that helps in maintaining the animal and ecological health systems and preserving the well-being of humans. At the time of shrinking resources, it is critical to examine the big picture first and design compartmental, integrated, and complementary approaches. We should examine the risk of zoonotic diseases to human health in the context of the whole ecosystem and then design a systematic approach that deals with the risk at the source or components of this ecosystem. The role of scientists in this regard is explaining the uncertainty in the process and the impact of this uncertainty in the recommendation for risk mitigation.

References

Baljer, G. and Wieler, L.H. 1999. Animals as a source of infections for humans—diseases caused by EHEC. *Dtsch. Tierarztl. Wochenschr.* 106, 339–343.

Bruce, B.B., Blass, M.A., Blumberg, H.M., Lennox, J.L., del Rio, C., and Horsburgh, C.R., Jr. 2000. Risk of *Cryptosporidium parvum* transmission between hospital roommates. *Clin. Infect. Dis.* 31, 947–950.

Covello, V.T. and. Merkhofer, M.W. 1993. *Risk Assessment Methods. Approaches for Assessing Health and Environmental Risks.* Plenum Press, New York.

Environmental Protection Agency (EPA). 1984. Risk Assessment and Management: Framework for Decision making. EPA/600/9-85/002.

Gupta, M. and Haas, C.N. 2004. The Milwaukee *Cryptosporidium* outbreak: Assessment of incubation time and daily attack rate. *J. Water Health* 2(2), 59–69.

Kahlor, L., Dunwoody, S., and Griffin, R.J. 2002. Attributions in explanations of risk estimates 27. *Public Underst. Sci.* 11, 243–257.

Naumova, E.N., Egorov, A.I., Morris, R.D., and Griffiths, J.K. 2003. The elderly and waterborne *Cryptosporidium* infection: Gastroenteritis hospitalizations before and during the 1993 Milwaukee outbreak. *Emerg. Infect. Dis.* 9, 418–425.

Pople, N.C., Allen, A.L., and Woodbury, M.R. 2001. A retrospective study of neonatal mortality in farmed elk. *Can. Vet. J.* 42, 925–928.

Preiser, G., Preiser, L., and Madeo, L. 2003. An outbreak of cryptosporidiosis among veterinary science students who work with calves. *J. Am. Coll. Health* 51, 213–215.

Schlesselman, J.J. 1982. *Case-Control Studies—Design Conduct, Analysis.* Oxford University Press, New York.

Schwabe, C.W. 1984. *Veterinary Medicine and Human Health*, 3rd ed. Williams & Wilkins, Baltimore, MD.

Wade, S.E., Mohammed, H.O., and Schaaf, S.L. 2000. Prevalence of Giardia sp. *Cryptosporidium parvum* and *Cryptosporidium andersoni* (syn. *C. muris*) correction of *Cryptosporidium parvum* and *Cryptosporidium muris* (*C. andersoni*) in 109 dairy herds in five counties of southeastern New York. *Vet. Parasitol.* 93, 1–11.

18

Codex Alimentarius:
What It Is and Why It Is Important

H. Michael Wehr

CONTENTS

18.1 Introduction

The Codex Alimentarius (meaning food code) Commission, or Codex as the organization is usually termed, is an international intergovernmental food standards organization whose importance increased substantially after the signing of the GATT Uruguay Round Trade Agreements and the implementation of the World Trade Organization (WTO). With the formal recognition given to Codex in the WTO Agreement on the Application of Sanitary and Phytosanitary Measures (SPS Agreement), Codex moved to the forefront of international science-based standards setting bodies associated with food safety and quality. Its standards, guidelines, and recommendations have substantial impact on food products that are internationally traded. The efforts of Codex in the areas of sound science and risk analysis have substantially affected the manner in which international food standards setting is undertaken. Codex additionally has the potential to significantly affect domestic food regulation because of the linkage of Codex to international trade agreements, and because of its impact on food regulatory bodies in individual member countries.

This chapter describes the history and organization of Codex, why it has become increasingly important, and how it develops and adopts food safety and quality standards. The policies Codex has established to undertake its scientific standards setting activities are described. The impact of the recently concluded Joint FAO/WHO Evaluation of the Codex Alimentarius and Other FAO and WHO Work on Food Standards on Codex management and operation is discussed. The chapter also outlines the work of Codex in the field of food hygiene, focusing on the Codex Committee on Food Hygiene (CCFH). The types of food hygiene codes of practice and other food hygiene texts that are developed by Codex are reviewed as is the work of CCFH in the field of microbiological risk assessment and microbiological risk management. The chapter briefly mentions the other noteworthy ongoing work in Codex.

18.2 What Is Codex?

The Codex Alimentarius Commission (CAC) is an international intergovernmental body that develops science-based food safety and commodity standards, guidelines, and recommendations to promote consumer protection and facilitate world trade.[1,2] Codex is a subsidiary body of two United Nations organizations, the Food and Agriculture Organization (FAO) and the World Health Organization (WHO). The Codex Secretariat's offices are located within the FAO offices in Rome, Italy. The work of the Codex Secretariat is funded through the FAO and WHO while much of the cost of operating the various committees of Codex is paid for by those countries that serve as hosts for the meetings of the committees (see below). Currently, Codex has 172 member countries. Full membership is also given to Regional Economic Integration Organizations (REIO).* Currently there is only one REIO, the European Commission.

Codex was established in 1962 when FAO and WHO recognized the need for international food standards to protect the health of consumers and to provide standards of identity and quality to facilitate in increasing global trade in foodstuffs. Under the General Principles of the Codex Alimentarius,[1] Codex is charged with developing food standards for adoption and use by member countries. The Codex Alimentarius itself is a collection of international food standards adopted by the CAC and presented in a uniform manner. The purpose of these standards is to protect the health of consumers and facilitate fair practices in food trade.[1] Codex texts are in the form of specific food standards, codes of practice, guidelines, and recommendations. The scope of the Codex Alimentarius includes standards for all principle foods, whether processed, semiprocessed, or raw, for distribution to the consumer. Materials to be used for further processing into foods are included in a standard to the extent necessary to achieve the purpose of the standard. The Codex Alimentarius includes provisions for food hygiene, food additives, pesticide residues, contaminants, food irradiation, labeling, and methods of analysis and sampling. It also includes provisions of an advisory nature in the form of codes of practice, guidelines, and recommended measures. Since its inception, Codex has adopted approximately 300 commodity or general standards and guidelines, more than 750 food additive provisions covering 222 food additives and almost 3000 pesticide and veterinary drug maximum residue limits covering 222 pesticides and 44 veterinary drugs.[2] The work and activities of Codex are available on the Internet through the FAO Home Page.†

18.3 Why Is Codex Important?

Although Codex has been recognized within the international food scientific and regulatory communities since its inception and has provided an important service in developing food safety and quality standards, it is only recently that Codex has emerged to become a key international standards setting body.

In 1994, the GATT Uruguay Round of International Trade Negotiations established the WTO and several trade agreements including the Agreement on the Application of Sanitary and Phytosanitary Measures (SPS Agreement) and the Agreement on Technical Barriers to Trade (TBT

---

* Regional Economic Integration Organization refers to an organization constituted by sovereign states of a given region which has legal competence in respect of specific matters.
† http://www.codexalimentarius.net

Agreement).[3] Article 3.1 of the SPS Agreement requires countries to base their sanitary and phytosanitary measures on international standards, guidelines, or recommendations unless they can scientifically justify a more stringent standard. Section 3 (a) of Annex A of the SPS Agreement states that, for food safety, certain standards, guidelines, and recommendations established by the CAC shall be recognized as international standards under the agreement. These include, among others, those relating to food additives, veterinary drug and pesticide residues, contaminants, methods of analysis and sampling, and codes and guidelines of hygienic practice. Article 3.2 of the SPS Agreement states that a country's sanitary and phytosanitary measures which conform to international standards, guidelines, or recommendations shall be presumed to be consistent with the relevant provisions of the SPS Agreement. Thus, although Codex standards are voluntary, countries have an obligation to base their own food safety standards on the work of Codex. Additionally, products produced in accordance with Codex standards essentially have safe harborage in international trade.

Codex is also important within the context of the TBT Agreement, which deals with product specifications not related to safety including commodity composition, packaging, and certain labeling standards. The TBT Agreement also requires countries to use international standards. While Codex as an organization is not specifically referenced in the TBT Agreement, the WTO has recognized Codex standards as those to be used preferentially in resolving technical trade disputes.

Codex thus becomes a true international focal point for food safety and quality with major impact on international trade and, potentially, on domestic food regulations. Its importance is therefore significantly greater than it was previously.

18.4   Structure of Codex

Codex undertakes its work through the CAC and a series of horizontal general subject committees, vertical commodity committees, task forces, and regional coordinating committees. Horizontal committees are those committees whose work applies to multiple commodities, such as the CCFH. Vertical committees are those that deal with a single commodity type or single commodity grouping (e.g., fish and fishery products) and whose work encompasses all aspects associated with that commodity (e.g., composition, food additives, pesticide residues, food hygiene, product labeling, and methods of analysis). An executive committee with international geographic representation acts for the commission between its meetings; the commission currently meets annually. The structure of Codex is shown in Figure 18.1.

Ten worldwide general subject or horizontal committees establish Codex standards, codes of practice, or guidelines that apply across all

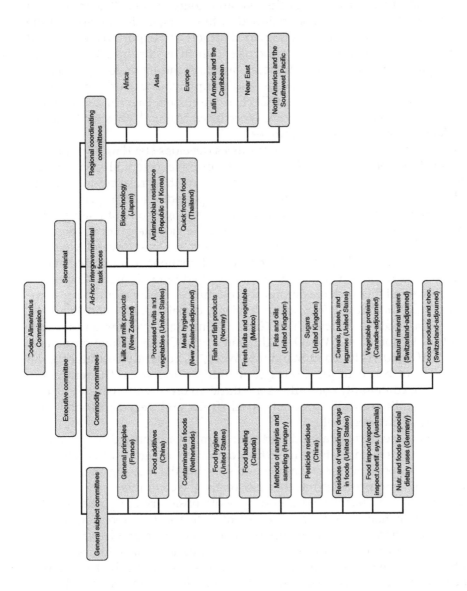

FIGURE 18.1

The structure of Codex Alimentarius.

commodities. Included in this category is the work of Codex committees that involve pesticide residue maximum residue limits (MRLs) (Committee on Pesticide Residues), veterinary drug MRLs (Committee on Residues of Veterinary Drugs in Foods), maximum permitted use levels for food additives (Committee on Food Additives), and contaminants (Committee on Contaminants in Foods). Also included in this category is the work of the Codex committees on food labeling, food import and export inspection and certification systems, general principles (which is the initial forum for Codex policy and procedural matters), nutrition and foods for special dietary uses, and methods of analysis and sampling. The work of the final general subject committee, the CCFH, is discussed later in the chapter. Readers are referred to the Codex Procedures Manual[1] for specific terms of reference for all Codex committees.

A series of Codex commodity committees develops standards specific for various food products. These standards provide essential composition information for product types as well as information relating to residues and contaminants (pesticides and other compounds as appropriate), food additives, food hygiene, labeling, packaging, and methods of analysis. For these latter areas, the commodity standards reference the general standards developed by the horizontal committees. Over the past several years, as Codex has completed much of the needed international commodity standards and as the interest and emphasis has shifted to food safety, Codex has de-emphasized the work of commodity committees. Many commodity committees have adjourned (e.g., meat hygiene, cereals, pulses and legumes, and cocoa/cocoa products). The Codex Alimentarius Commission, as a result of the Joint FAO/WHO Evaluation of the Codex Alimentarius and Other FAO and WHO Food Standards Work,[4] is currently considering the possibility of restructuring Codex commodity committees. Currently, the most active commodity committees are those involved with fish and fishery products, milk and milk products, fresh fruits and vegetables, and processed fruits and vegetables.

Each of these horizontal and vertical committees is hosted by a country (refer to countries indicated under the committee in Figure 18.1). The host country is responsible for arranging and securing the meeting site, pays for the meeting, and provides the chairperson for the committee.

Codex has also established a new type of subsidiary body, the Ad-Hoc Intergovernmental Task Force. The intent is to use task forces when the work is considered to be essentially of a one-time nature or when the task is limited and occasional. Currently, there are three active task forces dealing with foods derived from modern biotechnology, antimicrobial resistance, and quick frozen foods. Task forces on animal feeding and fruit and vegetable juices have also been established and adjourned.

A series of regional coordinating committees is also maintained by Codex. These committees at one time were primarily involved with the establishment of standards applicable only to the region. Today, they are primarily involved with reviewing and analyzing the broader Codex issues as they may affect the region. Regional coordinating committees also serve as a venue for establishing regional positions on proposed international standards.

Codex also utilizes the work and input of two other types of organizations. Joint WHO/FAO Expert Committees provide technical scientific risk assessment expertise for food additives, veterinary drugs, contaminants, and pesticide residues. The Joint Expert Committee on Food Additives (JECFA) provides this assistance for food additives, contaminants, and veterinary drugs, while the Joint Meeting on Pesticide Residues (JMPR) fills this role for pesticides. These committees are organizationally outside of Codex but, in large measure, their work is determined by the agenda of the Codex committees responsible for food additives, veterinary drugs, and pesticides. Risk assessments are evaluated by these expert committees according to established protocols, and their recommendations are utilized by the appropriate Codex committees to establish MRLs or maximum permitted use levels. A similar expert committee has been proposed for the field of microbiological risk assessment with the likelihood that the group will be established; currently, Codex is utilizing a series of meetings of experts to assess various microbiological risk assessments that have been done by individual countries (the Joint Expert Group on Microbiological Risk Assessment—JEMRA).

Also important to the work of Codex are international nongovernmental organizations (INGOs). These organizations have no vote in the adoption of standards (see below) but they can intervene in, and influence the discussion on, issues before the commission and its subsidiary bodies. There are many INGOs; examples of such organizations include the World Trade Organization, Consumers International, the International Organization for Standardization (ISO), AOAC International, International Council of Grocery Manufacturer Associations (ICGMA), the International Commission on Microbiological Specifications for Foods (ICMSF), and the International Dairy Federation (IDF). Some of the INGOs (e.g., ICMSF, IDF, and AOAC International) have served as technical advisors to appropriate Codex committees (e.g., ICMSF to the CCFH, and IDF to the Codex Committee on Milk and Milk Products). The role of INGOs is substantial in providing technical insight and important perspectives on the various issues under consideration by Codex.

Recent changes have been made to the management and operation of Codex as a result of the Joint FAO/WHO Evaluation of the Codex Alimentarius and Other FAO and WHO Food Standards Work.[4] Standards management was strengthened through the use of mandatory project documents for new work, a 5 year timeframe for standards development and adoption, and a periodic progress review. The Codex Executive Committee was enlarged and given a key role in standards management. Criteria for approving new work were revised and operating guidelines were established for committee chairpersons, committee host countries, and for the use of physical and electronic working groups. The commission also agreed to reestablish annual sessions of the commission in order to allow for faster adoption of standards. Work is continuing on revisions to Codex operations, particularly with respect to a review of the Codex committee structure and mandates of Codex committees and task forces.

18.5 Standards Development and Adoption Procedure of Codex

Codex utilizes an eight step procedure to elaborate and adopt standards and other texts.[1] The process is a purposefully deliberative, but time-managed system that ensures all member countries are given opportunity to consider the issues coming before any individual Codex committee. The eight-step procedure is summarized in Table 18.1.

New Codex standards, guidelines, codes of practice, and other texts may be proposed by any member government or by individual Codex committees. Proposals for new work must utilize a project document that includes the rationale for the new work, the main aspects of the work, and the need, if any, for expert scientific advice that is to be provided by FAO and WHO. New work must be approved by the commission or by the executive committee with subsequent confirmation by the commission.

Steps 1 and 2 of the Codex procedure involve the initial development processes for the elaboration of Codex texts. Step 1 involves the initial approval by the commission to proceed with new work. In some cases, especially in such areas as guidelines and codes of practice (including codes of hygienic practice), a discussion paper may be developed by the appropriate Codex committee on a proposed issue to determine whether the subject warrants further consideration by Codex. Step 1 also involves

TABLE 18.1

The Step Procedure of the Codex Alimentarius for the Development and Adoption of Standards and Other Texts

---

Steps 1–4: Codex Commission approves proposal for new standard or other text and assigns it to Committee. Secretariat arranges for draft of proposed standard or text. Proposed draft standard or text sent to countries for comments. Draft proposed standard or text and country comments initially reviewed by assigned Codex Committee.

Step 5: Initial review of proposed draft standard or text by the Codex Alimentarius Commission.

Steps 6–7: Draft proposed standard or text forwarded to member countries for second review. Second review, considering country comments, carried out by assigned Codex Committee.

Step 8: Final review of proposed standard or text by Codex Alimentarius Commission. Standard or text adopted, modified and adopted, or rejected by Commission.

Fast Track: Proposed standard or text adopted at Steps 5/8 when no objection exists.

an assignment by the executive committee or the commission to the appropriate Codex committee. Step 2 of the elaboration process involves the preparation of the draft proposed text, either by a member country or by the secretariat. In the case of residues of pesticides or veterinary drugs, the Codex Secretariat distributes the recommendations for MRLs, when available, from JMPR or JECFA.

Step 3 of the Codex step procedure involves the initial submission of the document to member countries for review and comment. Often, formal written comments on proposed Codex standards and texts are prepared by countries for consideration by the assigned Codex committee.

Step 4 is the first formal review of the proposed standard or text by the assigned Codex committee. At this stage, standards and texts are normally reviewed in depth and revisions are made as appropriate.

Step 5 is the first review by the full commission. This review is important because normally only 25%–30% of all member countries attend any specific meeting of a horizontal or vertical Codex committee. Total country participation at commission meetings is substantially higher, hence this initial review by the commission may be the first time that a country comments on a specific proposed Codex standard or text.

At Step 6, the now revised standard, including any comments made by the commission, is sent to all member countries for a second review. Again, as with Step 3, formal written comments are often prepared by a country for review by the assigned committee.

Step 7 is the second opportunity for the assigned Codex committee to review the revised proposed Codex standard or text. The committee has at hand the written country comments at Step 6.

Step 8 is the second and final review by the Codex Commission. The commission has the option of adopting the standard at this point, amending and adopting the standard, sending the standard back to the committee for further work, or rejecting the proposal. Normally, this review results in the adoption of the standard.

At any time during the process, a Codex committee or the commission can retain a document at any specific step, or can return a document to a previous step. Both of these instances frequently occur, particularly for proposed standards or texts that have difficult technical issues or in situations where consensus on a document cannot be reached.

The desire in Codex is for decisions to be reached by consensus, although provisions exist within the formal Codex operating procedures for voting on proposed standards and texts. Voting on decisions relating to the adoption of Codex texts has occurred very infrequently, and is usually associated with highly controversial issues (e.g., the elaboration of MRLs for growth promoting animal hormones).

An accelerated or "fast track" procedure is provided for in which Steps 6 and 7 are omitted. Thus, Steps 5 and 8 are combined and the proposed Codex standard or text may be adopted at the first consideration by the commission. A two-thirds majority vote is required to fast track a Codex standard or text. Normally, this process is used for noncontroversial items or items where early consensus is achieved.

Codex committees meet, on the average, once every 12–18 months. Hence, it takes some period of time to elaborate and adopt a Codex standard. As previously noted, such deliberations are important to ensure the development of appropriate and correct standards or texts, particularly in light of the impact of Codex under the SPS and TBT Agreements and the ramifications that these interrelationships have on international trade. Codex has, however, adopted a 5 year time frame for completion of work on any specific standard; extensions are possible for cause but must be approved by the executive committee.

18.6 National Delegations and Decision Making in Codex

Member countries of Codex maintain a Codex contact point; these points are listed on the Codex Internet Web site. They are the focal point for Codex operations within a country. Functions of national Codex contact points vary from country to country but activities include the management of national delegations to Codex committees, interaction with stakeholders, coordination or development of country positions on Codex documents, and receipt and distribution of Codex texts. Some Codex contact points maintain a library of Codex documents.

Representation at meetings of Codex committees and the commission is made through national delegations from each country. Since Codex is an intergovernmental body, the country delegate (and alternate delegate, if one is appointed) to any specific Codex committee and to meetings of the commission must be a governmental official. Delegations may also contain both governmental and nongovernmental advisors. Advisors are normally selected on the basis of the expertise and the assistance they can provide to the delegate on the technical and policy issues before the Codex committee or commission. Selection of nongovernmental advisors may also be based on the constituencies they represent. Countries limit the size of delegations and normally provide balance with respect to issues or needed expertise and constituency representations (e.g., industry, consumers).

In preparation for specific Codex meetings, countries prepare positions on issues (proposed standards and other texts) coming before the committees. These positions normally form the basis for a country's intervention (that is, verbally presenting a position or point of view) on the issue at the meeting of the committee. Countries often present draft positions at public meetings to ensure transparency and the broadest representation possible in determining final country positions. Countries may also share their national positions with other countries to develop support for their position on an issue. Countries may involve interested parties through public meetings and other mechanisms in the development, review, and comment activities carried out for proposed Codex standards and texts.

Codex meetings normally proceed through a set agenda, discussing all issues assigned to the committee on which it is working. Countries intervene in the discussion in an orderly fashion, providing their position. Consensus among the delegates is normally reached after several rounds of intervention and debate. As noted previously, Codex operates by intent and practice on a consensus basis although procedures for voting are maintained. Once discussion or debate is concluded on an issue, consensus on the standard or text is reached within the context of the step procedure. In the early stages of consideration, countries and the committee may agree to a preliminary consensus position, recognizing that the issue will be revised at a future meeting where the committee's final consensus decision may change. Ultimately, the committee either reaches a final consensus on the issue, a vote is taken (very rarely), or the committee agrees to cease work on the item. Countries wishing to record their opposition to a decision of a committee or the commission may do so. Should voting on an issue occur, each country is allotted one vote.

18.7   Codex and Science

From the beginning of Codex, its work has been science-based. Experts and specialists in a wide range of scientific disciplines have contributed to every aspect of Codex activities to ensure that Codex standards withstand scientific scrutiny. It is fair to say that the work of the CAC, and that of FAO and WHO in their supportive roles, has provided a focal point for food-related scientific research and investigation, and the commission itself has become a most important medium for the exchange of information about food.

The SPS Agreement provides the basis and driving force for the current policy on international food standards.

The SPS Agreement, which went into effect in 1995, includes provisions that require the use of science, including risk assessment, in standards setting. The specific provisions are as follows:

Article 2.2. Members shall ensure that any sanitary and phytosanitary measure is based on scientific principles.

Article 5.1. Members shall ensure that their sanitary and phytosanitary measures are based on an assessment, as appropriate to the circumstances, of the risks to human, animal, or plant life or health.

Codex, recognizing its role under the SPS Agreement as the reference international organization for food safety standards, initiated a process to strengthen its policies and operational practices with respect to the use of science in standards setting.

In 1995, the CAC established a set of four statements of principle concerning the role of science in the codex decision-making process and the extent to which other factors are taken into account[1] (Table 18.2), or "sound science principles" as they are commonly referred to by those involved with Codex. These four principles established the fundamental policy by which Codex will undertake its standards-setting work. The first principle clearly articulates that food standards, guidelines, and other recommendations of the Codex Alimentarius shall be based on the principle of sound scientific analysis and evidence. The second principle, relating to what are termed

TABLE 18.2

The Codex Alimentarius Statements of Principle Concerning the Role of Science in the Codex Decision-Making Process and the Extent to Which Other Factors Are Taken into Account

1. The food standards, guidelines, and other recommendations of Codex Alimentarius shall be based on the principle of sound scientific analysis and evidence, involving a thorough review of all relevant information, in order that the standards assure the quality and safety of the food supply.
2. When elaborating and deciding upon food standards Codex Alimentarius will have regard, where appropriate, to other legitimate factors relevant for the health protection of consumers and for the promotion of fair practices in food trade.
3. In this regard it is noted that food labeling plays an important role in furthering both of these objectives.
4. When the situation arises that members of Codex agree on the necessary level of protection of public health but hold differing views about other considerations, members may abstain from acceptance of the relevant standard without necessarily preventing the decision by Codex.

Criteria for the Consideration of the Other Factors Referred to in the Second Statement of Principle
    When health and safety matters are concerned, the *Statements of Principle Concerning the Role of Science* and the *Statements of Principle Relating to the Role of Food Safety Risk Assessment* should be followed;
    Other legitimate factors relevant for health protection and fair trade practices may be identified in the risk management process, and risk managers should indicate how these factors affect the selection of risk management options and the development of standards, guidelines, and related texts;
    Consideration of other factors should not affect the scientific basis of risk analysis; in this process, the separation between risk assessment and risk management should be respected, in order to ensure the scientific integrity of the risk assessment;
    It should be recognized that some legitimate concerns of governments when establishing their national legislation are not generally applicable or relevant worldwide;
    Only those other factors which can be accepted on a worldwide basis, or on a regional basis in the case of regional standards and related texts, should be taken into account in the framework of Codex;
    The consideration of specific other factors in the development of risk management recommendations of the Codex Alimentarius Commission and its subsidiary bodies should be clearly documented, including the rationale for their integration, on a case-by-case basis;
    The feasibility of risk management options due to the nature and particular constraints of the production or processing methods, transport, and storage, especially in developing countries, may be considered; concerns related to economic interests and trade issues in general should be substantiated by quantifiable data;
    The integration of other legitimate factors in risk management should not create unjustified barriers to trade; particular attention should be given to the impact on developing countries of the inclusion of such other factors.

"other legitimate factors," is more complex and states that Codex, in its standards setting activities, will have regard, where appropriate, to other legitimate factors relevant for the health protection of consumers and for the promotion of fair practices in food trade. There are differences of opinion among countries as to what constitutes an OLF. Countries generally accept that OLFs relating to the risk assessment process (e.g., good veterinary practices, good agricultural practices) are appropriate. Some countries may question, however, whether factors such as economic feasibility, environmental impact, impact on health status, and consumer perception of risk should be considered in international standards setting. Many countries might disagree with including such factors as animal welfare, consumer right to know, cost increases (or decreases) associated with technology, and relative risk (i.e., the risk associated with a product compared to other risks to which a consumer is exposed), and acceptance of these factors is likely to be difficult. Provisions of the SPS Agreement provide guidance as to factors countries can legitimately take into account when establishing sanitary and phytosanitary measures (e.g., economic factors including the relative cost effectiveness of alternative approaches to limiting risks, relevant processes and production methods, and relevant environmental conditions). These SPS provisions are likely to assist in clarifying the determination of acceptable OLFs for Codex standards setting. Additionally, the CAC, subsequent to the adoption of the sound science principles, adopted Criteria for the Consideration of the Other Factors Referred to in the Second Statement of Principle[1] (Table 18.2), which provides guidance to Codex committees and task forces in considering OLFs. WTO jurisprudence in trade dispute settlement is ultimately the probable method by which the most controversial and difficult OLFs will be determined.

Subsequently, the commission established the Statements of Principle Relating to the Role of Food Safety Risk Assessment[1] (Table 18.3).

At the request of Codex, FAO and WHO have undertaken a series of joint expert consultations[5-7] to elucidate the basic principles of risk analysis. Working from the findings of three joint expert consultations dealing with the three components of risk analysis (risk assessment, risk management, and risk communication) and from the discussions of several key Codex

TABLE 18.3

Codex Statements of Principles Relating to the Role of Food Safety
Risk Assessment

---

1. Health and safety aspects of Codex decisions and recommendations should be based on a risk assessment, as appropriate to the circumstances.
2. Food safety risk assessment should be soundly based on science, should incorporate the four steps of the risk assessment process, and should be documented in a transparent manner.
3. There should be a functional separation of risk assessment and risk management, while recognizing that some interactions are essential for a pragmatic approach.
4. Risk assessment should use available quantitative information to the greatest extent possible and risk characterizations.

---

horizontal committees (Food Hygiene, Pesticide Residues, Residues of Veterinary Drugs in Foods, and Food Additives and Contaminants), Codex has developed a comprehensive set of Working Principles of Risk Analysis for Application in the Framework of the Codex Alimentarius[1] (Table 18.4) that provides a further scientific foundation for the elaboration of Codex standards, guidelines, and recommendations.

Several Codex committees, including Food Hygiene, Food Additives and Contaminants, Residues of Veterinary Drugs in Foods, and Pesticide Residues, have also established various Codex texts relating to risk analysis (see below for the work of the CCFH in this regard).

TABLE 18.4

Working Principles for Risk Analysis for Application in the Framework of the Codex Alimentarius

---

Scope
1. These principles for risk analysis are intended for application in the framework of the Codex Alimentarius.
2. The objective of these Working Principles is to provide guidance to the Codex Alimentarius Commission and the joint FAO/WHO expert bodies and consultations, so that food safety and health aspects of Codex standards and related texts are based on risk analysis.
3. Within the framework of the Codex Alimentarius Commission and its procedures, the responsibility for providing advice on risk management lies with the Commission and its subsidiary bodies (risk managers), while the responsibility for risk assessment lies primarily with the joint FAO/WHO expert bodies and consultations (risk assessors).

Risk Analysis—General Principles
4. The risk analysis used in Codex should be
   applied consistently;
   open, transparent and documented;
   conducted in accordance with both the statements of principle concerning the role of science in the codex decision-making process and the extent to which other factors are taken into account and the statements of principle relating to the role of food safety risk assessment; and
   evaluated and reviewed as appropriate in the light of newly generated scientific data.
5. The risk analysis should follow a structured approach comprising the three distinct but closely linked components of risk analysis (risk assessment, risk management, and risk communication) as defined by the Codex Alimentarius Commission, each component being integral to the overall risk analysis.
6. The three components of risk analysis should be documented fully and systematically in a transparent manner. While respecting legitimate concerns to preserve confidentiality, documentation should be accessible to all interested parties.
7. Effective communication and consultation with all interested parties should be ensured throughout the risk analysis.
8. The three components of risk analysis should be applied within an overarching framework for management of food related risks to human health.
9. There should be a functional separation of risk assessment and risk management, in order to ensure the scientific integrity of the risk assessment, to avoid confusion over the functions to be performed by risk assessors and risk managers, and to reduce any conflict of interest. However, it is recognized that risk analysis is an iterative process, and interaction between risk managers and risk assessors is essential for practical application.

TABLE 18.4 (continued)

Working Principles for Risk Analysis for Application in the Framework
of the Codex Alimentarius

10. When there is evidence that a risk to human health exists but scientific data are insufficient or incomplete, the Codex Alimentarius Commission should not proceed to elaborate a standard but should consider elaborating a related text, such as a code of practice, provided that such a text would be supported by the available scientific evidence.
11. Precaution is an inherent element of risk analysis. Many sources of uncertainty exist in the process of risk assessment and risk management of food related hazards to human health. The degree of uncertainty and variability in the available scientific information should be explicitly considered in the risk analysis. Where there is sufficient scientific evidence to allow Codex to proceed to elaborate a standard or related text, the assumptions used for the risk assessment and the risk management options selected should reflect the degree of uncertainty and the characteristics of the hazard.
12. The needs and situations of developing countries should be specifically identified and taken into account by the responsible bodies in the different stages of the risk analysis.

Risk Assessment Policy
13. Determination of risk assessment policy should be included as a specific component of risk management.
14. Risk assessment policy should be established by risk managers in advance of risk assessment, in consultation with risk assessors and all other interested parties. This procedure aims at ensuring that the risk assessment is systematic, complete, unbiased, and transparent.
15. The mandate given by risk managers to risk assessors should be as clear as possible.
16. Where necessary, risk managers should ask risk assessors to evaluate the potential changes in risk resulting from different risk management options.

Risk Assessment
17. The scope and purpose of the particular risk assessment being carried out should be clearly stated and in accordance with risk assessment policy. The output form and possible alternative outputs of the risk assessment should be defined.
18. Experts responsible for risk assessment should be selected in a transparent manner on the basis of their expertise, experience, and their independence with regard to the interests involved. The procedures used to select these experts should be documented including a public declaration of any potential conflict of interest. This declaration should also identify and detail their individual expertise, experience, and independence. Expert bodies and consultations should ensure effective participation of experts from different parts of the world, including experts from developing countries.
19. Risk assessment should be conducted in accordance with the statements of principle relating to the role of food safety risk assessment and should incorporate the four steps of the risk assessment, i.e. hazard identification, hazard characterization, exposure assessment, and risk characterization.
20. Risk assessment should be based on all available scientific data. It should use available quantitative information to the greatest extent possible. Risk assessment may also take into account qualitative information.
21. Risk assessment should take into account relevant production, storage, and handling practices used throughout the food chain including traditional practices, methods of analysis, sampling and inspection, and the prevalence of specific adverse health effects.
22. Risk assessment should seek and incorporate relevant data from different parts of the world, including that from developing countries. These data should particularly include epidemiological surveillance data, analytical data, and exposure data. Where relevant data are not available from developing countries, the Commission should request that FAO/WHO initiate time-bound studies for this purpose. The conduct of the risk

(*continued*)

TABLE 18.4 (continued)

Working Principles for Risk Analysis for Application in the Framework
of the Codex Alimentarius

assessment should not be inappropriately delayed pending receipt of
these data; however, the risk assessment should be reconsidered when such data
are available.

23. Constraints, uncertainties, and assumptions having an impact on the risk assessment
    should be explicitly considered at each step in the risk assessment and documented in a
    transparent manner. Expression of uncertainty or variability in risk estimates may be
    qualitative or quantitative, but should be quantified to the extent that is scientifically
    achievable.

24. Risk assessments should be based on realistic exposure scenarios, with consideration of
    different situations being defined by risk assessment policy. They should include
    consideration of susceptible and high-risk population groups. Acute, chronic (including
    long-term), cumulative and/or combined adverse health effects should be taken into
    account in carrying out risk assessment, where relevant.

25. The report of the risk assessment should indicate any constraints, uncertainties,
    assumptions, and their impact on the risk assessment. Minority opinions should also be
    recorded. The responsibility for resolving the impact of uncertainty on the risk management
    decision lies with the risk manager, not the risk assessors.

26. The conclusion of the risk assessment including a risk estimate, if available, should be
    presented in a readily understandable and useful form to risk managers and made available
    to other risk assessors and interested parties so that they can review the assessment.

Risk Management

27. While recognizing the dual purposes of the Codex Alimentarius are protecting
    the health of consumers and ensuring fair practices in the food trade, Codex decisions
    and recommendations on risk management should have as their primary objective
    the protection of the health of consumers. Unjustified differences in the level of
    consumer health protection to address similar risks in different situations should be
    avoided.

28. Risk management should follow a structured approach including preliminary
    risk management activities, evaluation of risk management options, monitoring, and
    review of the decision taken. The decisions should be based on risk assessment,
    and taking into account, where appropriate, other legitimate factors relevant for the
    health protection of consumers and for the promotion of fair practices in food trade, in
    accordance with the Criteria for the Consideration of the Other Factors Referred to in
    the Second Statement of Principles.

29. The Codex Alimentarius Commission and its subsidiary bodies, acting as risk
    managers in the context of these Working Principles, should ensure that the conclusion
    of the risk assessment is presented before making final proposals or decisions on the
    available risk management options, in particular in the setting of standards or maximum
    levels, bearing in mind the guidance given in paragraph.

30. In achieving agreed outcomes, risk management should take into account
    relevant production, storage, and handling practices used throughout the food
    chain including traditional practices, methods of analysis, sampling and inspection,
    feasibility of enforcement and compliance, and the prevalence of specific adverse
    health effects.

31. The risk management process should be transparent, consistent, and fully
    documented. Codex decisions and recommendations on risk management should be
    documented, and where appropriate clearly identified in individual Codex standards
    and related texts so as to facilitate a wider understanding of the risk management
    process by all interested parties.

TABLE 18.4 (continued)

Working Principles for Risk Analysis for Application in the Framework
of the Codex Alimentarius

32. The outcome of the preliminary risk management activities and the risk assessment should
be combined with the evaluation of available risk management options in order to reach a
decision on management of the risk.
33. Risk management options should be assessed in terms of the scope and purpose of risk
analysis and the level of consumer health protection they achieve. The option of not
taking any action should also be considered.
34. In order to avoid unjustified trade barriers, risk management should ensure
transparency and consistency in the decision-making process in all cases.
Examination of the full range of risk management options should, as far as possible,
take into account an assessment of their potential advantages and disadvantages.
When making a choice among different risk management options, which are equally
effective in protecting the health of the consumer, the Commission and its subsidiary
bodies should seek and take into consideration the potential impact of such
measures on trade among its Member countries and select measures that are no
more trade-restrictive than necessary.
35. Risk management should take into account the economic consequences and the
feasibility of risk management options. Risk management should also
recognize the need for alternative options in the establishment of standards,
guidelines, and other recommendations, consistent with the protection of consumers'
health. In taking these elements into consideration, the Commission and its
subsidiary bodies should give particular attention to the circumstances of
developing countries.
36. Risk management should be a continuing process that takes into account all
newly generated data in the evaluation and review of risk management decisions.
Food standards and related texts should be reviewed regularly and updated
as necessary to reflect new scientific knowledge and other information relevant
to risk analysis.

Risk Communication
37. Risk communication should:
   i) promote awareness and understanding of the specific issues under consideration
   during the risk analysis;
   ii) promote consistency and transparency in formulating risk management options
   recommendations;
   iii) provide a sound basis for understanding the risk management decisions proposed;
   iv) improve the overall effectiveness and efficiency of the risk analysis;
   v) strengthen the working relationships among participants;
   vi) foster public understanding of the process, so as to enhance trust and confidence in
   the safety of the food supply;
   vii) promote the appropriate involvement of all interested parties; and
   viii) exchange information in relation to the concerns of interested parties about the risks
   associated with food.
38. Risk analysis should include clear, interactive, and documented communication amongst
risk assessors (Joint FAO/WHO expert bodies and consultations) and risk managers
(Codex Alimentarius Commission and its subsidiary bodies), and reciprocal
communication with member countries and all interested parties in all aspects of the
process.
39. Risk communication should be more than the dissemination of information. Its major
function should be to ensure that all information and opinion required for effective risk
management is incorporated into the decision making process.

This Codex effort in establishing the Sound Science Principles, the Working Principles of Risk Analysis for Application in the Framework of the Codex Alimentarius, and the various committee-specific risk analysis texts establish a comprehensive scientific framework for the work Codex undertakes in elaborating standards. This effort is also providing a framework for countries to use in their own individual food safety standards setting. As such the work of Codex extends far beyond the organization itself. This comprehensive sound science or risk analysis approach to standards setting, which is compatible with the provisions of the SPS Agreement, is beginning to be seen in new draft Codex standards. A good example is the Code of Hygienic Practice for Milk and Milk Products, which is discussed below.

18.8   Codex and Food Hygiene

The CCFH is primarily responsible for food hygiene matters within Codex. Food hygiene generally encompasses hygiene as it relates to good production, manufacturing, distribution, and marketing practices, the Hazard Analysis and Critical Control Point (HACCP) system, microbiological criteria for foods, and microbiological risk assessment and risk management. The terms of reference for CCFH[1] are fourfold. As an overarching responsibility, CCFH has the responsibility to suggest and prioritize where there is a need for microbiological risk assessment at the international level and to consider microbiological risk management matters related to food hygiene. This responsibility is applied through the remaining three terms of reference: (1) to draft basic provisions on food hygiene applicable to all food that, in practice, takes the form of the development (and revision when needed) of Codex Codes of Hygienic Practice for various food commodities and risk management guidelines to control specific foodborne pathogens; (2) to consider and review food hygiene provisions of Codex commodity standards or other texts; and (3) to consider specific hygiene problems assigned to it by the commission. These areas are described below.

18.8.1   Codes of Hygienic Practice

Codex Codes of Hygienic Practice provide guidance on the hygienic production and processing of foods. The base reference document in this area is the Recommended International Code of Practice: General Principles of Food Hygiene.[8] In addition to introductory sections on objectives and scope, this general food hygiene code of practice contains detailed recommended food hygiene practices for the following areas:

1. Primary production
2. Establishment: design and facilities

3. Control of operation
4. Establishment: maintenance and sanitation
5. Establishment: personal hygiene
6. Transportation
7. Product information and consumer awareness
8. Training

This General Principles document also contains a HACCP annex that presents the recommendations of Codex for the application of HACCP to food production. The Codex approach to HACCP utilizes the seven internationally recognized principles of HACCP. The annex presents a detailed discussion on the application of each principle including the establishment of critical control points (CCP) and critical limits for each CCP. Also presented is a flow diagram for the application of HACCP (Logic Sequence for Application of HACCP), an example of a decision tree to identify CCPs and an example of a HACCP worksheet. A recent revision to the HACCP annex provided additional guidance for small and lesser-developed businesses.

The CCFH also undertakes the development of commodity specific codes of hygienic practice. These commodity specific codes reference the Recommended International Code of Practice: General Principles of Food Hygiene and are constructed so that only hygiene provisions supplemental to those present in the general principles code and specific for the commodity type covered in the code are given. Examples of codes of hygienic practice include those for the following product areas:

- Canned fruit and vegetable products
- Milk and milk products
- Eggs and egg products
- Powdered formulae for infants and young children
- Fresh fruits and vegetable
- Packaged or bottled water other than natural mineral water
- Refrigerated packaged foods with extended shelf life
- Transport of foodstuffs in bulk and semipackaged foods

The Code of Hygienic Practice for Milk and Milk Products,[9] adopted by the commission in 2004, deserves special mention because the construction of this code is particularly reflective of the new responsibilities of Codex under the SPS Agreement. The development of this code arose from prior work of the CCFH dealing with soft cheeses and the difficulty experienced by the committee in dealing with complex microbiological risk issues associated with the production of soft unripened uncured cheeses made from raw milk. Countries differed as to the acceptable level of microbiological risk associated with this product type. The result was the development of a code that permits countries to manufacture products in multiple ways (in which the microbiological risks may be different). Countries have the right to accept or reject products based on their scientifically established Appropriate Level of Protection (ALOP). This code, for the first time, employs SPS terminology and concepts, relating the construct of a specific Codex document to the provisions of the SPS Agreement, and reflects the new and enhanced role of Codex under the SPS Agreement.

18.8.2   Hygiene Provisions of Commodity Standards

Codex develops recommended standards for a multitude of specific food commodities. The primary provisions of these codes are sections on essential composition (a basic standard of identity), packaging, and labeling. These standards also contain sections on maximum permitted residue levels for pesticides, veterinary drugs, contaminants, and maximum permitted use levels for food additives; each of these sections refers to general broad Codex standards for pesticide residue MRLs, veterinary drug MRLs, and food additive permitted use levels.

These commodity standards also contain a general section on food hygiene. The current recommended wording for the hygiene section of all commodity standards is as follows:[1]

- It is recommended that the products covered by the provisions of this standard be prepared and handled in accordance with the appropriate sections of the Recommended International Code of Practice–General Principles of Food Hygiene (CAC/RCP 1-1969, Rev. 4-2003) and other relevant Codex texts such as Codes of Hygienic Practice and Codes of Practice.
- The products should comply with any microbiological criteria established in accordance with the Principles for the Establishment and Application of Microbiological Criteria for Foods (CAC/GL 21-1997).

As the above-mentioned Codex commodity committees develop individual commodity standards, the CCFH has the responsibility to review the food hygiene section to ensure that the section's provisions are adequate for the product. This is normally a routine activity and the recommended wording noted above is approved. CCFH, however, has the capability to add specific additional provisions to the food hygiene section of commodity standards, should the committee deem them necessary to ensure the safe production and processing of the products covered by the specific commodity standard. The review of eight generic dairy product standards including that for cheese is a case in point.[10] Because of concern with potential microbiological risk issues associated with some product types (e.g., soft unripened uncured cheeses made from raw milk), the CCFH approved the following additional provision for the hygiene section of the eight dairy product standards.

- From raw material production to the point of consumption, the products covered by this standard should be subject to a combination of control measures, which may include, for example, pasteurization, and these should be shown to achieve the appropriate level of public health protection.

18.8.3   Other Food Hygiene Activities

In the context of its broad food hygiene responsibilities, the work of CCFH extends beyond the confines of specific Codex codes of hygienic practice and the hygiene provisions of specific Codex commodity codes. The work of CCFH is wide-ranging and significant, providing guidance to both Codex and countries, and affects the field of food microbiology generally. Work of CCFH in this broader context includes efforts in microbiological risk assessment and microbiological risk management, including the development of the concept of "microbiological metrics." This broader context also includes developing specific hygiene guidance for the control of specific foodborne pathogens.

18.8.4   Hygiene Guidance for Specific Foodborne Pathogens

Recognizing that the occurrence of certain foodborne pathogens (e.g., *Listeria monocytogenes*, enteropathogenic *Escherichia coli*) presents particular concern, and that similar control measures apply across commodities, CCFH has moved toward the development of pathogen-specific food hygiene risk management guidance documents. The format of these guidance documents has generally followed that of the Recommended International Code of Practice: General Principles of Food Hygiene; that is, sections on primary production, process control, product information, training, etc. To date, work has been undertaken or is being considered to develop guidance on *L. monocytogenes* in ready-to-eat foods; *Salmonella* and *Campylobacter* species in broiler chickens; enterohemorrhagic *E. coli* in ground beef and fermented sausages; and *Vibrio* species in seafood. Currently, the most advanced of these guidance documents is that for *Listeria*, the Codex Draft Guideline on the Application of the General Principles of Food Hygiene to the Control of *Listeria monocytogenes* in Ready to Eat Foods,[11] on which work has recently been completed by CCFH with a recommendation for the Commission to adopt the text at Step 8 of the Codex step procedure.

18.8.5   Microbiological Criteria

Recognizing the changing nature of regulatory control programs (e.g., from periodic inspection to HACCP) and the evolving thinking of the use of microbiological criteria (from an end-product application tool to a component of a risk management system), CCFH developed the document,

Principles for the Establishment and Application of Microbiological Criteria for Foods,[12] to provide guidance to both Codex and its member countries on the establishment and application of microbiological criteria for foods at any point in the food chain from primary production to final consumption.

The document defines a microbiological criterion to be an entity that defines the acceptability of a product or a food lot, based on the absence, presence, or number of microorganisms (including parasites), or the quantity of their toxins and metabolites, per unit of mass, volume, area, or lot.

The components of a criterion are specified to be

- a statement of the microorganism of concern and their toxins and metabolites and the reason for that concern,
- the food to which the criterion applies,
- the points in the food chain where the criterion applies,
- the analytical methods for detection or quantification,
- a plan defining the number of field samples to be taken and the size of the analytical unit,
- the number of analytical units that should conform to these limits, and
- the action to be taken when the criterion is not met.

The guidance describes the purposes for which microbiological criteria can be applied, specifically

- to formulate design requirements;
- to indicate the required microbiological status of raw materials, ingredients, and end-products at any stage of the food chain as appropriate;
- to examine foods (including raw materials and ingredients) of unknown origin or when other means of verifying the efficacy of HACCP-based systems and good manufacturing practices are not available; and,
- to determine that processes are consistent with the Codex General Principles of Food Hygiene.

The guidance notes that microbiological criteria can be applied by regulatory authorities to define and check compliance with microbiological requirements. Food business operators may use the microbiological criteria to ensure compliance with regulatory provisions, to formulate design requirements, and to examine end-products as one of the measures to verify or validate the efficacy of the HACCP plan.

The document outlines general considerations for establishing and applying microbiological criteria; e.g., evidence of an actual or potential public health hazard, the microbiological status of the raw material, the effect of processing, the category of consumers utilizing the product, the cost–benefit of implementing a criterion, and the intended use of the food. Also discussed is the rationale for establishing microbiological limits, sampling plans, and analytical methods.

Within CCFH, as part of the development of pathogen-specific hygiene guidance (see above), the use of microbiological criteria is evolving and is being viewed as one component of an overall risk-management program that may also include the use of various microbiological metrics including food safety objectives, performance objectives, performance criteria, and process criteria (see below).

18.9 Microbiological Risk Assessment and Risk Management

Codex, through the work of the CCFH, has developed a fundamental guidance document on microbiological risk assessment and has recently completed work on a companion document on microbiological risk management.

18.9.1 Microbiological Risk Assessment Guidance Document

Codex has established the first international intergovernmental guidance document for microbiological risk assessment, Principles and Guidelines for the Conduct of Microbiological Risk Assessment.[13] The scope of this document generally applies to risk assessment of microbiological hazards in food and is designed to ensure that sound science principles and practices are applied uniformly in evaluating microbiological hazards in foods. The document recognizes that microbiological risk assessment is a developing science, and that while the process should include quantitative information to the greatest extent possible, qualitative judgments will have to be made.

Eleven general principles applicable to the conduct of microbiological risk assessment (Table 18.5) are presented in the document. These principles state that microbiological risk assessment should be conducted according to the structured four step approach that is common to risk assessment generally (hazard identification, hazard characterization, exposure assessment, and risk characterization). The principles also incorporate provisions relating to performing a microbiological risk assessment, including the need for

- functional separation between risk assessment and risk management,
- a requirement for transparency in what is being done,

TABLE 18.5

The Codex Alimentarius General Principles of Microbiological Risk Assessment

1. Microbiological Risk Assessment should be soundly based on science.
2. There should be a functional separation between Risk Assessment and Risk Management.
3. Microbiological Risk Assessment should be conducted according to a structured approach that includes Hazard Identification, Hazard Characterization, Exposure Assessment and Risk Characterization.
4. A Microbiological Risk Assessment should clearly state the purpose of the exercise, including the form of Risk Estimate that will be the output.
5. The conduct of a Microbiological Risk Assessment should be transparent.
6. Any constraints that impact the Risk Assessment such as costs, resources, or time, should be identified and their possible consequences described.
7. The Risk Estimate should contain a description of uncertainty and where the uncertainty arose during the Risk Assessment process.
8. Data should be such that uncertainty in the Risk Estimate can be determined; data collection systems should, as far as possible, be of sufficient quality and precision that uncertainty in the Risk Estimate is minimized.
9. A Microbiological Risk Assessment should explicitly consider the dynamics of microbiological growth, survival, and death in foods and the complexity of the interaction (including sequelae) between human and agent following consumption as well as the potential for further spread.
10. Wherever possible, Risk Estimates should be reassessed over time by comparison with independent human illness data.
11. A Microbiological Risk Assessment may need reevaluation as new relevant information becomes available.

- identification of the limitation of data and resource constraints,
- consideration of the dynamics of microbial growth,
- specifying the uncertainties associated with each step of the risk assessment process, and
- reassessment as new data (e.g., new quantitative information on the occurrence of microorganisms in food, new dietary intake information).

Guidance is provided on the steps required to carry out a microbiological risk assessment. Each of the four structured steps of risk assessment is discussed in detail. Helpful information specific to the application of microbiological risk assessment is given. For example, influences that may affect the hazard characterization are detailed (e.g., replication rates of microorganisms, virulence and infectivity, delay of onset of clinical symptoms, effect of food attributes such as fat content). Similar information is described for the exposure assessment step (e.g., characteristics of the pathogenic agent, the microbial ecology of the food, the methods of packaging, processing, distribution, and storage).

The need for proper documentation and reassessment as new data develop (an important consideration in the comparatively new field of microbiological risk assessment) is stressed in the guidance document.

18.9.2 Joint Expert Group on Microbiological Risk Assessment

As noted above, FAO and WHO maintain two primary expert groups, the Joint Expert Committee for Food Additives and Contaminants (JECFA) and the Joint Meeting on Pesticide Residues (JEMA), which provide scientific technical risk assessment assistance and guidance to several Codex committees. The CCFH recommended and the CAC concurred with the establishment of similar joint expert group for food microbiological risk assessment. Although the group is yet to be formally established, a series of FAO/WHO Joint Expert Meetings on Microbiological Risk Assessment (JEMRA) have been held over several years. JEMRA has been undertaking a number of risk assessments associated with the CCFH's pathogen specific guidance (see above).

18.9.3 Microbiological Risk Management

The CCFH has recently completed work on a new document on Principles and Guidelines for the Conduct of Microbiological Risk Management,[14] recommending adoption by the CAC at Step 8 of the Codex step procedure. This document will be the first international guidance to both Codex committees and to countries on how to undertake and implement microbiological risk management activities.

The document builds on a series of risk management principles developed by the FAO/WHO Joint Expert Consultation on Risk Management and Food Safety[6] and provides a framework for undertaking microbiological risk management. The document contains guidance on four fundamental areas:

- Preliminary microbiological risk management activities consisting of
  - identification of the microbiological food safety issue,
  - development of a microbiological risk profile,
  - establishment of a risk assessment policy, and
  - commissioning appropriate risk assessments.
- Identification and selection of microbiological risk management options including guidance on
  - identification of options for Codex,
  - identification of options for countries, and
  - selection of microbiological risk management metrics (e.g., process criteria, microbiological criteria, performance criteria, performance objectives, and food safety objectives).
- Implementation of microbiological options, both with respect to Codex and countries.
- Monitoring and review of microbiological options.

A developing concept to utilize in the selection of appropriate microbiological options is that of "microbiological metrics" including food safety objectives and the related concepts of performance objective and performance criteria. On the basis of work carried out by CCFH, Codex recently adopted the following definitions for these three terms:[1]

Food Safety Objective (FSO): The maximum frequency or concentration of a hazard in a food at the time of consumption that provides or contributes to the appropriate level of protection (ALOP).

Performance Objective (PO): The maximum frequency or concentration of a hazard in a food at a specified step in the food chain before the time of consumption that provides or contributes to an FSO or ALOP, as applicable.

Performance Criterion (PC): The effect in frequency or concentration of a hazard in a food that must be achieved by the application of one or more control measures to provide or contribute to a PO or an FSO.

Extensive work on developing comprehensive guidance on these concepts for use in microbiological risk management is underway, both in CCFH and elsewhere. General information on the interrelated nature and application of FSOs, POs, PCs, and microbiological criteria is currently planned for inclusion as an annex to the Principles and Guidelines for the Conduct of Microbiological Risk Management. Additionally, specific application of these concepts will likely be incorporated into various Codex texts as they are developed or revised (e.g., the microbiological risk management texts on *Listeria* and other pathogens noted above). FSOs, POs, and PCs are likely to become important operational elements in future food safety programs.

18.10   Other Codex Work Areas

Recent important developments with Codex include the following.

18.10.1   Foods Derived from Modern Biotechnology

In 1999, the CAC, because of the increasingly important role of biotechnology, established an Ad-Hoc Intergovernmental Task Force on Foods Derived from Biotechnology. Over a 4 year time frame, the task force developed three important guidance documents; Principles for Risk Analysis of Foods Derived from Modern Biotechnology;[15] Guideline for the Conduct of Food Safety Assessment of Foods Derived from Recombinant-DNA Plants;[16] and Guideline for the Conduct of Food Safety Assessment of

Foods Produced from Recombinant-DNA Microorganisms.[17] During the development of these texts, a number of key issues were considered and incorporated into the document including a definition of modern biotechnology, the nature of food safety assessment of these foodstuffs; the use of comparators; assessing allergenicity; post-market monitoring; and traceability/product tracing. The CAC, at its 2005 session, reestablished the task force for a second 4 year lifetime. The reestablished task force has agreed to undertake work on the safety assessment of recombinant-r-DNA animals. The task force has also agreed to consider what, if any, additional guidance is needed to assess the safety of r-DNA plants developed for enhanced nutrient or health effects. Further, the task force has agreed to undertake new work to provide guidance on the extent of information required to perform a food safety assessment in situations of the low-level presence of r-DNA plant material in which the r-DNA plant has already been found to be safe and authorized for commercialization of food by one or more countries, but the importing country has not determined its food safety. This new work will also incorporate recommendations on the sharing of information used in the original food safety assessment.

18.10.2 Equivalence of Sanitary Measures Associated with Food Import and Export Inspection and Certification Systems

Following development by the Codex Committee on Food Import and Export Inspection and Certification Systems, the CAC, in 2003, adopted the Codex Guidelines on the Judgement of Equivalence of Sanitary Measures Associated with Food Inspection and Certification Systems.[18] This document provides essential guidance to countries for assessing two alternative measures or sets of measures intended to provide the same outcome with respect to the control of a hazard in a food. Subsequently, CCFICS agreed to undertake the development of additional detailed guidance in the form of an annex to the guidelines relating to several aspects of equivalence including the selection of measures, documentation for equivalence, the process of judging equivalence, and determining an "objective basis of comparison." This work is in progress.

18.10.3 Traceability/Product Tracing

Following discussions in the Codex Ad-Hoc Intergovernmental Task Force on Foods Derived from Biotechnology on the use of traceability/product tracing with respect to foods derived from modern biotechnology, and recognizing the general nature of traceability/product tracing, requested the Codex Committee on Food Import and Export Inspection and Certification Systems (CCFICS) to consider the development of guidance on the subject. Subsequently, CCFICS developed Principles for Traceability/Product Tracing within Food Import and Export Inspection and Certification Systems,[19] with adoption of the document by the CAC in 2006.

18.10.4   Inspection of Imported Foods Based on Risk

The Codex Committee on Food Import and Export Inspection and Certification, at its 14th (2005) session, completed work on Principles and Guidelines
for Imported Food Inspection Based on Risk.[20] As part of the new Codex
paradigm on developing risk-based guidance, the document provides guidance to governments on developing and operating a risk-based imported foods
inspection program. In addition to a set of principles for a risk-based inspection
program, the document contains sections on designing an imported food
inspection program, developing requirements and procedures, and implementing the import inspection program based on risk. This principles and
guideline document was adopted by the CAC at its 2006 Session.

18.10.5   Antimicrobial Resistance

Over the past several years, Codex has considered the issue of antimicrobial
resistance, particularly with respect to food safety. The CCFH developed an
advisory discussion paper[21] on the subject, which the committee provided
to the World Health Organization for information and considered how it
might deal with the matter of antimicrobial resistance. The Codex Committee on Residues of Veterinary Drugs in Foods has developed a Code of
Practice to Minimize and Contain Antimicrobial Resistance,[22] which has
been adopted by the CAC. Additionally, the Food and Agriculture Organization and the World Health Organization have competed two joint expert
consultations on the subject. During the course of these discussions, there
came forward recommendations to establish a Codex Ad-Hoc Task Force to
further consider the issue of antimicrobial resistance, particularly the
aspects of risk assessment and risk management with respect to key antimicrobial substances and foodborne pathogens. The CAC, at its 2006
session, agreed to establish a time-limited (four session) Task Force on
Antimicrobial Resistance with the following terms of reference: To develop
guidance on methodology and processes for risk assessment, its application
to the antimicrobials used in human and veterinary medicine as provided
by FAO/WHO through JEMRA, and in close cooperation with OIE, with
subsequent consideration of risk management options.

18.10.6   Principles for Risk Analysis for Application by Countries

As an outgrowth of its work on the development of the Codex Working
Principles for Risk Analysis for Application in the Framework of the Codex
Alimentarius,[1] the Codex Committee on General Principles has considered
the need for a companion document providing guidance to governments on
principles relating to undertaking risk analysis. The development of this
document has been controversial with respect to certain aspects of risk
management, which fall primarily to governments rather than to Codex,
especially the areas of the use of precaution and the use of other legitimate

factors. Discussions are continuing in CCGP as to whether such a Codex document should be developed and, if so, how the areas of difficulty can be appropriately addressed in a text that has WTO status.

_____

References

1. Codex Alimentarius Commission. *Procedural Manual*, 15th edition. Food and Agriculture Organization of the United Nations/World Health Organization, Rome, Italy, 2005, 162 pp.
2. Food and Agriculture Organization of the United Nations/World Health Organization. *Understanding the Codex Alimentarius*, Rome, Italy, 2005, 39 pp.
3. World Trade Organization. *The Results of the Uruguay Round of Multilateral Trade Negotiations, The Legal Texts*, Geneva, Switzerland, 1995, 558 pp.
4. Food and Agriculture Organization of the United Nations/World Health Organization. Report of the Evaluation of the Codex Alimentarius and Other FAO and WHO Food Standards Work, 15 November, 2002, 101 pp.
5. Food and Agriculture Organization of the United Nations/World Health Organization. *Application of Risk Analysis to Food Standards Issues: Report of the Joint FAO/WHO Consultation*, Geneva, Switzerland, 13–17 March, 1995.
6. Food and Agriculture Organization of the United Nations/World Health Organization. *Risk Management and Food Safety: Report of the Joint FAO/WHO Consultation*, Rome, Italy, 27–31 January, 1997.
7. Food and Agriculture Organization of the United Nations/World Health Organization. *The Application of Risk Communication to Food Standards and Safety Matters*, Rome, Italy, 2–6 February, 1998.
8. Food and Agriculture Organization of the United Nations/World Health Organization. Recommended international code of hygienic practice: General principles of food hygiene, CAC/RCP 1-1969, Rev 4 (2003). In *Food Hygiene, Basic Texts*, 3rd edition, Rome, Italy, 2003.
9. Food and Agriculture Organization of the United Nations/World Health Organization, Codex Committee on Food Hygiene, *Code of Hygienic Practice for Milk and Milk Products*, CAC/RCP 57-2004, Rome, Italy, 2004.
10. Codex Alimentarius Commission. *Report of the Thirtieth Session of the Codex Committee on Food Hygiene*, Washington, D.C. 20–24 October, 1997 (ALINORM 99/13), Appendix VII, *Hygiene Provisions of the Draft Revised Standards for Butter, Milk fat Products, Evaporated Milks, Sweetened and Condensed Milks, Milk and Cream Powders, Cheese, Whey Cheese, and the Draft Standard for Cheeses in Brine.*
11. Food and Agriculture Organization of the United Nations/World Health Organization, Draft: Guideline on the Application of the General Principles of Food Hygiene to the Control of *Listeria monocytogenes* in Ready to Eat Foods (at Step 8), ALINORM 07/30/13, Appendix III.
12. Food and Agriculture Organization of the United Nations/World Health Organization, Principles for the establishment and application of microbiological criteria for foods, CAC/GL 21-1997. In *Food Hygiene, Basic Texts*, 3rd edition, Rome, Italy, 2003.
13. Food and Agriculture Organization of the United Nations/World Health Organization, Principles and guidelines for the conduct of microbiological risk assessment, CAC/GL-30, 1999. In *Food Hygiene, Basic Texts*, 3rd edition, Rome, Italy, 2003.

14. Codex Alimentarius Commission, Joint FAO/WHO Food Standards Programme, Codex Committee on Food Hygiene, Draft: Principles and Guidelines for the Conduct of Risk Management (MRM), ALINORM 07/30/13, Appendix IV.
15. Food and Agriculture Organization of the United Nations/World Health Organization, Principles for risk analysis of foods derived from modern biotechnology, CAC/GL 44-2003, 2003. In *Foods Derived from Biotechnology*, Rome, Italy, 2004.
16. Food and Agriculture Organization of the United Nations/World Health Organization, Guideline for the conduct of food safety assessment of foods derived from recombinant-DNA plants, CAC/GL 45-2003, 2003. In *Foods Derived from Biotechnology*, Rome, Italy, 2004.
17. Food and Agriculture Organization of the United Nations/World Health Organization, Guideline for the conduct of food safety assessment of foods produced using recombinant-DNA microorganisms, CAC/GL 46-2003, 2003. In *Foods Derived from Biotechnology*, Rome, Italy, 2004.
18. Food and Agriculture Organization of the United Nations/World Health Organization, Guidelines on the judgment of equivalence of sanitary measures associated with food inspection and certification systems, CAC/GL 46-2003, 2003. In *Food Import and Export Inspection and Certification Systems, Combined Texts*, 2nd edition, Rome, Italy, 2005.
19. Codex Alimentarius Commission, Joint FAO/WHO Food Standards Programme, Proposed Draft: Principles for traceability/product tracing as a tool within a food inspection and certification system, CAC/GL 60, 2006.
20. Codex Alimentarius Commission, Joint FAO/WHO Food Standards Programme, Codex Committee on Food Import and Export Inspection and Certification Systems, Proposed Draft: Principles and guidelines for imported food inspection based on risk, ALINORM 06/29/30, Appendix II.
21. Food and Agriculture Organization of the United Nations/World Health Organization, Discussion paper on the risk profile for antimicrobial-resistant bacteria in food, CX/FH 01/12, Rome, Italy, 2001 (see also ALINORM 03/13, paras. 158–162).
22. Codex Alimentarius Commission, Joint FAO/WHO Food Standards Programme, Codex Committee on Food Import and Export Inspection and Certification Systems, Code of Practice to Minimize and Contain Antimicrobial Resistance, ALINORM 05/28/31, Appendix VIII.

19

The International Food Safety Authorities Network

Margaret Ann Miller, Kristin Viswanathan, and Jørgen Schlundt

CONTENTS

19.1 Background

The rapid globalization of food production and trade has increased the potential for international public health incidents involving food contaminated with pathogens or chemicals. In recent years, animal diseases, natural disasters, political unrest, and intentional and unintentional contamination of food have all caused food safety incidents of international concern.

Although effective prevention strategies throughout the entire farm-to-fork continuum are the most efficient way to produce safe food, it is impossible to completely eliminate food contamination events. Dealing with these events requires the rapid access and exchange of food safety information at both the national and international level. Clear, reliable, and authoritative information on food safety is essential not only for prevention and response measures, but also for maintaining international food trade and consumer confidence in the food supply. In response to this need the International Food Safety Authorities Network (INFOSAN) was created as an information network for the worldwide dissemination of important food safety information.[1]

INFOSAN has been set up as a global network in which each participating country has one or more INFOSAN Focal Points. The INFOSAN Focal Points are government officials in an agency related to the regulation of food. They are expected to receive INFOSAN information and disseminate it to the appropriate stakeholders in their country. Integrated within INFO-SAN is an emergency response system, INFOSAN Emergency, which is used to alert food safety authorities about foodborne disease outbreaks or food contamination events of international significance, i.e., international food safety incidents involving an imminent risk of serious injury or death to consumers. INFOSAN Emergency operates under the general public health umbrella of the World Health Organization's (WHO) International Health Regulations (IHR). Each country participating in INFOSAN has one INFOSAN Emergency Contact Point who is expected to notify INFOSAN of international food safety problems, accept notification and response responsibilities, and facilitate the communication of urgent messages during food safety emergencies. During a food safety emergency, the INFOSAN Emergency Contact Point is the authoritative source for information. As global food trade continues to flourish, worldwide information networks, like INFOSAN, are critical for the protection of the public health, the stability of international trade, and the promotion of consumer confidence.

19.2   The International Food Control System

19.2.1   Role of the World Health Organization Including International Health Regulations

The WHO is the United Nations agency for health. WHO's main goal is that all people attain the highest level of health possible, with health being defined as a state of complete physical, mental, and social well-being and not merely the absence of disease or infirmity.[2] To meet this goal, WHO strives to reduce the serious negative impact of foodborne diseases. Despite improvements over the last few decades, far too many people still suffer from poor health as a direct result of contaminated food. In both developing and developed countries, diseases linked to food production, including diseases caused by chemical or microbiological contamination and zoonotic diseases, represent a significant health problem with important social, economic, and political implications. WHO supports the use of science and technology to develop safer food production systems throughout the world. WHO works closely with the Food and Agriculture Organization of the United Nations (FAO) to improve food safety through scientific assessments of food-related risks including the assessment of food additives, chemical and microbiological contaminants, naturally occurring toxicants, residues of veterinary drugs, and foods derived from modern biotechnology. These assessments form a science-based foundation for risk reduction as well as public health-based international standards, which benefit both public health and economic development. WHO also supports, in collaboration with FAO and other relevant international organizations, the development of efficient food safety systems and science-based preventative efforts throughout the food production chain to lower the burden of zoonotic and foodborne diseases.

In 1969, the member states of WHO adopted IHR in agreement with the international community. These regulations represent the only regulatory framework for global public health. The IHR help prevent the international spread of infectious diseases by requiring national public health measures that are applicable to travelers and products at the point of entry. The current IHR require member states to notify WHO of only three diseases: cholera, plague, and yellow fever. However, the revised IHR (2005), which will go into effect in June 2007, will require all 192 member states to notify the WHO of any public health threat constituting a significant risk to other states through the global spread of disease.[3] In the event of such a threat, the IHR enable a coordinated international response as well as specific assistance to affected countries. The IHR (2005) set out the basic public health capacities that a member state must develop, strengthen, and maintain in order to detect, assess, notify, and respond to events that may constitute a public health emergency of international concern. International emergencies caused by contaminated food will fall within the scope of these regulations.

19.2.2 Role of the Food and Agriculture Organization of the United Nations

The mission of the Food and Agriculture Organization (FAO) is to defeat hunger.[4] FAO provides technical advice for food control systems and regulators at national and local levels, ensuring food quality and safety throughout the food chain. FAO promotes, in collaboration with WHO, the establishment and operation of national regulatory frameworks that are compatible with international requirements, in particular with those of the FAO/WHO Codex Alimentarius Commission (Codex).

19.2.3 Codex and International Food Safety Standards

The Codex was established by WHO and FAO to develop international food standards, guidelines, and recommendations to protect the health of consumers and ensure fair practices in food trade.[5] Codex has been most successful in achieving international harmonization of requirements for food quality and safety. It has formulated international standards for a wide range of food products and specific requirements covering pesticide residues, food additives, veterinary drug residues, hygiene, food contaminants, and labeling and certification systems. Following a recent evaluation of the Codex system, more emphasis is being placed on health. One important area of work now being strengthened is food microbiology. Codex is striving to decrease the microbiological contamination of food, and thereby decrease the burden of foodborne disease. Codex work has created worldwide awareness of food safety, quality, and consumer protection issues, and has achieved international consensus on how to deal with them scientifically through a risk-based approach. As a result, there has been a continuous appraisal of the principles of food safety and quality at the international level. The Codex food standards are the global reference point for consumers, food producers and processors, national food control agencies, and international food trade.

19.2.4 Food Safety and Global Food Trade

Ensuring that food is safe is an essential element of modern bilateral and multilateral trade agreements. The Sanitary and Phytosanitary (SPS) Agreement of the World Trade Organization (WTO) is the primary trade agreement dealing with the safety of food. The conclusion of the Uruguay Round of Multilateral Trade Negotiations in Marrakech led to the establishment of the WTO in 1995 and to the execution of the policies of the agreement on the application of Sanitary and Phytosanitary measures (SPS) and the agreement on Technical Barriers to Trade (TBT). Both these agreements are relevant in understanding the requirements for food protection measures at the national level, and the rules under which food is traded internationally. The SPS Agreement confirms the right of WTO member countries to apply measures to protect human, animal, and plant life and health.[6] The agreement covers all relevant laws, decrees, regulations; testing, inspection, certification, and approval procedures; and packaging and labeling requirements directly related to food safety.

The SPS Agreement sets out the basic measures that member countries can use to ensure that imported food is safe while ensuring that technical barriers are not used as an excuse to protect domestic producers. Member states are asked to apply only those measures for protection that are based on scientific principles, only to the extent necessary, and not in a manner that may constitute a disguised restriction on international trade. The agreement seeks to facilitate trade and protect health by encouraging the use of international standards, guidelines, or recommendations where they exist, and identifies those from Codex to be consistent with provisions of SPS. Thus, the Codex standards serve as a benchmark for the comparison of national sanitary and phytosanitary measures. Although it is not compulsory for member states to apply Codex standards, it is nevertheless in their best interests to harmonize their national food standards with those elaborated by Codex. A member country is permitted to establish a food safety measure that is more restrictive than the international standard provided the measure protects humans or animal life or health and is consistently applied to national products and imports.

The TBT Agreement requires that technical regulations on traditional quality factors, fraudulent practices, packaging, labeling, etc., imposed by countries will not be more restrictive on imported products than they are on products produced domestically.[7] It also encourages use of international standards.

19.2.5 Responsibilities of the SPS Notification Authority

The SPS agreement requires countries to notify the WTO of proposed modification to their sanitary and phytosanitary measures when (1) an international standard guideline or recommendation does not exist, (2) the content of the proposed SPS regulation is not the same as the international standard, or (3) the regulation may have a significant effect on trade of other countries.[8] Generally, changing an SPS measure requires notification of the WTO before implementation. However, in emergencies, which the SPS Agreement states as cases "where urgent problems of health protection arise or threaten to arise," a country can implement an emergency measure and notify the SPS authority either before or immediately after it comes into effect, with an explanation of why the country is resorting to emergency action. Notification of INFOSAN Emergency or the IHR Contact Points does not fulfill the notification requirements of the SPS agreement.

19.3 Mandate for the Development of INFOSAN

The rapid globalization of food production and trade has increased the potential for international incidents involving contaminated food. Food safety problems discovered in one country often are of interest or concern in other countries. Food safety authorities all over the world have acknowledged that ensuring food safety must not only be tackled at the national level but also through closer linkages among food safety authorities internationally. Although food safety authorities in some countries are easy to identify and access, this is certainly not the case for all countries.

A number of international conferences and resolutions have called for a coordinated approach for the effective management of public health emergencies, including those caused by contaminated food. International conferences including the Second FAO/WHO Global Forum for Food Safety Regulators and the FAO/WHO Pan-European Conference on Food Safety and Quality referred specifically to the need for effective sharing of food safety emergency information, with emphasis on developing countries.[9,10]

The World Health Assembly (WHA) has adopted a number of resolutions calling for improved communication among WHO and its member states on matters of food safety. In particular, in May 2002, the WHA, in expressing serious concern about health emergencies posed by natural, accidental, and intentional contamination of food, requested that WHO provide tools and support to member states to increase their capacity to respond to such emergencies (WHA55.16).[11] In January 2003, WHO published a report on the terrorist threats to food and guidance for establishing and strengthening prevention and response systems.[12] The report identified a food safety emergency network as one of the basic preparedness measures needed at the international level.

In July 2004, the Codex adopted a text entitled Principles and Guidelines for the Exchange of Information in Food Control Emergency Situations.[13] The document specifies that each country should designate a primary official contact point for food safety emergency situations, to act as the national contact point for information exchange. In the document, WHO is identified as being responsible for maintaining the list of primary official contact points for the exchange of information in food safety emergency situations.

19.4   The INFOSAN Network

In response to these requests, WHO developed the INFOSAN network to promote the exchange of food safety information and to improve collaboration among food safety authorities at the national and international level. The INFOSAN network provides a mechanism for the exchange of information on both routine and emerging food safety issues, in particular, rapid access to information in case of food safety emergencies. As most developing countries are food exporters or importers, their active participation in the network is essential.[1]

As of May 2006, 150 countries are members of the INFOSAN network. Each member country has designated one or several INFOSAN Focal Points. Although it may be desirable to have a single INFOSAN Focal Point, several focal points have been identified in countries where food safety authorities are located in several agencies. In this context, food safety authorities are broadly defined and include authorities involved in food legislation, risk assessment, food control and management, food inspection services, laboratory services for monitoring and surveillance, food safety information, trade officials, veterinary services, and education and communication, across the entire farm-to-fork continuum. Currently, INFOSAN Focal Points are located in several ministries, including ministries of health, commerce, agriculture, and trade.[1]

INFOSAN Focal Points receive INFOSAN notes and messages, WHO guidelines, and other important food safety information from INFOSAN

TABLE 19.1

INFOSAN Notes Published as of May 2006

Date Issued	Title
2006	Nutrient risk assessment
	Zoonotic diseases
2005	Avian influenza
	Global salm-surv
	Natural disasters
	Biotechnology
	Salmonella
	Acrylamide
	Enterobacter sakazakii
2004	Avian influenza
	Unusual sources of *Salmonella*

Source: The full text of all listed INFOSAN notes is available at http://www.who.int/foodsafety/fs_management/infosan_archives/en/index.html

(see Table 19.1).[14] The INFOSAN Focal Points are expected to disseminate INFOSAN information to interested parties and stakeholders in their country, as appropriate. The INFOSAN Focal Points are often asked to provide comments to INFOSAN on WHO guidelines and other topics of interest. INFOSAN Focal Points can similarly contact INFOSAN's secretariat and request the development of an INFOSAN informational note on a specific topic, the dissemination of material for comment, or information on a particular topic. Through the INFOSAN network these requests can be answered directly or routed to the appropriate national focal point. In many circumstances, the INFOSAN Focal Points communicate directly with other members of the network. INFOSAN similarly provides a forum in which developing countries can quickly learn about and more efficiently create food safety control systems. This crucial information sharing process ultimately benefits the entire international community in preventing and containing illness due to foodborne pathogens.

19.5 INFOSAN Emergency

As noted in the Codex text Principles and Guidelines for the Exchange of Information in Food Control Emergency Situations, communication during a food safety emergency is essential to minimize the potential adverse public health effects and to avoid unwarranted action with respect to trade.[13] INFOSAN Emergency responds to information about food contamination incidents by sending INFOSAN Alert messages to the INFOSAN emergency contact points in the affected countries. Information for potential INFOSAN emergency alerts includes information related to (1) microbiological, chemical, or other food contamination or (2) health events presumed to be associated with food consumption.

19.5.1 How INFOSAN Emergency Operates

Surveillance information on zoonotic diseases and food contamination problems is received by the WHO from a variety of sources, including WHO's surveillance networks, WHO's regional or country representatives, and members of the INFOSAN network. The copious amount of information received daily is reviewed to determine the priority with which each reported situation must be addressed. The decision to proceed with INFO-SAN emergency action is based upon three main criteria: (1) the distribution of the contaminated food item, (2) the potential for impact on health, and (3) the potential for impact on the economy. The INFOSAN Emergency network is activated only for food contamination events that are serious and involve international trade. The algorithm for deciding on whether or not additional action is needed is described in Table 19.2.

Once it is determined that further action is required, INFOSAN requests additional information by communicating directly with the INFOSAN Emergency Contact Point in the country of origin. If the INFOSAN Emergency Contact Point indicates that further involvement of INFOSAN is unnecessary, the event is closed. However, after verifying the extent of the problem and confirming the export of the contaminated food item, the INFOSAN Emergency Contact Point may request further assistance by INFOSAN. In this case, INFOSAN will send an official request, containing an offer to contact the exporting country's trading partners, as well as a draft of the formal INFOSAN alert message. After being approved by the INFOSAN Emergency Contact Point, this alert is e-mailed to the INFOSAN Emergency Contact Points in all affected countries. Table 19.3 summarizes the INFOSAN Emergency actions executed from 2005 through May 2006.

INFOSAN Emergency is closely linked to WHO's Global Outbreak Alert and Response Network (GOARN).[15] When a coordinated response is needed to contain a foodborne disease outbreak, GOARN ensures that appropriate technical assistance, including field teams of experts, reaches the affected member states rapidly. The cooperation of INFOSAN Emergency and GOARN aims to minimize the health impact and prevent further spread of the disease. INFOSAN is expanding the capabilities of GOARN by preparing a roster of not only food safety experts but of zoonoses specialists as well.

19.6 Linking INFOSAN to National Food Safety Systems

INFOSAN is designed to complement national food safety emergency systems. Although the government structures and agencies that deal with food

TABLE 19.2

Information Patterns Used to Classify INFOSAN Emergencies

Information Pattern	Further Action Required
Distribution	
Export is indicated or clearly stated	Yes
No information on export but the type of product is likely to be internationally distributed	Yes
No information on export but type of product is unlikely to be internationally distributed	Maybe—dependent on Public Health and Economic Impact
Local distribution only	Generally No
"No export" clearly stated	Generally No
Public Health Impact	
Information suggests a serious acute illness or death caused by the contaminated food item	Yes
No information on public health impact of the contaminated food item but the type of contamination is known to be associated with serious illness or death	Yes
No information on public health impact of the contaminated food item and the type of contamination is insufficiently specified or the association with serious illness is uncertain	Maybe—dependent upon Distribution and Economic Impact
The type of contamination is known not to be associated with serious illness or death	Generally No
Economic Impact	
Surveillance information indicates that inappropriate or widespread product embargos or mass panic, which could destabilize the country or the economy, could occur due to the presence of contaminated food items in the international marketplace	Yes

safety differ from one country to another, a modern national food control system must ensure the production and distribution of safe food. The term "food control system" refers to the essential integration of all parties involved in the production and distribution of safe food.

The FAO/WHO document, Assuring Food Safety and Quality: Guidelines for Strengthening National Food Control Systems, provides a detailed description of the elements of a national food control system and guidance on how to build the system.[16] The guidelines outline the building blocks of a food control system as (1) food laws and regulations, (2) food control management, (3) inspection service (4) laboratory services, and (5) information, education, communication, and training.

TABLE 19.3

Details of INFOSAN Alerts as of May 2006

2006

Dioxins in pig and poultry from Belgium
  No further INFOSAN action was required
Listeria in cheese from Australia
  No further INFOSAN action was required
Avian influenza in poultry from Nigeria
  No further INFOSAN action was required
Metal in powered milk from the United States
  No further INFOSAN action was required

2005

Salmonella Agona in infant formula from France
  Further INFOSAN action was required—INFOSAN Alerts were sent to 14 countries
  The majority of recipient countries reported that they received official information
    from INFOSAN only
Salmonella typhimurium in orange juice from the United States
  Further INFOSAN action was required—INFOSAN Alerts were sent to 4 countries
  The majority of recipient countries reported that they received official information
    from INFOSAN only
Salmonella in hens from Spain
  No further INFOSAN action was required
Escherichia coli 0157 in hamburger from France
  No further INFOSAN action was required
Listeria in meat from Australia
  No further INFOSAN action was required
E. coli 1026 in cheese from France
  No further INFOSAN action was required
Listeria in cheese from Switzerland
  No further INFOSAN action was required

The modern food control system shifts the focus of food safety strategies from response and recovery, following a contaminated food product reaching consumer markets, to strategies of prevention. Effective prevention strategies require the involvement of all stakeholders and the integration of scientifically based risk-assessments at all levels of the food production continuum. The primary responsibility for implementing and monitoring prevention strategies falls to industry. Primary preventive programs, such as Quality Assurance Programs and Hazard Analysis Critical Control Point (HACCP) Systems, aimed at preventing the initial contamination of food, not only improve consumer protection but are cost effective. Government regulators are responsible for developing national policies and standards that support the implementation of risk-based production control programs, monitoring and surveillance of these programs, and enforcement of legal standards. Similarly, industry is assigned a major role in secondary prevention by developing methods that are capable of rapidly detecting contaminated food products and preventing them from reaching consumer markets. Food recall plans, developed by industry and monitored by government, are an example of a secondary prevention strategy. It is essential that these recall plans include both national and international distribution. INFOSAN Emergency, through its Emergency Contact Points, can help industry and governments recall contaminated foods that have been distributed internationally.

When both primary and secondary prevention strategies fail to prevent consumer exposure to contaminated food, tertiary prevention plans, i.e., those that contain the contaminated food and thereby minimize the impact on public health, are needed. Access to timely and accurate information about the type of contamination, distribution of the product, and number of persons affected is critical for mounting a quick and appropriate emergency response that prevents the further spread of the product and disease. Integration of all stakeholders within the farm to fork continuum allows governments to access the information needed to rapidly detect potential or emerging food safety incidents, identify the affected food, and effectively remove the food from consumer access. INFOSAN Emergency is an essential component of tertiary prevention programs for situations where a contaminated food product has entered international commerce. INFOSAN Emergency can help countries identify and contain contaminated food with international distribution; therefore notification of INFOSAN should occur early in the recall process. Member states are encouraged to strengthen their National Food Control System as a basic means of preventing and controlling food safety emergencies.

19.7 Conclusion

The increased interconnectedness of global food markets necessitated the development of a global information and response network to protect the public health. As a network of food safety authorities aimed at preventing the international spread of contaminated food, the INFOSAN network possesses the unique ability to accumulate, analyze, and disseminate the information needed to monitor and effectively prevent or contain foodborne illness. While INFOSAN is designed to provide food safety authorities with timely and accurate information about critically important issues in food safety, INFOSAN Emergency, through its rapid response capabilities, is specifically tailored to detect emergency situations of food contamination and to utilize its privileged communication structure to minimize public health and economic impact. The adoption and implementation of the recently revised IHR (2005) will enhance the ability of the INFOSAN network to respond to foodborne contaminants by broadening the scope of national accountability to the WHO. In addition, the national preparedness plans recommended by the new IHR (2005) will provide a strong national infrastructure for the detection of potential food contamination. Through

INFOSAN, WHO will continue to work in cooperation and coordination with national governments to ensure that they develop the capability to practically decrease the burden of foodborne disease within the global community.

References

1. International Food Safety Authorities Network (INFOSAN). Department of Food Safety, Zoonoses, and Foodborne Diseases, World Health Organization, (July 2005). http://www.who.int/foodsafety/fs_management/infosan_0705_en.pdf (accessed May 2006).
2. WHO. *About WHO*. World Health Organization, United Nations (January 2006). http://www.who.int/about/en/ (accessed May 2006).
3. Revision of the International Health Regulations. Fifty-Eighth World Health Assembly, Agenda Item 13.1 (23 May 2005). http://www.who.int/csr/ihr/WHA58_3-en.pdf (accessed May 2006).
4. "FAO At Work." Food and Agriculture Organization of the United Nations, (May 2006). http://www.fao.org/UNFAO/about/index_en.html (accessed May 2006).
5. "Understanding the Codex Alimentarius." FAO Corporate Document Repository, originated by the Economic and Social Department (1999). http://www.fao.org/documents/show_cdr.asp?url_file=/docrep/w9114e/w9114e00.htm (accessed May 2006).
6. WTO. The WTO Agreement on the Application of Sanitary and Phytosanitary Measures (SPS Agreement). World Trade Organization (1 January 1995). http://www.wto.org/english/tratop_e/sps_e/spsagr_e.htm (accessed May 2006).
7. WTO. "Agreement on Technical Barriers to Trade. World Trade Organization (1 January 1995). http://www.wto.org/english/docs_e/legal_e/17-tbt.pdf (accessed May 2006).
8. WTO. Sanitary and Phytosanitary Measures. World Trade Organization (May 2006). http://www.wto.org/English/tratop_e/sps_e/sps_e.htm (accessed May 2006).
9. The United States of America. International Cooperation on Food Contamination and Foodborne Disease Surveillance. Second FAO/WHO Global Forum of Food Safety Regulators, Agenda Item 5.2 (12–14 October 2004). ftp://ftp.fao.org/docrep/fao/meeting/008/ae163e.pdf (accessed May 2006).
10. Pan-European Cooperation in Information and Communication Development. Pan-European Conference of Food Safety and Quality, Agenda Item 5 (25–28 February 2002). http://www.foodsafetyforum.org/paneuropean/ (accessed May 2006).
11. Resolutions and Actions by the Fifty-Fifth World Health Assembly of Interest to the Regional Committee. 26th Pan-American Sanitary Conference: 54th Session of the Regional Committee, p. 9 (23–27 September 2002). http://www.paho.org/english/gov/csp/csp26-26-e.pdf (accessed May 2006).
12. WHO. Terrorist Threats to Food: Guidance for Establishing and Strengthening Prevention and Response Systems. Food Safety Department, World Health Organization (2002). http://www.who.int/foodsafety/publications/general/en/terrorist.pdf (accessed May 2006).

13. CAC. Principles and Guidelines for the Exchange of Information in Food Control Emergency. Codex Alimentarius Commission, CAC/GL 19–1995, Rev. 1–2004 (July 2004). http://www.codexalimentarius.net/download/standards/36/CXG_019_2004e.pdf (accessed May 2006).
14. WHO. INFOSAN Information Note Archive. Department of Food Safety, World Health Organization, United Nations (May 2006). http://www.who.int/foodsafety/fs_management/infosan_archives/en/index.html (accessed May 2006).
15. WHO. Global Outbreak Alert and Response Network. Epidemic and Pandemic Alert Response, World Health Organization, United Nations (January 2006). http://www.who.int/csr/outbreaknetwork/en/ (accessed May 2006).
16. United Nations. Food and Agriculture Organization. World Health Organization. 2003. *Assuring Food Safety and Quality: Guidelines for Strengthening National Food Control Systems*. Rome: Food and Agriculture Organization.

Section V

Bioterrorism and Microbial Food Contamination

20

Biological Contamination of Food

Barbara Rasco and Gleyn E. Bledsoe

CONTENTS

Tommy G. Thompson, former secretary of Health and Human Services, said, he worried constantly about food poisoning. In a now famous statement he made before his resignation in December 2004, he said:

> "I, for the life of me, cannot understand why the terrorists have not, you know, attacked our food supply because it is so easy to do," he said. "And we are importing a lot of food from the Middle East, and it would be easy to tamper with that."

Although inspections of food imports have risen sharply in the past 4 years, "it still is a very minute amount that we're doing."[*]

His warning did much to promote the development of food defense programs throughout the private sector. In this chapter, we will discuss vulnerability assessments and risk assessment models as well as some of the microbes and toxins that could pose a threat for intentional food contamination.

---

[*] Branigin, W., Allen, M., and Mintz, J. 2004. Tommy Thompson Resigns From HHS. Bush Asks Defense Secretary Rumsfeld to Stay. *Washington Post*. Friday, December 3, p. A1, 2004.

20.1   Vulnerability Assessments

Bioterrorism refers to the use of a microbe or biological toxin that causes disease to harm people, to elicit widespread fear, or intimidation serving a political or ideological goal (NRC, 2006). Increased acts of politically motivated terrorism coupled with the easy acquisition and mass production of lethal microbes or toxins are thought by a number of experts to be inevitable (Atlas, 2001). The term "catastrophic terrorism" has been coined to describe the specific danger facing the United States from a bioterrorist attack. Unfortunately, the food supply is vulnerable to intentional criminal acts and to a wide spectrum of natural disasters that could cripple our capacity to deliver safe, affordable food in sufficient quantities to feed the nation. A further complication is that an attack using one or a combination of naturally occurring pathogens might at first be hard to define as an attack and not just a nonintentional incident. And the scope of an attack may also be difficult to determine as the targeting of a specific population such as first responders (Afton et al. 2005), military personnel, or transportation could be part of an isolated strike or part of a larger coordinated effort. Nor are the innocent excluded, as Al-Qaeda has stated the killing of American women and children is justified (Fouda and Fielding, 2004).

The primary purpose of intentional contamination of food is to terrorize people, not necessarily to kill them, although a few deaths would make a significant impact and would keep the issue fresh on people's minds. In fact, merely a false claim to have committed an intentional contamination act by a terrorist group could be almost as effective as an actual contamination event. The greatest impact to the food supply would most likely be from a relatively widespread but somewhat insidious contamination event affecting a large number of people in disparate markets and having wide-ranging impact in the agricultural sector. A recent study suggested that the U.S. food supply remains vulnerable to attack despite efforts over the past few years to improve preparedness and institute widespread preventive measures. U.S. officials are concerned that terrorist groups including Al-Qaeda may be plotting attacks against food and agricultural sectors (Drees, 2004). Evidence supporting this assertion included uncovering hundreds of documents targeting U.S. agricultural interests in the caves of Afghanistan and safe houses of terrorist groups. Home-based labs producing incendiary devices, ricin, anthrax, pathogens, and components for chemical contaminant or explosives have been uncovered in numerous locations throughout the world, including the United States. Although explosive devices have been the favorite tool of environmental, animal rights and political terrorists to date, a number of different agents have been used to contaminate consumer goods and foods across the world (Rasco and Bledsoe, 2005) and illicit drugs, including allegations of botulinum toxin contamination in black tar heroin in the northern United States in August 2006.

Three important points must be considered when analyzing the use of biological preparations to contaminate food. First, biological agents are easy to conceal. A small amount may be sufficient to harm large populations and cause epidemics over a broad geographic region. Second, the contagious nature of some infectious diseases means that once a person has been exposed and infected it may be possible for him/her to continue to spread the disease to others depending upon the agent used. Third, in the most worrisome scenario of a surreptitious attack, the first responders are likely to be health professionals in emergency rooms, physician offices, and out-patient clinics rather than law enforcement and other traditional first responders. The longer the terrorist-induced epidemic goes unrecognized and undiagnosed, the longer the delay in initiating treatment and other control efforts.

Foods are effective targets for intentional contamination because there are several chemical, radiological, and biological agents that could be success-fully employed, many of which are difficult to isolate and detect in complex matrices like food. Many of contaminants have little effect on the sensory properties of a food and would not create suspicion for food sellers or con-sumers. Food products at the greatest risk include those that are perishable, ready-to-eat, and which would be distributed and consumed before there had been time to detect the hazard. Furthermore, food is distributed rapidly, often over great distances, and to large numbers of people in different loca-tions, creating the potential for widespread impact. The systems in place for producing and distributing food also create risks. For example, food and agriculture products are commonly accessible to terrorists at some point during growing, harvesting, processing, storage, and distribution. The unit operations involved in food production such as mixing, blending in minor components, diluting, or size reduction could spread a toxic material throughout a larger batch or numerous batches of product or spread con-tamination throughout a facility to such an extent that the facility could not be used until it had been decontaminated, often at considerable cost. The extensive and costly measures imposed upon rendering plants to clean and decontaminate facilities to reduce the risk of distributing prions from infected bovine tissue into the food and animal feed supply resulting from the possibility or actual processing of a single bovine spongiform enceph-alopathy (BSE)-infected cow provides an example of the types of measures that may be required of a food processing operation following an intentional contamination event.

This BSE example is a situation in which the perceived risk of a human health impact led to an inappropriate and excessive response because of a lack of reliable information about what the real health impact could possibly be. As a result, many rendering facilities were driven out of business because of the excessive cost of the government-mandated cleanups. The negative impact of these 2003 events continued and in 2006 there was not enough rendering capacity remaining in the West Coast to handle the thousands of dairy cattle, roughly 2% of the entire herd, and other livestock died in California from a protracted spell of abnormally high temperatures exceeding 110°F (Anon, 2006).

BSE also provides another example of the costs of contamination, albeit in this case unintentional, of just one sector of the food supply where damages in excess of $7 billion were absorbed by the beef industry in the United Kingdom in the late 1990s (Manning et al. 2005). A similar situation faces the food industry with the risk assessment and evaluation of mitigation strategies associated with the intentional contamination of food. It is likely that there will be overzealous government action taken in response to any incident of intentional contamination unless we get a better handle on the actual public health risk such an incident would pose and develop guidelines for reactions appropriate to the magnitude of the actual hazard.

A great deal of emphasis has been placed by the federal government on risk assessment and control strategies for exotic agents that could be used to contaminate food and water. This emphasis is justifiable in the case of the introduction of zoonotic disease, and for developing scientific data on the inactivation and removal of contaminants from food and the food processing environment, public health measures for detection and response to an incident, and analytical methods for detection of agents in food and environmental samples. The recent emphasis on exotic agents as a vehicle for contamination of processed food is necessary to obtain the scientific and technical information to improve detection, control, and response in case these materials are used; however, in the long term, focus on exotic agents may be unwarranted as the risk posed by more conventional microbes and toxins is more likely and this continued focus creates the possibility that attention and limited private and public sector resources will be diverted away from the development of effective controls and mitigation strategies for more likely risks to the food supply.

The U.S. Department of Agriculture (USDA) and Food and Drug Administration (FDA) have conducted numerous vulnerability assessments of our food supply, including a recent study released in June 2006 (FDA, 2006) involving the agency and a number of state and private sector participants. The agency's attention has remained focused on risk assessment and threat agent detection with the use of the CARVER + Shock model being the most recent iteration of risk assessment models promoted by the agency within the past 5 years. As both the FDA and USDA are encouraging businesses to conduct vulnerability assessments and to develop food safety plans, it will be important for the agencies to release their findings to the private sector so that appropriate mitigation and control strategies can be developed at the corporate and facility level. Unfortunately, these agencies have not been forthcoming in releasing many of their specific findings claiming that to do so would be to assist potential terrorists to identify vulnerable targets, a situation reminiscent of the failure of intelligence agencies to advise the commanders in Pearl Harbor of the eminent threat of a Japanese attack in December 1941.

In response to the threat, many companies are using Hazard Analysis Critical Control Point (HACCP)-based risk assessment models to perform these tasks because they are familiar with HACCP risk assessment models and the development of HACCP plans, and have been able to expand the application of HACCP successfully from food safety to the food defense arena. Others are using Operational Risk Management (ORM), or CARVER, or CARVER + Shock models for this purpose or a combination, employing the ORM and CARVER models within the hazard analysis component of a HACCP-based plan.

The primary objective for developing and implementing a food defense plan for a company must be developing the ability to differentiate between a real and a perceived risk and to determine quickly and be able to prove when presented with an incident, whether the incident is a result of an intentional act of contamination or not, and if the alleged incident is a hoax. The basic strategy for risk assessment should be as follows: how likely is it that the type of contamination could occur, how bad would the outcome be of a contamination event (severity), what realistic preventive measures can be implemented, and what response measures should an organization take if food is intentionally contaminated (Ryan, 2005). Selection of preventive and response strategies, by necessity, must also be based upon a cost-benefit analysis, but the most important task is for a company to develop a guided process for food defense. The needs of the organization should drive the selection of a model for risk assessment. Broad industry concerns are often too difficult to use because of a lack of data on actual risks to a product or an operation as well as threat agents, agent–food matrix interactions, toxicity of threat agents in a food system and capabilities of terrorists to obtain or produce agents affective for foods (Ryan, 2005). Developing food defense programs for the very diverse food industry in the United States with over 1.2 million retail food facilities (including restaurants and groceries), 57,000 food processing companies and at least an additional 100,000 registered food handling and processing facilities is a daunting task. To complicate matters further, over 150,000 imported food shipments are received each week in the United States.

The recent FDA study has been able to produce some useful distinctions between points within a process (or nodes) for different foods and agricultural production processes evaluated to date (Table 20.1). This study has also show commonalities across sectors and provides some protective measures and mitigation strategies that could be useful for food defense plans.

In general from these recent government studies, the greatest vulnerability for production agriculture exists from a highly transmissible or contagious plant or animal disease. A disease outbreak can have a significant impact on the national economy, even if introduced in a small number (possibly a single animal or plant) near our borders or in an imported shipment. Zoonotic diseases pose considerable risk as threat agents. The highest concern in food processing is for products where there is direct human contact

TABLE 20.1

Industries Proposed and Completed for USDA and FDA Site Visits (SPPA Study)

USDA Proposed Site Visits	USDA Completed Site Visits (2006) (States Listed)[a]	FDA Proposed Site Visits	FDA Completed Site Visits (2006) (States Listed)
Preharvest		Animal by-products	
Aquaculture production		Animal foods/feeds	
Beef cattle feedlot	NE	Baby food	MI (applesauce, jarred)
Cattle stockyard/auction barn	MO, KS	Breaded food, frozen, raw	
Citrus production facility		Canned food, low acid	
Corn farm		Cereal, whole grain not heat treated	
Dairy farm	ID	Deli salads	
Grain elevator and storage facility		Dietary supplement, botanical, tablets	
Grain export handling facility	LA	Entrees, fully cooked	
Poultry farm		Flour	
Rice mill		Frozen packaged entrees	FL, WI (pizza)
Seed production facility		Fruit juice	NH (apple)
Soybean farm		Gum arabic	
Swine production facility	IA	High-fructose corn syrup	
Veterinary biologics firm		Honey	
Postharvest		Ice cream	
Deli meat processing facility		Infant formula	AZ
Ground beef processing facility	KS	Milk, fluid	NY
Hot dog/Frankfurter processing		Peanut butter	
Import reinspection facility		Produce, fresh	
Liquid egg processing	PA	Produce, cut, modified atmosphere packaged	CA (bagged salad)
Poultry processing	AR	Retail setting	
Retailers (further processing on-site)		Seafood, cooked, refrigerated, ready-to-eat	
School food service central kitchen	NC	Soft drink, carbonated	
Related industries		Spices	
Transportation companies		Vitamins/microingredient, premixes, flavors	
Warehouses		Water, bottled	PA
		Yogurt	MN, TN

Source: Adapted from FDA. 2006. Strategic Partnership Program Agroterrorism (SPPA) Initiative. First Year Status Report September 2005–2006.

[a] California, Illinois, Iowa, Nebraska, and Texas account for one-third of total U.S. agricultural production.

with a large volume of product such as a bulk raw ingredient or a large amount of mixed ingredients, particularly when human access is a normal operational step such as is the case when manual addition of a smaller amount of secondary ingredients is involved. The handling of secondary ingredients is also a concern because these are usually dispersed and mixed into larger amounts of product during further processing.

Unfortunately, the responsibility for developing preventive measures for food defense plans and mitigation strategies remains with the private sector. Both the FDA and USDA are incorporating food defense components into inspections and, although neither agency is "writing up" food defense infarctions in and of themselves, they will do so when such a factor would be considered to otherwise violate a food safety regulation.

Developing a model for risk assessment for a terrorist attack against the food supply will depend first on the ability of a terrorist to carry out an attack, the intent of the terrorist to carry out a particular attack, and the opportunity to conduct an attack. This creates a threat. Risk is the threat coupled with vulnerability. Vulnerability is the accessibility of the targeted food or food production operation to attack. The role of the food industry is to reduce the opportunity for an attack.

20.2 Developing Food Defense Plans

Hazard Analysis Critical Control Point (HACCP) is commonly used for food safety risk assessment. A HACCP-based assessment has the flexibility to address both food safety and food defense concerns and has been promoted as a reasonable model for food defense by the World Health Organization (WHO, 2002) as well as by numerous other experts (Rasco and Bledsoe, 2005). HACCP in this context would involve the development and implementation of preventive measures to reduce the risk of intentional contamination of a food product within a food facility and during its distribution after the most probable hazards of intentional contamination have been identified. An effective security plan within a facility would be built upon a foundation that includes and integrates an already effective HACCP plan, security, and food safety aspects of good manufacturing practices (GMPs) (e.g., under 21 CFR Part 110), a workable and effective sanitation standard operating procedure and an up-to-date product recall program (21 CFR Part 7). A food defense plan would have to be compatible with these programs regardless of the model that might be used to develop it.

Hazard Analysis Critical Control Point provides the underlying theoretical basis for the development of food defense plans in cases where either an ORM- or CARVER-based risk assessment has been used. How a critical control point is determined is similar for both HACCP and ORM. Risk analysis under a HACCP-based food defense model uses objective and subjective criteria to determine whether intentional contamination would be reasonably likely to occur at any particular point in an operation and whether a preventive measure could be instituted to prevent or eliminate the risk, or reduce it to acceptable levels. When the hazard analysis is conducted, criteria such as severity and shock could be factored in. Critical controls would be established for the food defense program in a similar manner as in a HACCP-based food safety program; certain points in the operation where control as well as a monitoring system for these would have to be established. Critical control points (known as nodes or risk or critical nodes in CARVER + Shock) denote points in a process that present a high risk for food contamination. Critical limits would have to be determined at each of these nodes for controlling the risk, and corrective actions developed to fix the underlying food defense problem if a critical limit is not met and control is lost. A confidential records system and verification program should also be established as part of a HACCP-based food defense system. As with any HACCP program, it is critical to reevaluate the food defense plan when there is a change in production practices, logistics, shipping or distribution, suppliers, or employee practices that may alter how a product could be intentionally contaminated.

Critics of using a HACCP-based model for food defense claim that it is not designed to address the risk of intentional contamination and that predetermined corrective actions for food defense have not been incorporated into HACCP models, for example, components outside of a conventional food unit operations such as in plant surveillance, employee screening, training and monitoring, and physical security functions. Although this may be true, it does not undermine the usefulness of a HACCP-based model for development of a food defense program, since HACCP in theory is rigorous enough to be adapted for these applications. The flexibility of the HACCP-based risk assessment is often easier for a company to use. Unfortunately, HACCP has been undermined by an overlay of regulatory controls that have resulted from the forced adoption of agency-defined hazards, critical control points and monitoring requirements, and from mandatory controls proscribed in guidance documents that have morphed into de facto regulations for meat, poultry, juice, and seafood HACCP programs. This has led to the misunderstanding on the part of some that HACCP is an inappropriate base for food defense risk assessment. However, the primary benefit of using a HACCP-based approach remains—that is HACCP allows an organization to focus its attention on the points where the risk is greatest and to adapt existing monitoring and verification strategies that are already in place as part of food safety programs for implementation to food defense. A simple example of how HACCP could be applied to a particular food is outlined here and in the tables below (Tables 20.2 through 20.4).

A number of risk assessment models have been created that use more formalized scales or ratings than HACCP to characterize different risks. One of the most useful of these models is "Risk Ranger," a program to

TABLE 20.2

An Example of a HACCP-Based Food Defense Application. Production
and Distribution of Frozen Pacific Cod (*Gadus morhua*) Fillets

This is a description of the steps that could be involved in a food defense program for a frozen,
wild-harvested ocean aquatic food product. These steps may need to be modified as each
operation is unique:

1. Harvest and primary processing: Fishes are harvested, using trawl or longline gear from the
   Pacific Ocean off the coast of Alaska, headed, gutted, and filleted using automated equipment
   on board. Fish fillets are layered by hand between sheets of colored plastic inside a plastic
   lined fiberboard box (roughly 17 lb of product) that has been placed within a metal plate
   freezer frame (shatter pack). After filling, the box is closed and frozen at –30°C, which takes
   approximately 3 h. After freezing, the boxes are "broken out" from the freezer frames, the
   flaps of the boxes sealed with tape that has the company logo on it, and three boxes placed
   within a preprinted cardboard master carton. The master carton has the company name,
   address, and contact information along with places for the following information to be written
   in indelible marker: approximate weight, product identification (country of origin, product
   from, size, and species), lot code, harvest location, and name of processing vessel. The master
   cartons are stacked onto pallets, shrink wrapped, labeled with product identification (same as
   above), and the pallets placed into a storage freezer (–20°C). Package is tamper evident only to
   the extent that removal of the tape on the master carton could be detected.
2. Transit to secondary processing facility: After the ship arrives at port, the pallets are loaded
   onto a refrigerated truck with a forklift or hoist and shipped to a secondary processing
   facility for storage before further processing. Loads are sealed and seal numbers recorded on
   shipping documentation. Temperature recorders are included in each shipment.
3. Receipt at secondary processor: Product is received within 8 h of the ship being unloaded.
   Product is transferred from the trucks to the storage freezer in the processing facility with a
   forklift. Seal integrity and seal numbers, package integrity, quantity shipped, and
   temperatures are verified.
4. Storage at processing facility: Product is held frozen until needed. Product flow is first in,
   first out. There is a continuous temperature recorder on the freezer and freezer checks are
   made every 4 h when the plant is operating.
5. Processing—slack out: Pallets are removed from the freezer and moved to the production
   floor to thaw. The number of units and weight from each lot and the lot number are
   recorded. Temperatures are taken intermittently and when the product core temperature
   reaches 28°F, the master cartons are transferred to processing tables.
6. Repackaging: Master cartons are opened and approximately 5 lb of product is transferred
   manually into preprinted plastic heat-sealable, frozen product retail bags. Since the product
   for sale is whole fillets, this will be an approximate weight. Bags are heat sealed. Package is
   tamper evident to the extent that it is easy to tell the bag has been torn or an attempt has been
   made to break the seal. Product is weighed and a bar code readable label with the weight is
   applied to the bag. Package information also includes: lot code (with encoded information on
   production line, facility, and production time), use by date, food preparation tips, recipes,
   allergen information, ingredients, country of origin, and company contact information
   (name, address, web site with e-mail and phone).
7. Freezing and frozen storage: Ten bags of product are placed into a master carton which is in
   turn sealed, palleted, shrink wrapped, and then refrozen. A label is applied to the master
   which has the same information as the retail pack. A similar identifying label is wrapped
   within each pallet.
8. Distribution to retailer: Pallets are transferred from the storage freezer with a fork lift to a
   refrigerated van (common carrier) that is capable of holding the temperature at –20°C. The
   truck makes multiple deliveries within the same metropolitan area. Retailers receive both
   full and partial pallets of product. Product is transferred from the van by forklift or hand
   truck to the retailer's store and transferred to the product storage freezer.

(*continued*)

TABLE 20.2 (continued)

An Example of a HACCP-Based Food Defense Application. Production
and Distribution of Frozen Pacific Cod (*Gadus morhua*) Fillets

9. Retail sale: Personnel from the frozen food department replace stock on sales shelf as
necessary and use a first-in, first-out product rotation. Consumers remove product from the
retail case for purchase. Any product returned by a consumer is not restocked.

The points at which this product is most susceptible to intentional contamination is during
production, at one of the numerous transfer points, or at retail point of sale.

Source: Adapted from Rasco, B.A., and Bledsoe, G.E., 2005, pp. 187.

calculate food risks and can be easily used by individuals with little experience in risk modeling. It is a useful tool for helping food safety managers to
think in terms of risk and possible strategies that can be used to control risk.
Risk Ranger employs a simple statistical risk calculation to aid in determining relative risks from different products, pathogens, and processing combinations. It was developed by the Australian Food Safety Centre
(http://www.foodsafetycentre.com.au/riskranger.html) based on the work
of Ross and Sumner (2002). Risk Ranger uses a generic but robust model
based upon all elements of food safety to generate the risk calculations and
rates risk from negligible risk (e.g., 0—mild food borne illness in 1 of 10
billion people) to extremely high risk (e.g., 100—every member of the
population eats a meal containing a lethal dose every day). The model
includes 11 key questions relating to the severity of the hazard, likelihood
of a disease causing dose of the hazardous material being present in a meal
and the probability of exposure as well as the size of the population affected
and specific risk factors for a certain targeted populations, products, or
operations. In addition to ranking risks, Risk Ranger helps to focus the
attention of the users on the interplay between factors that contribute to
foodborne disease. The model can be used to explore the effect of different
risk-reduction strategies, or the extent of the change required to bring about
a desired reduction in risk. Factors for Risk Ranger assessment are:

1. Susceptibility and hazard
    a. Hazard severity
    b. Susceptibility of the population of interest
2. Probability of exposure to food
    a. Frequency of consumption
    b. Percent of population consuming the food
    c. Size of the consuming population
3. Probability of the food containing an infective dose
    a. Probability of contamination of raw product on a per serving
       basis
    b. Effect of processing

TABLE 20.3

A Model Food Defense Plan Based upon a HACCP Model—Hazard Analysis Worksheet
Product Description: Frozen Cod Fish Fillets, Retail Pack (Heat Sealed Plastic Bag)
Intended Use/Consumer: Retail Sale to General Public

Item, Step, or Function	Are Any Hazards Significant (Reasonably) Likely to Occur?	What Controls or Preventive Measures Can Be Applied to Prevent, Eliminate or Reduce a Significant Hazard?	Is Control at This Point Critical?
Harvesting and primary processing	Yes	Certification of lot by vendor/supplier guarantee for packaging material	Yes
		Tamper-evident packaging	Yes
		Periodic testing	No
Transit to secondary processing facility	Yes	All openings, doors, vents, etc., on truck or conveyance locked and sealed by vendor	Yes
		Time and temperature recording included in shipment	
		Automated trip recorder/report	Yes
		Vehicle in secured facility when unattended	No
		Vehicle secured when driver absent	Yes
Receiving at processing facility	Yes	Verifying seals, seal integrity, and paperwork at receipt, check lot, product type, quantity, number of units, origin	Yes
		Check product temperature and package integrity	Yes
Storage at processing facility	Yes	Ensure that product is secure and access to it is limited to authorized individuals only	Yes
Processing—slacking out	No	Product remains in original packaging; process is short and poses little risk	No
Repackaging	Yes	Individual fish are handled and placed into packaging in which contamination would not be evident to retail purchaser	Yes
Freezing and frozen storage	Yes	Product coded for traceability at retail level	Yes
		Product properly inventoried	No

(continued)

TABLE 20.3 (continued)

A Model Food Defense Plan Based upon a HACCP Model–Hazard Analysis Worksheet

Product Description: Frozen Cod Fish Fillets, Retail Pack (Heat Sealed Plastic Bag)

Intended Use/Consumer: Retail Sale to General Public

Item, Step, or Function	Are Any Hazards Significant (Reasonably Likely to Occur)?	What Controls or Preventive Measures Can Be Applied to Prevent, Eliminate or Reduce a Significant Hazard?	Is Control at This Point Critical?
Distribution to retailer	Yes	Tamper-evident seals present on unitized packs	Yes
		Traceability features present	Yes
		All openings, doors, vents, etc. on truck or conveyance locked and sealed by vendor	Yes
		Data and temperature recording devices included with shipment	Yes
		Automated trip recorder/report	Yes
Retail sale	Yes	Control receipt and storage of inventory	Yes
		Control stock rotation	No
		Ensure that all foods are properly and legibly labeled and have lot codes and other traceability features	Yes
		Do not restock or sell food items found in other areas of the store, of which have been returned by a consumer	Yes
		Check package integrity of products on shelf	Yes
		Watch for suspicious activity	Yes

Company name: Capitol Fish Co.
Address: 1600 Penn Ave.
Western, WA 98103
Prepared by: Bill Frost

Bill Frost

Date: November 4, 2006

TABLE 20.4

A Model Food Defense Plan Based upon a HACCP Model—Food Defense Plan Form

Product Description: Frozen Cod Fish Fillets, Retail Pack (Heat Sealed Plastic Bag)

Intended Use/Consumer: Retail Sale to General Public

Critical Control Point	Critical Limit	Monitoring				Corrective Action	Verification	Records
		What	How	Frequency	Who			
Harvesting and primary processing	Vendor certification received at shipment	Certification received	Check against shipping documents	Each lot	Receiving QC	Isolate and investigate if required records verification is possible, accept; if not, reject	Daily record review	Production record
	Lot ID numbers	Lot identification	Check product ID against shipping documents	Each lot		Isolate and investigate, reject if safety cannot be assured		
	All units have functional tamper-evident packaging; packaging intact	Package integrity	Visual	Each unit		Isolate and investigate; if cannot adequately ID lots, reject Reject and isolate; retain product if criminal activity is suspected and contact law enforcement		

(continued)

TABLE 20.4 (continued)

A Model Food Defense Plan Based upon a HACCP Model—Food Defense Plan Form
Product Description: Frozen Cod Fish Fillets, Retail Pack (Heat Sealed Plastic Bag)
Intended Use/Consumer: Retail Sale to General Public

Critical Control Point	Critical Limit	Monitoring				Corrective Action	Verification	Records
		What	How	Frequency	Who			
Transit to secondary processing facility	Seals intact and ID numbers match	Seals intake and ID numbers match	Seals and ID numbers	Visual and match against shipping records	Shipper	Isolate product and investigate. Retain product if criminal activity is suspected and contact law enforcement, release if discrepancies in paperwork can be rectified	Daily record review	Shipping records
	Time and temperature recorders in each shipment	Time-temperature recorder in shipment	Recorder is present and functional	Visual		Isolate product and inspect for quality and safety; install and calibrate functional recorder into shipment	Shipping document review with each shipment	
	Vehicle secure when driver is absent	Vehicle secure	Driver log or report	Each shipment		Isolate and investigate; if product may have been	Driver log review with each shipment	

Receiving at processing facility	Time temperature recorder is in shipment	No unexplained deviations	Visual and recorder printout	Each shipment	Receiving QC	tampered with, reject and isolate; retain product if criminal activity is suspected and contact law enforcement	Daily review of shipping documents and recorder printouts	Receiving records
						Isolate and investigate; if deviation cannot be explained, reject		
	Trip report received	Trip record	Visual	Each shipment		Obtain trip report and review current procedures with shipper		
	Product and package integrity	Visual	Visual	Each unit		Document product or packaging defect; isolate and examine product; if suspicious, reject; if criminal activity suspected, retain product and contact law enforcement		

(continued)

TABLE 20.4 (continued)

A Model Food Defense Plan Based upon a HACCP Model—Food Defense Plan Form

Product Description: Frozen Cod Fish Fillets, Retail Pack (Heat Sealed Plastic Bag)

Intended Use/Consumer: Retail Sale to General Public

Critical Control Point	Critical Limit	Monitoring				Corrective Action	Verification	Records
		What	How	Frequency	Who			
	Lot numbers match	Lot identification	Check product identifiers against shipping documents	Each lot		Isolate product and investigate; if required records verification is possible accept; if not reject; of criminal activity suspected, retain product and contact law enforcement		
Storage at processing facility	No unauthorized access	Access to stored product	Locked storage with keys issued to authorized individuals only	Weekly	Production supervisor	Keys marked do not duplicate; collect keys from ex-employees and those no longer authorized; if cannot account for all issued keys, re-key, and issue new keys	Weekly review of safety inspection and employment records	Safety inspection log; employee or contractor log
Repackaging	Product integrity	Product handled by trusted individuals only	Two-person rule; employee vigilance for	Each lot	Packaging lead	Isolate suspicious product and evaluate; if tampering is	Daily records review	Packaging log

			suspicious activity			possible, reject and destroy; if criminal activity is suspected, isolate, and retain product and contact law enforcement		
	Package integrity	Package properly sealed	Visual	Each unit	Line worker	Reject, then isolate damaged product		
	Package coded for traceability	Package properly sealed	Visual	Each unit	Line worker	Isolate and relabel uncoded product; if this is not possible, reject and destroy product	Daily records review, review of deviation reports for relabeled goods	
Freezing and frozen storage	Tamper-evident seals present and intact on unitized packages	Seals present and intact	Visual	Each unit	Warehouse supervisor	If product is damaged. Isolate and examine; if it may be contaminated, destroy it		Freezer log
	Traceability features incorporated into unitized packages	Traceability features present and functional	Visual	Each unit		Replace tamper-evident packaging if possible; apply new traceability features		
Distribution to retailer	All openings, vents doors, etc., on truck or conveyance are locked and sealed before shipment. Seal numbers are recorded	Seals are present and numbers are recorded	Check numbers against vendor documents	Each shipment	Receiving QC	If seals and related documentation not consistent, reject shipment	Daily review of shipping records	Shipping records

(continued)

TABLE 20.4 (continued)

A Model Food Defense Plan Based upon a HACCP Model—Food Defense Plan Form
Product Description: Frozen Cod Fish Fillets, Retail Pack (Heat Sealed Plastic Bag)
Intended Use/Consumer: Retail Sale to General Public

Critical Control Point	Critical Limit	Monitoring				Corrective Action	Verification	Records
		What	How	Frequency	Who			
	Date and temperature recorder device(s) are included in shipment and are functional	Data and temperature logger are present and functional	Check for any unexplained variations			Reject shipment for which there is an unexplained deviation		
	Automated trip recorder or report	Trip recorder set	Recover and review report			Isolate shipments for which there is questionable information; reject if suspicious activity is possible; if criminal activity is suspected, retain product and contact law enforcement		
Retail sale	Receipt and storage of product is controlled	Product delivered to secure area and unloaded under supervision of retailer	Offload monitored by retail personnel	Each shipment	Receiving QC	Isolate shipment. Do not offload into retail facility until security issues have been adequately addressed.	Daily review of shipping and receiving records and security inspection report	Shipping and receiving records. Reports of security inspections

					Reject if security cannot be guaranteed and retain product if criminal activity is suspected		
All food is properly labeled and has traceability features	Examine master cases at unload for labeling and traceability features	Visual	Each shipment	Receiving QC	Isolate any food not properly labeled and note defect. Reject. If criminal activity is suspected, contact law enforcement	Daily review of inventory control reports	Inventory control reports
	Examine units while stocking		Each unit	Inventory control staff	Isolate unit and note defect. Labeling is not clear and traceability or tamper evident features are damaged or absent. Reject if criminal activity is suspected, retain product and contact law enforcement	Daily review of inventory control report	Inventory control reports
Perishable foods are not restocked; returned perishable food items are not resold	Restocked or returned perishable food items	Product recovery location and sale history	Any affected item	Any employee	Isolate and discard	Review of inventory control and departmental shift reports	Inventory control and security inspection reports

(continued)

TABLE 20.4 (continued)

A Model Food Defense Plan Based upon a HACCP Model—Food Defense Plan Form

Product Description: Frozen Cod Fish Fillets, Retail Pack (Heat Sealed Plastic Bag)

Intended Use/Consumer: Retail Sale to General Public

| Critical Control Point | Critical Limit | Monitoring | | | | Corrective Action | Verification | Records |
		What	How	Frequency	Who			
	Package integrity is checked for products on shelf	Examine products on shelf during shift and when stocking shelves	Visual	Any affected item	Department manager	Isolate, report defect, and discard. Retain product if criminal activity is suspected and contact law enforcement	Review of inventory control and departmental shift reports	Inventory control and security inspection reports
	No suspicious activity that could jeopardize food safety is observed	Monitor customers and employee behavior	Visual or via surveillance system	Any individual	All employees	Question suspicious individuals. If criminal activity is suspected, contact law enforcement	Daily review of security report	Security inspection reports

Company Name: Capitol Fish Co.
Address: 1600 Penn Ave.
Western, WA 98103
Prepared by Bill Frost
Bill Frost
Date: November 4, 2006

    c. Likelihood of food recontamination after processing

    d. Effectiveness of postprocessing control system

    e. Increase in the postprocessing contamination level that would cause infection or intoxication in the average consumer

    f. Effect of consumer preparation before eating

The underlying assumptions as well as the equations underlying this risk model are provided and can be modified for unique applications. The output is a ranking relative to a control value providing a means to compare different risks and risk scenarios. Although not specifically designed for food defense, Risk Ranger can be modified for risk assessments in this area.

Probably the most familiar risk ranking model in this area in the United States are ORM-based models that use scales and ratings allowing for easy categorization of different risks. The problem with ORM is that the risk characterizations are often based on assumptions that may not be valid. The matrix developed for ORM is overly simplistic for business use (Ryan, 2005) and traditional ORM does not permit an organization to assign either an unknown likelihood or unknown severity to a particular risk (Rasco and Bledsoe, 2005). Despite these flaws, ORM has proven to be a good model for simple operations and has been promoted for use in restaurants and when subjective analysis can be overlaid on reliable scientific information, the model is useful. A modification of the conventional ORM model is presented in Table 20.5 which could be useful for risk assessments in the food industry.

Implementation of ORM is similar to HACCP and involves the following steps: (1) identify the hazards, (2) assess the risk, (3) analyze possible risk control measures, (4) make control decisions, (5) implement risk controls (this would include monitoring), and (6) supervise and review the ORM plan for effectiveness. The objective of ORM is to make the risk control decision at the most appropriate levels. This establishes clear accountability and accepts no unnecessary risk. There are a number of risk control options for an ORM-based model. Reducing the hazard is a common feature between food safety and food defense plans and requires that systems and operations are designed and function to minimize risk through the incorporation of preventive measures, the addition of safety and monitoring and warning devices, and by verifying hazard control programs, training, and exercises. Rejecting the product or refusing to take the risk is also appropriate if the overall cost of the risk exceeds its benefits to the business or operation. Another alternative is to avoid the risk altogether by canceling a job, unit operation or production, or sale of a specific product. Delaying the risk is another possible strategy if timing is not critical to the operation or if taking a particular product off the market for a short period when there are indications that risk levels are high is an option, the business could incorporate, for example, removing self-serve deli or salad lines and replacing these with prepackaged items. Also it may be

TABLE 20.5

An Operational Risk Management Matrix for Food Defense

		Probability					
		Frequent-A	Likely-B	Occasional-C	Seldom-D	Unlikely-E	Unknown-F
Severity							
Catastrophic	I	Extremely high	Extremely high	High	High	Medium	Unknown
Critical	II	Extremely high	High	High	Medium	Low	Unknown
Moderate	III	High	Medium	Medium	Low	Low	Unknown
Negligible	IV	Medium	Low	Low	Low	Low	Unknown
Unknown	V	Unknown	Unknown	Unknown	Unknown	Unknown	Unknown

Notes:

Severity:

Catastrophic—food contamination incident that could cause total business failure. Fatalities and numerous serious illnesses or injuries would result.

Critical—food contamination incident that could cause a major loss of business. Serious illnesses or injuries would result.

Moderate—food contamination incident that could cause some loss of business. No serious illness or injuries would be likely.

Negligible—food contamination incident that could cause a small loss in business. Unlikely to cause serious illnesses or injuries.

Unknown—food contamination incident with a severity that is difficult to predict.

Probability:

Frequent—food contamination incident that occurs often. Specific individuals or the general population would be continuously exposed.

Likely—food contamination incident that has occurred several times. Specific individuals or the general population would regularly be exposed.

Occasional—food contamination incident that occurs occasionally. Exposure would be sporadic.

Seldom—food contamination incident that may occur. Exposure would be low.

Unlikely—food contamination incident that is not likely to occur. Exposure would be rare.

Unknown—food contamination incident that may or may not occur. Probability of occurrence is difficult to predict. Exposure of targeted individuals or the population at large is difficult to predict.

possible to transfer the risk to others by forming a cooperative or through insurance, if this is available, to reduce the overall impact of a loss if one should occur. Spreading the risk is often possible by increasing the exposure distance or deliveries in time and between different suppliers and carriers. Compensating for a risk is one of the most common methods to control risk and involves creating redundant capacity and backup systems for critical equipment, materials, staff, and logistic support. ORM and the following described CARVER + Shock approaches can best be employed in the hazard analysis portion of a comprehensive plan based upon HACCP.

CARVER + Shock-like ORM is a model derived from the military to assess risk. It can be adaptable to business applications but may have to be modified to be useful. The most useful feature as well as the greatest flaw with CARVER models is that they are based on the perspective of the attacker and not up on the intrinsic vulnerabilities of the facility or the inherent risks of a particular food product or consuming population. CARVER covers the risk assessment component only, so from there, either a HACCP or ORM-based plan would have to be developed.

For CARVER to be useful, one has to know who the attacker is likely to be. In practice, most food facilities using CARVER consider two types of attacker, a politically motivated "outsider," and a disgruntled "insider," and conduct the analysis using both of these scenarios. A new type of attack should also be considered as part of a CARVER analysis, and that is a conspiracy between an insider and one or more outsiders, particularly in light thwarted attempt in August 2006 to blow up airliners flying from the United Kingdom to the United States. This involved a conspiracy between an insider and outsiders, the former an airline security employee with full access to the entire airport and the latter, a number of suicide bombers trained to assemble liquid components into explosives on board and then to activate the detonator with a cell phone or other electronic devices to blow up airplanes.

CARVER models have six steps with an additional factor of shock added. These are: criticality, accessibility, recuperability, vulnerability, effect, recognizability, and shock and are defined as follows:

- Criticality—considers the public health and economic impacts of a successful attack. Criticality is evaluated from the attacker's perspective and whether an attack on facility meets the goal of the attacker to cause economic, psychological, and physical damage. Criticality requires some knowledge of the attackers and their motivation. This CARVER factor makes the model difficult to use in a private sector context unless there is an understanding of who the attacker might be. Therefore, the best strategy is to conduct an analysis using generic attackers of the types described above.

- Accessibility—relates to the attacker's physical access to the target. The target is accessible when the attacker has sufficient resources and the physical ability to reach a specific location and achieve the desired effect. Accessibility also infers that the attacker has the ability to escape following the attack (if that is their intent and perhaps not a valid assumption). Reducing target accessibility should be the primary focus of a food defense plan for a food business, as it is often the only factor over which a business has significant control. Accessibility for a specific type of attack, the method of the attack, and controls in place to deter such an attack are also all critical for determining if an incident is a hoax.

Security analyses are conducted to determine exposure and evaluate weaknesses within a business operation. Questions to ask are as follows:

1. Could the attacker reach the product without detection?
2. Could an attacker bring enough material through the conventional security infrastructure at the facility?
3. Could an attacker introduce enough material at a point in the process to successfully contaminate the product at levels high enough to cause harm without this action being detected?
4. Could the contaminant be detectable in the product by a simple test?

Having appropriate detection and mitigation strategies in place are important. A facility must be able to assure law enforcement, government regulators, and the media that enough barriers had been established within the facility to deter the alleged attack and that these barriers could not have been breached without detection. In the case of a hoax, a company must be able to say with certainty that the contamination did not happen, and making a statement that it is likely that it did not happen is not good enough anymore (Ryan, 2005).

- Recuperability—is the ability to recover from an attack financially and emotionally and to rebuild the physical assets and customer base for the business. The level of shock from an attack can impact how fast a company can recover because of the effect an attack has on employees, their families, customers, shareholders, and the broader community. Recuperability factors in the time necessary for recovery. This time can be shortened if sufficient redundancies have been built into the company operations to meet customer needs until the attacked facility can fully recover. A company must prioritize the use of resources to recover from an attack. A company will never make money from spending funds on security and these expenditures must be justified as rational business decisions (Ryan, 2005). However, security expenditures can reduce the time it takes to recover from an attack, reduce liability, mitigate damages, and protect company value.

- Vulnerability—evaluates whether the attacker has the means and resources to accomplish an attack with the desired effect, and the ease of accomplishing the attack. The federal government has conducted vulnerability assessments of a number of products and product categories (Table 20.1) focusing on contamination risk and is developing models to assess overall food supply. Vulnerability assessment is an area where cooperation is necessary among scientific, regulatory, and business communities to provide realistic evaluations of vulnerabilities and to ascertain which types of attacks are most likely, and of alleged attacks, which are credible and which are not.

- Effect—relates to the actual, direct, and immediate impact of an attack. The effect of an attack is a major factor considered in a security analysis and includes financial losses (e.g., product losses, physical damage to assets, cost for repair, rebuilding and decontamination, costs to return workforce to normal levels, and contract and liability losses). Security measures such as surveillance can reduce the effect by making it possible to determine what and how much product may have been affected.

- Recognizability—is the ease of identifying a target. The political motivation of the attacker and the symbolic or iconoclastic significance of a particular target play a role in how easy targets are recognized. This is a significant factor for outside attackers more so than insiders. Factors affecting recognizability are whether the desired target could be confused with other targets, size, and complexity of the target, and unique features of the target. It is unlikely that a terrorist would not want publicity about an attack; however, this is possible if a particular attack is part of a strategic long-term plan and the attack is the first of a series of broader based ones. Because product tampering may not be easily recognized, it is important for a facility to have a good handle on vulnerability assessments to determine whether or not a target has been attacked.

- Shock—is the psychological effect of an attack and incorporates both the short- and long-term behavioral changes that may be precipitated by an attack. Attacking a significant or well-known target, a target with broad geographic scope, or a target with high-emotional impact such products for young children, would add to the shock value. Some attackers may take advantage of the cascading effect throughout the food supply chain and understand the broad-ranging impact that an attack on a key food product may have across the population or over a long course of time. There has been much emphasis in the WMD community placed upon the number of deaths and serious injuries resulting from an attack and the shock value of such an incident. However, a greater risk from an attack on the food supply would result from a series of ongoing repeated attacks and contamination hoaxes that undermine consumer confidence in the safety of the food supply. The economic impact to an industry from a series of attacks such as this would be severe.

20.3 Mitigation Strategies

Basic tenets of threat assessment take into consideration the value of the asset to be attacked, the vulnerability of the asset, the likelihood of an attack, and the intent and capability of the attacker. Food businesses face the task of reducing the capability and likelihood of an attack by addressing foreseeable risks and developing effective and efficient means to reduce the risk, which work and can be implemented within a facility. Table 20.5 provides some possible mitigation strategies that may be useful in a food processing operation.

20.4 Intentionally Contaminating Food

Intentional contamination with toxic items that are relatively easy to obtain remain the greatest threat to the food supply and a number of warnings have been issued by the FBI and others noting that terrorists may try to contaminate food or the environment. Currently there are 72 agents not including plant pathogens regulated by either the Center for Disease Control (CDC) or the USDA (NRC 2006), some of which are included in addition to more conventional food contaminants in Table 20.6. Although the focus of the media has been upon sensational incidents with purified biotoxins or relatively exotic agents, isolating, and culturing crude preparations of bacteria is fairly straightforward for individuals with modest scientific ability and pose a significant threat, particularly if the overarching objective for the contamination is to cause an economic or political impact. The wider reaching politically motivated attack targeting voters in central Oregon by the religious cult of the Bagwan Shree Rashneesh in 1984, used relatively crude preparations of *Salmonella enteritidis* Typhimurium (Rasco and Bledsoe, 2005; Miller, 2001), sickened at least 750 people and provides evidence that effective attacks are possible using easily obtainable substances. Numerous food contamination incidents using toxic metals, industrial chemicals, and pesticides during the protracted Zimbabwean civil war (Rasco and Bledsoe, 2005) and Israeli-Palestinian conflict (Manning et al. 2005) indicate that terrorists may resort to materials that are relatively easy to obtain most recently (Spring 2007) with deaths of hundreds of companion animals from contaminated food (wheat flour with malamine). In other confirmed bioterrorism incidents, *Shigella dysenteriae* type 2 was used in an incident in 1996 in Texas by a disgruntled coworker to infect laboratory workers who ate pastries during work breaks. Identical strains of *S. dysenteriae* were isolated from stool culture of a patient, from a recovered muffin, and from laboratory stock cultures, some of which were missing. In 1997, seven laboratory workers were infected with *Salmonella sonnei* in New Hampshire. In 1998, a number of anthrax hoaxes were received by CDC involving letters sent to health clinics in Indiana, Kentucky, Tennessee, and a private business in Tennessee. Along with these incidents, telephoned hoaxes involving anthrax contamination of ventilation systems in a number of public and private premises were also made. *Brucella* sp. was implicated in the mysterious death of a 38 year old New Hampshire woman in 1999. In the same year a suspicious cluster of encephalitis in New York City occurred at the same time as an outbreak of West Nile-like virus (Ashford et al. 2003).

Agroterrorism involves the intentional introduction of a plant or animal disease. Spreading a livestock viral disease such as foot and mouth disease, avian viruses (exotic Newcastle disease [END]), or high-pathogenicity avian flu (HPAI) would have a devastating effect on agriculture systems and have been proposed by combatants during the Iran–Iraq war in the 1980s and in more recent conflicts as a strategy to influence the outcome of long and protracted regional conflicts. Projections indicate that introduction of disease into a single animal in an important dairy productions area such as Southern Idaho or California could spread through out the entire western United States within a few short weeks. An outbreak of such a disease in the United Kingdom in 2001 led to the slaughter of hundreds of animals and $4–5 billion in damages, including $1.6 billion simply to destroy the animals. National elections were delayed in 2001 and the government restructured to better respond to an introduction of foreign animal disease into the food supply (Manning et al. 2005). Costly outbreaks in Taiwan (1997) involved the destruction of 3.8 million pigs, and cost roughly $5 billion.

Avian flu is the zoonotic which has received the greatest attention recently because of the potential the virus has to mutate to highly pathogenic forms. The virus can survive in cold conditions and when protected by organic matter such as nasal secretions, liquid manure, and feces. The H5N1 virus, in particular can survive 1–7 days at around 70°F and in feces for 7 days at 68°F, 6 days at 98°F, over 30 days in water at 32°F or 30–35 days at 39°F in feces and an indefinite period under frozen storage. The virus is no longer viable following treatment for 10 min at 140°F and 90 min at 133°F (EPA, 2006) and increasing salinity or pH decrease viability of the virus in fresh surface water. Known highly pathogenic forms of avian influenza can be contracted by humans by direct contact with airborne aerosols, a disease that has a 57% fatality rate. Of the 227 individuals in 10 countries diagnosed with the disease, 129 have died. Reported incidents have been traced back to an initial 1959 incident in Scotland.

Avian flu has also caused billions of dollars of losses in the past 10 years. The most recent scares being 1997–1999 in Hong Kong where 18 people became ill and six died (H5N1) and all of the local 1.4 million poultry

TABLE 20.6

Possible Mitigation Strategies Based upon Site-Specific Vulnerability Assessments

Improve physical security measures	Add deterrents at highly accessible or vulnerable nodes: surveillance, additional supervision, restricted access, physical barriers, limiting personal items at work place.
Conduct site-specific vulnerability assessments	Conduct assessment and periodic reviews. Develop and evaluate risk assessment models and other tools to find the most useful ones for your business.
Evaluate process and design changes	Design physical layout of facility and production lines to position the critical nodes in the process so that they can be easily monitored and traffic can be controlled. Consider incorporating processing steps to eliminate or reduce risk of threat agents as data become available on how these can be best controlled.
Evaluate security plan	Use penetration audits to assess and validate security measures to determine effectiveness of current plan.
Modify operating procedures	Incorporate food defense measures into standard operating procedures or manufacturing practices. Focus on raw material inspection procedures as well as manufacturing operations.
Improve vendor programs	Have vendors and suppliers incorporate food defense measures into their programs. Add food defense criteria to procurement selection processes for vendors. Conduct food defense training with vendors.
Adopt biosecurity best practices	Support best practices for protecting plant and animals from disease and for isolation and quarantine of contaminated animals and plants. Screen water, feed, and transportation providers. When appropriate, provide decontamination facilities for clothing, people, and vehicles. For food processing operations, the primary functions in biosecurity would be (1) rapid notification of contamination to authorities, (2) containment, and (3) removal or destruction of product.
Consider an employee peer monitoring program	Emphasize food defense with employees and encourage them to focus on security, being on the alert for suspicious activity, having employees only work in teams at specific critical nodes, have employees verify or oversee the production of other individuals.
Provide awareness training	Educate employees, vendors, and customers about food defense with materials and programs appropriate for the particular audience.
Support trade industry group practices	Support activities within industry groups to develop uniform, appropriate food defense strategies and promote their adoption. This will show leadership and promote consumer confidence in food safety.
Develop threat indicators	Early warnings of suspicius activity include the following: employees, visitors, vendors, and contractors observed in areas where they have no legitimate reason to be there; individuals expressing an unusual interest in business practices, production or sales practices; unusual employee attendance or health patterns relating to a particular job function or work area; delays in deliveries, deviations from delivery schedules, or evidence of product tampering.

TABLE 20.6 (continued)

Possible Mitigation Strategies Based upon Site-Specific Vulnerability Assessments

Responding to a contamination incident	Detection of an agent may not be rapid, reliable or within the capability of a company to conduct. The type of response a company will take will depend upon how likely it is that the product is to be contaminated. The best strategy for defense against a hoax will be to show that it was unlikely that product safety was breached at the point where the alleged contamination occurred.
Communicating risk	Improving communication between industry, first responders, law enforcement, and regulators will be critical in response to a contamination incident. Consolidating and sharing resources among these groups should be promoted. Companies should maintain a simplified, up-to-date point of contact list and procedures to follow in case of an incident. Government should develop clearer protocols of whom to contact and when, besides law enforcement, in case of an incident.

Source: Adapted from FDA 2006. Strategic Partnership Program Agroterrorism (SPPA) Initiative. First Year Status Report September 2005–2006. www.fda.gov

were killed. Hong Kong was struck again in 2003 resulting in the death of 2.5 million birds, with three human cases and one fatality (H5N1). Avian flu swept through Europe in 2003 where one quarter of the flocks in The Netherlands, Belgium, and Germany were destroyed, resulting in 89 cases of human illness and one fatality (H7N7). Again in 2004, avian flu (H5N1) struck Southeast Asia; 100 million birds were killed with 34 human cases reported and 24 deaths (Manning et al. 2005). Later in 2005–2006, the disease resulted in the decimation of poultry stock in eastern, southern, and central Asia through western Europe creating huge scares in markets where poultry is a major source of dietary protein and a primary source of cash income for women and their families. It should be noted that infected poultry is safe if cooked properly (to 165°F) and if conventional food preparation practices are used to prevent cross-contamination. The virus can be inactivated within 30 min on clean food-contact surfaces with 5.25% sodium hypochlorite, 2% sodium hydroxide, phenolic compounds, acidified ionophore compounds, chlorine dioxide, strong oxidizing agents, and 4% sodium carbonate/0.1% sodium silicate (EPA, 2006).

Carcass disposal is a major issue and the EPA recommends on-site composting within 24 h of death or secure transport to an off-site treatment or disposal facility (EPA, 2006) for landfill disposal, composting, incineration, rendering, or alkaline hydrolysis. Recommendations for controlling avian influenza viruses in the environment include proper sanitation and holding the buildings at 90°F–100°F for 1 week.

The effective use of food contamination agents depends upon the following:

1. Potential impact to human, animal, or plant health;
2. The type of food material contaminated;
3. How easy it would be to detect contamination of the food through discernible changes in appearance, odor or flavor;
4. The point in the food supply chain where the contamination was introduced;
5. The potential for widespread contamination; and
6. The fear people would have from the use of the contaminant or the particular food to spread illness or disease.

Intentional contamination should be suspected when (1) unusual or not easily explained outbreaks occur that are more likely to be caused by intentional contamination, (2) outbreaks result from bioengineered pathogens that may have unusual or unexpected characteristics, and (3) bioengineered pathogens that may not be easily detected by existing assays (Ashford et al. 2003).

Biological agents, specifically microbes or toxins can be dispersed into liquids or solid media and as aerosols or airborne particles. Microbes, unlike chemical agents, tend to be highly target specific. The primary difficulty with the use of microbes to contaminate food is with their control. Environmental conditions for effectively transmitting microbes have to be managed, e.g., nutrients, temperature, water activity, and pH; and for spores, air movement. Factors affecting the viability of a particular strain or its toxic properties by oral transmission in food matrices is often not well understood, even for the common foodborne disease agents, and most of the technical literature in the biological warfare area using microbes as the agent has involved the dissemination of pure or relatively pure materials into well-defined media, most often with inhalation or consumption at a high concentration being the application studied. Also, limiting the impact of the biological agent to a specific target may be difficult with secondary transmission from people to people or through other vectors such as insects, rodents, or birds.

Although almost any pathogen could be used to intentionally spread disease, the Centers for Disease Control and Prevention have developed a list of high-risk biological agents, many of which are listed in Table 20.7. Based upon investigative studies to date, the most likely agents, in order of frequency of outbreaks, are as follows: unknown infectious agent, *Vibrio cholerae*, *Yersinia pestis*, viral hemorrhagic fever viruses, *Bacillus anthracis*, *Clostridium botulinum*, *Coxiella burnetii*, and *Francisella tularensis* (Ashford et al. 2003). A short description of some of these agents is provided below.

Biological toxins are more like chemical agents than microbes and are effective upon delivery without the requirement that they grow or survive within either the food or the host to cause injury. Toxins can be dispersed as aerosols or in a liquid or solid. Biological toxins are highly toxic and can kill or debilitate at levels as low as 1–10 parts per 1,000,000,000,000,000 (10^{15}) and commonly at the part per million or part per billion level. Many biological toxins would have little if any effect on the sensory properties of food at effective levels. A successful agent would be is water soluble, stable over a relatively wide pH range, and have limited susceptibility to thermal inactivation. In general, the residual effects of a biological toxin within the environment are similar too or less than a chemical agent, and clearly less so than a radiological agent. The most important exception to this would be *Bacillus* sp. and *Clostridium* sp. spores which can persist in soil and the estuarine environment for years and could similarly persist inside insulation, wood, carpet, and other building materials for a long period. Biological agents have the unfortunate characteristic of low visibility, high potency, substantial accessibility, and relative ease of delivery (Atlas, 2001).

Viruses, bacteria (and their toxins), fungi (and their toxins), and rickettsia have been proposed as food adulterants. Viruses and retroviruses do not survive well outside the host; however, rhinoviruses that cause the common cold, can survive well in humid environments and are highly contagious. Examples commonly cited as potential biological warfare agents include some types of encephalitis, psittacosis, yellow fever, and dengue fever; however, the likelihood that these would be an agent of choice for contaminating food is somewhat low. However, the introduction of a much more common virus, such as hepatitis A, can cause substantial economic havoc such as that associated with the 2003 outbreak around Christmas involving green onions from Mexico which resulted in at least one large nationwide warehouse store discontinuing this product permanently, despite its popularity, in part because of concerns over food safety and the inability to economically detect this pathogen in this product.

Bacteria, bacterial spores, and bacterial toxins are among the most likely contaminating agents and have been used to intentionally contaminate food or initiate bioterrorism attacks. Certain bacteria can enter a dormant state and form spores when challenged by heat, low moisture conditions, or chemicals such as chlorine or other sanitizers. Bacteria act either by causing an infection or by producing a toxin that causes illness. Many of the potential agents are present in the environment and can have legitimate uses, such as botulinum toxin for treatment of neurological disorders and cosmetic applications. Transmission of these materials through the air has the potential of impacting the greatest number of people. Canadian researchers confirmed the effectiveness of dispersing powdered anthrax spores and aerosol through paper envelopes in an indoor environment, with rapid delivery of a highly localized concentration of spores. Indoor airflows, activity patterns, and heating and cooling systems further dispersed spores throughout other parts of the building. The porosity of common paper products is greater than the diameter of the spores. Spores can settle on surfaces or inside porous material and then disperse (secondary aerosolization) at a later

TABLE 20.7

Possible Biological Agents for Food Contamination

	Potential Agents					
	Food Safety	Food Safety and Food Defense	Food Defense or Bioterrorism Agent	Vaccine Available	Natural Reservoirs	Potential Mode of Transmission
Food or Water Associated						
Aeromonas hydrophila	x	—	—	—	Freshwater environments and in brackish water. Some strains of *A. hydrophila* cause illness in fish and amphibians. Humans may acquire infections through open wounds or by ingestion of a sufficient number of the organisms in food or water. Water, worldwide distribution	Water or food
Avian influenza viruses	—	x	—	Yes	Soil and water	Airborne, contact with nasal secretions
Bacillus anthracis	—	—	x	Yes	Soil, worldwide distribution	Soil, food, water
Bacillus cereus	x	—	—	—	Soil	Food, water, animal contact (cutaneous or mucosal abrasion)
Brucella sp. (*B. melitensis, suis, abortus, canis*) (undulant or Malta fever)	—	x	—	Yes	Cattle, swine, goats, sheep, camels, dogs, coyotes	

Organism					Reservoir / Source	Transmission
Campylobacter jejuni	—	x	—	—	Healthy cattle, chickens, birds, and even flies. It is sometimes present in nonchlorinated water sources such as streams and ponds	Food, animal contact
Chlamydia psittaci (psittacosis)	—	x	—	—	Birds, poultry	Inhalation of dust from infected droppings, and secretions, aerosols, water
Clostridium botulinum	—	x	—	Yes	Organism and its spores are widely distributed in nature: cultivated and forest soils, bottom sediments of streams, lakes, and coastal waters, and in the intestinal tracts of fish and mammals, and in the gills and viscera of crabs and other shellfish	Soil and food
Clostridium perfringens	x	—	—	—	Frequently occurs in the intestines of humans and many domestic and feral animals. Spores of the organisms persist in soil, sediments, and areas subject to human or animal fecal pollution. Soil, gastrointestinal tract of humans and animals	Soil and food
Coxiella burnetii, Q fever	—	—	x	Yes	Sheep, goats, cattle, dogs, cats, some wild animals, ticks, birds	Airborne. Inhalation of dust from infected tissues, direct contact with infected animals, food, water
Cryptosporidium parvum, and other species	x	—	—	—	Human, diverse range of animals, including cattle and other domestic animals	Food, water, person-to-person, animal-to-person, airborne

(continued)

TABLE 20.7 (continued)

Possible Biological Agents for Food Contamination

	Potential Agents				
	Food Safety	Food Safety and Food Defense	Food Defense or Bioterrorism Agent	Vaccine Available	Natural Reservoirs	Potential Mode of Transmission
Escherichia coli, hemorrhagic	—	x	—	—	Soil, water, gastrointestinal tract of humans and animals	Water and food
Hepatitis A virus	—	x	—	Yes	Humans	Water, food, person-to-person
Listeria monocytogenes	—	x	—	—	Some studies suggest that 1%–10% of humans may be intestinal carriers of *L. monocytogenes*. It has been found in at least 37 mammalian species, both domestic and feral, as well as at least 17 species of birds and possibly some species of fish and shellfish. It can be isolated from soil, silage, and other environmental sources. Fresh and estuarine waters, soil, gastrointestinal tract of humans and animals	Water and food
Plesiomonas shigelloides	x	—	—	—	Freshwater, freshwater fish, and shellfish and from many types of animals, including cattle, goats, swine, cats, dogs, monkeys, vultures, snakes, and toads	Water

Rickettsia prowazekii (typhus)	x	—	—	Rodents, humans	Louse, infective rat fleas contaminate fresh skin wounds or the flea bite site, aerosol
Salmonella sp.	x	—	—	Wide range of domestic and wild animals, poultry, and swine. Environmental sources of the organism include water, soil, insects, factory surfaces, kitchen surfaces, animal feces, raw meats, raw poultry, and raw seafoods, to name only a few	Water and food, person-to-person and animal-to-person contact, aerosols
Shigella sp.	x	—	—	Principally a disease of humans except other primates such as monkeys and chimpanzees. The organism is frequently found in water polluted with human feces, water, and gastrointestinal tract of humans and animals	Water, food, person-to-person
Staphylococcus aureus	x	—	Experimental	Air, dust, sewage, water, milk, and food or on food equipment, environmental surfaces, humans, and animals. Humans and animals are the primary reservoirs. Staphylococci are present in the nasal passages and throats and on the hair, and skin of 50 percent or more of healthy individuals. Skin, nasal secretions, and gastrointestinal tract of humans and animals	Water and food
Streptococcus sp.	x	—	—	Skin, nasal secretions, and gastrointestinal tract of humans and animals	Water and food

(continued)

TABLE 20.7 (continued)

Possible Biological Agents for Food Contamination

	Potential Agents				Natural Reservoirs	Potential Mode of Transmission
	Food Safety	Food Safety and Food Defense	Food Defense or Bioterrorism Agent	Vaccine Available		
Vibrio cholerae	—	x	—	Yes	Aquatic environments worldwide	Water, food, wound infection from exposure to contaminated water
Vibrio parahaemolyticus	x	—	—	—	Estuarine and marine environments	Water, food, wound infections from exposure to contaminated water
Vibrio vulnificus	—	x	—	—	Coastal waters	Water, food, wound infections from exposure to contaminated water
Yersinia enterocolitica	—	x	—	—	Soil, water, animals (e.g. beavers, pigs, and squirrels)	Food, water
Yersinia pestis	—	—	x	Yes	Wild and domestic rodents, lagomorphs	Vector borne, airborne, contaminated water, and food
Yersinia pseudotuberculosis	x	—	—	—	Soil and water, various animal reservoirs	Airborne, contaminated water, and food
Toxins						
α-Amanitin	—	x	—	—	Amanita species mushrooms	Consuming amanita species mushrooms

					Source	Route of exposure
Abrin, jequirity bean (*Abrus precatorius*)	—	x	—	—	Seeds	Consuming seeds or toxin extract, food, water, aerosols, skin, dermal, parenteral, skin-to-eye contact, injection
Aflatoxin	—	x	—	—	Tree nuts, peanuts, other oilseeds, corn, and cottonseed, animal feed, excreted in the milk and urine of dairy cattle and other mammalian species that have consumed aflatoxin-contaminated food or feed	Food, aerosols
Anatoxin, *Anabaena flos-aquae*	—	x	—	—	Freshwater cyanobacteria	Water
Bovine spongiform encephalopathy (prion)	—	x	—	No	Brain, nerve, and distal ileal tissues of cattle	Consumption of prion-containing materials
Clostridium botulinum	—	x	—	Yes	Soil, animals including fish	Food, water, wound infection from exposure to toxic spores
Clostridium perfringens epsilon toxin	—	x	—	No	Soil, animals	Food, water, wound infection from exposure to toxic spores
Conotoxins	—	—	x	—	Cone snail venom *Conus geographus*, *C. magus*, and *C. ermineus*	Consumption of fish predating on cone snails, toxin consumption, exposure to aerosols
Microcystins, *Microcystis* spp.	—	x	—	—	Freshwater cyanobacteria water	Water

(continued)

TABLE 20.7 (continued)

Possible Biological Agents for Food Contamination

	Potential Agents					
	Food Safety	Food Safety and Food Defense	Food Defense or Bioterrorism Agent	Vaccine Available	Natural Reservoirs	Potential Mode of Transmission
Mushroom toxins: gyromitrin, orellanine, muscarine, muscimol, psilocybin, coprine	—	x	—	—	Various mushrooms	Food, oral, inhalation, or skin contact with toxin
Ricin, castor bean, (*Ricinus communis*)	—	x	—	Experimental	Castor bean	Consuming seeds or toxin extract, airborne, injection, food, water, skin, dermal, parenteral, skin-to-eye contact
Saxitoxin, from the marine dinoflagellate, *Alexandrium* sp. formerly *Gonyaulax* sp.	—	x	—	No	Dinoflagellates, shellfish, and other marine species	Food, water, injection
Shiga toxin (*Escherichia coli* or *Shigella* sp.)	—	x	—	—	Soil, water, gastrointestinal tract of humans and animals	Food, water
Staphylococcal enterotoxin B (*Staphylococcus aureus*)	—	x	—	Experimental	Human, contaminated milk, and milk products	Food, water

			Infected grain	Oral, skin contact, aerosols		
Trichothecene mycotoxins, e.g., x	—	No	—	Oral, skin contact, aerosols	diacetoxyscirpenol from *Fusarium roseum* and other *Fusarium* sp.	—
Tetrodotoxin	—	x	—	—	Puffer fish, California Newt, parrot fish, frogs of the genus *Atelopus*, the blue-ringed octopus, starfish, angelfish, and xanthid crabs	Food, water, aerosols
Other Sources						
Burkholderia mallei, formerly *Pseudomonas mallei* (glanders)	—	—	x	No	Horses, donkeys and mules, possibly dogs and cats.	Direct contact with infected animals, infection through mucosal surfaces of the eyes and nose and abraded or lacerated skin. Sporadic cases have been documented in veterinarians, horse caretakers, and laboratory workers. Aerosols, water, food, person-to-person
Burkholderia pseudomallei, formerly *Pseudomonas pseudomallei* (melioidosis)	—	—	x	No	Soil and water worldwide	Inoculation of skin lesion from contaminated soil or water, inhalation of contaminated dust, aerosol
Cercopithecine herpesvirus 1 (herpes B virus)	—	—	x	—	Macaque monkeys and possible in other Old World monkeys	Contact with monkey saliva, secretions, or tissues; bites and

(continued)

TABLE 20.7 (continued)

Possible Biological Agents for Food Contamination

	Potential Agents			Vaccine Available	Natural Reservoirs	Potential Mode of Transmission
	Food Safety	Food Safety and Food Defense	Food Defense or Bioterrorism Agent			
						scratches or splashes; person-to-person transmission
Coccidioides immiti, Rift Valley fever	—	—	x	Yes	Cattle, buffalo, sheep, goats, camels, and humans	Animal-to-person, aerosols
Coccidioides posadasii	—	—	x	—	Alkaline soil in rodent burrows in desert-like areas (Southwest United States)	Inhalation of infected dust
Crimean-Congo hemorrhagic fever virus	—	—	x	Yes	Rodent	Contact with urine, feces, or saliva of infected rodents, infected ticks, direct handling and preparation of fresh carcasses of infected animals, usually domestic livestock. Nosocomial transmission
Ebola virus	—	—	x	—	Unknown	Through open wounds, injection, aerosol
Equine encephalitis virus (eastern, Venezuelan)	—	—	x	Yes	Rodents, mosquitos, horses, and amplifying host	Arthropod borne Aerosol exposure

Agent				Reservoir	Transmission
Francisella tularensis	—	x	Yes	Diverse mammalian and tick reservoirs, rodent mosquito cycle possible	Vector borne, food, water, air
Hendra virus	—	x	—	Flying foxes (bats of the genus *Pteropus*)	Direct exposure to tissues and secretions from infected horses, aerosols
Lassa fever virus	—	x	—	Rodent	Animal-to-person, aerosol
Marburg virus	—	x	—	Unknown	Through open wounds, injection, aerosol
Monkeypox virus	—	x	—	Squirrels possibly mice, and rabbits	Bites from infected animals, contact with infected animal's blood, body fluids, or skin rash; person-to-person through large respiratory droplets during long periods of face-to-face contact, touching body fluids of a sick person or contaminated objects such as bedding or clothing
Nipah virus	—	x	—	Unknown	Transmission to humans, cats, and dogs through close contact with infected pigs
Reconstructed 1918 influenza virus	—	x	Experimental	None	Person-to-person
Smallpox, variola major virus	—	x	Yes	Humans (eradicated) only in designated laboratories	Person-to-person airborne, direct contact with skin lesion or contaminated objects

(continued)

TABLE 20.7 (continued)

Possible Biological Agents for Food Contamination

	Potential Agents			Vaccine Available	Natural Reservoirs	Potential Mode of Transmission
	Food Safety	Food Safety and Food Defense	Food Defense or Bioterrorism Agent			
South American hemorrhagic fever viruses (New World arenaviruses) (Flexal, Guanarito, Junin, Machupo, Sabia)	—	—	x	—	Rodents, mosquitos, ticks, primates	Arthropod borne aerosol or fomites from slaughtering infected animals, aerosols
Tick-borne encephalitis complex (flavi) virus (Central European tick-borne	—	—	x	Yes	Tick vector and reservoir. The main hosts are small rodents, with humans being accidental hosts	Vector borne, raw milk from goats, sheep, or cows. Laboratory infections, aerosols, person-to-person transmission has not

Agent				Reservoir	Transmission
encephalitis, far eastern tick-born encephalitis, Kyasanur forest disease, Omsk hemorrhagic fever, Russian spring and summer encephalitis)					been reported. Vertical transmission from an infected mother to fetus has occurred
Variola minor virus (alastrim)	—	x	—	Rodents	Animal-to-person, person-to-person, airborne, direct contact with skin lesion or contaminated objects
Yellow fever	—	x	Yes	Mosquito (*Aedes aegypti*)	Person-to-person by mosquito vector

Sources: From National Research Council. 2006. National Academies of Science, Engineering and Medicine. Overcoming Challenges to Develop Countermeasures against Aerosolized Bioterrorism Agents; Appropriate Use of Animal Models. Committee on Animal Models for Testing Interventions against Aerosolized Bioterrorism Agents. ISBN:0-309-66102-1. 90 pp. http://eww.nap.edu/catalog/11640.html; Centers for Disease Control and Prevention, United States, www.cdc.gov<http://www.cdc.gov>. Accessed December 2006; Rasco, B.A. and Bledsoe, G.E. in *Bioterrorism and Food Safety*, Boca Raton, FL, 2005, 1–32; FDA 2005. Bad Bug Book. Fda.gov; Takhistov, P. and Bryant. C.M., *Food Technol.*, 60, 34,2006; Tierno, P.M. in *The Secret Life of Germs*, Simon & Schuster Inc., New York, 2001, 240.

x denotes possibility for use as an agent.

time, making further recontamination possible. Secondary aerosolization poses a limited risk as long as spore density remained below one million spores per square meter (Rasco and Bledsoe, 2005).

Infection of water or food and the use of insect vectors or animal hosts are other possible methods of transmission. Many bacteria can adapt to the environment once released and can grow readily with victims of the attack not being aware of exposure to an infective agent until days or weeks following an attack. Before diagnosis, an infection could be widely spread through the air or by direct contact with the victim. Illnesses may initially be mild, and flu-like delaying proper diagnosis.

Infection of a food with fungal cells or spores poses a particular threat to commercial agriculture and there are a number of different rusts, smuts, and easy-to-grow agents, for example, the rice blast fungus *Pyricularia oryzae* that have been proposed as a biological warfare agent. Use of fungal toxins in an impure form (such as aflatoxin-contaminated grain) could cause an acute illness at low levels in domesticated poultry and aquacultured fish and causes liver damage to humans.

Among one of the most closely studied agents recently is anthrax. Anthrax is classified as a bioterrorism category A threat agent. There are a small number of cases of anthrax reported each year, generally associated with hunting, animal slaughter, and consumption of contaminated meat. In September and October 2001, however, letters containing *Bacillus anthracis* spores were sent through the U.S. mail to individuals in the print media, broadcast journalists, and a number of politicians. Five years following the incident, delivery of mail in the Washington DC area is not back to normal. Eleven inhalation and 11 cutaneous cases resulted, mostly among postal workers and of these, five of the 11 inhalation infections were fatal. The illnesses were spread across the Eastern United States in Connecticut (one), Florida (two), Maryland (three), New Jersey (five), New York City (eight), Pennsylvania (one), and Virginia (two). Twenty-two other bioterrorism-related cases were reported in Texas in 2001. A later incident in 2003 targeted members of Congress and others. None of the perpetrators of these attacks have been apprehended or even positively identified.

Advances have been made to treat individuals and the environment including food contact surfaces in case of a contamination incident involving food. Most recently, a bacteriophage enzyme (PlyPH) that causes *Bacillus anthracis* to lyse at a wide range of pH and temperatures (Amato, 2006) was isolated. A mouse model of an anthrax-like infection indicated that PlyPH is safe and can save roughly half of the animals treated. Bacterial cells do not appear to develop resistance.

Environmental remediation following an anthrax-contamination incident is difficult because the spores are highly resistant to chemical and physical treatment (Erickson and Kornacki, 2003). Resistance is dependent upon strain, circumstances surrounding sporulation and characteristics of the medium in which the spores are present. D values (decimal reduction times) range from 2.5–7.5 min at 90°C to 1.7–4.5 min at 95°C. Spores are more sensitive at pH less than 5. Recommended treatments include heating at 110°C for 15 min, autoclaving (120°C) for 10 min, microwaving (>112°C) or dry heat treatment for 3 h (140°C). Spores can be inactivated by ultraviolet radiation (280–315 nm) and survive for only 20–30 min in nutrient agar when exposed to direct sunlight. Ionizing radiation is also effective at 15 kGy which is currently higher than the level permitted for treating fresh red meat (4.5 kGy) or frozen red meat (7 kGy). Anthrax spores are not killed by common cleaners and disinfectants, including alcohols, phenols, quaternary ammonium compounds, ionic, and nonionic detergents, acids, or alkalis. Effective compounds include formaldehyde (5%) glutaraldehyde (2%, pH 8–8.5), hydrogen peroxide (3%), and peracetic acid (0.6%) with treatment times taking up to 4 h (Erickson and Kornacki, 2003).

Tularemia (*Francisella tularensis*) is another agent of great concern which was reinstated as a notifiable disease in 2000 due in part to potential terrorist threats. On average, there are six cases per 10,000,000 population in the United States annually, a substantial reduction since the 1950s when the rate was six times higher. Tularemia was one of the agents studied by the Japanese during World War II and the microbe may have been disseminated by the Japanese as a weapon in Manchuria during the war. Similarly, tularemia outbreaks affecting tens of thousands of Russian and German soldiers on the eastern European front point to a deliberate release of this organism. In the 1950s and 1960s, the United States reportedly developed an aerosol delivery system for tularemia and stockpiled it. Estimates of the economic impact of an aerosol-dispersed incident with tularemia are $5.4 billion for every 100,000 individuals exposed. Reports of terrorist attempts with this microbe are limited, but cannot be ruled out.

One of the most notable bacterial biowarfare agents is plague. *Yersinia pestis* is an organism that has raised fear from antiquity to the present day. Although there is an average of less than 10 cases per year in the United States, it is considered by some to be one of the most likely choices for weaponization by terrorists and has been a component of numerous weapons arsenals. In World War II, the Japanese dropped plague-infested fleas over population centers in China causing numerous sporadic outbreaks of disease. Following the war, the United States and Soviet Union developed technologies to aerosolize plague to increase the reliability of dispersion. The former USSR developed the capability of weaponizing large quantities of plague with thousand of scientists at 10 institutes reported to have experience with the agent. Through the 1990s cultures of plague bacteria and other potential biological weapons agents were commercially shipped to suspicious purchases before stricter federal controls were instituted. In one incident, a microbiologist with suspicious motives was arrested after fraudulently obtaining *Y. pestis* cultures through the mail (Inglesby et al. 2001) in a form considered to be an agent that could be subject to aerosol release. In a World Health Organization study, 50 kg of plague bacteria released as an aerosol over a city of five million people could cause 150,000 cases of pneumonic plague and result in 36,000 deaths. The agent would remain viable for at least an hour and could be dispersed over an area of up to 10 km^2.

Viruses are potential agents that pose new and different threats, not only in regard to genetically engineered variants of influenza and small pox but also recovery and dispersion of hemorrhagic viruses from animals to humans as development encroaches into more remote areas reaching the natural, and until recently relatively undisturbed, reservoirs of these agents. These viruses have a high mortality and morbidity at very low-infective doses. Most are highly infectious, can be dispersed by aerosols, human-to-human contact, nosocomial transmission, animal-to-human contact, and insect vectors making widespread outbreaks a possibility. There is no reliable treatment for most of these conditions. Fortunately, large-scale deployment of hemorrhagic viruses is not yet technically feasible because of the difficulty of working with these viruses although both the United States and the former Soviet Union have been able to weaponize hemorrhagic viruses. In the early 1990s, the USSR had stocks of Marburg, Ebola, Lassa, Junin, and Marchupo viruses. The United States has weaponized both yellow fever and Rift Valley fever viruses. North Korea may currently have yellow fever-based weapons (Rasco and Bledsoe, 2005). A possible scenario to employ such pathogens would be to infect humans and animals by infecting livestock via an insect vector.

Bacterial and plant toxins include a wide range of compounds and have been used to intentionally poison people. Ricin is recovered using a relatively simple procedure from the castor bean (*Ricinus communis*). It is a water soluble, heat sensitive globular protein of approximately 64,000 Da consisting of two peptide chains, each 32,000 Da linked by a disulfide bond. Abrin is a similar toxin recovered from *Abrus precatorius* seed (common names: jequirity bean, Indian licorice seed, rosary pea, mienie-mienie) (NIOSH, 2003). There are no antidotes for either of these. Both are highly toxic by inhalation or ingestion. A lethal dose can be as little as 500 ng by injection. Both abrin and ricin inhibit protein synthesis and have potential medical application for treating bone marrow transplant and cancer patients. Ricin has been used as a bioterrorist agent and had been weaponized in the late 1980s in Iraq where it was tested in animal experiments and artillery field trials (Audi et al. 2005). Ricin was discovered both in home-based laboratories in Britain in 2003 in the hands of suspected terrorists and in a South Carolina mail-sorting room, serving the offices of former Tennessee senator and majority leader, William Frist, Maryland (2003 and 2004) as well as in the possession of individuals linked with terrorist organizations (id). Initial symptoms resemble gastroenteritis (1–4 h onset) or respiratory illness. Moderate to severe illness has gastrointestinal symptoms such as persistent vomiting and voluminous diarrhea (bloody or nonbloody) typically leading to substantial fluid loss. This can result in dehydration and hypovolemic shock. In severe cases, liver, and renal failure result.

Botulinum toxin has a notorious history as a biological weapon. Recent examples include development of botulinum delivery systems by the Aum Shinrikyo cult in Japan, which isolated the toxin from soil samples. Cultures of the organism were used by the Japanese in the World War II occupation of China to kill Manchurian prisoners. In addition, Germany had a weapons program in place during World War II. In anticipation of possible use in Normandy, the allied troops had over one million doses of botulinum toxoid prepared. The former Soviet Union and Iraq had the most recent and sophisticated programs employing botulinum toxin, including several tests by the former conducted at the Aralsk-7 site on Vozrozhdeniye Island (now Kazakhstan) through the 1980s. Soviet scientists reported attempts to splice the gene for botulinum toxin into other bacteria and this expertise has reportedly been hired out over the past 20 years following the collapse to Syria, North Korea, Iran, and possibly others. A point-source aerosol release could kill or incapacitate 10% of the people within a 0.5 km radius (Arnon et al. 2001).

Capabilities to produce botulinum have increased recently as the material has been approved for medical uses (at concentration of 0.3% of the estimated human lethal injection dose) to treat headache, pain, stroke, traumatic brain injury, cerebral palsy, achalasia, and various dystonias. It is also widely used to temporarily remove wrinkles, crow's feet, and laugh lines.

Saxitoxin is back on the radar screen as a biological agent, and has had a colorful history both in the foodborne illness realm and as a potential agent. Saxitoxin is one of several toxins produced by either a dinoflagellate or a bacterial symbiont associated with it, as it is still not clear whether or not the implicated marine microalga with which it is most closely associated can be produced in axenic culture. Saxitoxin is the most potent, nonprotein, naturally occurring toxin known and 1000 times more toxic than the nerve gas sarin, and along with ricin are the only two naturally occurring schedule 1 chemical warfare agents. It is highly selective and blocks ion transport through sodium channels of plasma membranes on nerve cells. It has no effect on potassium or calcium channels, chloride ion flux, or acetylcholine release making it an extremely valuable compound for physiological and neurological experiments. Various derivations such as adding a carbamate group increases its toxicity. Saxitoxin is water soluble, heat, and pH stable, affording it the ability to withstand cooking without losing toxicity (Edwards, 2006).

The U.S. government began experimenting with saxitoxin as a covert agent in the 1950s and developed injection devices using it, one of which was reportedly provided to U-2 pilot Francis Gary Powers, who was shot down in a reconnaissance flight over the Soviet Union. Much saxitoxin was isolated from butter clams (*Saxidomus giganteus*) harvested in the Pacific Northwest and Alaska for governmental use during this period. This mollusk can selectively concentrate the toxin in its siphon and store it for years. Illnesses associated with saxitoxin have afflicted travelers through the region, native and nonnative alike throughout recorded history, with the most notable being the loss of several Aleut members of the Russian trader Baranov's crew at the subsequently christened "Poison Bay" located between Sitka and Hoonah, Alaska in 1793. Remaining stores of the toxin are held by the National Institute of Health where it is used as an analytical standard for monitoring paralytic shellfish poisoning toxins in harvested shellfish by state and tribal authorities and is used in neurological research.

20.5   Conclusion

Food and agriculture are part of the critical infrastructure and it behooves us to establish a coordinated strategy at the regional and national level to protect the food supply by conducting reasonable risk assessments and developing defensive strategies (Goodman, 2006) to address intentional contamination. Food has been targeted in the past, and is a relatively soft target. The food industry needs to have the support of government at the local and national levels to develop realistic and workable food defense programs without the imposition of additional regulatory burdens and costs. The role of governmental entities remains to ensure that food safety, food security, prevention, and response efforts are coordinated in such a way as to avoid confusion and unnecessary duplication of effort. It remains our greatest hope as food science professionals that we will never experience a large-scale intentional contamination incident involving the food supply but if such an attack should occur, we will be prepared to respond to it.

References

Afton, M.K., Nakata, M., Ching-Lee, M., and Effler, P.V. 2005. Food safety for first responders. *Emerg. Infect. Dis.* 11(3):508–509. http://www.cdc.gov/eid
Amato, I. 2006. Bacterial control anthrax destroyer. *Chem. Eng. News* May 1, 2006. p. 9. www.cen-oline.org
Anonymous. 2006. Heat stresses rendering plants. *Capital Press*. August 4, 2006. p. A12.
Arnon, S.S., Schechter, R., Inglesby, T.V., Henderson, D.A., Bartlett, J.G., Ascher, M.S, Eitzen, E., Fine, A.D., Hauer, J., Layton, M., Lillibridge, S.R., Osterholdm, M.T., O' Toole, T., Parker, G., Perl, T.M., Russell, P.K., Swerdlow, D.L., and Tonat, K. 2001. Botulinum toxin as a biological weapon. Medical and public health management. *JAMA* 285:1059–1070.
Ashford, D.A., Kaiser, R.M., Bales, M.E., Shutt, K., Patrawala, A., McShan, A., Tappero, J.W., Perkins, B.A., and Dannenberg, A.L. 2003. Planing against bio-

logical terrorism: Lessons from outbreak investigations. *Emerg. Infect. Dis.* 9(5):515–519.

Atlas, R.M. 2001. Bioterrorism before and after September 11. *Crit. Rev. Microbiol.* 27(4):355–379.

Audi, J., Belson, M., Patel, M., Schier, J., and Osterloh, J. 2005. Ricin poisoning: A comprehensive review. *JAMA* 294(18):2342–2351.

Centers for Disease Control and Prevention, United States, www.cdc.gov<http://www.cdc.gov>. Accessed December 2006.

DHHS. 2001. Statement of Tommy G. Thompson, Secretary U.S. Department of Health and Human Services. Topic: Bioterrorism Preparedness. Before the Subcommittee on Labor, Health and Human Services, Education, and Related Agencies Committee on Appropriations. United States Senate. October 3, 2001.

Drees, C. 2004. U.S. food sector may be vulnerable to attack. February 24. Citing: Yim, RA Combatting Terrorism: Evaluation of Selected Characteristics of National Strategies Related to Terrorism. GAO-04-408T. Presented February 3 before the Subcommittee on National Security, Emerging Threat and International Relations, House Committee on Government Reform. http://www.gao.gov/news.items/d04408t.pdf

Edwards, N. 2006. Saxitoxin from food poisoning to chemical warfare. University of Suffex at Brighton. http://www.chm.bris.ac.uk. August 30, 2006.

EPA. 2006. Disposal of Domestic Birds Infected by Avian Influenza: An Overview of Considerations and Options US Environmental Protection Agency. August 11, 2006, EPA530-R-06-009. 30 pp.

Erickson, M.C. and Kornacki, J.L. 2003. *Bacillus anthracis*: Current knowledge in relation to contamination of food. *J. Food Prot.* 66(4):691–699.

FDA. 2005. Bad Bug Book. Fda.gov.

FDA. 2006. Strategic Partnership Program Agroterrorism (SPPA) Initiative. First Year Status Report September 2005–2006. http://www.fda.gov

Fouda, Y. and Fielding, N. 2004. *Masterminds of Terror: The Truth Behind the Most Devastating Terrorist Attack the World Has Ever Seen*. Arcade Publishing, NY.

Goodman, T. 2006. Connecting food safety and food security. Presentation to the Association of Food and Drug Officials. Public Health Administration and Food Security Specialist. Division of Food Protection, Indiana State Department of Health.

Inglesby, T.V., Dennis, D.T, Henderson, D.A., Bartlett, J.G., Ascher, M.S., Eitzen, E., Fine, A.D., Friedlander, A.M., Hauer, J., Koerner, J.F., Layton, M., Lillibridge, S.R., McDade, J.E., Osterholm, M.T., O'Toole, T., Parker, G., Perl, T.M., Russell, P.K., Shoch-Spana, M., and Tonat, K. 2001. Plague as a biological weapon, medical and public health management. *JAMA* 283:2281–2290.

Manning, L., Baines, R.N., and Chadd, S.A. 2005. Deliberate contamination of the food supply chain. *Br. Food J.* 107(4/5):225–245.

Meinhardt, P.L. 2005. Water and bioterrorism. Preparing for the potential threat to U.S. water supplies and public health. *Annu. Rev. Public Health* 26:213–237.

Miller, J., Engelberg, S., and Broad, W. 2001. Chapter 1–The Attack. In: *Germs: Biological Weapons and America's Secret War*. Simon & Schuster, Inc., New York, pp. 15–24.

NRC. 2006. National Academies of Science, Engineering and Medicine. Overcoming Challenges to Develop Countermeasures against Aerosolized Bioterrorism

Agents; Appropriate Use of Animal Models. Committee on Animal Models for Testing Interventions against Aerosolized Bioterrorism Agents. ISBN:0-309-66102-1. 90 pp. http://eww.nap.edu/catalog/11640.html

NIOSH. 2003. Emergency response card. Biotoxin Abrin. Cdc.gov/agent/abrin. Accessed August 2006.

Rasco, B.A. and Bledsoe, G.E. 2005. *Bioterrorism and Food Safety*. Boca Raton, FL, pp. 1–32.

Ross, T. and Sumner, J.L. 2002. A simple spread-sheet based food safety risk assessment tool. *Int. J. Food Microbiol.* 77:39–53.

Ryan, R. 2005. Risk assessment to drive research on contaminant detection. Proceedings of the Institute of Food Technologist's First Annual Food Protection and Defense Research Conference. November 3–4, 2005. http://www.ift.org

Takhistov, P. and Bryant, C.M. 2006. Protecting the food supply. *Food Technol.* 60:34–43.

Tierno, P.M. 2001. Germ warfare and terrorism. In: *The Secret Life of Germs*. Simon & Schuster, Inc., New York, p. 240.

Western Institute for Food Safety and Security. 2005. Understanding the Dangers of Agroterrorism. An Agroterrorism Awareness Course for Frontline Responders. Davis, CA. http://wifss.ucdavis.edu

WHO. 2002. Food Safety Issues. Terrorist Threats to Food. Guidance for Establishing and Strengthening Prevention and Response Systems. World Health Organization, Food Safety Department, Geneva, Switzerland.

Index

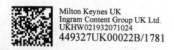